BUCK'S

2026
HCPCS Level II

Jackie L. Koesterman, CPC
Lead Technical Collaborator
Coding and Reimbursement Specialist
JDK Medical Coding EDU
Grand Forks, North Dakota

INCLUDES NETTER'S ANATOMY ART

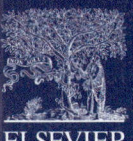
ELSEVIER

Elsevier
3251 Riverport Lane
St. Louis, Missouri 63043

BUCK'S 2026 HCPCS LEVEL II   ISBN: 978-0-443-40944-8

Copyright © 2026 by Elsevier, Inc. All rights reserved, including those for text and data mining, AI training, and similar technologies.

Publisher's note: Elsevier takes a neutral position with respect to territorial disputes or jurisdictional claims in its published content, including in maps and institutional affiliations.

No part of this publication may be reproduced or transmitted in any form or by any means, electronic or mechanical, including photocopying, recording, or any information storage and retrieval system, without permission in writing from the publisher. Details on how to seek permission, further information about the Publisher's permissions policies and our arrangements with organizations such as the Copyright Clearance Center and the Copyright Licensing Agency, can be found at our website: www.elsevier.com/permissions.

This book and the individual contributions contained in it are protected under copyright by the Publisher (other than as may be noted herein).

Notice

Practitioners and researchers must always rely on their own experience and knowledge in evaluating and using any information, methods, compounds or experiments described herein. Because of rapid advances in the medical sciences, in particular, independent verification of diagnoses and drug dosages should be made. To the fullest extent of the law, no responsibility is assumed by Elsevier, authors, editors or contributors for any injury and/or damage to persons or property as a matter of products liability, negligence or otherwise, or from any use or operation of any methods, products, instructions, or ideas contained in the material herein.

Previous editions copyrighted 2025, 2024, 2023, 2022, 2021, 2020, 2019, 2018, 2017, 2016, 2015, 2014, 2013, 2012, 2011, 2010, 2009, 2008, 2007, 2006, 2005, 2004, 2003, 2002, 2001, 2000

International Standard Book Number: 978-0-443-40944-8

Senior Content Strategist: Luke Held
Content Development Manager: Danielle Frazier
Senior Content Development Specialist: Joshua S. Rapplean
Publishing Services Manager: Deepthi Unni
Project Manager: Nayagi Anandan
Senior Book Designer: Maggie Reid

Printed in Canada

Last digit is the print number: 9   8   7   6   5   4   3   2   1

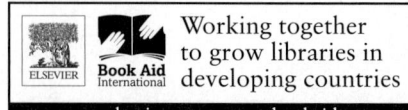

DEDICATION

To all who require of themselves the highest level of accuracy, integrity, and professionalism. You enhance our profession and are a tremendous asset to health care. May this manual be of assistance to you.
With Greatest Admiration.

Carol J. Buck, MS

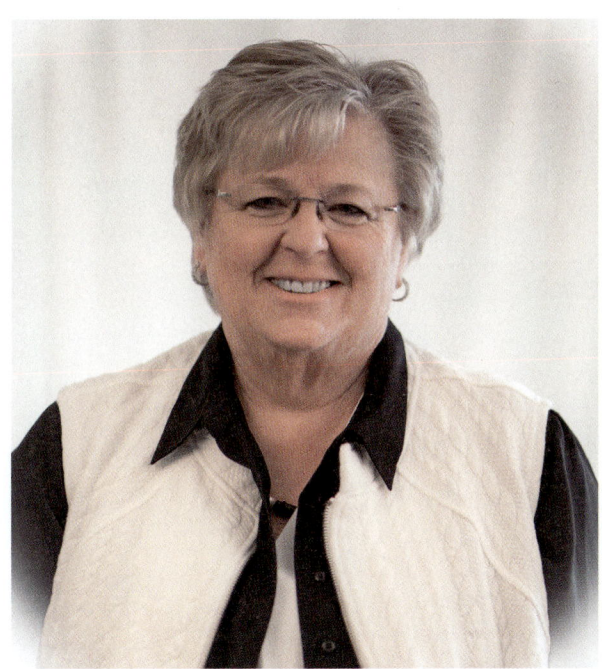

DEVELOPMENT OF THIS EDITION

Lead Technical Collaborator

Jackie L. Koesterman, CPC
Coding and Reimbursement Specialist
JDK Medical Coding EDU
Grand Forks, North Dakota

CONTENTS

INTRODUCTION vi

GUIDE TO USING THE 2026 HCPCS LEVEL II CODES vii

SYMBOLS AND CONVENTIONS viii

2026 HCPCS UPDATES xiv

ANATOMY ILLUSTRATIONS xvi

2026 HCPCS INDEX 1

2026 TABLE OF DRUGS 43

2026 HCPCS LEVEL II MODIFIERS 101

2026 HCPCS LEVEL II NATIONAL CODES 113

Appendix A—Jurisdiction List for DMEPOS HCPCS Codes 423

Appendix B—General Correct Coding Policies: Medicare National Correct Coding Initiative Policy Manual 431

Figure Credits 447

Updates will be posted on codingupdates.com when available.

Check codingupdates.com for Practitioner and Facility Medically Unlikely Edits (MUEs) and Column 1 and Column 2 Edits.

Check the Centers for Medicare & Medicaid Services (www.cms.gov/Manuals/IOM/list.asp) website and codingupdates.com for full and select IOMs.

Notice: 2026 DMEPOS updates were unavailable at the time of printing. Check codingupdates.com for updates and DMEPOS Modifiers in January.

INTRODUCTION

Each quarter CMS will post an update to the HCPCS code set to their website. A direct link to all the quarterly updates can also be found on our companion website (codingupdates.com)

The Centers for Medicare & Medicaid Services (CMS) (formerly Health Care Financing Administration [HCFA]) Healthcare Common Procedure Coding System (HCPCS) is a collection of codes and descriptors that represent procedures, supplies, products, and services that may be provided to Medicare beneficiaries and to individuals enrolled in private health insurance programs. The codes are divided as follows:

Level I: Codes and descriptors copyrighted by the American Medical Association's (AMA's) Current Procedural Terminology, ed. 4 (CPT-4). These are five-position numeric codes representing physician and nonphysician services.

Level II: Includes codes and descriptors copyrighted by the American Dental Association's current dental terminology, seventh edition (CDT-7/8). These are five-position alpha-numeric codes comprising the D series. All other Level II codes and descriptors are approved and maintained jointly by the alpha-numeric editorial panel (consisting of CMS, the Health Insurance Association of America, and the Blue Cross and Blue Shield Association). These are five-position alpha-numeric codes representing primarily items and nonphysician services that are not represented in the Level I codes.

Level III: The CMS eliminated Level III local codes. See Program Memorandum AB-02-113.

Headings are provided as a means of grouping similar or closely related items. The placement of a code under a heading does not indicate additional means of classification, nor does it relate to any health insurance coverage categories.

HCPCS also contains modifiers, which are two-position codes and descriptors used to indicate that a service or procedure that has been performed has been altered by some specific circumstance but not changed in its definition or code. Modifiers are grouped by the levels. Level I modifiers and descriptors are copyrighted by the AMA. Level II modifiers are HCPCS modifiers. Modifiers in the D series are copyrighted by the ADA.

HCPCS is designed to promote uniform reporting and statistical data collection of medical procedures, supplies, products, and services.

HCPCS Disclaimer

Inclusion or exclusion of a procedure, supply, product, or service does not imply any health insurance coverage or reimbursement policy.

HCPCS makes as much use as possible of generic descriptions, but the inclusion of brand names to describe devices or drugs is intended only for indexing purposes; it is not meant to convey endorsement of any particular product or drug.

Updating HCPCS

The primary updates are made annually. Quarterly updates are also issued by CMS.

GUIDE TO USING THE 2026 HCPCS LEVEL II CODES

Medical coding has long been a part of the health care profession. Through the years medical coding systems have become more complex and extensive. Today, medical coding is an intricate and immense process that is present in every health care setting. The increased use of electronic submissions for health care services only increases the need for coders who understand the coding process.

2026 HCPCS Level II was developed to help meet the needs of today's coder.

All material adheres to the latest government versions available at the time of printing.

Annotated

Throughout this text, revisions and additions are indicated by the following symbols:

- ▶ **New:** Additions to the previous edition are indicated by the color triangle.
- ↺ **Revised:** Revisions within the line or code from the previous edition are indicated by the color arrow.
- ✓ **Reinstated** indicates a code that was previously deleted and has now been reactivated.
- ✱ ~~Deleted~~ words have been removed from this year's edition.

HCPCS Symbols

- ✪ **Special coverage instructions** apply to these codes. Usually these special coverage instructions are included in the Internet Only Manuals (IOM). References to the IOM locations are given in the form of Medicare Pub. 100 reference numbers listed below the code. IOM select references are located at codingupdates.com.
- ⊘ **Not covered or valid by Medicare** is indicated by the "No" symbol. Usually the reason for the exclusion is included in the Internet Only Manuals (IOM) select references at codingupdates.com.
- ✱ **Carrier discretion** is an indication that you must contact the individual third-party payers to find out the coverage available for codes identified by this symbol.
- *Other* Drugs approved for Medicare Part B and other FDA-approved drugs are listed as Other.
- A2-Z3 **ASC Payment Indicators** identify the 2026 final payment for the code. A list of Payment Indicators is listed in the front matter of this text.
- A-Y **OPPS Status Indicators** identify the 2026 final status assigned to the code. A list of Status Indicators is listed in the front matter of this text.
- Ⓑ Bill Part B MAC.
- Ⓑ Bill DME MAC.
- *Coding Clinic* Indicates the American Hospital Association *Coding Clinic®* for HCPCS references by year, quarter, and page number.
- ♿ DMEPOS identifies durable medical equipment, prosthetics, orthotics, and supplies that may be eligible for payment from CMS.
- ♀ Indicates a code for female only.
- ♂ Indicates a code for male only.
- Ⓐ Indicates a code with an indication of age.
- Indicates a code included in the MIPS Quality Measure Specifications.
- Qp Indicates there is a maximum allowable number of units of service, per day, per patient for physician/provider services (*see* codingupdates.com for Practitioner Medically Unlikely Edits).
- Qh Indicates there is a maximum allowable number of units of service, per day, per patient in the outpatient hospital setting (*see* codingupdates.com for Hospital Medically Unlikely Edits).

Red, green, and blue typeface terms within the Table of Drugs and tabular section are terms added by the publisher and do not appear in the official code set. Information supplementing the official HCPCS Index produced by CMS is *italicized*.

SYMBOLS AND CONVENTIONS

HCPCS Symbols

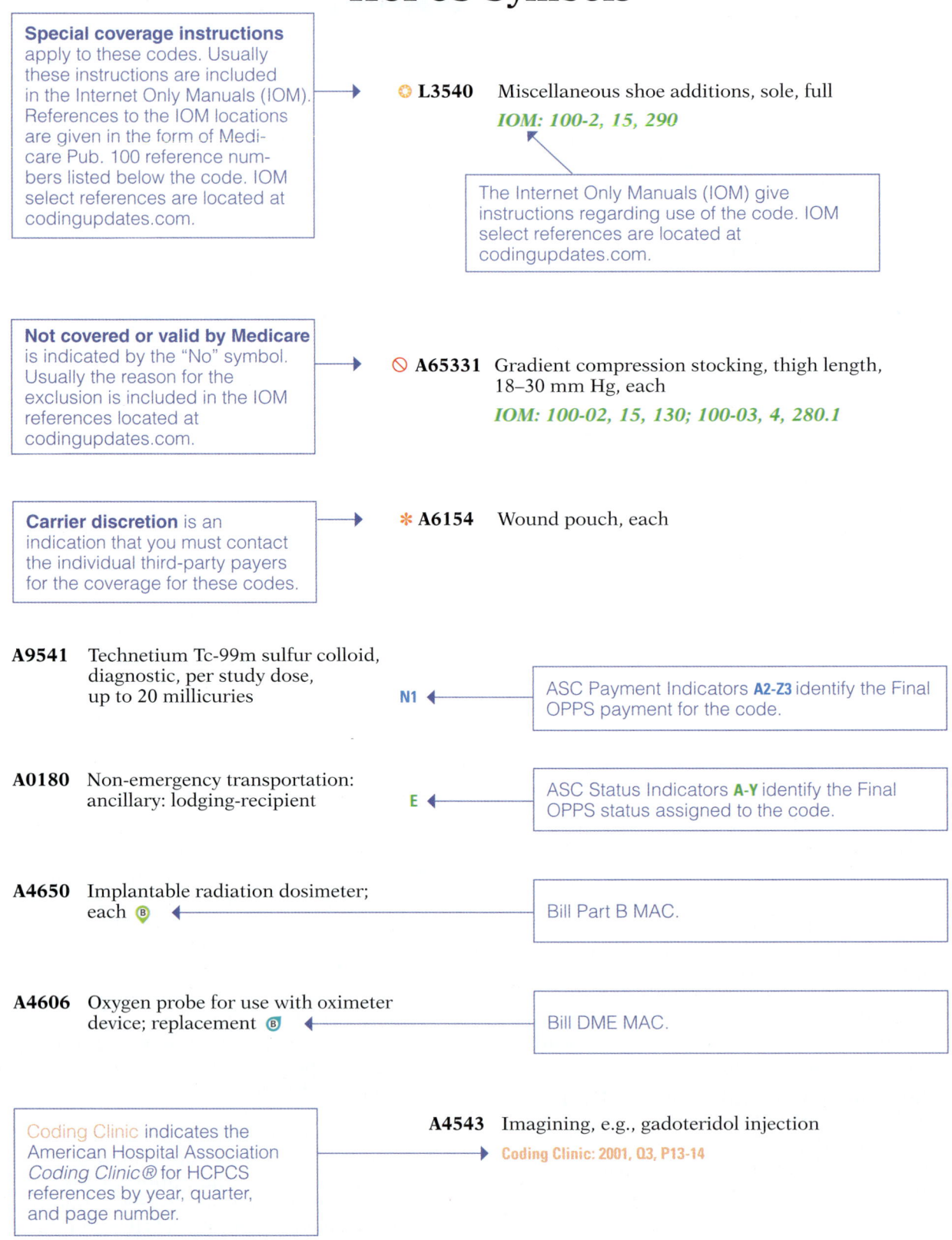

Special coverage instructions apply to these codes. Usually these instructions are included in the Internet Only Manuals (IOM). References to the IOM locations are given in the form of Medicare Pub. 100 reference numbers listed below the code. IOM select references are located at codingupdates.com.

○ **L3540** Miscellaneous shoe additions, sole, full
IOM: 100-2, 15, 290

The Internet Only Manuals (IOM) give instructions regarding use of the code. IOM select references are located at codingupdates.com.

Not covered or valid by Medicare is indicated by the "No" symbol. Usually the reason for the exclusion is included in the IOM references located at codingupdates.com.

⊘ **A65331** Gradient compression stocking, thigh length, 18–30 mm Hg, each
IOM: 100-02, 15, 130; 100-03, 4, 280.1

Carrier discretion is an indication that you must contact the individual third-party payers for the coverage for these codes.

∗ **A6154** Wound pouch, each

A9541 Technetium Tc-99m sulfur colloid, diagnostic, per study dose, up to 20 millicuries **N1**

ASC Payment Indicators **A2-Z3** identify the Final OPPS payment for the code.

A0180 Non-emergency transportation: ancillary: lodging-recipient **E**

ASC Status Indicators **A-Y** identify the Final OPPS status assigned to the code.

A4650 Implantable radiation dosimeter; each ⓑ

Bill Part B MAC.

A4606 Oxygen probe for use with oximeter device; replacement ⓑ

Bill DME MAC.

Coding Clinic indicates the American Hospital Association *Coding Clinic®* for HCPCS references by year, quarter, and page number.

A4543 Imagining, e.g., gadoteridol injection
Coding Clinic: 2001, Q3, P13-14

Codes shown are for illustration purposes only and may not be current codes.

Symbols and Conventions ix

DMEPOS symbol identifies durable medical equipment, prosthetics, orthotics, and supplies that may be eligible for payment from CMS.

E2210 Wheelchair accessory, bearings, any type, replacement only, each ♿

✱ **A4233** Replacement battery, alkaline (other than J cell), for use with medically necessary home blood glucose monitor owned by patient, each ♿

If "incident to" physician service, do not bill; otherwise bill DME MAC

On DMEPOS Fee Schedule.

❂ **B9000** Enteral nutrition infusion pump - without alarm **Qp** Y

Pump will be denied as not medically necessary if medical necessity of pump is not documented

IOM: 100-02, 15, 120; 100-03, 3, 180.2; 100-04, 20, 100.2.2

PEN: On Fee Schedule

On the Parenteral and Enteral Nutrition Items or Services (PEN) with modifier(s) from current PEN Fee Schedule.

A4261 Cervical cap for contraceptive use ♀

Indicates for female only.

A4267 Contraceptive supply, condom, male, each ♂

Indicates for male only.

Indicates a **reinstated** code.

✔ **D2970** Temporary crown (fractured tooth)

Indicates **new** information or a new code.

▶ **A4614** Peak expiratory flow rate meter, hand-held

Indicates a **revision** within the line or code.

↺ **J0270** Injection alprostadil, per 1.25 mcg

Codes shown are for illustration purposes only and may not be current codes.

Symbols and Conventions

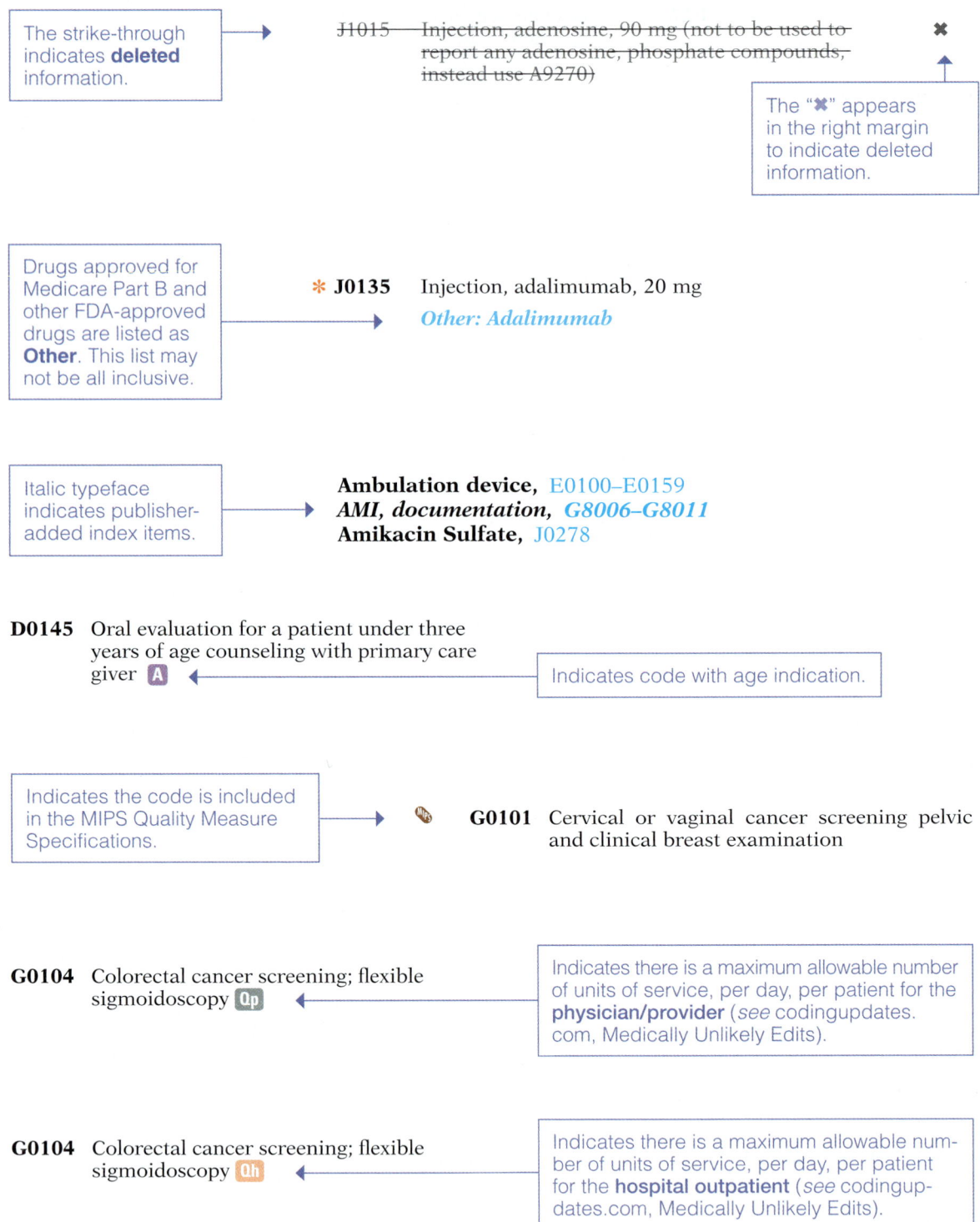

Codes shown are for illustration purposes only and may not be current codes.

A2-Z3 ASC Payment Indicators

Final ASC Payment Indicators for CY 2026	
Payment Indicator	**Payment Indicator Definition**
A2	Surgical procedure on ASC list in CY 2007; payment based on OPPS relative payment weight.
B5	Alternative code may be available; no payment made.
D1	Ancillary dental service/item; no separate payment made.
D2	Non office-based dental procedure added in CY 2024 or later.
D5	Deleted/discontinued code; no payment made.
F4	Corneal tissue acquisition, hepatitis B vaccine; paid at reasonable cost.
G2	Non-office-based surgical procedure added in CY 2008 or later; payment based on OPPS relative payment weight.
H2	Brachytherapy source paid separately when provided integral to a surgical procedure on ASC list; payment OPPS rate.
J7	OPPS pass-through device paid separately when provided integral to a surgical procedure on ASC list; payment contractor-priced.
J8	Device-intensive procedure; paid at adjusted rate.
K2	Drugs, biologicals, and radiopharmaceuticals paid separately when provided integral to a surgical procedure on ASC list; payment based on OPPS rate.
K5	Items, codes, and services for which pricing information and claims data are not available. No payment made.
K7	Unclassified drugs and biologicals; payment contractor-priced.
L1	Influenza vaccine; pneumococcal vaccine. Packaged item/service; no separate payment made.
L6	Special payment; New Technology Intraocular Lens (NTIOL) or qualifying non-opioid device.
N1	Packaged service/item; no separate payment made.
P2	Office-based surgical procedure added to ASC list in CY 2008 or later with MPFS nonfacility PE RVUs; payment based on OPPS relative payment weight.
P3	Office-based surgical procedure added to ASC list in CY 2008 or later with MPFS nonfacility PE RVUs; payment based on MPFS nonfacility PE RVUs.
R2	Office-based surgical procedure added to ASC list in CY 2008 or later without MPFS nonfacility PE RVUs; payment based on OPPS relative payment weight.
Z2	Radiology or diagnostic service paid separately when provided integral to a surgical procedure on ASC list; payment based on OPPS relative payment weight.
Z3	Radiology or diagnostic service paid separately when provided integral to a surgical procedure on ASC list; payment based on MPFS nonfacility PE RVUs.
Final Changes to the ASC Payment System and CY 2026 Payment Rates, http://www.cms.gov/Medicare/Medicare-Fee-for-Service-Payment/ASCPayment/ASC-Regulations-and-Notices.html.	

A-Y OPPS Status Indicators

	Final OPPS Payment Status Indicators for CY 2026	
Indicator	**Item/Code/Service**	**OPPS Payment Status**
A	Services furnished to a hospital outpatient that are paid under a fee schedule or payment system other than OPPS,* for example:	Not paid under OPPS. Paid by MACs under a fee schedule or payment system other than OPPS. Services are subject to deductible or coinsurance unless indicated otherwise.
	• Ambulance Services	
	• Separately Payable Clinical Diagnostic Laboratory Services	Not subject to deductible or coinsurance.
	• Separately Payable Non-Implantable Prosthetics and Orthotics	
	• Physical, Occupational, and Speech Therapy	
	• Diagnostic Mammography	
	• Screening Mammography	Not subject to deductible or coinsurance.
	Unclassified drugs and biologicals reportable under HCPCS code C9399 and not otherwise classified FDA-approved prescription drugs for HIV PrEP reported under code J0799	Contractor priced at 95 percent of drug or biological's average wholesale price (AWP) using Red Book or an equivalent recognized compendium and paid under OPPS.
B	Codes that are not recognized by OPPS when submitted on an outpatient hospital Part B bill type (12x and 13x)	Not paid under OPPS. • May be paid by MACs when submitted on a different bill type, for example, 75x (CORF), but not paid under OPPS. • An alternate code that is recognized by OPPS when submitted on an outpatient hospital Part B bill type (12x and 13x) may be available.
C	Inpatient Procedures	Not paid under OPPS. Admit patient. Bill as inpatient.
D	Discontinued Codes	Not paid under OPPS or any other Medicare payment system.
E1	Items, Codes, and Services: • Not covered by any Medicare outpatient benefit category • Statutorily excluded by Medicare • Not reasonable and necessary	Not paid by Medicare when submitted on outpatient claims (any outpatient bill type).
E2	Items, Codes, and Services: For which pricing information and claims data are not available	Not paid by Medicare when submitted on outpatient claims (any outpatient bill type).
F	Corneal Tissue Acquisition; Certain CRNA Services	Not paid under OPPS. Paid at reasonable cost.
G	Pass-Through Drugs and Biologicals	Paid under OPPS; separate APC payment.
H	Pass-Through Device Categories	Separate cost-based pass-through payment; not subject to co-payment.
H1	Non-opioid Medical Devices for Post-Surgical Pain Relief	Separate payment based on hospital's charges adjusted to cost. Subject to criteria and payment limitation under Section 4132 of the CAA, 2023.
J1	Hospital Part B services paid through a comprehensive APC	Paid under OPPS; all covered Part B services on the claim are packaged with the primary "J1" service for the claim, except the Comprehensive APC payment exclusions found in the most recent Addendum J.
J2	Hospital Part B Services That May Be Paid Through a Comprehensive APC	Paid under OPPS; Addendum B displays APC assignments when services are separately payable. (1) Comprehensive APC payment based on OPPS comprehensive-specific payment criteria. Payment for all covered Part B services on the claim is packaged into a single payment for specific combinations of services, except the Comprehensive APC payment exclusions found in the most recent Addendum J. (2) Packaged APC payment if billed on the same claim as a HCPCS code assigned status indicator "J1." (3) In other circumstances, payment is made through a separate APC payment or packaged into payment for other services.

A-Y OPPS Status Indicators—cont'd

Final OPPS Payment Status Indicators for CY 2026

Indicator	Item/Code/Service	OPPS Payment Status
K	NonPass-Through Drugs and Non-Implantable Biologicals, including Therapeutic Radiopharmaceuticals	Paid under OPPS: separate APC payment.
K1	Non-Opioid Drugs and Biologicals For Post-Surgical Pain Relief	Paid under OPPS; separate APC payment. Subject to criteria and payment limitation under Section 4132 of the CAA, 2023.
L	Influenza Vaccine; Pneumococcal Pneumonia Vaccine; Hepatitis B Vaccines; Covid-19 Vaccine; Monoclonal Antibody Therapy Product	Not paid under OPPS. Paid at reasonable cost; not subject to deductible or coinsurance.
M	Items and Services Not Billable to the MAC	Not paid under OPPS.
N	Items and Services Packaged into APC Rates	Paid under OPPS; payment is packaged into payment for other services. Therefore, there is no separate APC payment.
P	Partial Hospitalization or Intensive Outpatient Program	Paid under OPPS; per diem APC payment.
Q1	STV-Packaged Codes	Paid under OPPS; Addendum B displays APC assignments when services are separately payable. (1) Packaged APC payment if billed on the same claim as a HCPCS code assigned status indicator "S," "T," or "V." (2) Composite APC payment if billed with specific combinations of services based on OPPS composite-specific payment criteria. Payment is packaged into a single payment for specific combinations of services. (3) In other circumstances, payment is made through a separate APC payment.
Q2	T-Packaged Codes	Paid under OPPS; Addendum B displays APC assignments when services are separately payable. (1) Packaged APC payment if billed on the same claim as a HCPCS code assigned status indicator "T." (2) In other circumstances, payment is made through a separate APC payment.
Q3	Codes That May Be Paid Through a Composite APC	Paid under OPPS; Addendum B displays APC assignments when services are separately payable. Addendum M displays composite APC assignments when codes are paid through a composite APC. (1) Composite APC payment based on OPPS composite-specific payment criteria. Payment is packaged into a single payment for specific combinations of service. (2) In other circumstances, payment is made through a separate APC payment or packaged into payment for other services.
Q4	Conditionally Packaged Laboratory Tests	Paid under OPPS or CLFS. (1) Packaged APC payment if billed on the same claim as a HCPCS code assigned published status indicator "J1," "J2," "S," "T," "V," "Q1," "Q2," or "Q3." (2) In other circumstances, laboratory tests should have a status indicator of "A" and payment is made under the CLFS.
R	Blood and Blood Products	Paid under OPPS; separate APC payment.
S	Procedure or Service, Not Discounted when Multiple	Paid under OPPS; separate APC payment.
T	Procedure or Service, Multiple Procedure Reduction Applies	Paid under OPPS; separate APC payment.
U	Brachytherapy Sources	Paid under OPPS; separate APC payment.
V	Clinic or Emergency Department Visit	Paid under OPPS; separate APC payment.
Y	Non-Implantable Durable Medical Equipment	Not paid under OPPS. All institutional providers other than home health agencies bill to a DME MAC.

* Note — Payments "under a fee schedule or payment system other than OPPS" may be contractor priced.

Final Changes to the ASC Payment System and CY 2026 Payment Rates, http://www.cms.gov/Medicare/Medicare-Fee-for-Service-Payment/HospitalOutpatientPPS/Hospital-Outpatient-Regulations-and-Notices.html.

2026 HCPCS UPDATES

2026 HCPCS New/Revised/Deleted Codes and Modifiers

Each quarter CMS will post an update to the HCPCS code set to their website. A direct link to all the quarterly updates can also be found on our companion website (codingupdates.com)

NEW CODES/MODIFIERS

January	G0540	J1414	M1401	Q5145	J1299	Q5147	Q4371
A9615	G0541	J1552	M1402	Q5146	J1308	Q5148	Q4372
C1735	G0542	J2290	M1403	Q9996	J1808	Q5149	Q4373
C1736	G0543	J2472	M1404	Q9997	J1938	Q5150	Q4375
C1737	G0544	J2802	M1405	Q9998	J2351	Q5151	Q4376
C1738	G0545	J3392	M1406		J2428	Q5152	Q4377
C1739	G0546	J7514	M1407	**April**	J2804	Q9999	Q4378
C7562	G0547	J7601	M1408	A2030	J2865	S4024	Q4379
C7563	G0548	J9026	M1409	A2031	J7521		Q4380
C7564	G0549	J9028	M1410	A2032	J9024	**July**	Q4382
C7565	G0550	J9076	M1411	A2033	J9038	C9174	Q5098
C8001	G0551	J9292	M1412	A2034	J9054	C9175	Q5099
C8002	G0552	M1371	M1413	A2035	J9161	J0165	Q5100
C8003	G0553	M1372	M1414	A6515	L0720	J0166	Q5153
C9173	G0554	M1373	M1415	A6516	L1933	J0167	
C9610	G0555	M1374	M1416	A6517	L1952	J0168	**October**
C9804	G0556	M1375	M1417	A6518	L5827	J0169	A2036
C9806	G0557	M1376	M1418	A6519	L6028	J0616	A2037
C9807	G0558	M1377	M1419	A6611	L6029	J0618	A2038
C9808	G0559	M1378	M1420	A9154	L6030	J1163	A2039
C9809	G0560	M1379	M1421	A9611	L6031	J1326	A4288
E1803	G0561	M1380	M1422	C8004	L6032	J2312	A9612
E1804	G0562	M1381	M1423	C8005	L6033	J2313	A9616
E1807	G0563	M1382	M1424	C9300	L6037	J3373	C1740
E1808	G0564	M1383	M1425	C9301	L6700	J3374	C1741
E1813	G0565	M1384	Q0155	C9302	L7406	J3375	C1742
E1814	H0052	M1385	Q0521	C9303	Q2057	J3391	C8006
E1822	H0053	M1386	Q4346	C9304	Q4354	J7172	C9305
E1823	J0139	M1387	Q4347	E0201	Q4355	J7356	C9306
E1826	J0601	M1388	Q4348	E1022	Q4356	J9174	E0150
E1827	J0602	M1390	Q4349	E1023	Q4357	J9220	E0658
E1828	J0603	M1391	Q4350	E1032	Q4358	J9275	E0659
E1829	J0605	M1392	Q4351	E1033	Q4359	J9276	J0163
G0532	J0607	M1393	Q4352	E1034	Q4360	J9289	J0164
G0533	J0608	M1394	Q4353	E1832	Q4361	J9341	J0458
G0534	J0609	M1395	Q5139	G0183	Q4362	J9342	J0462
G0535	J0615	M1396	Q5140	G0566	Q4363	J9382	J0525
G0536	J0666	M1397	Q5141	G0567	Q4364	Q2058	J0582
G0537	J0870	M1398	Q5142	J0281	Q4365	Q4368	J0614
G0538	J0901	M1399	Q5143	J1072	Q4366	Q4369	J0668
G0539	J1307	M1400	Q5144	J1271	Q4367	Q4370	J0675

J0681	J2151	L5657	M0238	Q4388	Q4396	
J0738	J2291	L6034	Q0235	Q4389	Q4397	
J0752	J3290	L6035	Q0237	Q4390	Q5154	
J0759	J3402	L6036	Q4383	Q4391	Q5155	
J1370	J3403	L6038	Q4384	Q4392	Q5156	
J1612	J7173	L6039	Q4385	Q4393	Q5157	
J1807	J7174	M0235	Q4386	Q4394	Q5158	
J1809	J9011	M0236	Q4387	Q4395	Q5159	
J1834	L1007	M0237				

REVISED CODES/MODIFIERS

January	G2101	G9247	M1150	M1344	A6586	L1951	C1982
TB	G2107	G9254	M1176	M1345	A6587	L1971	E0765
E1800	G2116	G9255	M1177	M1346	A6588	L6692	E0986
E1805	G2126	G9321	M1179	M1347	C1739	L6698	J1961
E1810	G8577	G9322	M1211	M1348	C9793		J7300
E1815	G8578	G9659	M1212	M1349	E1028	**July**	J9072
E1825	G8694	G9660	M1259		E1801	C8005	L5673
E1830	G8842	G9999	M1260	**April**	E1811	J1954	L5679
G2069	G8843	J2468	M1267	A4453	E1816	J9292	L5783
G2076	G8844	J9033	M1268	A4459	E1818	Q9998	L6028
G2077	G8923	J9072	M1272	A6549	E1841		L7406
G2091	G8934	L8720	M1292	A6583	J9073	**October**	
G2099	G9246	M0004	M1343	A6585	L1932	C1739	

DELETED CODES/MODIFIERS

January	C9795	G1020	G9458	M0003	J1890	Q0243	G9038
JG	G0106	G1021	G9459	M1154	J1940	Q0244	J0171
MA	G0120	G1022	G9460	M1155	J9037	Q0245	J0173
MB	G0122	G1023	G9707	M1219	J9247	Q0247	J2310
MC	G1001	G1024	G9751	M1264	L8010	Q4231	J2311
MD	G1002	G2012	G9760	Q0516	M0220	Q5139	J3370
ME	G1003	G2070	G9892	Q0517	M0221	S0017	J3371
MF	G1004	G2071	G9893	Q0518	M0222	S0028	J3372
MG	G1007	G2072	G9921	Q0519	M0223	S0032	J9340
MH	G1008	G8482	G9974	Q0520	M0240	S0039	M0248
QQ	G1010	G8483	G9975	Q5131	M0241	S4988	
C7558	G1011	G8484	G9990	Q5132	M0243		**October**
C9169	G1012	G8965	G9991		M0244	**July**	C9088
C9170	G1013	G8966	J0135	**April**	M0245	C9173	C9174
C9171	G1014	G9402	J0570	A9155	M0246	C9300	C9175
C9172	G1015	G9403	J2796	G0564	M0247	C9301	C9248
C9290	G1016	G9404	J2806	G0565	Q0220	C9302	J2150
C9769	G1017	G9405	J9058	J1094	Q0221	C9303	J2503
C9786	G1018	G9406	J9059	J1300	Q0222	C9304	S0074
C9794	G1019	G9407	J9259	J1810	Q0240	G9037	

NEW, REVISED, AND DELETED DENTAL CODES

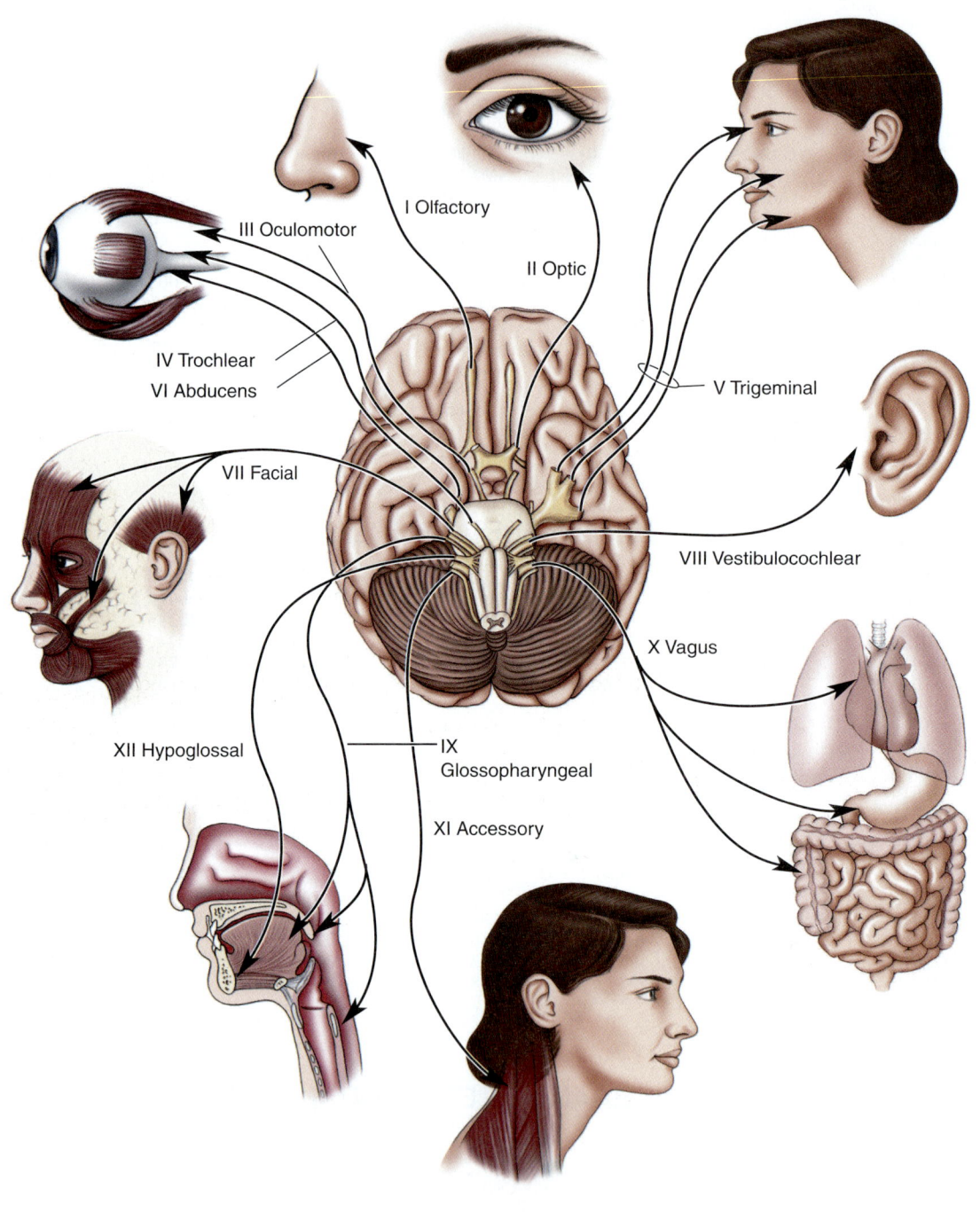

Plate 1 Cranial Nerves (12 pairs) are known by their numbers (Roman numerals) and names. (Herlihy BL: The Human Body in Health and Illness, ed 6, St. Louis, 2018, Elsevier.)

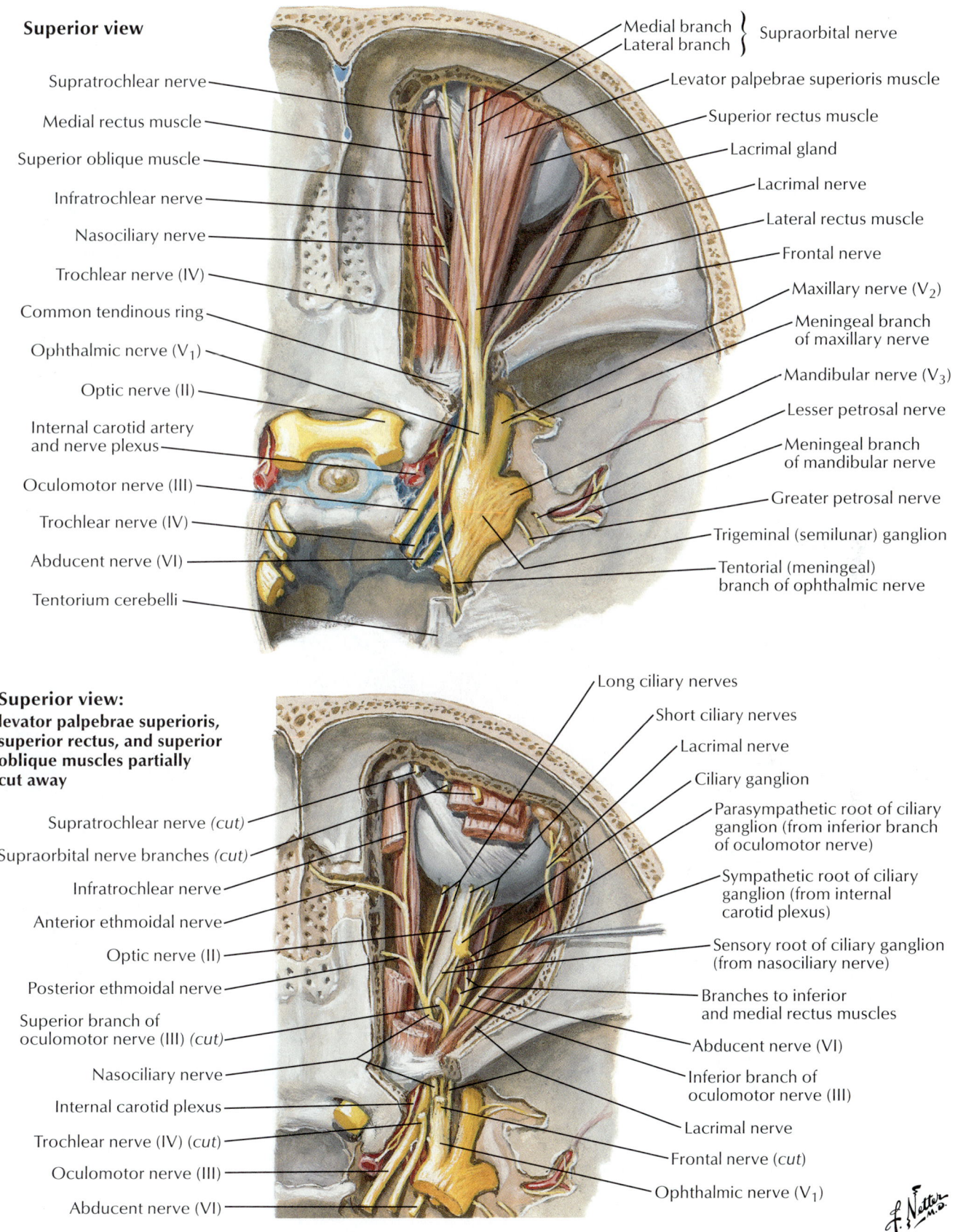

Plate 2 Nerves of Orbit.

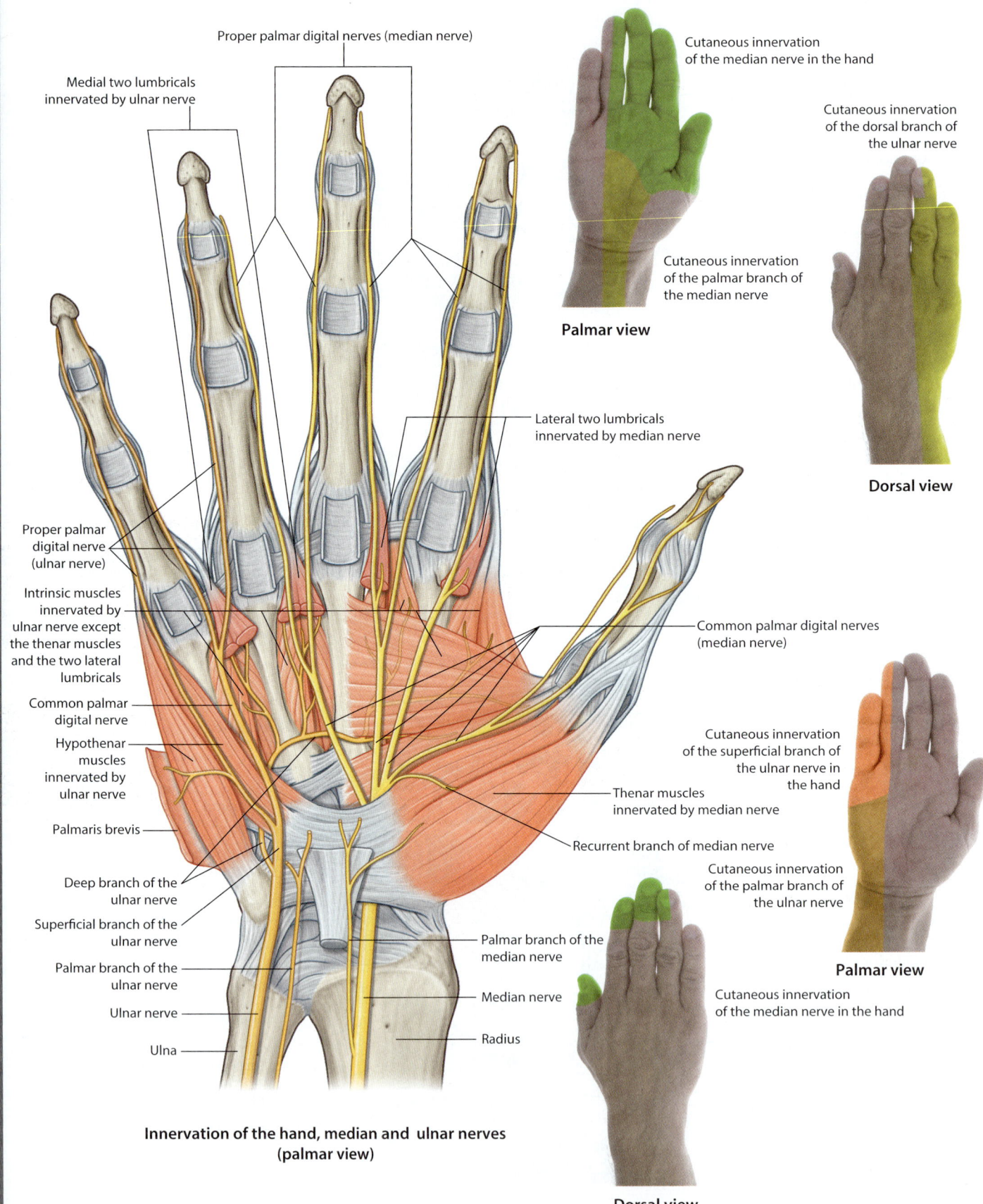

Plate 3 Innervation of the Hand: Median and Ulnar Nerves (From Drake RL, Vogl AW, Mitchell AWM, Tibbitts RM, Richardson PE: Gray's Atlas of Anatomy, ed 2, Philadelphia, 2015, Churchill Livingstone.)

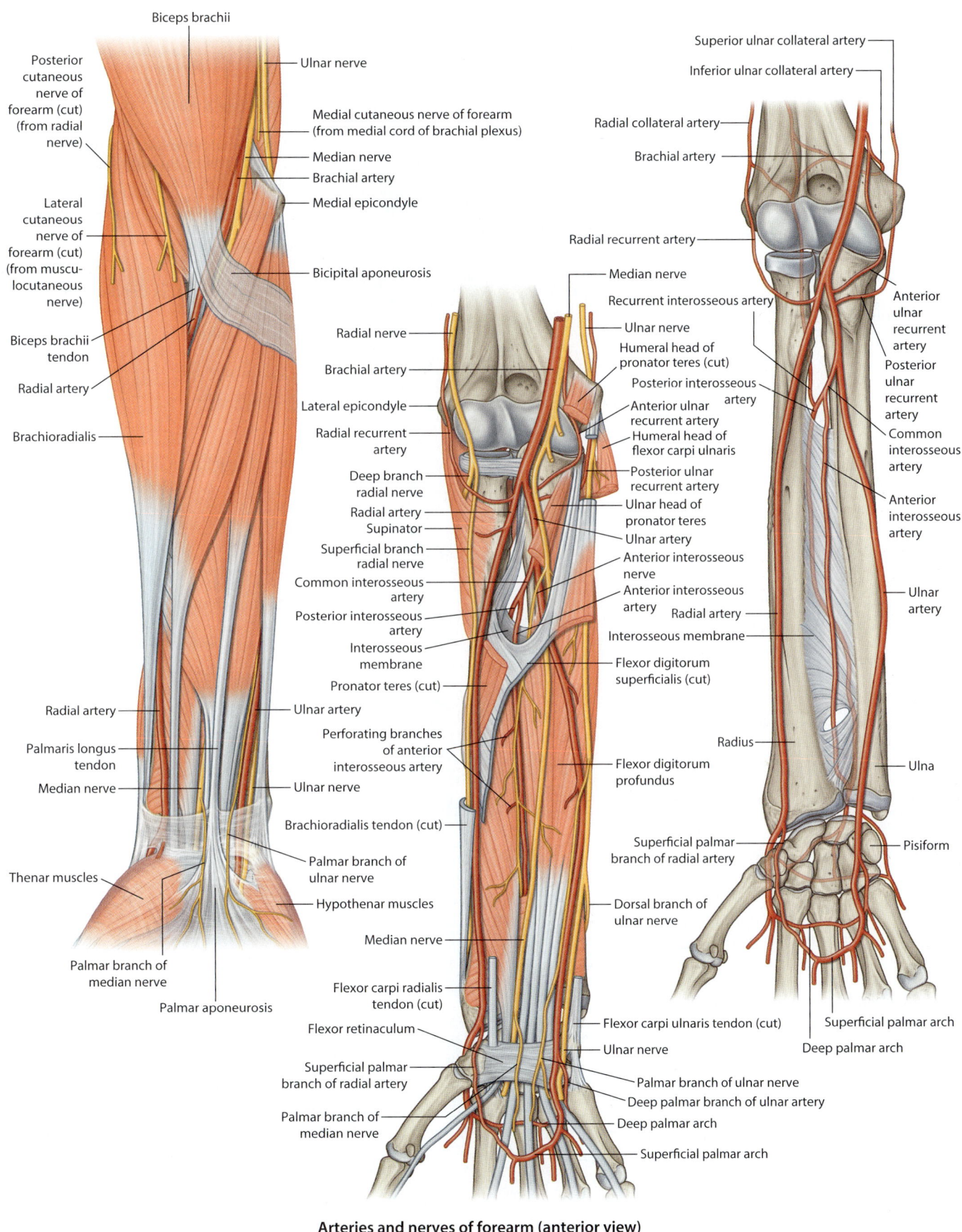

Arteries and nerves of forearm (anterior view)

Plate 4 Arteries and Nerves of the Forearm (Anterior View) (From Drake RL, Vogl AW, Mitchell AWM, Tibbitts RM, Richardson PE: Gray's Atlas of Anatomy, ed 2, Philadelphia, 2015, Churchill Livingstone.)

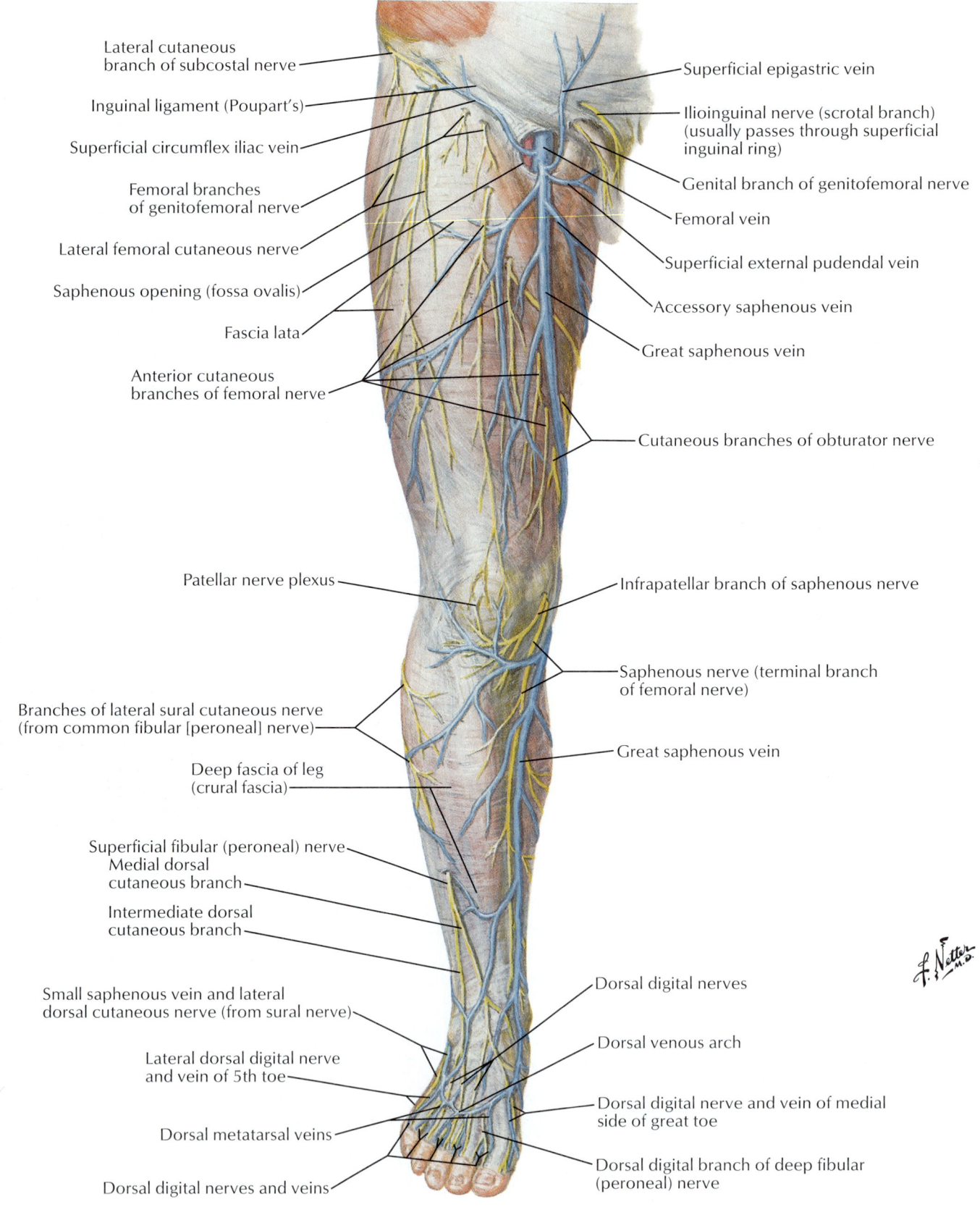

Plate 5 Superficial Nerves and Veins of Lower Limb: Anterior View. (Copyright 2025 Elsevier Inc. All rights reserved. www.netterimages.com. Image ID: 4846.)

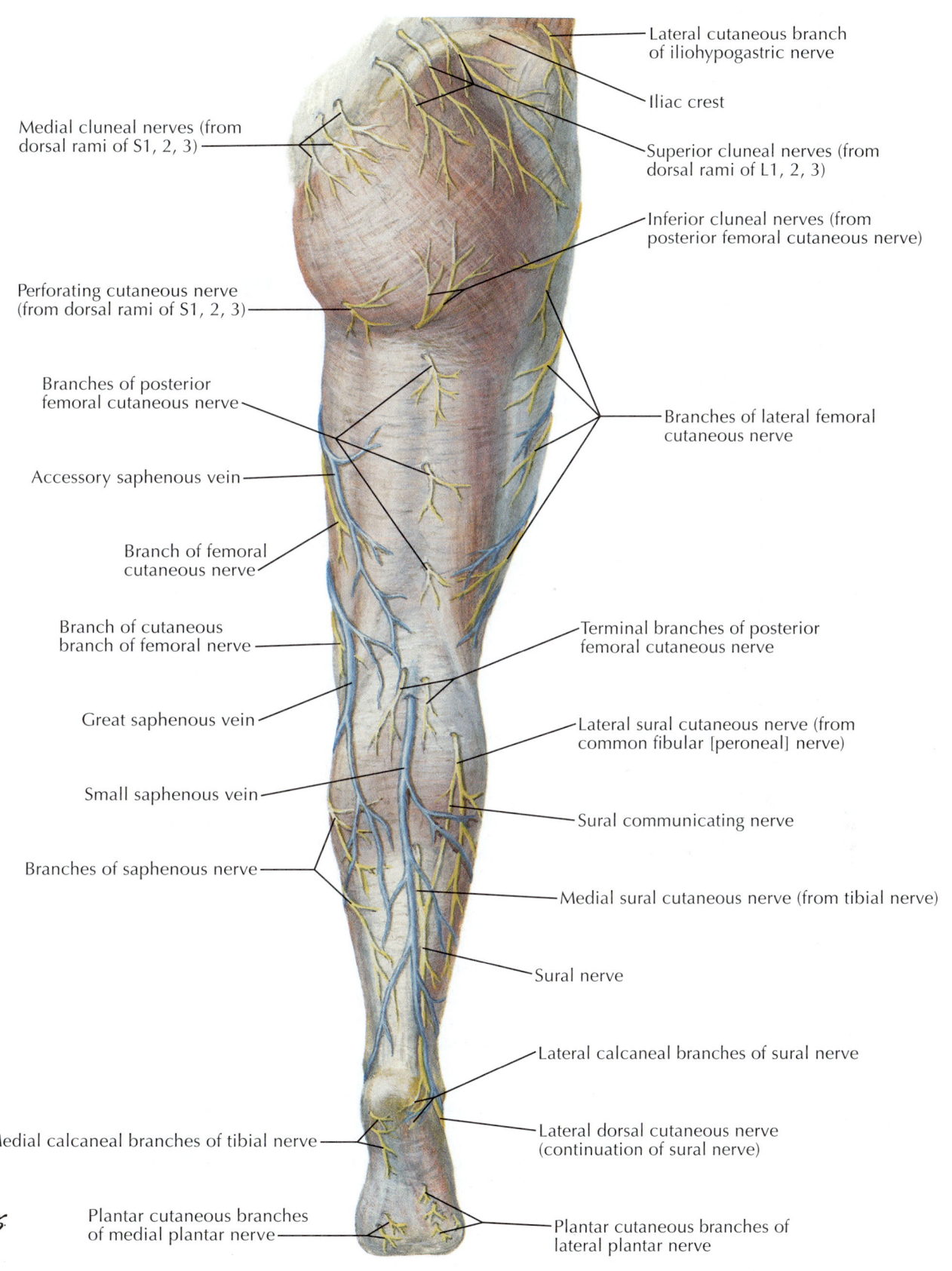

Plate 6 Superficial Nerves and Veins of Lower Limb: Posterior View. (Copyright 2025 Elsevier Inc. All rights reserved. www.netterimages.com. Image ID: 4669.)

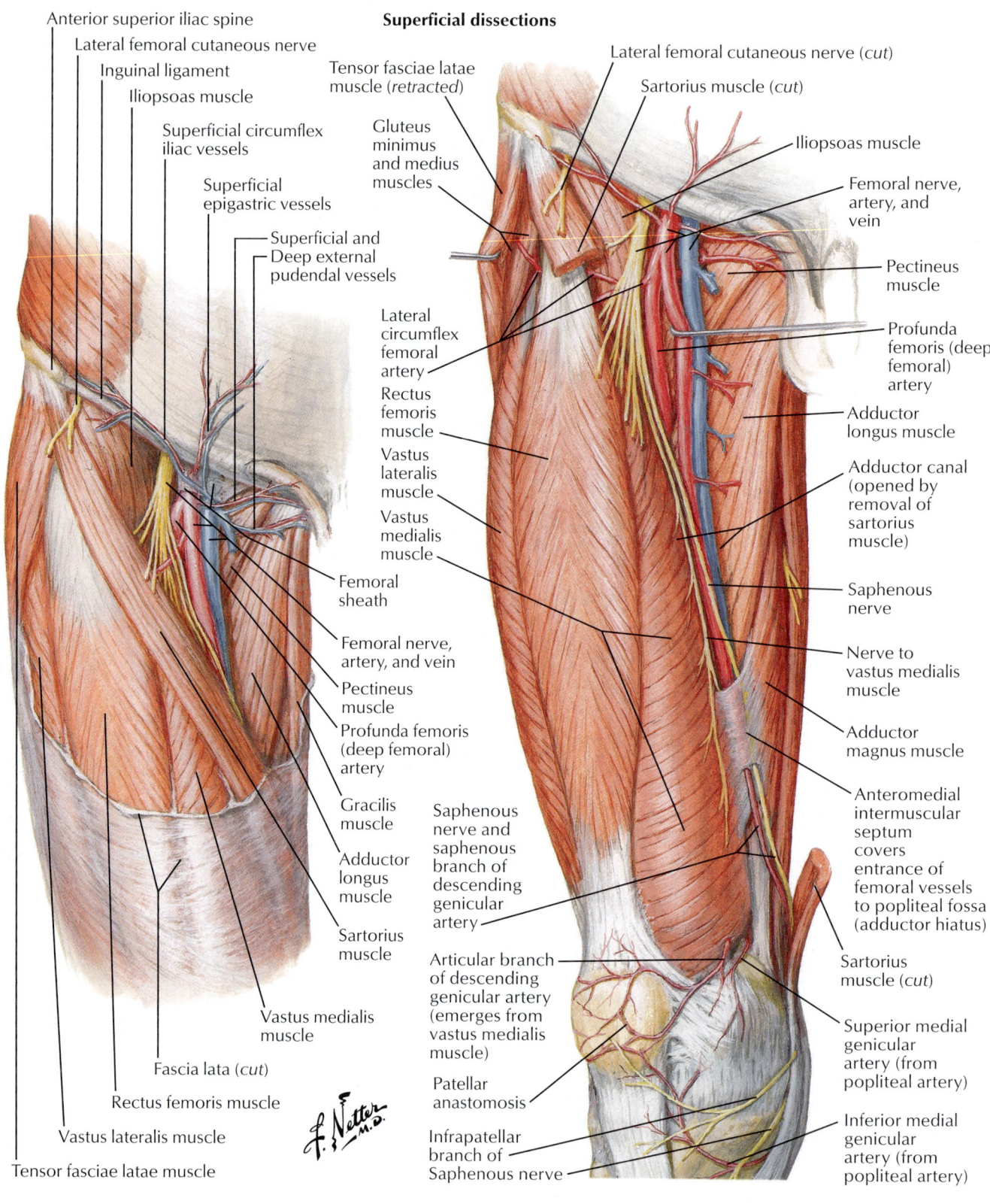

Plate 7 Arteries and Nerves of Thigh: Anterior Views. (Copyright 2025 Elsevier Inc. All rights reserved. www.netterimages.com. Image ID: 4475.)

Deep dissection

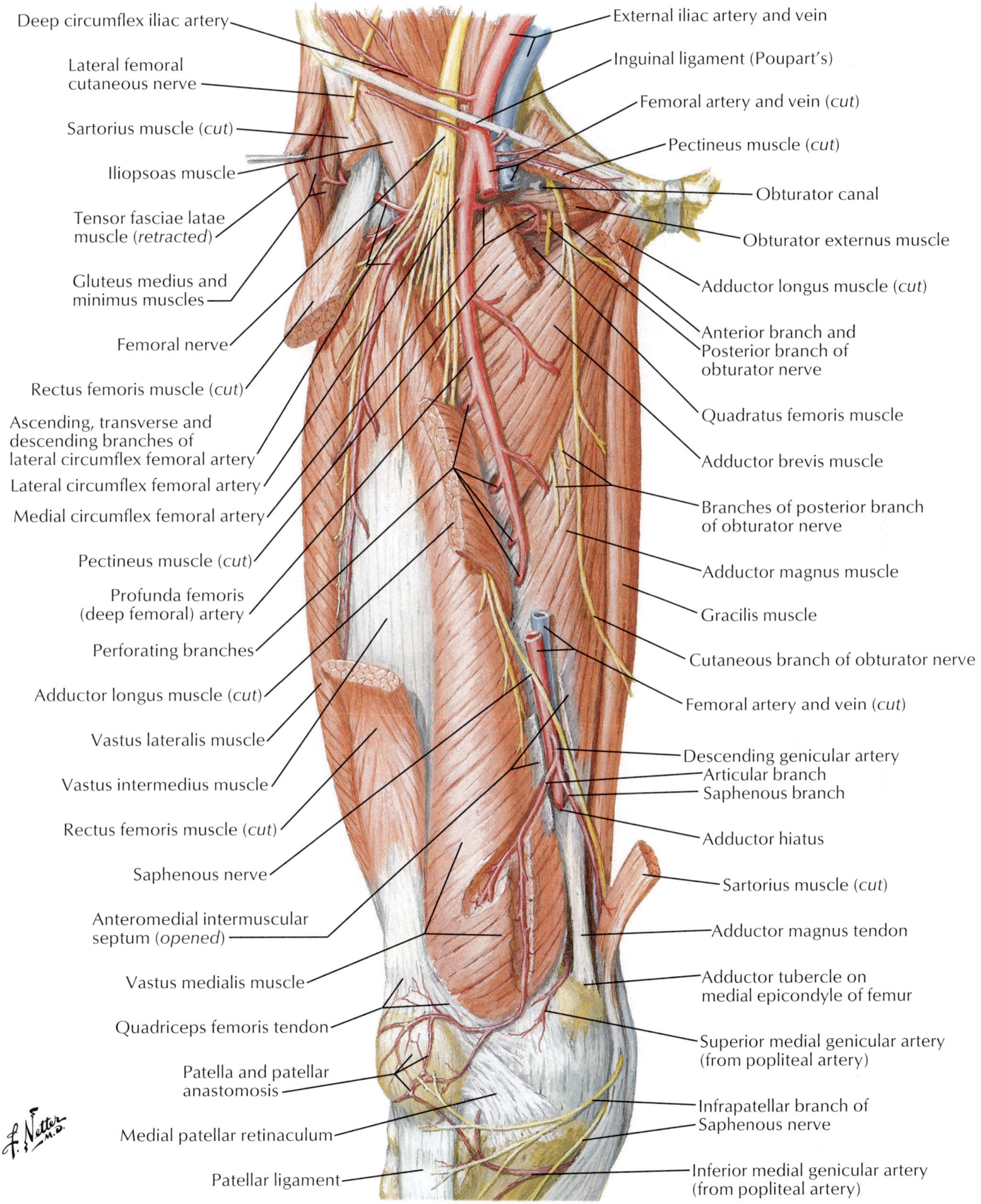

Plate 8 Arteries and Nerves of Thigh: Posterior View. (Copyright 2025 Elsevier Inc. All rights reserved. www.netterimages.com. Image ID: 49316.)

Deep dissection

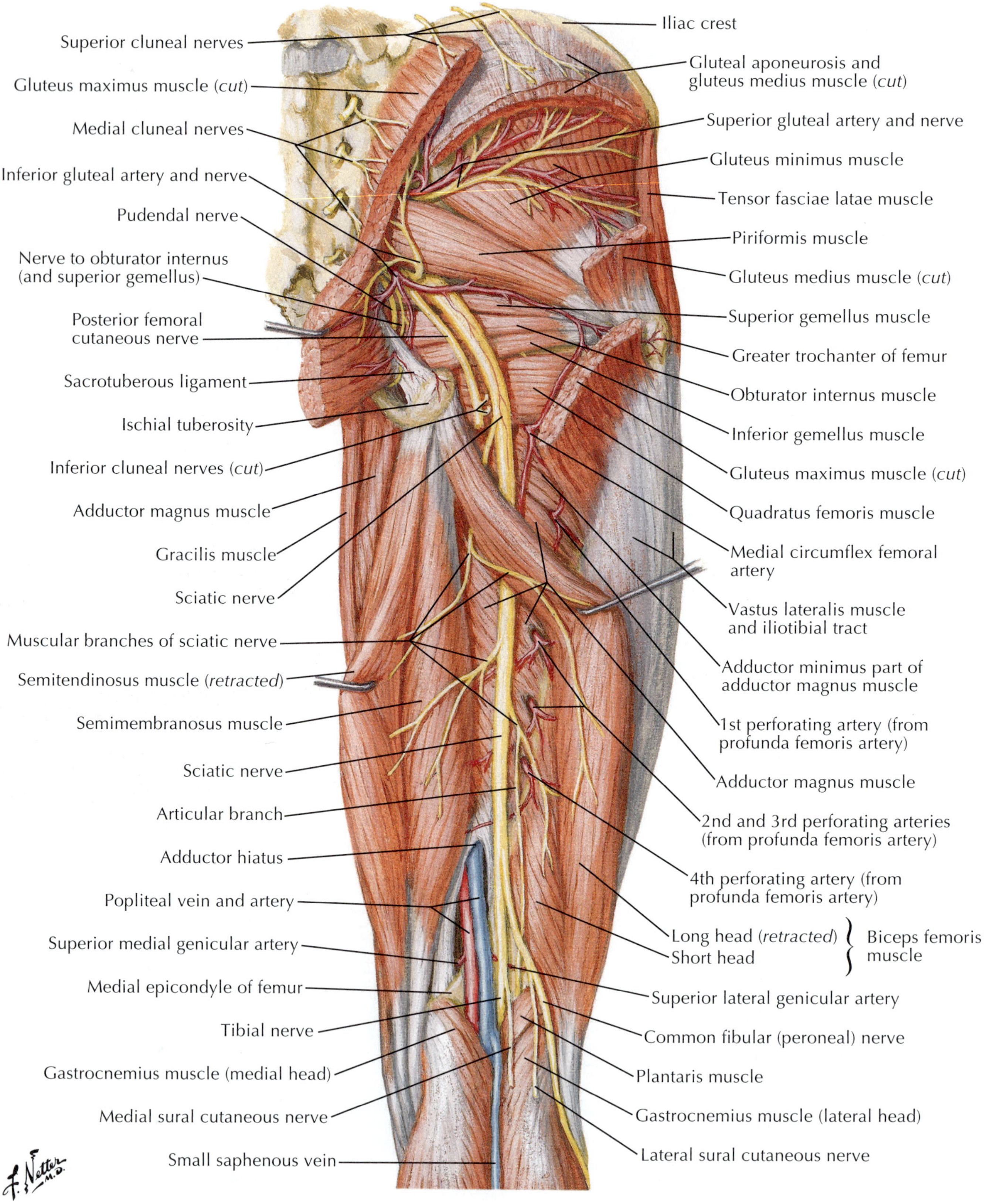

Plate 9 Arteries and Nerves of Thigh: Posterior View. (Copyright 2025 Elsevier Inc. All rights reserved. www.netterimages.com. Image ID: 49317.)

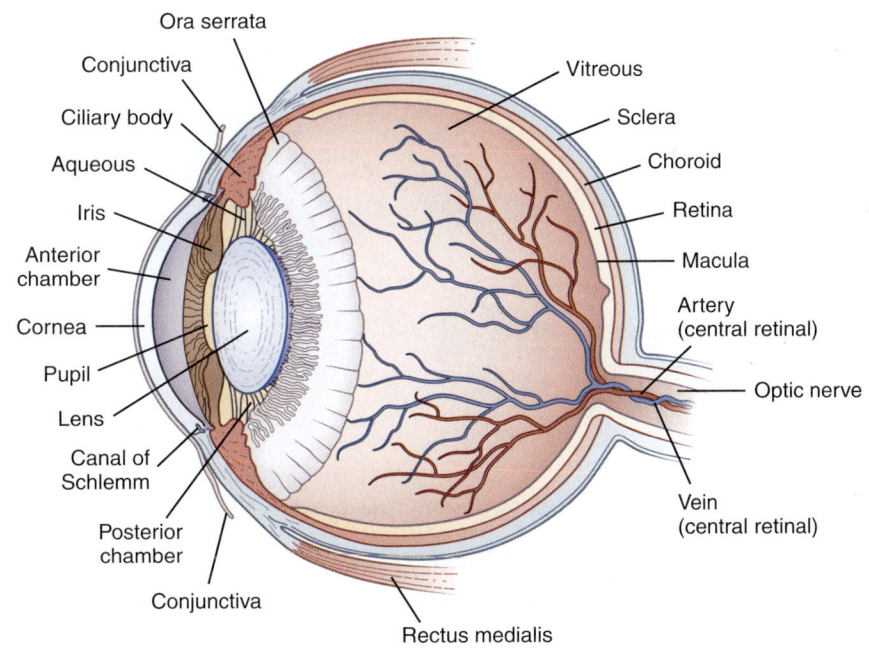

Plate 10 Anatomy of the Eye. (Dehn RW, Asprey DP: Essential Clinical Procedures, ed 3, Philadelphia, 2013, Saunders.)

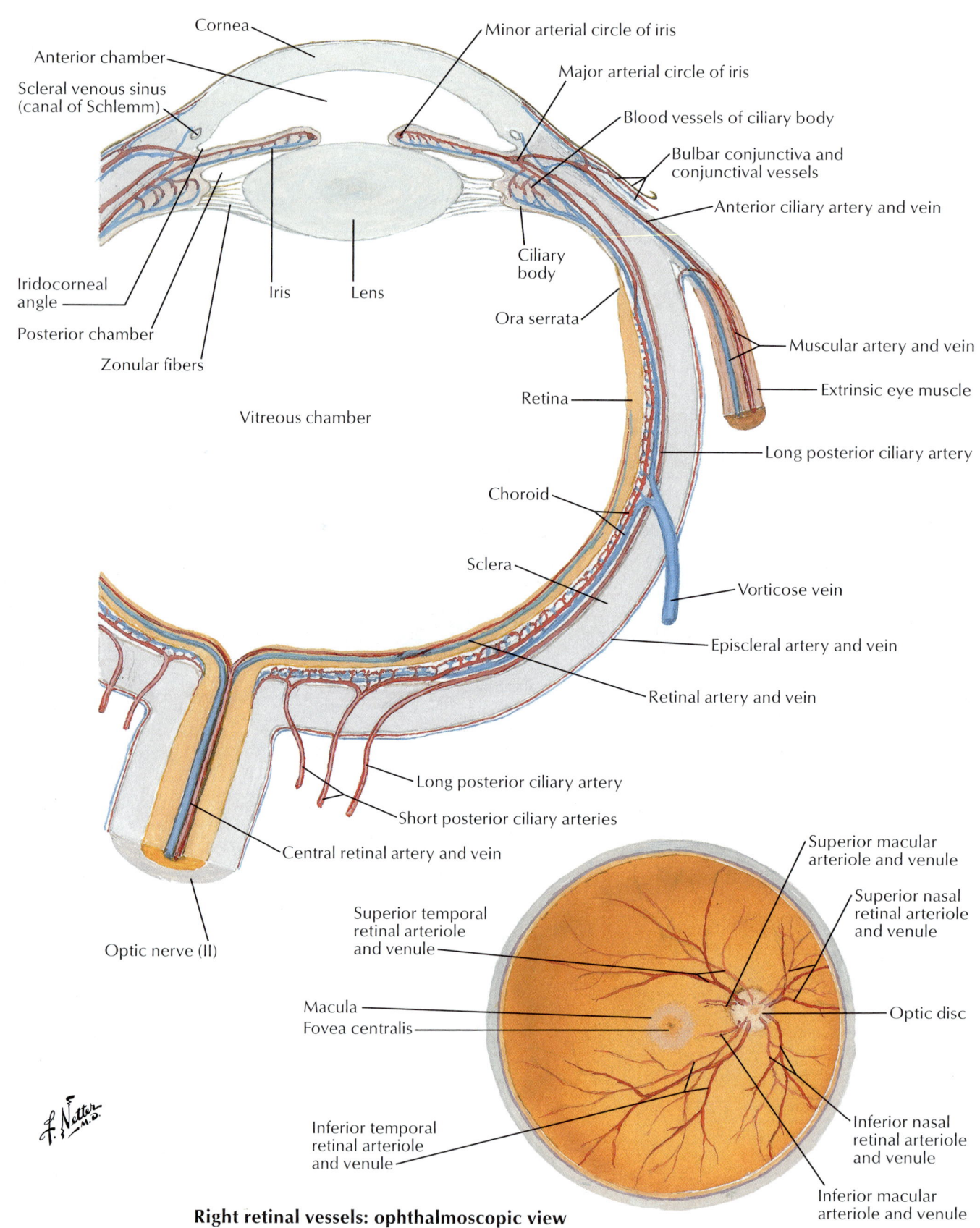

Right retinal vessels: ophthalmoscopic view

Plate 11 Intrinsic Arteries and Veins of Eye. (Copyright 2025 Elsevier Inc. All rights reserved. www.netterimages.com. Image ID: 49107.)

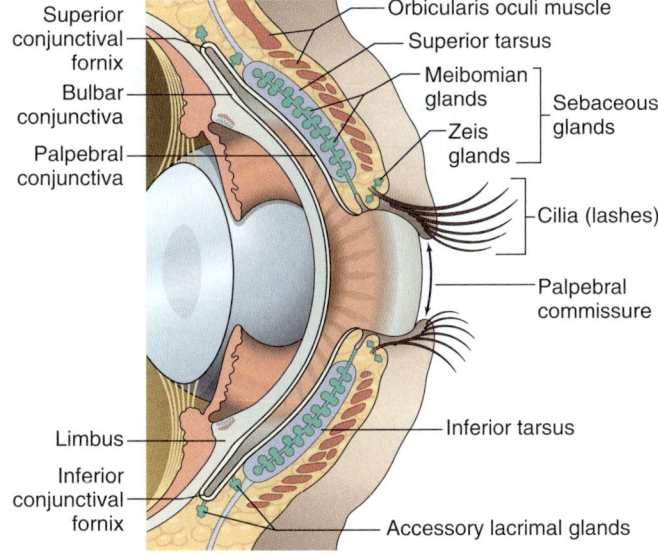

Plate 12 Anatomy of the Conjunctiva and Eyelids. (Kumar V, Abbas AK, Aster JC: Robbins and Cotran Pathologic Basis of Disease, ed 9, Philadelphia, 2015, Saunders.)

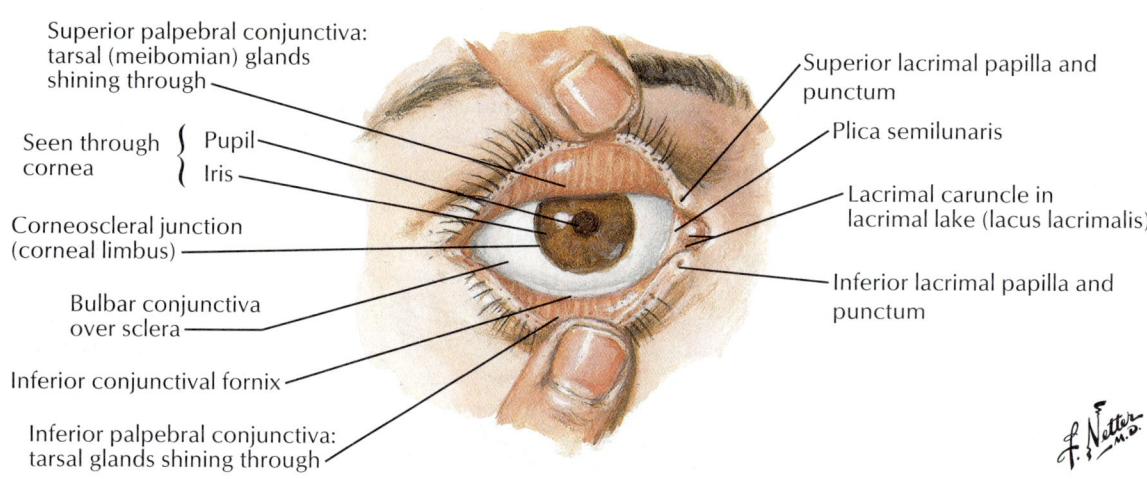

Plate 13 Eyelid. (Copyright 2025 Elsevier Inc. All rights reserved. www.netterimages.com. Image ID: 4557.)

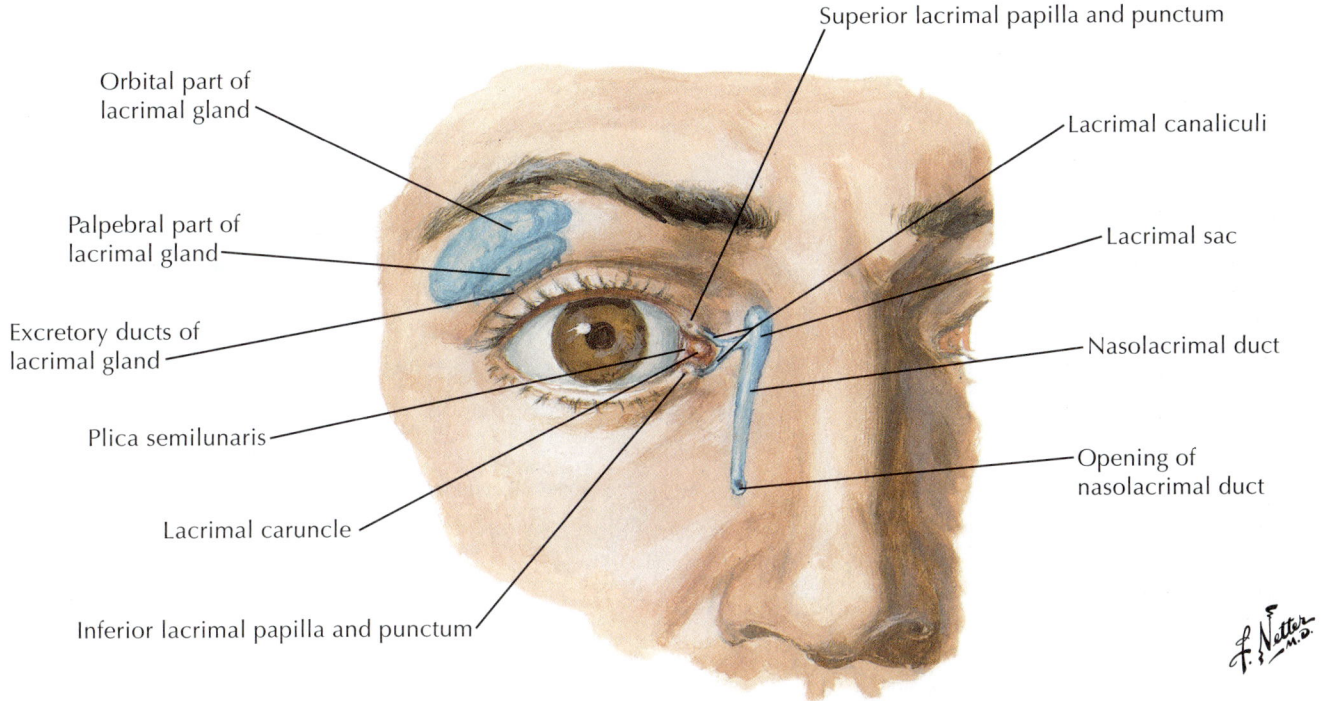
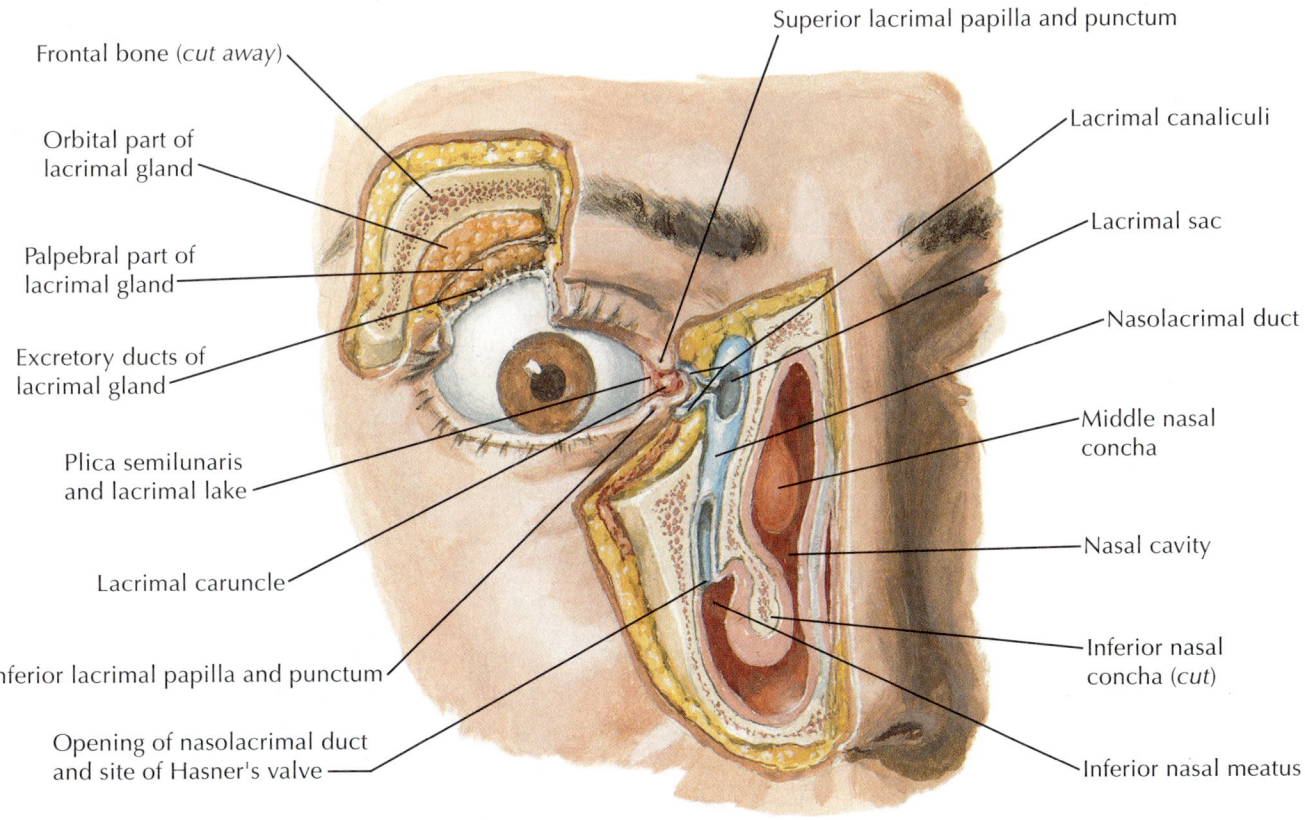

Plate 14 Lacrimal Apparatus. (Copyright 2025 Elsevier Inc. All rights reserved. www.netterimages.com. Image ID: 49103.)

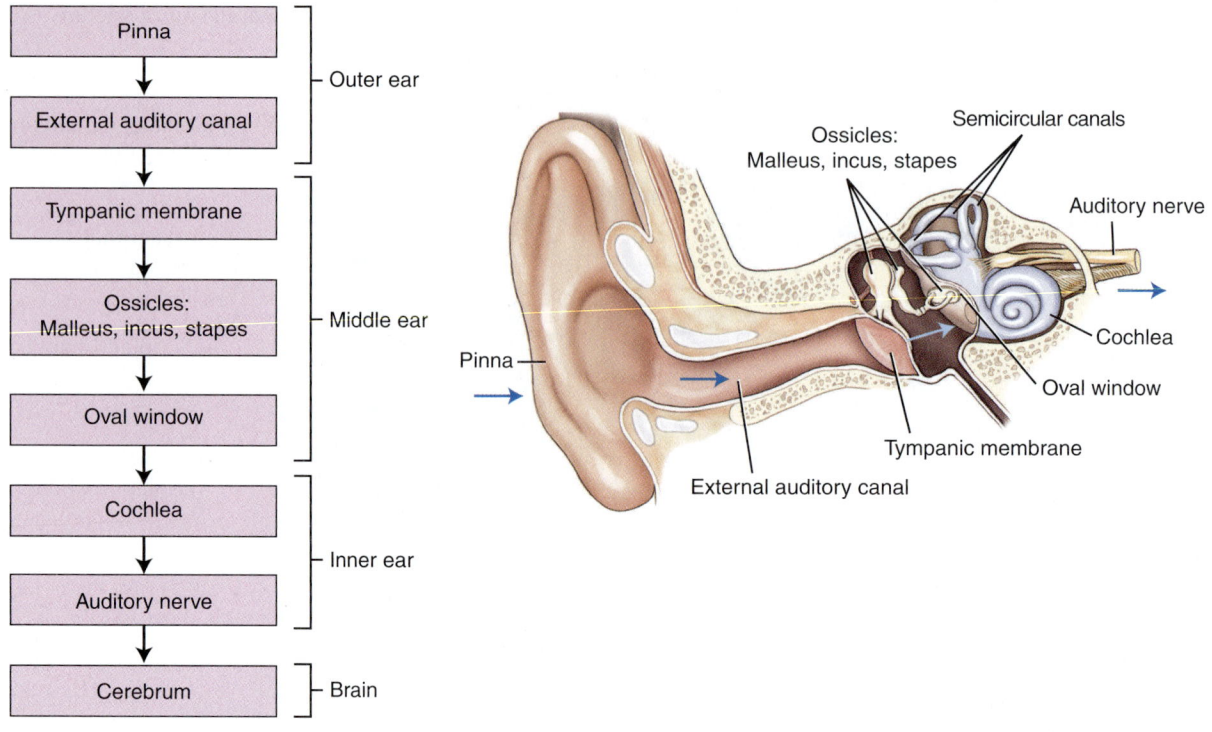

Plate 15 Pathway of Sound. (LaFleur Brooks D, LaFleur Brooks M: Basic Medical Language, ed 4, St. Louis, 2013, Mosby.)

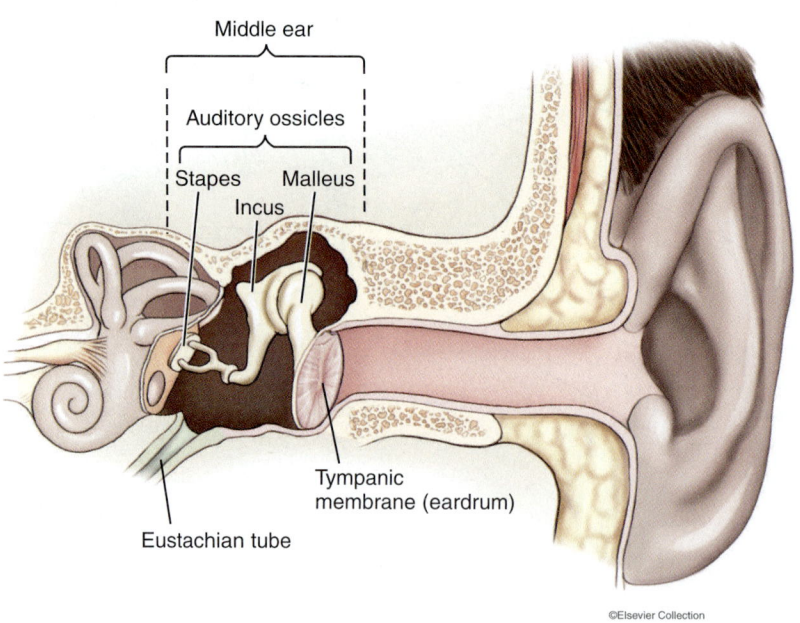

Plate 16 Middle Ear Structures. (©Elsevier Collection.)

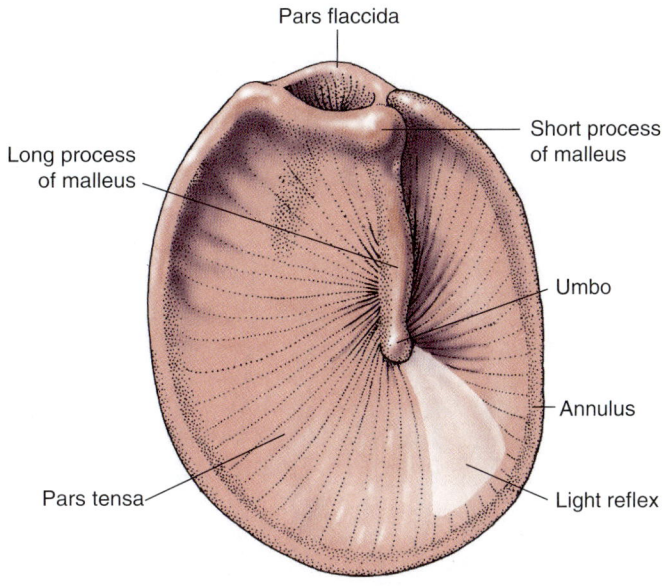

Plate 17 Structural Landmarks of Tympanic Membrane. (Ignatavicius DD, Workman ML: Medical-Surgical Nursing: Patient-Centered Collaborative Care, ed 7, St. Louis, 2013, Saunders.)

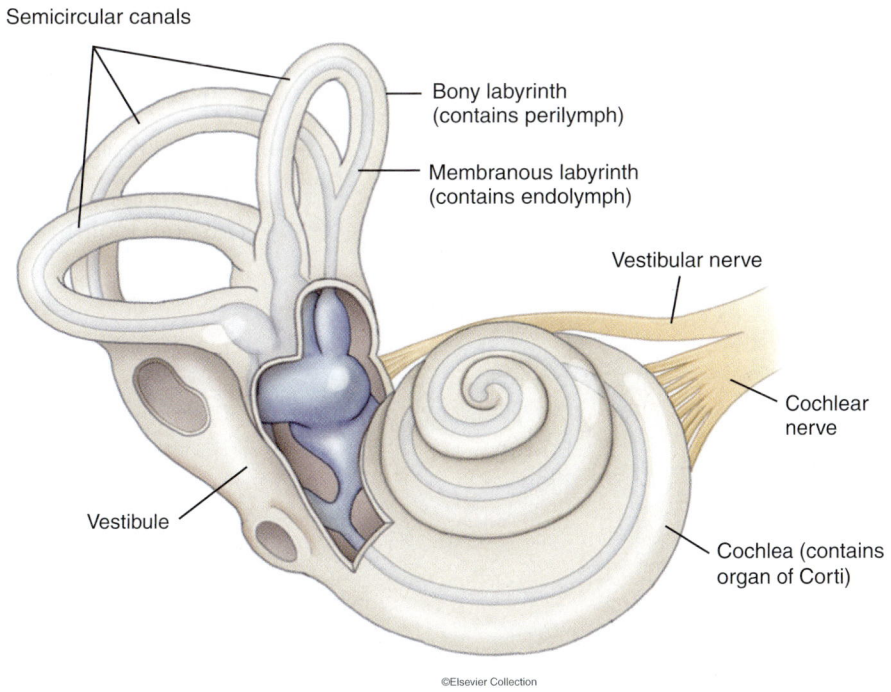

Plate 18 Inner Ear Structures. (©Elsevier Collection.)

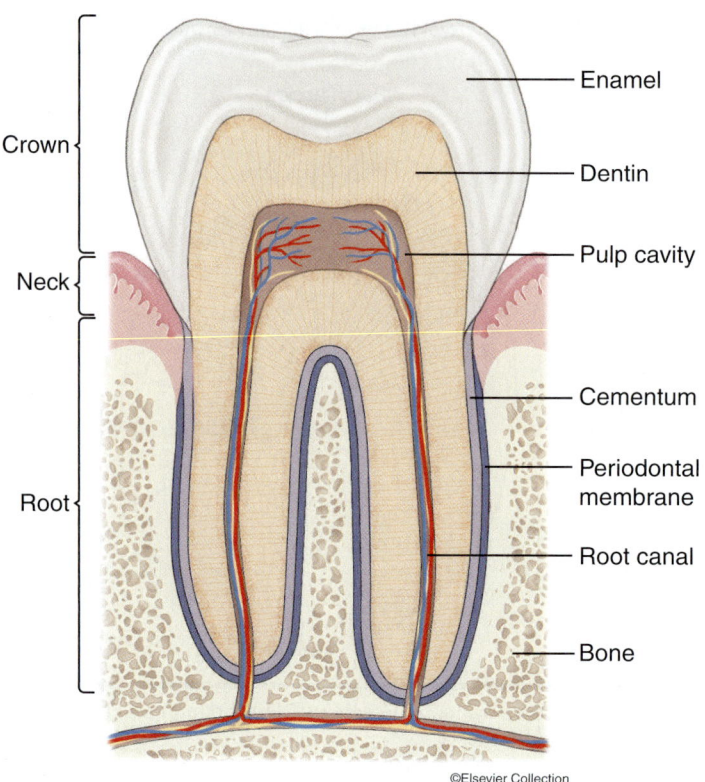

Plate 19 The Tooth. (©Elsevier Collection).

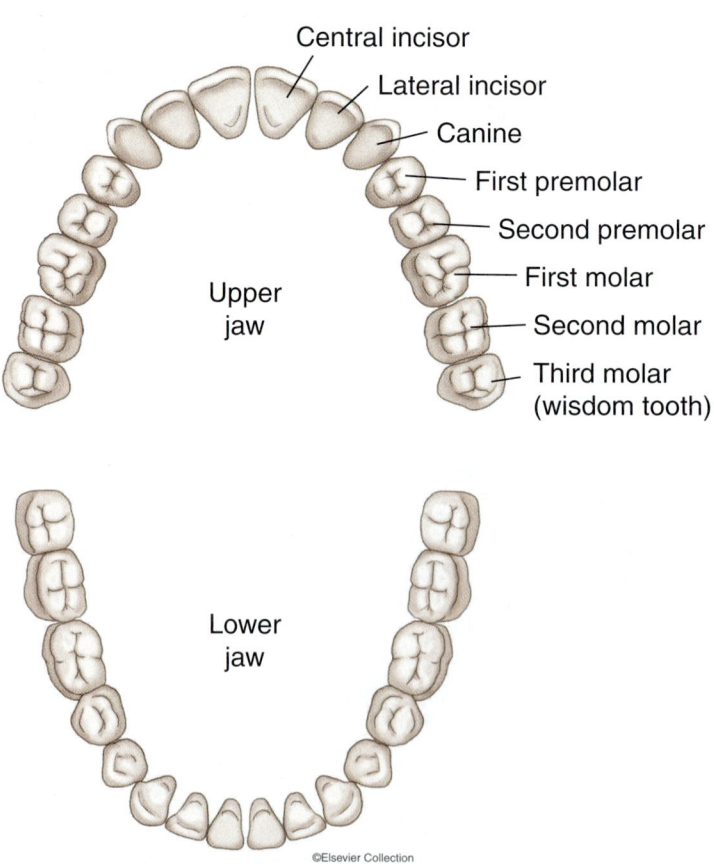

Plate 20 Adult Teeth. (©Elsevier Collection).

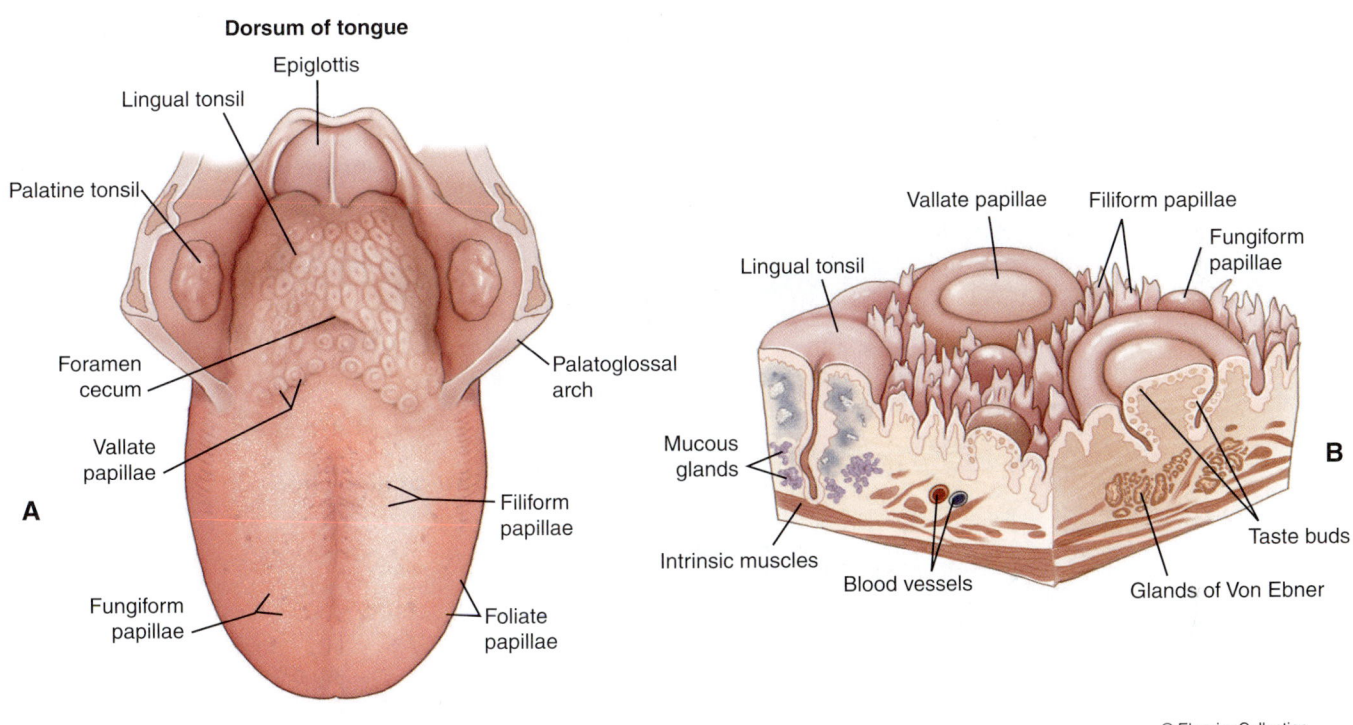

Plate 21 A, Dorsal view of tongue showing the roughened large lingual tonsils on the posterior of the tongue and the foliate papillae on the side. B, Section of dorsal of the tongue showing a cutaway through lingual papillae and showing von Ebner's glands at the base of the vallate papilla. (Brand RW, Isselhard DE: Anatomy of Orofacial Structures: A Comprehensive Approach, ed 8, St. Louis, 2019, Elsevier.)

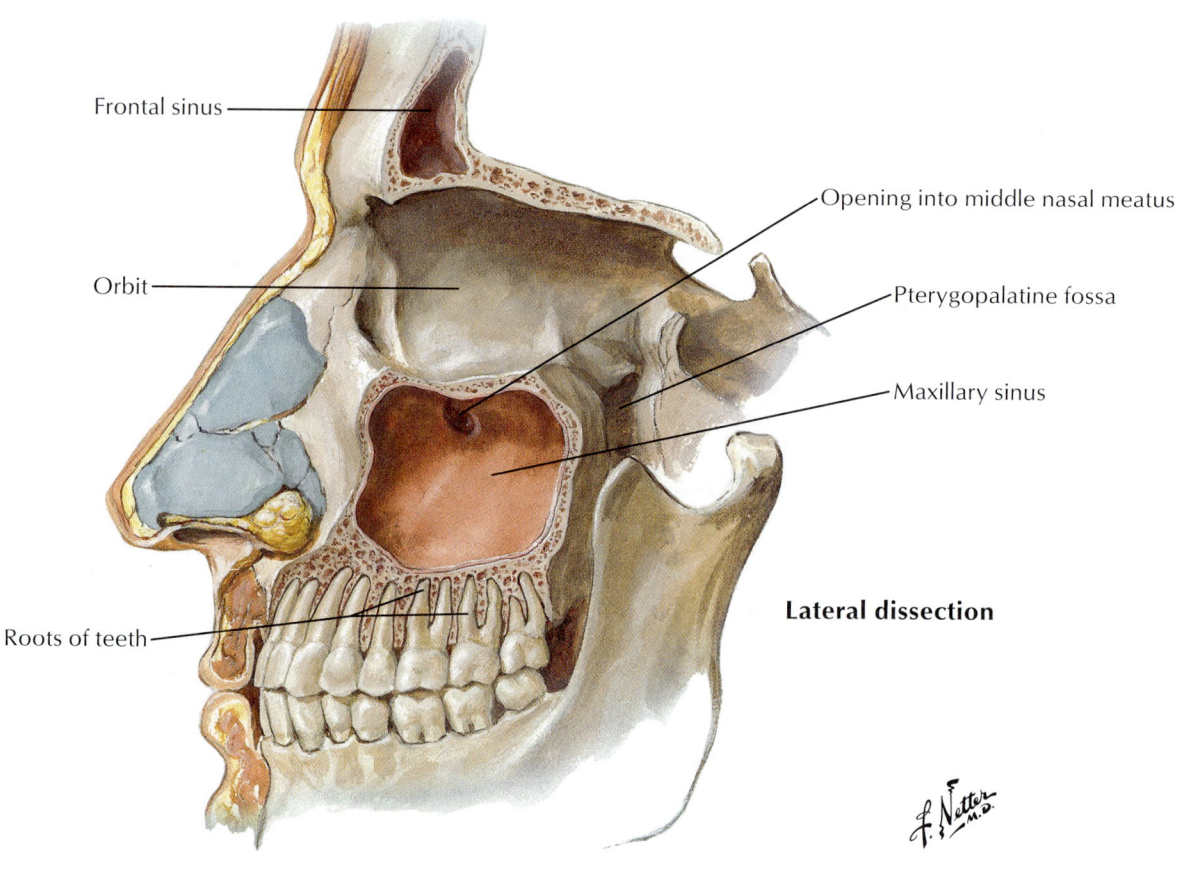

Plate 22 Paranasal Sinuses. (Copyright 2025 Elsevier Inc. All rights reserved. www.netterimages.com. Image ID: 8427.)

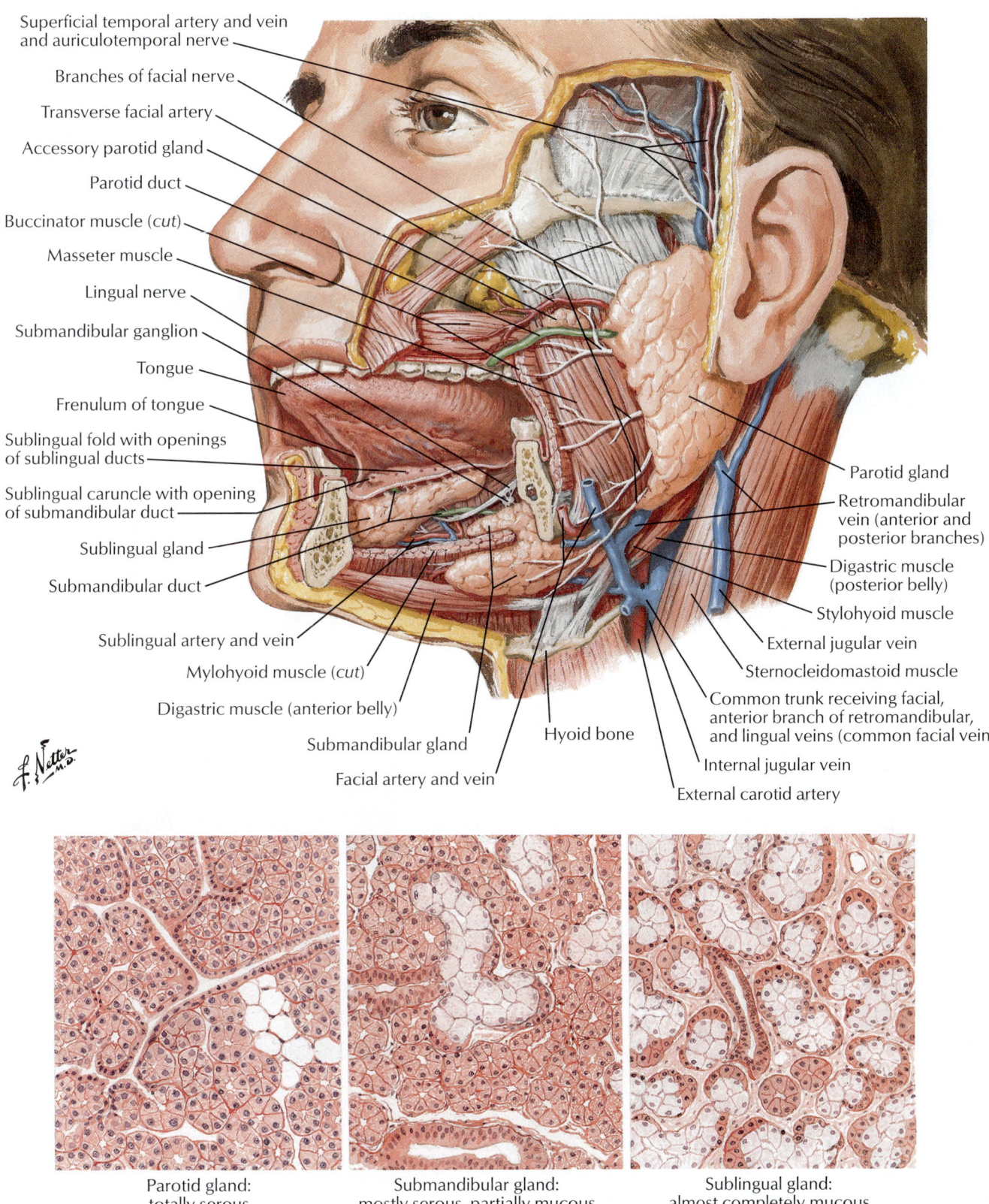

Plate 23 Salivary Glands. (Copyright 2025 Elsevier Inc. All rights reserved. www.netterimages.com. Image ID: 4396.)

Coronary Arteries: Arteriographic Views

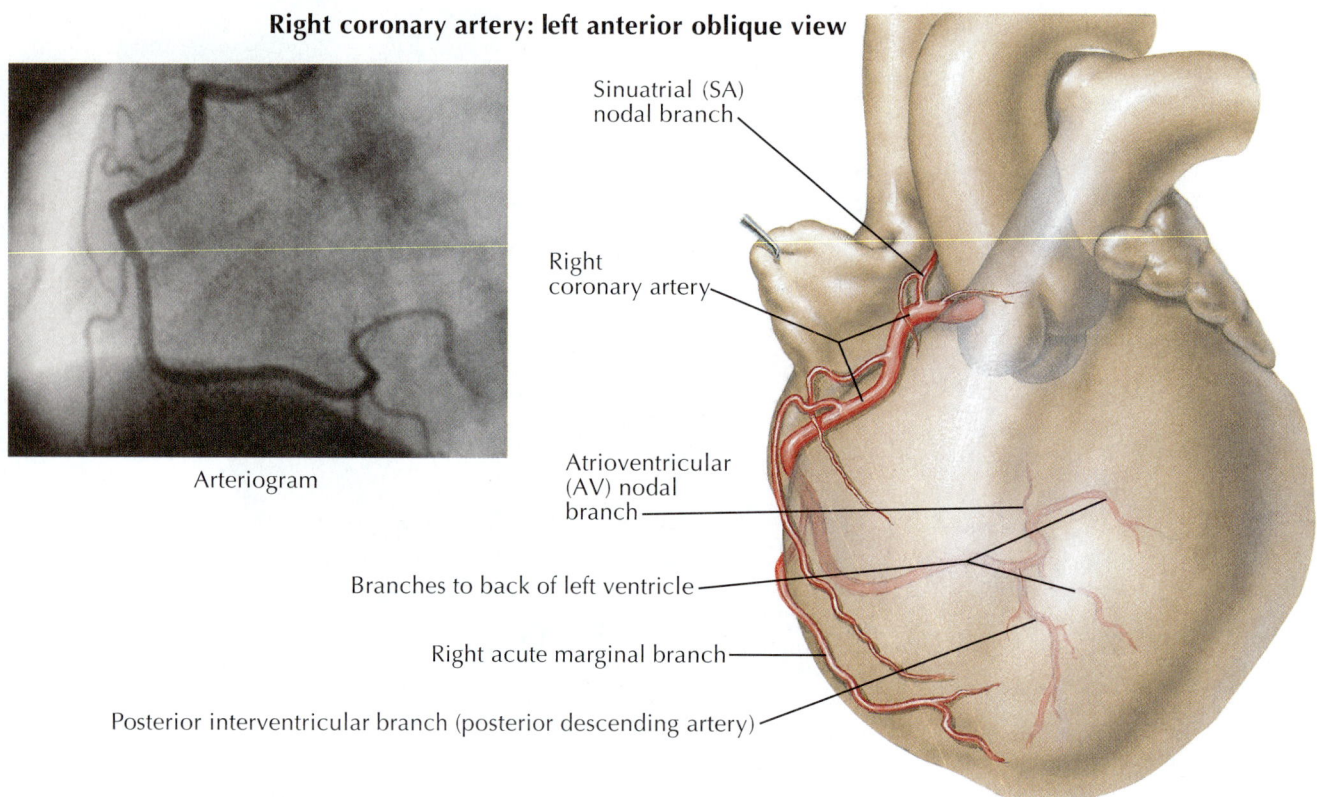

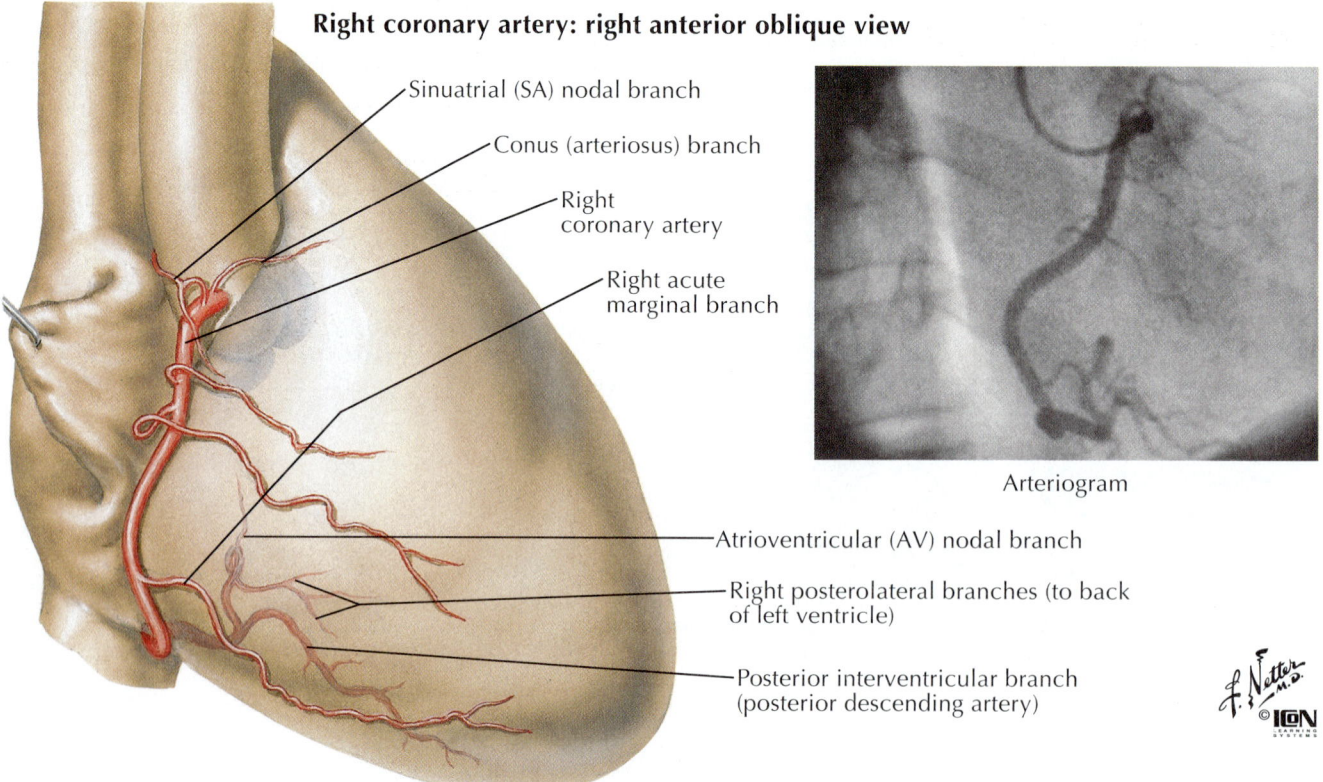

Plate 24 Coronary Arteries: Arteriographic Views. (Copyright 2025 Elsevier Inc. All rights reserved. www.netterimages.com. Image ID: 4725.)

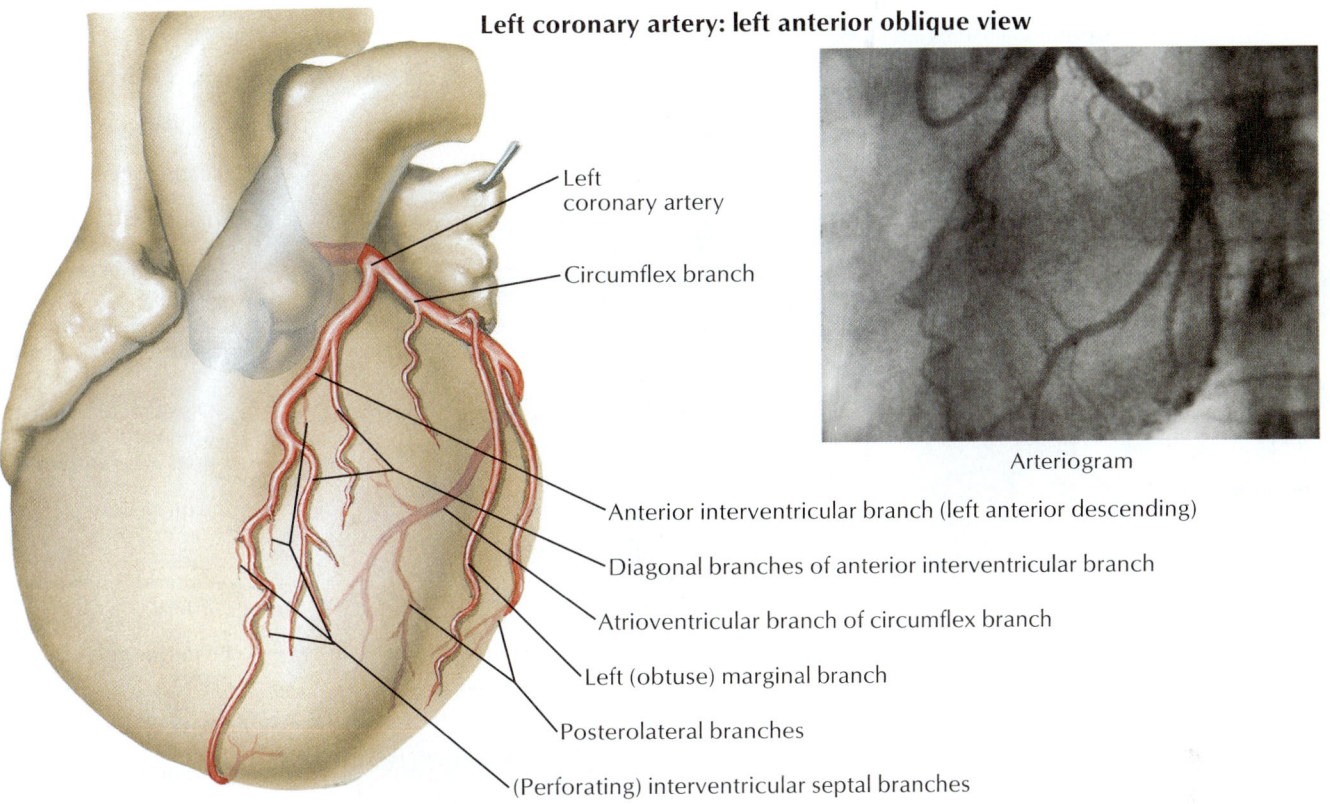

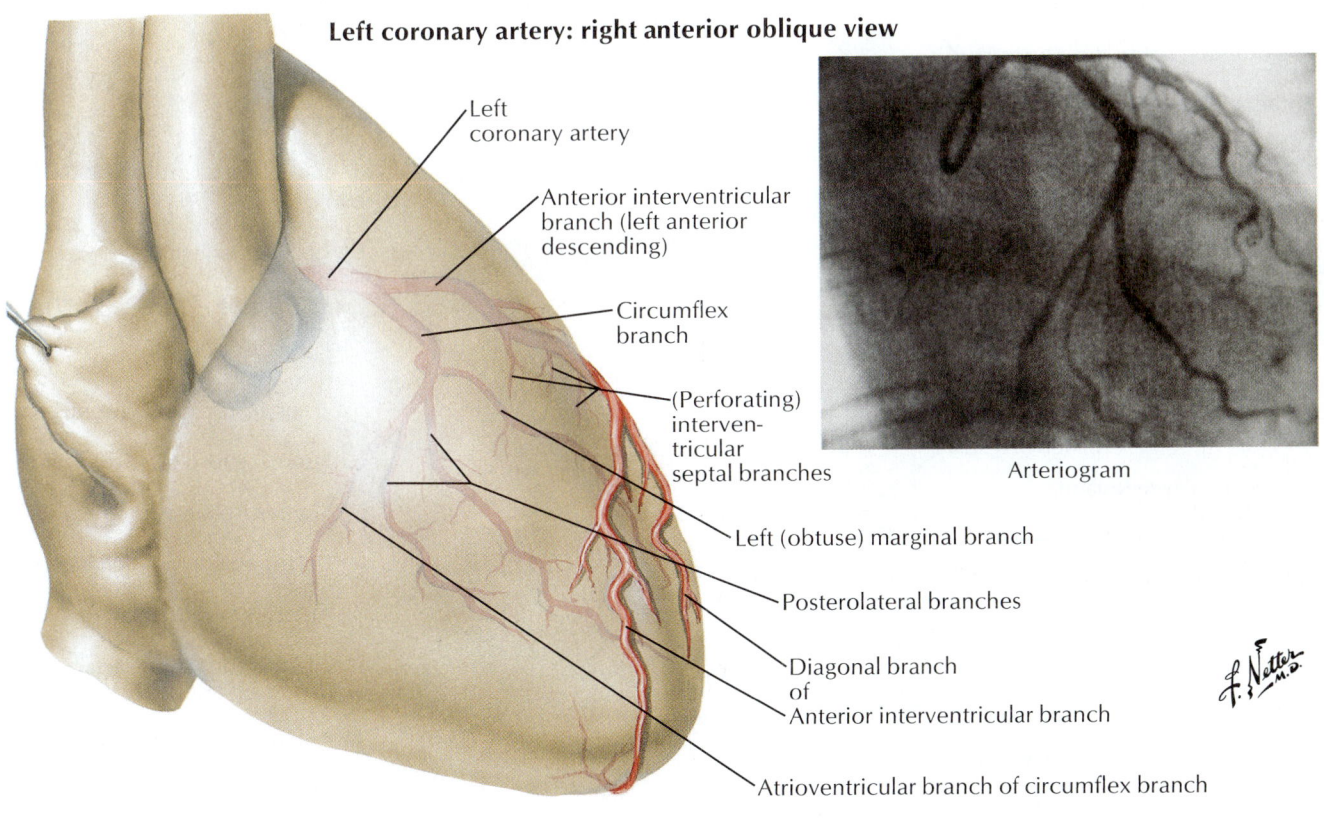

Plate 25 Coronary Arteries: Arteriographic Views. (Copyright 2025 Elsevier Inc. All rights reserved. www.netterimages.com. Image ID: 4542.)

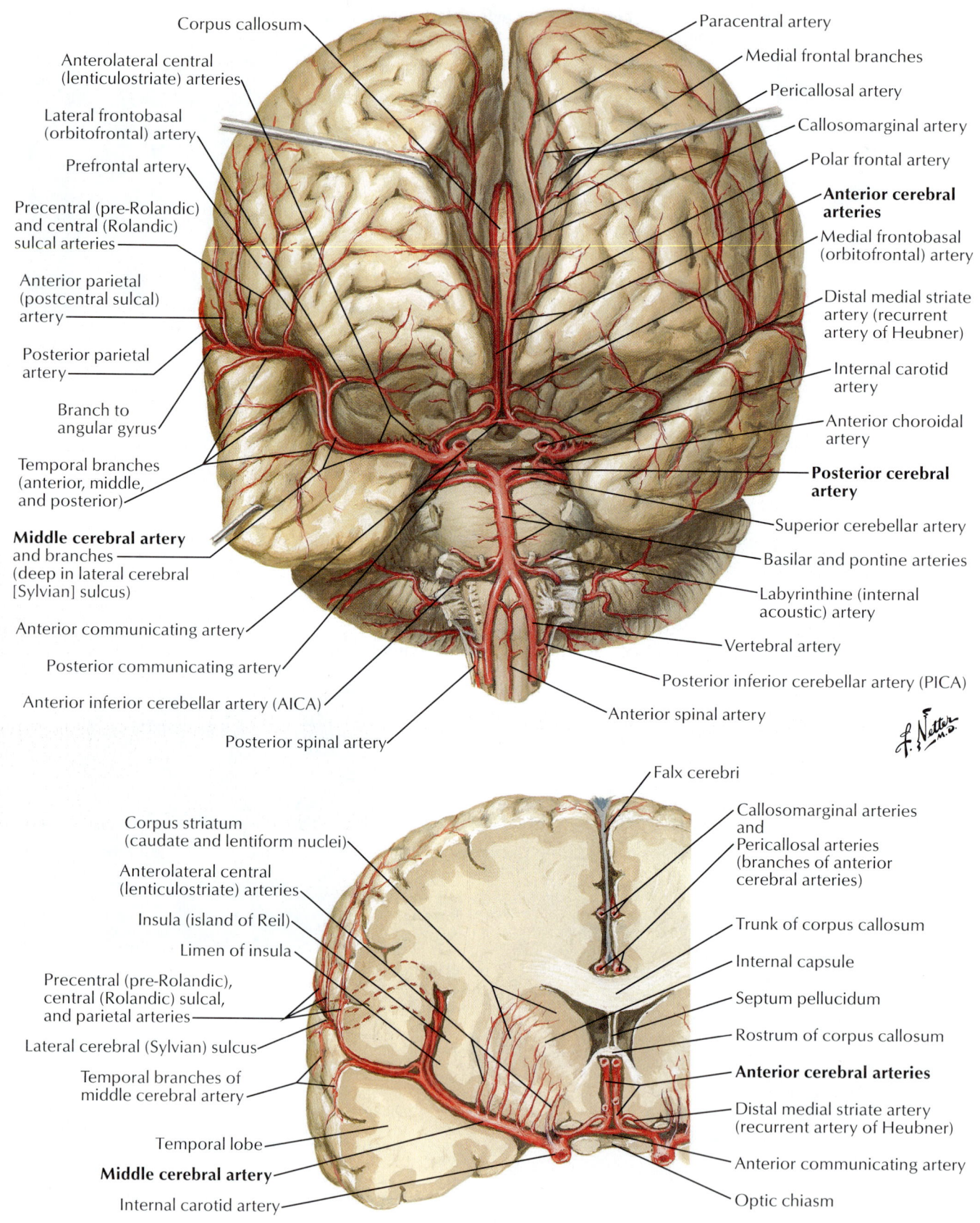

Plate 26 Arteries of Brain: Frontal View and Section. (Copyright 2025 Elsevier Inc. All rights reserved. www.netterimages.com. Image ID: 4588.)

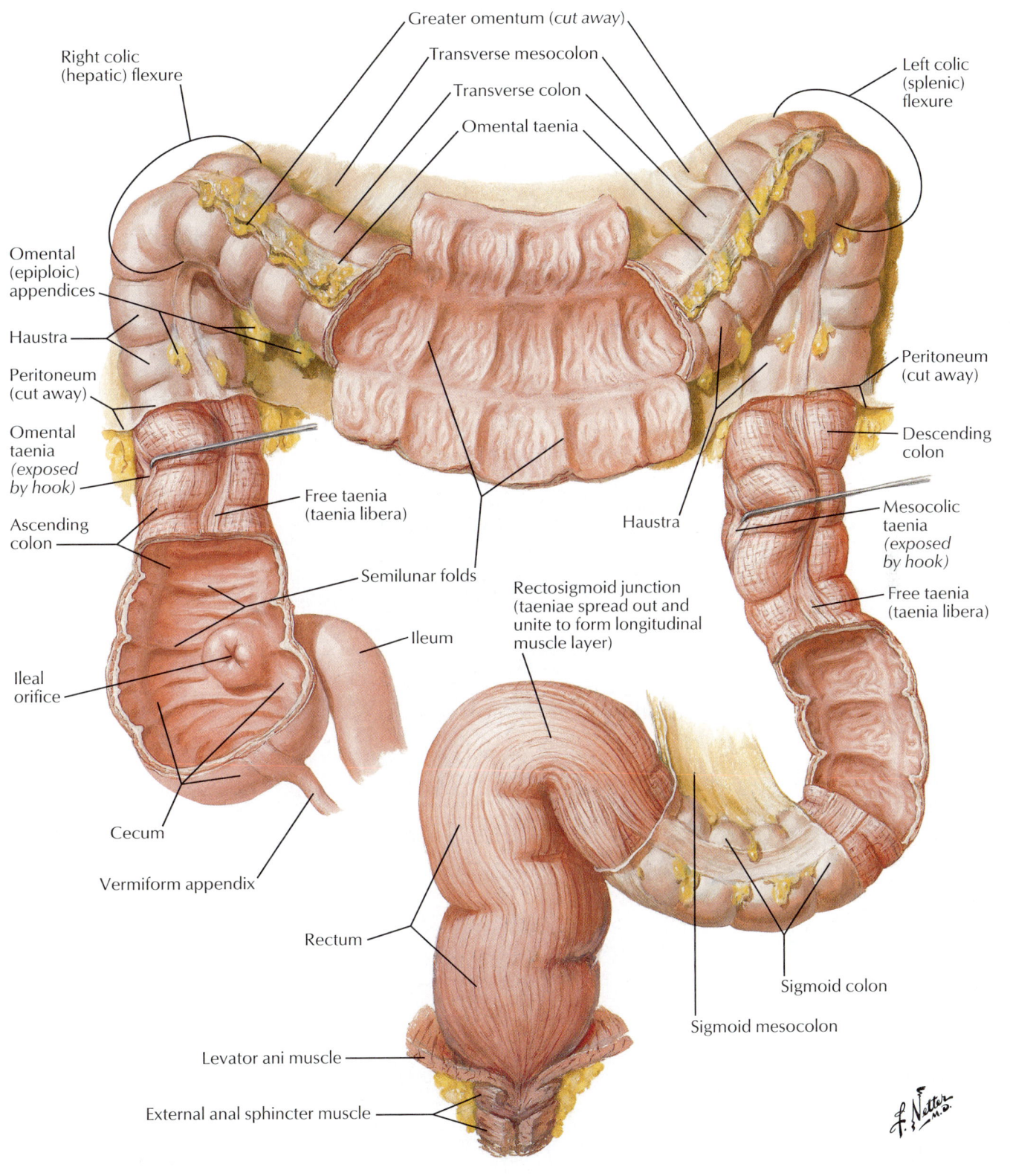

Plate 27 Mucosa and Musculature of Large Intestine. (Copyright 2025 Elsevier Inc. All rights reserved. www.netterimages.com. Image ID: 4778.)

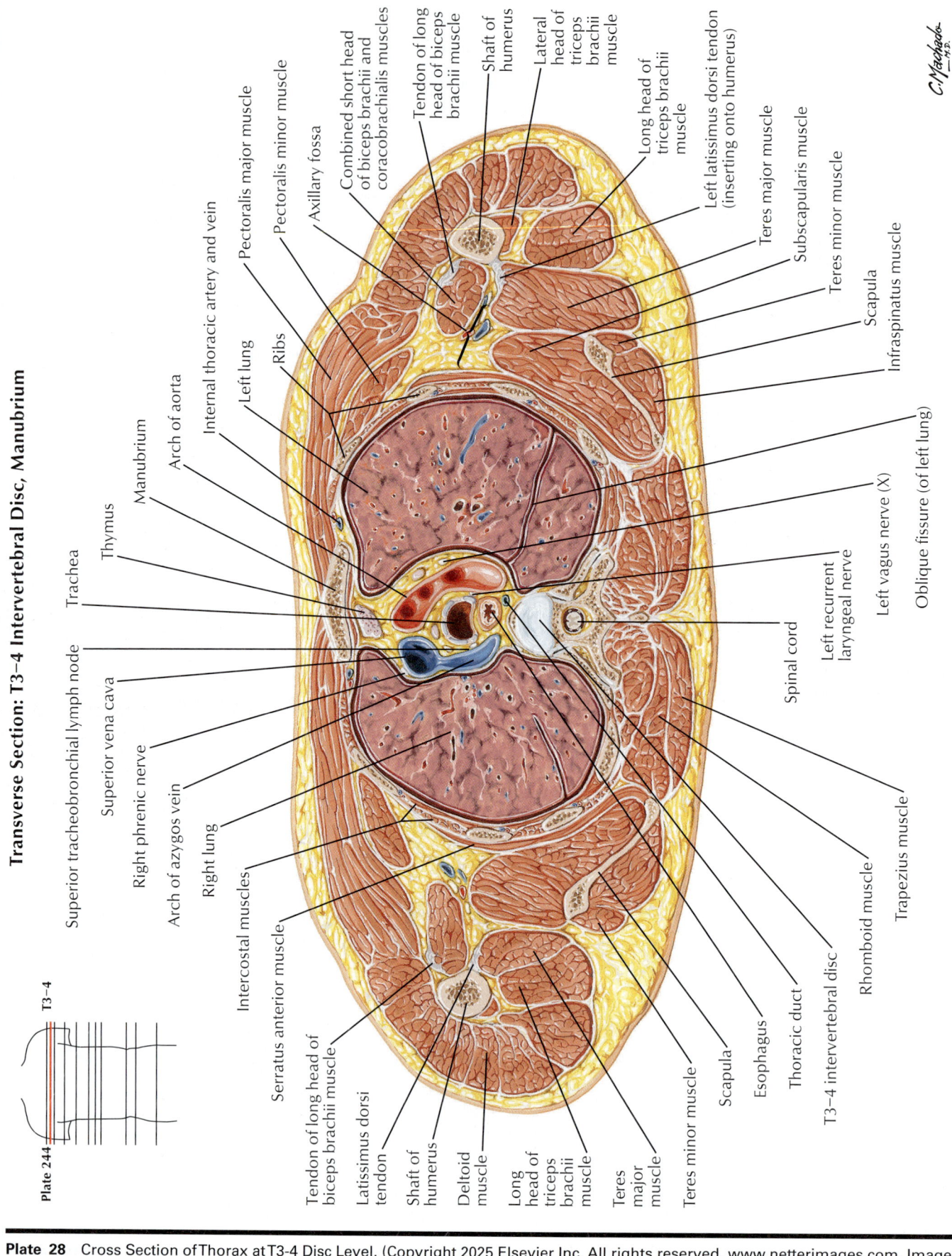

Transverse Section: T3–4 Intervertebral Disc, Manubrium

Plate 28 Cross Section of Thorax at T3-4 Disc Level. (Copyright 2025 Elsevier Inc. All rights reserved. www.netterimages.com. Image ID: 4880.)

xl

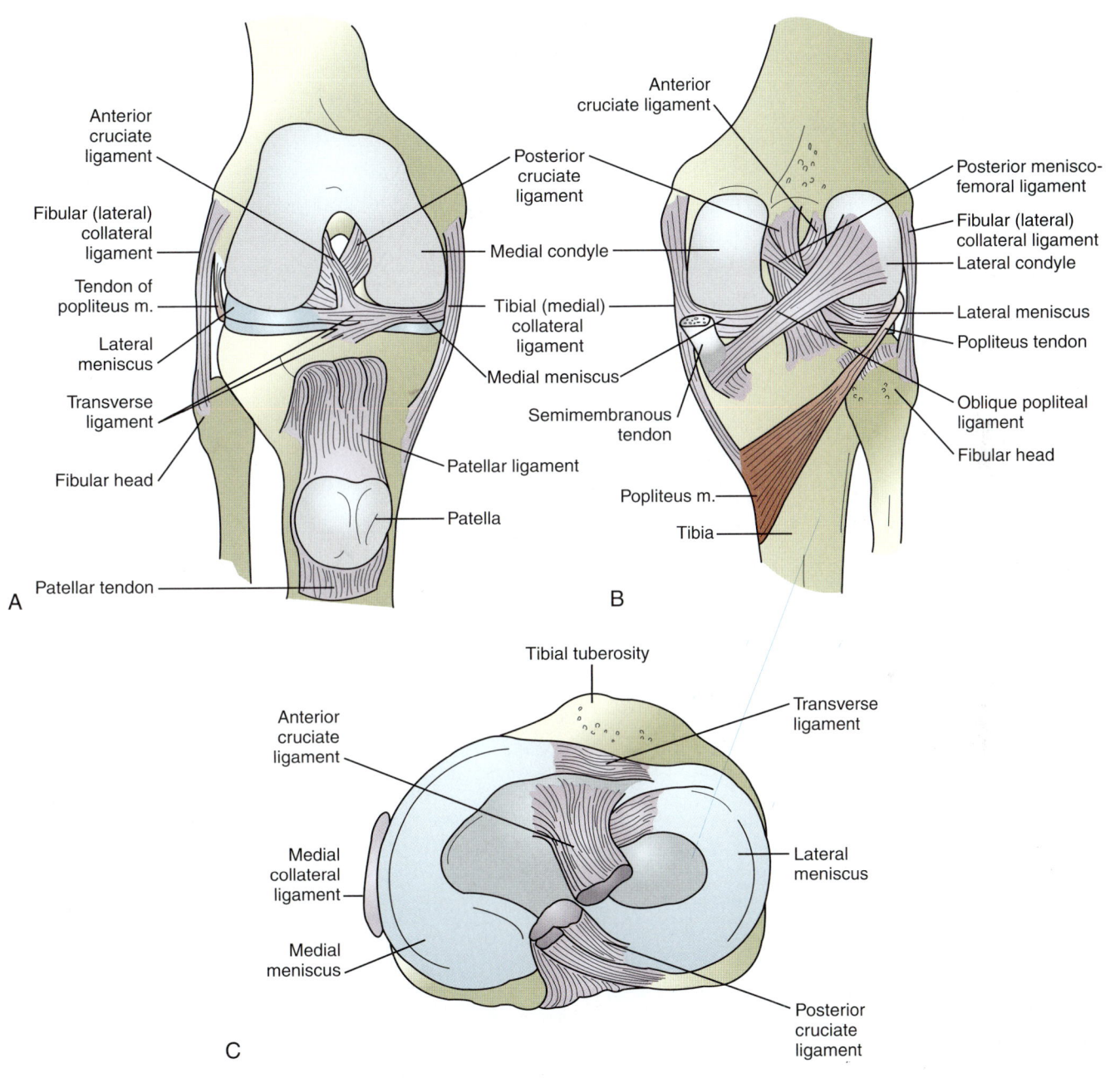

Plate 29 Knee joint opened; anterior, posterior, and proximal views. A, Anterior view of the knee joint, opened by folding the patella and patellar ligament inferiorly. On the lateral side is the fibular collateral ligament, separated by the popliteal tendon from the lateral meniscus. On the medial side, the tibial collateral ligament is attached to the medial meniscus. The anterior and posterior cruciate ligaments are seen between the femoral condyles. B, Posterior view of the opened knee joint with a more complete view of the posterior cruciate ligament. C, The femur is removed, showing the proximal (articular) end of the right tibia. On the medial side is the gently curved medial meniscus; on the lateral side is the more tightly curved lateral meniscus. The anterior end of the medial meniscus is anchored to the surface of the tibia by the transverse ligament. The cut ends of the anterior and posterior cruciate ligaments are shown, as well as the meniscofemoral ligament. (Fritz S: Mosby's Essential Sciences for Therapeutic Massage: Anatomy, Physiology, Biomechanics, and Pathology, ed 5, St. Louis, 2017, Elsevier.)

HCPCS 2026

INDEX

A

Abatacept, J0129
Abciximab, J0130
Abdomen
  dressing holder/binder, A4461, A4463
  pad, low profile, L1270
Abduction control, each, L2624
Abduction restrainer, A4566
Abduction rotation bar, foot, L3140–L3170
  adjustable shoe style positioning device, L3160–L3161
  including shoes, L3140
  plastic, heel-stabilizer, off-shelf, L3170
  without shoes, L3150
Abecma, Q2055
AbobotulinumtoxinA, J0586
Absorption dressing, A2001–A2010, A2015–A2021, A6251–A6256
Access, site, occlusive, device, G0269
Access system, A4301
Acesso trifaca, Q4386 ◀
Accessories
  ambulation devices, E0153–E0159
    crutch attachment, walker, E0157
    forearm crutch, platform attachment, E0153
    leg extension, walker, E0158
    replacement, brake attachment, walker, E0159
    seat attachment, walker, E0156
    walker, platform attachment, E0154
    wheel attachment, walker, per pair, E0155
  artificial kidney and machine; (see also ESRD), E1510–E1699
    adjustable chair, ESRD patients, E1570
    automatic peritoneal dialysis system, intermittent, E1592
    bath conductivity meter, hemodialysis, E1550
    blood leak detector, hemodialysis, replacement, E1560
    blood pump, hemodialysis, replacement, E1620
    cycler dialysis machine, peritoneal, E1594
    deionizer water system, hemodialysis, E1615
    delivery/installation charges, hemodialysis equipment, E1600
    hemodialysis machine, E1590
    hemostats, E1637
    heparin infusion pump, hemodialysis, E1520
    kidney machine, dialysate delivery system, E1510
    peritoneal dialysis clamps, E1634
    portable travel hemodialyzer, E1635
    reciprocating peritoneal dialysis system, E1630
    replacement, air bubble detector, hemodialysis, E1530
    replacement, pressure alarm, hemodialysis, E1540
    reverse osmosis water system, hemodialysis, E1610
    scale, E1639
    sorbent cartridges, hemodialysis, E1636
    transducer protectors, E1575
    unipuncture control system, E1580
    water softening system, hemodialysis, E1625
    wearable artificial kidney, E1632
  beds, E0271–E0280, E0300–E0326
    bed board, E0273

Accessories (Continued)
  bed, board/table, E0315
  bed cradle, E0280
  bed pan, standard, E0275
  bed side rails, E0305–E0310
  bed-pan fracture, E0276
  hospital bed, extra heavy duty, E0302, E0304
  hospital bed, heavy duty, E0301–E0303
  hospital bed, pediatric, electric, E0329
  hospital bed, safety enclosure frame, E0316
  mattress, foam rubber, E0272
  mattress, innerspring, E0271
  over-bed table, E0274
  pediatric crib, E0300
  powered pressure-reducing air mattress, E0277
  wheelchairs, E0950–E1030, E1032–E1034, E1050–E1298, E2301, E2399, K0001–K0109 ◀
    accessory tray, E0950
    arm rest, E0994
    back upholstery replacement, E0982
    calf rest/pad, E0995
    commode seat, E0968
    detachable armrest, E0973
    elevating leg rest, E0990
    headrest cushion, E0955
    headrest hardware, E1033 ◀
    joystick, E1032 ◀
    lateral trunk/hip support, E0956
    loop-holder, E0951–E0952
    manual swingaway, E1028
    manual wheelchair, adapter, amputee, E0959
    manual wheelchair, anti-rollback device, E0974
    manual wheelchair, anti-tipping device, E0971
    manual wheelchair, hand rim with projections, E0967
    manual wheelchair, headrest extension, E0966
    manual wheelchair, lever-activated, wheel drive, E0988
    manual wheelchair, one-arm drive attachment, E0958
    manual wheelchair, power add-on, E0983–E0984
    manual wheelchair, push activated power assist, E0986
    manual wheelchair, solid seat insert, E0992
    medial thigh support, E0957
    modification, pediatric size, E1011
    narrowing device, E0969
    No. 2 footplates, E0970
    oxygen related accessories, E1352–E1406
    positioning belt/safety belt/pelvic strap, E0978
    power-seating system, E1002–E1010
    reclining back addition, pediatric size wheelchair, E1014
    residual limb support system, E1020
    safety vest, E0980
    seat lift mechanism, E0985
    seat upholstery replacement, E0981 ◀
    securement system, E1022–E1023 ◀
    shock absorber, E1015–E1018
    shoulder harness strap, E0960
    truck, hip support, E1034 ◀

◀ New   ↻ Revised   ✔ Reinstated   ~~deleted~~ Deleted

Accessories (Continued)
  wheelchairs (Continued)
    ventilator tray, E1029–E1030
    wheel lock brake extension, manual, E0961
    wheelchair, amputee, accessories, E1170–E1200
    wheelchair, fully inclining, accessories, E1050–E1093
    wheelchair, heavy duty, accessories, E1280–E1298
    wheelchair, lightweight, accessories, E1240–E1270
    wheelchair, semi-reclining, accessories, E1100–E1110
    wheelchair, special size, E1220–E1239
    wheelchair, standard, accessories, E1130–E1161
  whirlpool equipment, E1300–E1310

Ace type, elastic bandage, A6448–A6450
Acelagraft, Q4395 ◀
Acetaminophen, J0131, J0134, J0136–J0138
Acetazolamide sodium, J1120
Acetylcysteine
  inhalation solution, J7604, J7608
  injection, J0132
Activity, therapy, G0176
Acyclovir, J0133
Adalimumab, Q5140–Q5145 ~~J0135, Q5131–Q5132~~ ◀
Additions to
  fracture orthosis, L2180–L2192
    abduction bar, L2300–L2310
    adjustable motion knee joint, L2186
    anterior swing band, L2335
    BK socket, PTB and AFO, L2350
    disk or dial lock, knee flexion, L2425
    dorsiflexion and plantar flexion, L2220
    dorsiflexion assist, L2210
    drop lock, L2405
    drop lock knee joint, L2182
    extended steel shank, L2360
    foot plate, stirrup attachment, L2250
    hip joint, pelvic band, thigh flange, pelvic belt, L2192
    integrated release mechanism, L2515
    lacer custom-fabricated, L2320–L2330
    lift loop, drop lock ring, L2492
    limited ankle motion, L2200
    limited motion knee joint, L2184
    long tongue stirrup, L2265
    lower extremity orthrosis, L2200–L2397
    molded inner boot, L2280
    offset knee joint, L2390
    offset knee joint, heavy duty, L2395
    Patten bottom, L2370
    pelvic and thoracic control, L2570–L2680
    plastic shoe insert with ankle joints, L2180
    polycentric knee joint, L2387
    pre-tibial shell, L2340
    quadrilateral, L2188
    ratchet lock knee extension, L2430
    reinforced solid stirrup, L2260
    rocker bottom, custom fabricated, L2232
    round caliper/plate attachment, L2240
    split flat caliper stirrups, L2230
    straight knee joint, heavy duty, L2385

Additions to (Continued)
  fracture orthosis (Continued)
    straight knee, or offset knee joints, L2405–L2492
    suspension sleeve, L2397
    thigh/weight bearing, L2500–L2550
    torsion control, ankle joint, L2375
    torsion control, straight knee joint, L2380
    varus/valgus correction, L2270–L2275
    waist belt, L2190
  general additions, orthosis, L2750–L2999
    lower extremity, above knee section, soft interface, L2830
    lower extremity, concentric adjustable torsion style mechanism, L2861
    lower extremity, drop lock retainer, L2785
    lower extremity, extension, per extension, per bar, L2760
    lower extremity, femoral length sock, L2850
    lower extremity, full kneecap, L2795
    lower extremity, high strength, lightweight material, hybrid lamination, L2755
    lower extremity, knee control, condylar pad, L2810
    lower extremity, knee control, knee cap, medial or lateral, L2800
    lower extremity orthrosis, non-corrosive finish, per bar, L2780
    lower extremity orthrosis, NOS, L2999
    lower extremity, plating chrome or nickel, per bar, L2750
    lower extremity, soft interface, below knee, L2820
    lower extremity, tibial length sock, L2840
    orthotic side bar, disconnect device, L2768

Adenosine, J0151, J0153
Adhesive, A4364
  bandage, A6413
  disc or foam pad, A5126
  remover, A4455, A4456
  support, breast prosthesis, A4280
  wound, closure, G0168
Administration, chemotherapy, Q0083–Q0085
  both infusion and other technique, Q0085
  infusion technique only, Q0084
  other than infusion technique, Q0083
Administration, Part D
  vaccine, hepatitis B, G0010
  vaccine, influenza, G0008
  vaccine, pneumococcal, G0009
Administrative, Miscellaneous and Investigational, A9000–A9999
  alert or alarm device, A9280
  ~~artificial saliva, A9155~~
  artificial saliva, A9154 ◀
  DME delivery set-up, A9901
  exercise equipment, A9300
  external ambulatory insulin delivery system, A9274
  foot pressure off loading/supportive device, A9283
  helmets, A8000–A8004
  home glucose disposable monitor, A9275
  hot-water bottle, ice cap, heat wrap, A9273
  miscellaneous DME, NOS, A9999
  miscellaneous DME supply, A9900

◀ New   ⤺ Revised   ✔ Reinstated   ~~deleted~~ Deleted

Administrative, Miscellaneous and Investigational
(Continued)
  monitoring feature/device, stand-alone or integrated, A9279
  multiple vitamins, oral, per dose, A9153
  non-covered item, A9270
  non-prescription drugs, A9150
  pediculosis treatment, topical, A9180
  radiopharmaceuticals, A9500–A9700
  reaching grabbing device, A9281
  receiver, external, interstitial glucose monitoring system, A9278
  sensor, invasive, interstitial continuous glucose monitoring, A9276
  single vitamin/mineral trace element, A9152
  spirometer, non-electronic, A9284
  transmitter, interstitial continuous glucose monitoring system, A9277
  wig, any type, A9282
  wound suction, disposable, A9272
Admission, observation, G0379
Ado-trastuzumab, J9354
~~**Adrenalin,** J0171~~
Aducanumab-avwa, J0172
Aduhelm, J0172
Advanced life support, *A0390, A0426, A0427, A0433*
  ALS2, A0433
  ALS emergency transport, A0427
  ALS mileage, A0390
  ALS, non-emergency transport, A0426
Advograft dual, Q4382 ◀
Advograft one, Q4380 ◀
Adzynma, J7171
Aeroguard, Q4370 ◀
Aerosol
  compressor, E0571–E0572
  compressor filter, A7013–A7014, K0178–K0179
  mask, A7015, K0180
Afamelanotide implant, J7352
Afamitresgene autoleucel, Q2057 ◀
Aflibercept, J0177–J0178, Q5147, Q5149–Q5150, Q5155 ◀
AFO, E1815, E1830, L1900–L1990, L4392, L4396
Afstyla, J7210
Agalsidase beta, J0180
Aggrastat, J3245
A-hydroCort, J1710
Aid, hearing, *V5030–V5263*
Aide, home, health, *G0156, S9122, T1021*
  home health aide/certified nurse assistant, in home, S9122
  home health aide/certified nurse assistant, per visit, T1021
  home health or hospital setting, G0156
Air bubble detector, dialysis, E1530
Air fluidized bed, E0194
Air pressure pad/mattress, E0186, E0197
Air travel and nonemergency transportation, A0140
Alarm
  not otherwise classified, A9280
  pressure, dialysis, E1540

Alatrofloxacin mesylate, J0200
Albumin, human, P9041, P9042
Albuterol
  all formulations, inhalation solution, J7620
  all formulations, inhalation solution, concentrated, J7610, J7611
  all formulations, inhalation solution, unit dose, J7609, J7613
Alcohol, A4244
Alcohol wipes, A4245
Alcohol/substance, assessment, *G0396, G0397, H0001, H0003, H0049*
  alcohol abuse structured assessment, greater than 30 min., G0397
  alcohol abuse structured assessment, 15–30 min., G0396
  alcohol and/or drug assessment, Medicaid, H0001
  alcohol and/or drug screening; laboratory analysis, Medicaid, H0003
  alcohol and/or drug screening, Medicaid, H0049
Aldesleukin (IL2), J9015
Alefacept, J0215
Alemtuzumab, J0202
Alert device, A9280
Alfentanil hydrochloride, J0216
Alginate dressing, A6196–A6199
  alginate, pad more than 48 sq. cm, A6198
  alginate, pad size 16 sq. cm, A6196
  alginate, pad size more than 16 sq. cm, A6197
  alginate, wound filler, sterile, A6199
Alglucerase, J0205
Alglucosidase, J0220
Alglucosidase alfa, J0221
Allogen, Q4212
Allopurinol sodium, J0206
Alphanate, J7186
Alpha-1–proteinase inhibitor, human, J0256, J0257
Alprostadil
  injection, J0270
  urethral suppository, J0275
ALS mileage, *A0390*
Alteplase recombinant, J2997
Alternating pressure mattress/pad, A4640, E0180, E0181, E0277
  overlay/pad, alternating, pump, heavy duty, E0181
  powered pressure-reducing air mattress, E0277
  replacement pad, owned by patient, A4640
Alymsys, Q5126
Ambulance, A0021–A0999
  air, A0430, A0431, A0435, A0436
    conventional, transport, one way, fixed wing, A0430
    conventional, transport, one way, rotary wing, A0431
    fixed wing air mileage, A0435
    rotary wing air mileage, A0436
  disposable supplies, A0382–A0398
    ALS routine disposable supplies, A0398
    ALS specialized service disposable supplies, A0394
    ALS specialized service, esophageal intubation, A0396
    BLS routine disposable, A0832
    BLS specialized service disposable supplies, defibrillation, A0384, A0392

Ambulance (Continued)
   non-emergency transport, fixed wing, S9960
   non-emergency transport, rotary wing, S9961
   oxygen, A0422

Ambulation device, E0100–E0159
   brake attachment, wheeled walker replacement, E0159
   cane, adjustable or fixed, with tip, E0100
   cane, quad or three prong, adjustable or fixed, with tip, E0105
   crutch attachment, walker, E0157
   crutch forearm, each, with tips and handgrips, E0111
   crutch substitute, lower leg platform, with or without wheels, each, E0118
   crutch, underarm, articulating, spring assisted, each, E0117
   crutches forearm, pair, tips and handgrips, E0110
   crutches, underarm, other than wood, pair, with pads, tips and handgrips, E0114
   crutches, underarm, other than wood, with pad, tip, handgrip, with or without shock absorber, each, E0116
   crutches, underarm, wood, each, with pad, tip and handgrip, E0113
   leg extensions, walker, set (4), E0158
   platform attachment, forearm crutch, each, E0153
   platform attachment, walker, E0154
   seat attachment, walker, E0156
   walker, enclosed, four-sided frame, wheeled, posterior seat, E0144
   walker, folding, adjustable or fixed height, E0135
   walker, folding, wheeled, adjustable or fixed height, E0143, E0150 ◄
   walker, heavy duty, multiple braking system, variable wheel resistance, E0147
   walker, heavy duty, wheeled, rigid or folding, E0149
   walker, heavy duty, without wheels, rigid or folding, E0148
   walker, rigid, adjustable or fixed height, E0130
   walker, rigid, wheeled, adjustable or fixed height, E0141
   walker, with trunk support, adjystable or fixed height, any, E0140
   wheel attachment, rigid, pick up walker, per pair, E0155

Amchoslast excel, Q4372 ◄
Amchothick, Q4368 ◄
Amikacin Sulfate, J0278
Aminocaproic acid, J0281 ◄
Aminolevulinate, J7309
Aminolevulinic acid HCl, J7308
Aminophylline, J0280
Aminolevulinic
   Ameluz, J7345
Amiodarone HCl, J0282, J0283
Amisulpride, J0184
Amitriptyline HCl, J1320
Ammonia N-13, A9526
Ammonia test paper, A4774
Amniodefent matrix, Q4379 ◄
Amnioiwrap2, Q4221
Amnion Bio, Q4211
Amnioplast, Q4369, Q4391 ◄
Amniotic membrane, V2790
Amobarbital, J0300

Amphotericin B, J0285
   Lipid Complex, J0287–J0289
Ampicillin
   sodium, J0290
   sodium/sulbactam sodium, J0295
Amputee
   adapter, wheelchair, E0959
   prosthesis, L5000–L7510, L7520, L7900, L8400–L8465
     above knee, L5200–L5230
     additions to exoskeletal knee-shin systems, L5710–L5782
     additions to lower extremity, L5610–L5617
     additions to socket insert and suspension, L5654–L5699
     additions to socket variations, L5630–L5653
     additions to test sockets, L5618–L5629
     additions/replacements feet-ankle units, L5700–L5707
     ankle, L5050–L5060
     below knee, L5100–L5105
     component modification, L5785–L5795
     endoskeletal, L5810–L5999
     endoskeleton, below knee, L5301–L5312
     endoskeleton, hip disarticulation, L5331–L5341
     fitting endoskeleton, above knee, L5321
     fitting procedures, L5400–L5460
     hemipelvectomy, L5280
     hip disarticulation, L5250–L5270
     initial prosthesis, L5500–L5505
     knee disarticulation, L5150–L5160
     male vacuum erection system, L7900
     partial foot, L5000–L5020
     preparatory prosthesis, L5510–L5600
     prosthetic socks, L8400–L8485
     repair, prosthetic device, L7520
     tension ring, vacuum erection device, L7902
     upper extremity, battery components, L7360–L7368
     upper extremity, other/repair, L7400–L7510
     upper extremity, preparatory, elbow, L6584–L6586
     upper limb, above elbow, L6250
     upper limb, additions, L6600–L6700 ◄
     upper limb, below elbow, L6100–L6130
     upper limb, elbow disarticulation, L6200–L6205
     upper limb, endoskeletal, above elbow, L6500
     upper limb, endoskeletal, below elbow, L6400
     upper limb, endoskeletal, elbow disarticulation, L6450
     upper limb, endoskeletal, interscapular thoracic, L6570
     upper limb, endoskeletal, shoulder disarticulation, L6550
     upper limb, external power, device, L6920–L6975
     upper limb, interscapular thoracic, L6350–L6370
     upper limb, partial hand, L6000–L6025
     upper limb, postsurgical procedures, L6380–L6388
     upper limb, preparatory, shoulder, interscapular, L6588–L6590
     upper limb, preparatory, wrist, L6580–L6582
     upper limb, shoulder disarticulation, L6300–L6320
     upper limb, terminal devices, L6703–L6915, L7007–L7261
     upper limb, wrist disarticulation, L6050–L6055

Amputee (Continued)
  stump sock, L8470–L8485
    single ply, fitting above knee, L8480
    single ply, fitting, below knee, L8470
    single ply, fitting, upper limb, L8485
  wheelchair, E1170–E1190, E1200, K0100
    detachable arms, swing away detachable elevating footrests, E1190
    detachable arms, swing away detachable footrests, E1180
    detachable arms, without footrests or legrest, E1172
    detachable elevating legrest, fixed full length arms, E1170
    fixed full length arms, swing away detachable footrest, E1200
    heavy duty wheelchair, swing away detachable elevating legrests, E1195
    without footrests or legrest, fixed full length arms, E1171

Amygdalin, J3570
Anadulafungin, J0348
Anacaulase-bcdb, J7353
Analysis
  semen, G0027
Anaphylaxis, due to vaccine, M1160–M1161, M1163
Angiography, iliac, artery, G0278
Angiography, renal, non-selective, G0275
  non-ophthalmic fluorescent vascular, C9733
  reconstruction, G0288
Angioplasty, C7531–C7535
Anistreplase, J0350
Ankle splint, recumbent, K0126–K0130
Ankle-foot orthosis (AFO), L1900–L1990, L2106–L2116, L4361, L4392, L4396
  ankle gauntlet, custom fabricated, L1904
  ankle gauntlet, prefabricated, off-shelf, L1902
  double upright free plantar dorsiflexion, olid stirrup, calf-band/cuff, custom, L1990
  fracture orthosis, tibial fracture, thermoplastic cast material, custom, L2106
  multiligamentus ankle support, prefabricated, off-shelf, L1906
  plastic or other material, custom fabricated, L1940
  plastic or other material, prefabricated, fitting and adjustment, L1932, L1933, L1951, L1952 ◀
  plastic or other material, with ankle joint, prefabricated, fitting and adjustment, L1971
  plastic, rigid anterior tibial section, custom fabricated, L1945
  plastic, with ankle joint, custom, L1970
  posterior, single bar, clasp attachment to shoe, L1910
  posterior, solid ankle, plastic, custom, L1960
  replacement, soft interface material, static AFO, L4392
  single upright free plantar dorsiflection, solid stirrup, calf-band/cuff, custom, L1980
  single upright with static or adjustable stop, custom, L1920
  spiral, plastic, custom fabricated, L1950
  spring wire, dorsiflexion assist calf band, L1900
  static or dynamic AFO, adjustable for fit, minimal ambulation, L4396

Ankle-foot orthosis (Continued)
  supramalleolar with straps, custom fabricated, L1907
  tibial fracture cast orthrosis, custom, L2108
  tibial fracture orthrosis, rigid, prefabricated, fitting and adjustment, L2116
  tibial fracture orthrosis, semi-rigid, prefabricated, fitting and adjustment, L2114
  tibial fracture orthrosis, soft prefabricated, fitting and adjustment, L2112
  walking boot, prefabricated, off-the-shelf, L4361
Anterior-posterior-lateral orthosis, L0700, L0710, L0720 ◀
Antibiotic, G8708–G8712
  antibiotic not prescribed or dispensed, G8712
  patient not prescribed or dispensed antibiotic, G8708
  patient prescribed antibiotic, documented condition, G8709
  patient prescribed or dispensed antibiotic, G8710
  prescribed or dispensed antibiotic, G8711
Antidepressant, documentation, G8126–G8128
Anti-emetic, oral, J8498, J8597, Q0163–Q0181
  antiemetic drug, oral NOS, J8597
  antiemetic drug, rectal suppository, NOS, J8498
  diphenhydramine hydrochloride, 50 mg, oral, Q0163
  dolasetron mesylate, 100 mg, oral, Q0180
  dronabinol, 2.5 mg, Q0167
  granisetron hydrochloride, 1 mg, oral, Q0166
  hydroxyzine pomoate, 25 mg, oral, Q0177
  perphenazine, 4 mg, oral, Q0175
  prochlorperazine maleate, 5 mg, oral, Q0164
  promethazine hydrochloride, 12.5 mg, oral, Q0169
  thiethylperazine maleate, 10 mg, oral, Q0174
  trimethobenzamide hydrochloride, 250 mg, oral, Q0173
  unspecified oral dose, Q0181
Anti-hemophilic factor (Factor VIII), J7190–J7192
Anti-inhibitors, per I.U., J7198
Antimicrobial, prophylaxis, documentation, G8201
Anti-neoplastic drug, NOC, J9999
Antithrombin III, J7197
Antithrombin recombinant, J7196
Apollo ft, Q4385 ◀
Apomorphine, J0364
Aponvie, C9145
Appliance
  cleaner, A5131
  pneumatic, E0655–E0673
    non-segmental pneumatic appliance, E0655, E0660, E0665, E0666
    segmental gradient pressure, pneumatic appliance, E0671–E0673
    segmental pneumatic appliance, E0656–E0659, E0667–E0670 ◀
Application, heat, cold, E0200–E0239
  electric heat pad, moist, E0215
  electric heat pad, standard, E0210
  heat lamp with stand, E0205
  heat lamp without stand, E0200
  hydrocollator unit, pads, E0225
  hydrocollator unit, portable, E0239
  infrared heating pad system, E0221
  non-contact wound warming device, E0231

Application, heat, cold (Continued)
  paraffin bath unit, E0235
  phototherapy (bilirubin), E0202
  pump for water circulating pad, E0236
  therapeutic lightbox, E0203
  warming card, E0232
  water circulating cold pad with pump, E0218
  water circulating heat pad with pump, E0217
Aprotinin, J0365
Aqueous
  shunt, L8612
  sterile, J7051
ARB/ACE therapy, G8473–G8475
Arbutamine HCl, J0395
Arch support, L3040–L3100
  hallus-valgus night dynamic splint, off-shelf, L3100
  intralesional, J3302
  non-removable, attached to shoe, longitudinal, L3070
  non-removable, attached to shoe, longitudinal/metatarsal, each, L3090
  non-removable, attached to shoe, metatarsal, L3080
  removable, premolded, longitudinal, L3040
  removable, premolded, longitudinal/metatarsal, each, L3060
  removable, premolded, metatarsal, L3050
Arformoterol, J7605
Argatroban, J0883–J0884, J0891–J0892, J0898–J0899
Aripiprazole, J0400, J0401
Aripiprazole, (abilify asimtufii), J0402
Aripiprazol lauroxil, (aristada), J1944
  aristada initio, H1943
Arm, wheelchair, E0973
Arsenic trioxide, J9017
Artacent cord, Q4216
Artesunate, J0391
Arthrography, injection, sacroiliac, joint, G0259, G0260
Arthroscopy, knee, surgical, G0289, S2112
  chondroplasty, different compartment, knee, G0289
  harvesting of cartilage, knee, S2112
Arthroscopy, shoulder, C9781
Artificial
  cornea, L8609
  heart system, miscellaneous component, supply or accessory, L8698
  kidney machines and accessories (see also Dialysis), E1510–E1699
  larynx, L8500
  saliva, A9155
Ascendion, Q4390 ◀
Ascent, Q4213
Asparaginase, J9019–J9021
Aspirator, VABRA, A4480
Assessment
  alcohol/substance (see also Alcohol/substance, assessment), G0396, G0397, H0001, H0003, H0049
  assessment for hearing aid, V5010
  audiologic, V5008–V5020
  cardiac output, M0302
  conformity evaluation, V5020
  fitting/orientation, hearing aid, V5014

Assessment (Continued)
  health care tool, G0136
  hearing screening, V5008
  itch severity, M1197–M1198, M1205–M1206
  repair/modification hearing aid, V5014
  speech, V5362–V5364
Assistive listening devices and accessories, V5281–V5290
  FMlDM system, monaural, V5281
Astramorph, J2275
Atezolizumab, J9022, J9024 ◀
Atherectomy, PTCA, C9602, C9603
Atidarsagene autotemcel, J3391 ◀
Atropine
  inhalation solution, concentrated, J7635
  inhalation solution, unit dose, J7636
Atropine sulfate, J0461, J0462 ◀
Attachment, walker, E0154–E0159
  brake attachment, wheeled walker, replacement, E0159
  crutch attachment, walker, E0157
  leg extension, walker, E0158
  platform attachment, walker, E0154
  seat attachment, walker, E0156
  wheel attachment, rigid pick up walker, E0155
Audiologic assessment, V5008–V5020
Auditory osseointegrated device, L8690–L8694
Aurothioglucose, J2910
Avacincaptad pegol, J2782
Avalglucosidase alfa-ngpt, J0219
Avelumab, J9023
Axatilimab-csfr, J9038 ◀
Axobiomembrane, Q4211
Axolotl ambient or axolotl cryo, Q4215, Q4383–Q4384 ◀
Azacitidine, J9025
Azathioprine, J7500, J7501
Azithromycin injection, J0456
Azmiro, J1072 ◀
Aztreonam, J0457
Aztreonam/Avibactam, J0458 ◀

B

Back supports, L0621–L0861, L0960
  lumbar orthrosis, L0625–L0627
  lumbar orthrosis, sagittal control, L0641–L0648
  lumbar-sacral orthrosis, L0628–L0640
  lumbar-sacral orthrosis, sagittal-coronal control, L0640, L0649–L0651
  sacroiliac orthrosis, L0621–L0624
Baclofen, J0475, J0476
Bacterial sensitivity study, P7001
Bag
  drainage, A4357
  enema, A4458
  irrigation supply, A4398
  urinary, A4358, A5112
Bandage, conforming
  elastic, >5", A6450
  elastic, >3", <5", A6449

◀ New ⮂ Revised ✓ Reinstated ~~deleted~~ Deleted

Bandage, conforming (Continued)
　elastic, load resistance 1.25 to 1.34 foot pounds, >3", <5", A6451
　elastic, load resistance <1.35 foot pounds, >3", <5", A6452
　elastic, <3", A6448
　non-elastic, non-sterile, >5", A6444
　non-elastic, non-sterile, width greater than or equal to 3", <5", A6443
　non-elastic, non-sterile, width <3", A6442
　non-elastic, sterile, >5", A6447
　non-elastic, sterile, >3" and <5", A6446
Bamlan and etesev, M0245
Bamlanivimab and etesevima, Q0245
Basiliximab, J0480
Bath, aid, E0160–E0162, E0235, E0240–E0249
　bath tub rail, floor base, E0242
　bath tub wall rail, E0241
　bath/shower chair, with/without wheels, E0240
　pad for water circulating heat unit, replacement, E0249
　paraffin bath unit, portable, E0235
　raised toilet seat, E0244
　sitz bath chair, E0162
　sitz type bath, portable, with faucet attachment, E0161
　sitz type bath, portable, with/without commode, E0160
　toilet rail, E0243
　transfer bench, tub or toilet, E0248
　transfer tub rail attachment, E0246
　tub stool or bench, E0245
Bathtub
　chair, E0240
　stool or bench, E0245, E0247–E0248
　transfer rail, E0246
　wall rail, E0241–E0242
Battery, L7360, L7364–L7368
　charger, E1066, L7362, L7366
　replacement for blood glucose monitor, A4233–A4236
　replacement for cochlear implant device, L8618, L8623–L8625
　replacement for TENS, A4630
　ventilator, A4611–A4613
Bebtelovimab, M0222–M0224–M0238, ~~Q0222~~ ◀
Beclomethasone inhalation solution, J7622
Bed
　accessories, E0271–E0280, E0300–E0326
　　bed board, E0273
　　bed cradle, E0280
　　bed pan, fracture, metal, E0276
　　bed pan, standard, metal, E0275
　　mattress, foam rubber, E0272
　　mattress innerspring, E0271
　　over-bed table, E0274
　　power pressure-reducing air mattress, E0277
　air fluidized, E0194
　cradle, any type, E0280
　drainage bag, bottle, A4357, A5102
　hospital, E0250–E0270, E0300–E0329
　pan, E0275, E0276
　rail, E0305, E0310
　safety enclosure frame/canopy, E0316

Behavioral, health, treatment services (Medicaid), H0002–H2037
　activity therapy, H2032
　alcohol/drug services, H0001, H0003, H0005–H0016, H0020–H0022, H0026–H0029, H0049–H0050, H2034–H2036
　assertive community treatment, H0040
　community based wrap-around services, H2021–H2022
　comprehensive community support, H2015–H2016
　comprehensive medication services, H2010
　comprehensive multidisciplinary evaluation, H2000
　crisis intervention, H2011
　day treatment, per diem, H2013
　day treatment, per hour, H2012
　developmental delay prevention activities, dependent child of client, H2037
　family assessment, H1011
　foster care, child, H0041–H0042
　health screening, H0002
　hotline service, H0030
　medication training, H0034
　mental health clubhouse services, H2030–H2031
　multisystemic therapy, juveniles, H2033
　non-medical family planning, H1010
　outreach service, H0023
　partial hospitalization, H0035
　plan development, non-physician, H0033
　prenatal care, at risk, H1000–H1005
　prevention, H0024–H0025
　psychiatric supportive treatment, community, H0036–H0037
　psychoeducational service, H2027
　psychoscial rehabilitation, H2017–H2018
　rehabilitation program, H2010
　residential treatment program, H0017–H0019
　respite care, not home, H0045
　self-help/peer services, H0039
　sexual offender treatment, H2028–H2029
　skill training, H2014
　supported employment, H2024–H2026
　supported housing, H0043–H0044
　therapeutic behavioral services, H2019–H2020
Behavioral, counseling, diabetes prevention, G9886–G9887
Behavioral therapy, cardiovascular disease, G0446
Belatacept, J0485
Belimumab, J0490
Bellacell, Q4220
Belt
　belt, strap, sleeve, garment, or covering, any type, A4467
　exsufflation, A4468
　extremity, E0945
　ostomy, A4367
　pelvic, E0944
　safety, K0031
　wheelchair, E0978, E0979
Bench, bathtub; (see also Bathtub), E0245
Bendamustine HCl
　~~Apotex, J9058~~
　~~Baxter, J9059~~

◀ New　↻ Revised　✓ Reinstated　~~deleted~~ Deleted

Bendamustine HCl *(Continued)*
    Bendeka, 1 mg, J9034
    Hydrochloride, 1 mg, J9033 ↩
    Vivimusta, J9056
Bendamustine HCl (Belrapzo/bendamustine), J9036
Benesch boot, L3212–L3214
Benztropine, J0515
~~Beqvez, C9172~~
Beremagene, J2401
Beta-blocker therapy, *G9188–G9191*
Betadine, A4246, A4247
Betameth, J0704
Betamethasone
    acetate and betamethasone sodium phosphate, J0702
    inhalation solution, J7624
Bethanechol chloride, J0520
Betibeglogene, J3393
Bevacizumab, J9035, Q2024
    adcd (Vegzelma), Q5129
    bvzr (Zirabez), Q5118
Bezlotoxuman, J0565
Bifocal, glass or plastic, V2200–V2299
    aniseikonic, bifocal, V2218
    bifocal add-over 3.25 d, V2220
    bifocal seg width over 28 mm, V2219
    lenticular, bifocal, myodisc, V2215
    lenticular lens, V2221
    specialty bifocal, by report, V2200
    sphere, bifocal, V2200–V2202
    spherocylinder, bifocal, V2203–V2214
Bilirubin (phototherapy) light, E0202
Binder, A4465
Biofeedback device, E0746
Bioimpedance, electrical, cardiac output, M0302
Biosimilar (infliximab), Q5102–Q5124
BioWound, Q4217
Biperiden lactate, J0190
Bitolterol mesylate, inhalation solution
    concentrated, J7628
    unit dose, J7629
Bivalirudin, J0582, J0583 ◄
Bivigam, 500 mg, J1556
Bladder calculi irrigation solution, Q2004
Bleomycin sulfate, J9040
Blinded procedure, C9782-C9783
Blood
    count, G0306, G0307, S3630
        complete CBC, automated, without platelet count, G0307
        complete CBC, automated without platelet count, automated WBC differential, G0306
        eosinophil count, blood, direct, S3630
    component/product not otherwise classified, P9099
    fresh frozen plasma, P9017
    glucose monitor, E0607, E2100–E2102, S1030, S1031, S1034
        blood glucose monitor, integrated voice synthesizer, E2100
        blood glucose monitor with integrated lancing/blood sample, E2101

Blood *(Continued)*
    glucose monitor *(Continued)*
        continuous noninvasive device, purchase, S1030
        continuous noninvasive device, rental, S1031
        home blood glucose monitor, E0607
    glucose test, A4253
    glucose, test strips, dialysis, A4772
    granulocytes, pheresis, P9050
    ketone test, A4252
    leak detector, dialysis, E1560
    leukocyte poor, P9016
    mucoprotein, P2038
    platelets, P9019
    platelets, irradiated, P9032
    platelets, leukocytes reduced, P9031
    platelets, leukocytes reduced, irradiated, P9033
    platelets, pheresis, P9034, P9072, P9073, P9100
    platelets, pheresis, irradiated, P9036
    platelets, pheresis, leukocytes reduced, P9035
    platelets, pheresis, leukocytes reduced, irradiated, P9037
    pressure monitor, A4660, A4663, A4670
    pump, dialysis, E1620
    red blood cells, deglycerolized, P9039
    red blood cells, irradiated, P9038
    red blood cells, leukocytes reduced, P9016
    red blood cells, leukocytes reduced, irradiated, P9040
    red blood cells, washed, P9022
    strips, A4253
    supply, P9010–P9022
    testing supplies, A4770
    tubing, A4750, A4755
Blood collection devices accessory, A4257, E0620
BMI, G8417–G8422
Body jacket
    scoliosis, L1300, L1310
Body mass index, G8417–G8422
Body sock, L0984
Bond or cement, ostomy skin, A4364
Bone
    density, study, G0130
Boot
    pelvic, E0944
    surgical, ambulatory, L3260
Bortezomib, J9041, J9046, J9048–J9049, J9051, J9054 ◄
Brachytherapy radioelements, Q3001
    brachytherapy, LDR, prostate, G0458
    brachytherapy planar source, C2645
    brachytherapy, source, hospital outpatient, C1716–C1717, C1719
Breast prosthesis, L8000–L8035, L8600
    adhesive skin support, A4280
    custom breast prosthesis, post mastectomy, L8035
    garment with mastectomy form, post mastectomy, L8015
    implantable, silicone or equal, L8600
    mastectomy bra, with integrated breast prosthesis form, unilateral, L8001
    mastectomy bra, with prosthesis form, bilateral, L8002

◄ New   ↩ Revised   ✓ Reinstated   ~~deleted~~ Deleted

Breast prosthesis (Continued)
  mastectomy bra, without integrated breast prosthesis form, L8000
  mastectomy form, L8020
  mastectomy sleeve, L8010
  nipple prosthesis, L8032
  silicone or equal, with integral adhesive, L8031
  silicone or equal, without integral adhesive, L8030

Breast pump
  accessories, A4281–A4287
    adapter, replacement, A4282
    cap, breast pump bottle, replacement, A4283
    disposable collection, storage bag, A4287
    locking ring, replacement, A4286
    polycarbonate bottle, replacement, A4285
    shield and splash protector, replacement, A4284
    tubing, replacement, A4281
    value, replacement, A4288 ◄
  electric, any type, E0603
  heavy duty, hospital grade, E0604
  manual, any type, E0602

Breathing circuit, A4618
Brentuximab Vedotin, J9042
Brexanolone, J1632
Bronchoscopy, C7509–C7512, C7556
Brolucizumab-dbll, J0179
Brompheniramine maleate, J0945
Budesonide inhalation solution, J7626, J7627, J7633, J7634
Bulking agent, L8604, L8607
Bumetanide, J1939
Bupivacaine, C9144, J0665–J0666, J0668 ◄
Buprenorphine hydrochlorides, J0592
Buprenorphine/Naloxone, J0571–J0578
Buprenorphone, G0533 ◄
Burn, compression garment, A6501–A6513
  bodysuit, head-foot, A6501
  burn mask, face and/or neck, A6513
  chin strap, A6502
  facial hood, A6503
  foot to knee length, A6507
  foot to thigh length, A6508
  glove to axilla, A6506
  glove to elbow, A6505
  glove to wrist, A6504
  lower trunk, including leg openings, A6511
  trunk, including arms, down to leg openings, A6510
  upper trunk to waist, including arm openings, A6509

Bus, nonemergency transportation, A0110
Busulfan, J0594, J8510
Butorphanol tartrate, J0595
Bypass, graft, coronary, artery
  surgery, S2205–S2209

C

C-1 Esterase Inhibitor, J0596–J0598
Cabazitaxel, J9043, J9064
Cabergoline, oral, J8515

Cabinet/System, ultraviolet, E0691–E0694
  multidirectional light system, 6 ft. cabinet, E0694
  timer and eye protection, 4 foot, E0692
  timer and eye protection, 6 foot, E0693
  ultraviolet light therapy system, treatment area 2 sq ft., E0691

Cabote rilpivir J0741
Cabotegravir, J0739
Caffeine citrate, J0706
Cage, interbody, C1831
Calaspargase pegol injection-mknl, J9118
Calcitonin-salmon, J0630
Calcitriol, J0636, S0169
Calcium
  acetate, J0615 ◄
  chloride, J0618 ◄
  disodium edetate, J0600
  gluconate, J0612, J0613
  glycerophosphate and calcium lactate, J0620
  lactate and calcium glycerophosphate, J0620
  leucovorin, J0640

Calibrator solution, A4256
Camcevi, J1952
Canakinumab, J0638
Cancer, screening
  cervical or vaginal, G0101
  colorectal, G0104–G0105, G0121, G0328 ⤴
    alternative to screening colonoscopy, barium enema, G0120
    alternative to screening sigmoidoscopy, barium enema, G0106
    barium enema, G0122
    colonoscopy, high risk, G0105
    colonoscopy, not at high-risk, G0121
    fecal occult blood test, 1-3 simultaneous, G0328
    flexible sigmoidoscopy, G0104
  prostate, G0102, G0103

Cane, E0100, E0105
  accessory, A4636, A4637

Canister
  disposable, used with suction pump, A7000
  non-disposable, used with suction pump, A7001

Cannula, nasal, A4615
Cantharidin, J7354
Capecitabine, oral, J8522
Capsaicin patch, J7336
Carbidopa 5 mg/levodopa 20 mg enteral suspension, J7340
Carbon filter, A4680
Carboplatin, J9045
Carboprost tromethamine, J0675 ◄
Cardia Event, recorder, implantable, E0616
Cardiokymography, Q0035
Cardiovascular services, M0300–M0301
  Fabric wrapping abdominal aneurysm, M0301
  IV chelation therapy, M0300

Cardioverter-defibrillator, G0448
Care
  cancer, M0001
  optimal, M0002–M0003
  supportive, M0004

◄ New   ⤴ Revised   ✔ Reinstated   deleted Deleted

Care, coordinated, G9001–G9011, H1002
  coordinated care fee, home monitoring, G9006
  coordinated care fee, initial rate, G9001
  coordinated care fee, maintenance rate, G9002
  coordinated care fee, physician coordinated care oversight, G9008
  coordinated care fee, risk adjusted high, initial, G9003
  coordinated care fee, risk adjusted low, initial, G9004
  coordinated care fee, risk adjusted maintenance, G9005
  coordinated care fee, risk adjusted maintenance, level 3, G9009
  coordinated care fee, risk adjusted maintenance, level 4, G9010
  coordinated care fee, risk adjusted maintenance, level 5, G9011
  coordinated care fee, scheduled team conference, G9007
  prenatal care, at-risk, enhanced service, care coordination, H1002
Care plan, G0162
Carfilzomib, J9047
Carmustine, J9050, J9052
Case management, T1016, T1017
  behavioral health, G0323
Casimersen J1426
Caspofungin acetate, J0637
Cast
  hand restoration, L6900–L6915
  materials, special, A4590
  supplies, A4580, A4590, Q4001–Q4051
    body cast, adult, Q4001–Q4002
    cast supplies (e.g., plaster), A4580
    cast supplies, unlisted types, Q4050
    finger splint, static, Q4049
    gauntlet cast, adult, Q4013–Q4014
    gauntlet cast, pediatric, Q4015–Q4016
    hip spica, adult, Q4025–Q4026
    hip spica, pediatric, Q4027–Q4028
    long arm cast, adult, Q4005–Q4006
    long arm cast, pediatric, Q4007–Q4008
    long arm splint, adult, Q4017–Q4018
    long arm splint, pediatric, Q4019–Q4020
    long leg cast, adult, Q4029–Q4030
    long leg cast, pediatric, Q4031–Q4032
    long leg cylinder cast, adult, Q4033–Q4034
    long leg cylinder cast, pediatric, Q4035–Q4036
    long leg splint, adult, Q4041–Q4042
    long leg splint, pediatric, Q4043–Q4044
    short arm cast, adult, Q4009–Q4010
    short arm cast, pediatric, Q4011–Q4012
    short arm splint, adult, Q4021–Q4022
    short arm splint, pediatric, Q4023–Q4024
    short leg cast, adult, Q4037–Q4038
    short leg cast, pediatric, Q4039–Q4040
    short leg splint, adult, Q4045–Q4046
    short leg splint, pediatric, Q4047–Q4048
    shoulder cast, adult, Q4003–Q4004
    special casting material (fiberglass), A4590
    splint supplies, miscellaneous, Q4051
  thermoplastic, L2106, L2126

Caster
  front, for power wheelchair, K0099
  wheelchair, E0997, E0998
Catheter, A4300–A4355
  anchoring device, A4333, A4334, A5200
  cap, disposable (dialysis), A4860
  convert, C7547
  coronary artery, C7516–C7529, C7552–C7553, C7557–C7558
  exchange, C7548
  external collection device, A4327–A4330, A4347–A7048
  female external, A4327–A4328
  indwelling, A4338–A4346
  insertion tray, A4354
  insulin infusion catheter, A4224
  intermittent with insertion supplies, A4353
  irrigation supplies, A4355
  male external, A4324, A4325, A4326, A4348
  nephroureteral, C7546
  oropharyngeal suction, A4628
  starter set, A4329
  trachea (suction), A4609, A4610, A4624
  transluminal angioplasty, C2623
  transtracheal oxygen, A4608
  vascular, A4300–A4301
Catheterization, specimen collection, P9612, P9615
CBC, G0306, G0307
Cefazolin sodium, J0687–J0690, J0694
Cefepime HCl, J0692, J0701, J0703
Cefiderocol, J0699
Cefotaxime sodium, J0698
Cefotentan disodium, J0525 ◀
Ceftaroline fosamil, J0712
Ceftazidime, J0713, J0714
Ceftizoxime sodium, J0715
Ceftobiprole medocaril sodium, J0681 ◀
Ceftolozane 50 mg and tazobactam 25 mg, J0695
Ceftriaxone sodium, J0696
Cefuroxime sodium, J0697
Celera, Q4259
CellCept, K0412
Cellesta cord, Q4214
Cellesta or cellesta duo, Q4184
Cellular therapy, M0075
Cement, ostomy, A4364
Cemiplimab injection-rwlc, J9119
Centrifuge, A4650
Centruroides Immune F(ab), J0716
Cephalin Floculation, blood, P2028
~~Cephalothin sodium,~~ ~~J1890~~
Cephapirin sodium, J0710
Certification, physician, home, health (per calendar month), G0179–G0182
  Physician certification, home health, G0180
  Physician recertification, home health, G0179
  Physician supervision, home health, complex care, 30 min or more, G0181
  Physician supervision, hospice 30 min or more, G0182
Certolizumab pegol, J0717
Cerumen, removal, G0268

◀ New   ↻ Revised   ✔ Reinstated   ~~deleted~~ Deleted

Cervical
  cancer, screening, G0101
  cytopathology, G0123, G0124, G0141–G0148
    screening, automated thin layer, manual rescreening, physician supervision, G0145
    screening, automated thin layer preparation, cytotechnologist, physician interpretation, G0143
    screening, automated thin layer preparation, physician supervision, G0144
    screening, by cytotechnologist, physician supervision, G0123
    screening, cytopathology smears, automated system, physician interpretation, G0141
    screening, interpretation by physician, G0124
    screening smears, automated system, manual rescreening, G0148
    screening smears, automated system, physician supervision, G0147
  halo, L0810–L0830
  head harness/halter, E0942
  orthosis, L0100–L0200
    cervical collar molded to patient, L0170
    cervical, flexible collar, L0120–L0130
    cervical, multiple post collar, supports, L0180–L0200
    cervical, semi-rigid collar, L0150–L0160, L0172, L0174
    cranial cervical, L0112–L0113
  traction, E0855, E0856
Cervical cap contraceptive, A4261
Cervical-thoracic-lumbar-sacral orthosis (CTLSO), L0700, L0710, L0720 ◄
Cetuximab, J9055
Chair
  adjustable, dialysis, E1570
  lift, E0627
  rollabout, E1031
  sitz bath, E0160–E0162
  transport, E1035–E1039
    chair, adult size, heavy duty, greater than 300 pounds, E1039
    chair, adult size, up to 300 pounds, E1038
    chair, pediatric, E1037
    multi-positional patient transfer system, extra-wide, greater than 300 pounds, E1036
    multi-positional patient transfer system, up to 300 pounds, E1035
Change
  ureterostomy tube, C7549
Chaplain Services, Q9001–Q9003
Chelation therapy, M0300
Chemical endarterectomy, M0300
Chemistry and toxicology tests, P2028–P3001
Chemotherapy
  administration (hospital reporting only), Q0083–Q0085
  drug, oral, not otherwise classified, J8999
  drugs; (see also drug by name), J9000–J9999
Chest shell (cuirass), E0457
Chest Wall Oscillation System, E0483
  hose, replacement, A7026
  vest, replacement, A7025

Chest wrap, E0459
Chin cup, cervical, L0150
Chloramphenicol sodium succinate, J0720
Chlordiazepoxide HCl, J1990
Chloromycetin sodium succinate, J0720
Chloroprocaine HCl, J2401–J2402
Chloroprocaine hcl ophthalmic, J2403
Chloroquine HCl, J0390
Chlorothiazide sodium, J1205
Chlorpromazine HCl, J3230
  Chlorpromazine HCL, 5 mg, oral, Q0161
Chorionic gonadotropin, J0725
Choroid, lesion, destruction, G0186
Chromic phosphate P32 suspension, A9564
Chromium CR-51 sodium chromate, A9553
Cidofovir, J0740
Cilastatin sodium, imipenem, J0743
Ciltacabtagene, Q2056
Cinacalcet, J0604
Cipaglucosidase, J1203
Ciprofloxacin
  for intravenous infusion, J0744
  octic suspension, J7342
Cisplatin, J9060
Cladribine, J9065
Clamp
  dialysis, A4918
  external urethral, A4356
Cleanser, wound, A6260
Cleansing agent, dialysis equipment, A4790
Clevidipine butyrate, J0759 ◄
Clindamycin phosphate, J0736, J0737
Clinical care for indigenous persons, H0052–H0053 ◄
Clofarabine, J9027
Clonidine, J0735
Closure, wound, adhesive, tissue, G0168
Clotting time tube, A4771
Clubfoot wedge, L3380
Cocaine, C9143
Cochlear prosthetic implant, L8614
  accessories, L8615–L8617, L8618
  batteries, L8621–L8624
  replacement, L8619, L8627–L8629
    external controller component, L8628
    external speech processor and controller, integrated system, L8619
    external speech processor, component, L8627
    transmitting coil and cable, integrated, L8629
Cocoon, membrane, Q4264
Codeine phosphate, J0745
Cold/Heat, application, E0200–E0239
  bilirubin light, E0202
  electric heat pad, moist, E0215
  electric heat pad, standard, E0210
  heat lamp with stand, E0205
  heat lamp, without stand, E0200
  hydrocollator unit, E0225
  hydrocollator unit, portable, E0239
  infrared heating pad system, E0221
  non-contact wound warming device, E0231

Cold/Heat, application (Continued)
  paraffin bath unit, E0235
  pump for water circulating pad, E0236
  therapeutic lightbox, E0203
  warming card, non-contact wound warming device, E0232
  water circulating cold pad, with pump, E0218
  water circulating heat pad, with pump, E0217
Colistimethate sodium, J0770
Collagen
  meniscus implant procedure, G0428
  skin test, G0025
  urinary tract implant, L8603
  wound dressing, A2006–A2014, A6020–A6024
Collagenase, Clostridium histolyticum, J0775
Collar, cervical
  multiple post, L0180–L0200
  nonadjust (foam), L0120
Colorectal, screening, cancer, G0104–G0105, G0121, G0328 ↩
Coly-Mycin M, J0770
Comfort items, A9190
Commode, E0160–E0175
  chair, E0170–E0171
  lift, E0172, E0625
  pail, E0167
  seat, wheelchair, E0968
Complete, blood, count, G0306, G0307
Composite dressing, A6200–A6205
Compressed gas system, E0424–E0446
  oximeter device, E0445
  portable gaseous oxygen system, purchase, E0430
  portable gaseous oxygen system, rental, E0431
  portable liquid oxygen, rental, container/supplies, E0434
  portable liquid oxygen, rental, home liquefier, E0433
  portable liquid oxygen system, purchase, container/refill adapter, E0435
  portable oxygen contents, gaseous, 1 month, E0443
  portable oxygen contents, liquid, 1 month, E0444
  stationary liquid oxygen system, purchase, use of reservoir, E0440
  stationary liquid oxygen system, rental, container/supplies, E0439
  stationary oxygen contents, gaseous, 1 month, E0441
  stationary oxygen contents, liquid, 1 month, E0442
  stationary purchase, compressed gas system, E0425
  stationary rental, compressed gaseous oxygen system, E0424
  topical oxygen delivery system, NOS, E0446
Compression
  arm sleeve, A6576–A6578
  arm sleeve/glove combination, A6574–A6575
  bandage, A4460, A6594–A6609
  burn garment, A6501–A6513 ◀
  garment, A6515–A6529, A6565–A6573, A6610 ◀
  gauntlet, A6582
  glove, A6579–A6581
  stockings, A6530–A6549, A6552–A6564
  wrap, A6583–A6589, A6593, A6611 ◀
Compressor, E0565, E0570, E0571, E0572, E0650–E0652

Concizumab-mtci, J7173 ◀
Conductive gel/paste, A4558
Conductivity meter, bath, dialysis, E1550
Conference, team, G0175, G9007, S0220, S0221
  coordinate care fee, scheduled team conference, G9007
  medical conference/physician/interdisciplinary team, patient present, 30 min, S0220
  medical conference physician/interdisciplinary team, patient present, 60 min, S0221
  scheduled interdisciplinary team conference, patient present, G0175
Congo red, blood, P2029
Consultation, S0285, S0311, T1040, T1041
  Telehealth, G0425–G0427
Contact layer, A6206–A6208
Contact lens, V2500–V2599
Continent device, A5081, A5082, A5083
Continuous glucose monitoring system
  receiver, A9278, E2103, *S1037*
  sensor, A9276, *S1035*
  transmitter, A9277, *S1036*
Continuous passive motion exercise device, E0936
Continuous positive airway pressure device(CPAP), E0601
  compressor, K0269
Contraceptive
  cervical cap, A4261
  condoms, A4267, A4268
  diaphragm, A4266
  intratubal occlusion device, A4264
  intrauterine, copper, J7300
  intrauterine, levonorgestrel releasing, J7296–J7298, J7301
  patch, J7304
  spermicide, A4269
  supply, A4267–A4269
  vaginal ring, J7303
Contracts, maintenance, ESRD, A4890
Contrast, Q9951–Q9969
  HOCM, Q9958–Q9964
  injection, iron based magnetic resonance, per ml, Q9953
  injection, non-radioactive, non-contrast, visualization adjunct, Q9968
  injection, octafluoropropane microspheres, per ml, Q9956
  injection, perflexane lipid microspheres, per ml, Q9955
  injection, perflutren lipid microspheres, per ml, Q9957
  LOCM, Q9965–Q9967
  LOCM, 400 or greater mg/ml iodine, per ml, Q9951
  oral magnetic resonance contrast, Q9954
  Tc-99m per study dose, Q9969
Contrast material
  injection during MRI, A4643
  low osmolar, A4644–A4646
Coordinated, care, G0534, G9001–G9011 ◀
  CORF, registered nurse- face-face, G0128
Corneal tissue processing, V2785

Corset, spinal orthosis, L0970–L0976
  LSO, corset front, L0972
  LSO, full corset, L0976
  TLSO, corset front, L0970
  TLSO, full corset, L0974
Corticorelin ovine triflutate, J0795
Corticotropin (acthar gel), J0801
Corticotropin (ani), J0802
Corvert (see Ibutilide fumarate)
Cosibelimab-ipdl, J9275 ◄
Cosyntropin, J0833, J0834
Cough stimulating device, A7020, E0482
Counseling
  alcohol misuse, G0443
  cardiovascular disease, G0448
  immunization, G0310–G0315
  obesity, G0447
  sexually transmitted infection, G0445
Count, blood, G0306, G0307
Counterpulsation, external, G0166
Cover, wound
  alginate dressing, A6196–A6198
  foam dressing, A6209–A6214
  hydrogel dressing, A6242–A6248
  non-contact wound warming cover, and accessory,
    A6000, E0231, E0232
  specialty absorptive dressing, A6251–A6256
Covid-19 convalescent plasma, C9507
Covid test, K1034
**CPAP (continuous positive airway pressure)
    device,** E0601
  headgear, K0185
  humidifier, A7046
  intermittent assist, E0452
Cradle, bed, E0280
Crib, E0300
Cromolyn sodium, inhalation solution, unit dose,
    J7631, J7632
Crotalidae polyvalent immune fab, J0840
Crovalimab-akkz, J1307 ◄
Crutches, E0110–E0118
  accessories, A4635–A4637, K0102
  crutch substitute, lower leg, E0118
  forearm, E0110–E0111
  underarm, E0112–E0117
Cryoprecipitate, each unit, P9012
CTLSO, L0700, L0710, L0720, L1000–L1120 ◄
  addition, axilla sling, L1010
  addition, cover for upright, each, L1120
  addition, kyphosis pad, L1020
  addition, kyphosis pad, floating, L1025
  addition, lumbar bolster pad, L1030
  addition, lumbar rib pad, L1040
  addition, lumbar sling, L1090
  addition, outrigger, L1080
  addition, outrigger bilateral, vertical extensions, L1085
  addition, ring flange, L1100
  addition, ring flange, molded to patient model, L1110
  addition, sternal pad, L1050
  addition, thoracic pad, L1060
  addition, trapezius sling, L1070

CTLSO *(Continued)*
  *anterior-posterior-lateral control, molded to patient
    model (CTLSO),* L0710
  *cervical, thoracic, lumbar, sacral orthrosis
    (CTLSO),* L0700
  furnishing initial orthrosis, L1000
  immobilizer, infant size, L1001
  *sagittal-coronal control, rigid lateral frame, axilla to
    trochanter,* L1006, L1007 ◄
  tension based scoliosis orthosis, fitting, L1005
Cuirass, E0457
Culture sensitivity study, P7001
Cushion, wheelchair, E0977
Cutaquig, J1551
Cyanocobalamin Cobalt C057, A9559
Cycler dialysis machine, E1594
Cyclophosphamide, J9071–J9076 ◄
  oral, J8530
Cyclosporine, J7502, J7515, J7516
Cygnus matrix, Q4199
Cystourethroscopy, C7550, C7554, C9761
Cytarabine, J9100
  liposome, J9098
Cytomegalovirus immune globulin (human), J0850
Cytopathology, cervical or vaginal, G0123, G0124,
    G0141–G0148

D

Dacarbazine, J9130
Daclizumab, J7513
Dactinomycin, J9120
Dalalone, J1100
Dalbavancin, 5mg, J0875
Dalteparin sodium, J1645
Daprodustat, oral, J0889
Daptomycin, J0872–J0874, J0877, J0878
Daratumumab, J9144, J9145
Darbepoetin Alfa, J0881–J0882
Datopotamab deruxtecan-dlnk, J9011 ◄
Daunorubicin
  Citrate, J9151
  HCl, J9150
DaunoXome (see Daunorubicin citrate)
Daxibotulinumtoxina-lanm, J0589
Debridement
  bone, C7500
Decitabine, J0893, J0894
Decubitus care equipment, E0180–E0199
  air fluidized bed, E0194
  air pressure mattress, E0186
  air pressure pad, standard mattress, E0197
  dry pressure mattress, E0184
  dry pressure pad, standard mattress, E0199
  gel or gel-like pressure pad mattress, standard, E0185
  gel pressure mattress, E0196
  heel or elbow protector, E0191
  positioning cushion, E0190
  *power pressure reducing mattress overlay, with
    pump,* E0181, E0183
  powered air flotation bed, E0193

Decubitus care equipment (Continued)
  pump, alternating pressure pad, replacement, E0182
  synthetic sheepskin pad, E0189
  water pressure mattress, E0187
  water pressure pad, standard mattress, E0198
Deferoxamine mesylate, J0895
Defibrillator, external, E0617, K0606
  battery, K0607
  electrode, K0609
  garment, K0608
Degarelix, J9155
Deionizer, water purification system, E1615
Delandistrogene, J1413
Delivery/set-up/dispensing, A9901
Denileukin diftitox-cxdl, J9161 ◀
Denosumab, J0897, Q5136, Q5157–Q5159 ◀
Density, bone, study, G0130
Depo-estradiol cypionate, J1000
Dermacell, dermacell awn or dermacell awn porous, Q4122
Dermal filler injection, G0429
Desmopressin acetate, J2597
Destruction, lesion, choroid, G0186
Detector, blood leak, dialysis, E1560
Developmental testing, G0451
Devise, support, fistula, C8000
Devices, other orthopedic, E1800–E1841
  assistive listening device, V5267–V5290
Dexamethasone
  ~~acetate, J1094~~
  inhalation solution, concentrated, J7637
  inhalation solution, unit dose, J7638
  intravitreal implant, J7312
  lacrimal ophthalmic insert, J1096
  oral, J8540, J8541
  sodium phosphate, J1100
Dexmedetomidine, J1105
Dextran, J7100
Dextrose
  saline (normal), J7042
  water, J7060, J7070
Dextrose, 5% in lactated ringers infusion, J7121
Dextrostick, A4772
Diabetes
  evaluation, G0245, G0246
  shoes (fitting/modifications), A5500–A5508
    deluxe feature, depth-inlay shoe, A5508
    depth inlay shoe, A5500
    molded from cast patient's foot, A5501
    shoe with metatarsal bar, A5505
    shoe with off-set heel(s), A5506
    shoe with rocker or rigid-bottom rocker, A5503
    shoe with wedge(s), A5504
    specified modification NOS, depth-inlay shoe, A5507
  training, outpatient, G0108, G0109
Diagnostic
  copper, A9592
  florbetaben, Q9983
  flutemetamol F18, Q9982
  mammography, digital image, G9899, G9900
  radiology services, R0070–R0076

Dialysate
  concentrate additives, A4765
  solution, A4720–A4728
  testing solution, A4760
Dialysis
  air bubble detector, E1530
  bath conductivity, meter, E1550
  chemicals/antiseptics solution, A4674
  circuit, C7513–C7515, C7530
  disposable cycler set, A4671
  emergency, G0257
  equipment, E1510–E1702
  extension line, A4672–A4673
  filter, A4680
  fluid barrier, E1575
  home, S9335, S9339
  kit, A4820
  pressure alarm, E1540
  shunt, A4740
  supplies, A4650–A4927
  tablo hemodialysis system, E1629
  tourniquet, A4929
  unipuncture control system, E1580
  unscheduled, G0257
  venous pressure clamp, A4918
Dialyzer, A4690
Diaper, T1500, T4521–T4540, T4543, T4544
  adult incontinence garment, A4520, A4553
  incontinence supply, rectal insert, any type, each, A4337
  disposable penile wrap, T4545
Diathermy low frequency ultrasonic treatment device for home use, K1004
Diazepam, J3360
Diazoxide, J1730
Diclofenac, J1130
Dicyclomine HCl, J0500
Diethylstilbestrol diphosphate, J9165
Difelikefalin (for ESRD on dialysis), J0879
Digital behavioral therapy, A9291
Digoxin, J1160
Digoxin immune fab (ovine), J1162
Dihydroergotamine mesylate, J1110
Diltiazem hydrochloride, J1163 ◀
Dimenhydrinate, J1240
Dimercaprol, J0470
Dimethyl sulfoxide (DMSO), J1212
Diphenhydramine HCl, J1200
Dipyridamole, J1245
Disarticulation
  lower extremities, prosthesis, L5000–L5999
    above knee, L5200–L5230
    additions exoskeletal-knee-shin system, L5710–L5782
    additions to lower extremities, L5610–L5617
    additions to socket insert, L5654–L5699
    additions to socket variations, L5630–L5653
    additions to test sockets, L5618–L5629
    additions/replacements, feet-ankle units, L5700–L5707
    ankle, L5050–L5060
    below knee, L5100–L5105

◀ New   ↻ Revised   ✓ Reinstated   ~~deleted~~ Deleted

Disarticulation (Continued)
  lower extremities, prosthesis (Continued)
    component modification, L5785–L5795
    endoskeletal, L5810–L5999
    endoskeletal, above knee, L5321
    endoskeletal, hip disarticulation, L5331–L5341
    endoskeleton, below knee, L5301–L5312
    hemipelvectomy, L5280
    hip disarticulation, L5250–L5270
    immediate postsurgical fitting, L5400–L5460
    initial prosthesis, L5500–L5505
    knee disarticulation, L5150–L5160
    partial foot, L5000–L5020
    preparatory prosthesis, L5510–L5600
  upper extremities, prosthesis, L6000–L6692
    above elbow, L6250
    additions to upper limb, L6600–L6700 ◄
    below elbow, L6100–L6130
    elbow disarticulation, L6200–L6205
    endoskeletal, below elbow, L6400
    endoskeletal, interscapular thoracic, L6570–L6590
    endoskeletal, shoulder disarticulation, L6550
    immediate postsurgical procedures, L6380–L6388
    interscapular/thoracic, L6350–L6370
    partial hand, L6000–L6039 ◄
    shoulder disarticulation, L6300–L6320
    wrist disarticulation, L6050–L6055
Disease
  status, oncology, G9063–G9139
Dispensing, fee, pharmacy, G0333, Q0510–Q0514, S9430
  dispensing fee inhalation drug(s), 30 days, Q0513
  dispensing fee inhalation drug(s), 90 days, Q0514
  inhalation drugs, 30 days, as a beneficiary, G0333
  initial immunosuppressive drug(s), post transplanr, G0510
  oral anti-cancer, oral anti-emetic, immunosuppressive, first prescription, Q0511
  oral anti-cancer, oral anti-emetic, immunosuppressive, subsequent preparation, Q0512
Disposable supplies, ambulance, A0382, A0384, A0392–A0398
DME
  miscellaneous, A9900–A9999
    DME delivery, set up, A9901
    DME supple, NOS, A9999
    DME supplies, A9900
DMSO, J1212
Dobutamine HCl, J1250
Docetaxel, J9171–J9172, J9174 ◄
Documentation
  antidepressant, G8126–G8128
  blood pressure, G8476–G8478
  bypass, graft, coronary, artery, documentation, G8160–G8163
  CABG, G8160–G8163
  dysphagia, G8232
  dysphagia, screening, G8232, V5364
  ECG, 12–lead, G8705, G8706
  eye, functions, G8315–G8333

Documentation (Continued)
  influenza, immunization, ~~G8482–G8484,~~ M1169
  kidney health evaluation, M1189–M1190
  medical reason, M1178, M1183–M1185, M1194, M1201–M1202
  pharmacologic therapy for osteoporosis, G8635
  physician for DME, G0454
  prophylactic antibiotic, G8702, G8703
  prophylactic parenteral antibiotic, G8629–G8632
  prophylaxis, DVT, G8218
  prophylaxis, thrombosis, deep, vein, G8218
  urinary, incontinence, G8063, G8267
  vaccine, immunization, M1172
Dolasetron mesylate, J1260
Dome and mouthpiece (for nebulizer), A7016
Donanemab, J0175
Dopamine HCl, J1265
Doripenem, J1267
Dornase alpha, inhalation solution, unit dose form, J7639
Dostarlimab-gxly, J9272
Doxercalciferol, J1270
Doxil, J9001
Doxorubicin HCl, J9000, J9002
Doxycycline hyclate, J1271 ◄
Drainage
  bag, A4357, A4358
  board, postural, E0606
  bottle, A5102
Dressing
  alginate, A6196–A6199
  collagen, A6020–A6024
  composite, A6200–A6205
  contact layer, A6206–A6208
  foam, A6209–A6215
  gauze, A6216–A6230, A6402–A6406
  holder/binder, A4462
  hydrocolloid, A6234–A6241
  hydrogel, A6242–A6248
  specialty absorptive, A6251–A6256
  transparent film, A6257–A6259
  tubular, A6457
  wound, K0744–K0746
Dronabinol, Q0155 ◄
Droperidol, J1790
  ~~and fentanyl citrate, J1810~~
Dropper, A4649
Drugs; (see also Table of Drugs)
  administered through a metered dose inhaler, J3535
  antiemetic, J8498, J8597, Q0163–Q0181
  chemotherapy, J8500–J9999
  disposable delivery system, 50 ml or greater per hour, A4305
  disposable delivery system, 5 ml or less per hour, A4306
  immunosuppressive, J7500–J7599
  infusion supplies, A4221, A4222, A4230–A4232
  inhalation solutions, J7608–J7699
  non-prescription, A9150
  not otherwise classified, J3490, J7599, J7699, J7799, J7999, J8499, J8999, J9999

◄ New ↻ Revised ✓ Reinstated ~~deleted~~ Deleted

Drugs (Continued)
  oral, NOS, J8499
  prescription, oral, J8499, J8999
Dry pressure pad/mattress, E0179, E0184, E0199
Duel layer impax membrane, Q4262
Duograft aa, Q4376 ◄
Duograft ac, Q4375 ◄
Durable medical equipment (DME), E0100–E1830, K Codes
  additional oxygen related equipment, E1352–E1406
  arm support, wheelchair, E2626–E2633
  artificial kidney machines/accessories, E1500–E1699
  attachments, E0156–E0159
  bath and toilet aides, E0240–E0249
  canes, E0100–E0105
  commodes, E0160–E0175
  crutches, E0110–E0118
  decubitus care equipment, E0181–E0199
  DME, respiratory, inexpensive, purchased, A7000–A7509
  gait trainer, E8000–E8002
  heat/cold application, E0200–E0239
  hospital beds and accessories, E0250–E0373
  humidifiers/nebulizers/compressors, oxygen IPPB, E0550–E0585
  infusion supplies, E0776–E0791
  IPPB machines, E0500
  jaw motion rehabilitation system, E1700–E1702
  miscellaneous, E1902–E2120
  monitoring equipment, home glucose, E0607
  negative pressure, E2402
  non-pneumatic compressor, E0677–E0683
  other orthopedic devices, E1800–E1841
  oxygen/respiratory equipment, E0424–E0487
  pacemaker monitor, E0610–E0620
  patient lifts, E0621–E0642
  pneumatic compressor, E0650–E0676
  rollout chair/transfer system, E1031–E1039
  safety equipment, E0700–E0705
  speech device, E2500–E2599
  suction pump/room vaporizers, E0600–E0606
  temporary DME codes, regional carriers, K0000–K9999
  TENS/stimulation device(s), E0720–E0770
  traction equipment, E0830–E0900
  trapeze equipment, fracture frame, E0910–E0948
  walkers, E0130–E0155
  wheelchair accessories, E2201–E2397
  wheelchair, accessories, E0950–E1030
  wheelchair, amputee, E1170–E1200
  wheelchair cusion/protection, E2601–E2621
  wheelchair, fully reclining, E1050–E1093
  wheelchair, heavy duty, E1280–E1298
  wheelchair, lightweight, E1240–E1270
  wheelchair, semi-reclining, E1100–E1110
  wheelchair, skin protection, E2622–E2625
  wheelchair, special size, E1220–E1239
  wheelchair, standard, E1130–E1161
  whirlpool equipment, E1300–E1310
Duraclon, (see Clonidine)
Dyphylline, J1180
Dysphagia, screening, documentation, G8232, V5364
Dystrophic, nails, trimming, G0127

E

Ear mold, V5264, V5265
Ecallantide, J1290
~~Echocardiography image,~~ ~~C9786~~
Echocardiography injectable contrast material, A9700
  ECG, 12–lead, G8704
~~Eculizumab,~~ ~~J1300~~
Eculizumab, J1299, Q5151–Q5152 ◄
ED, visit, G0380–G0384
Edetate
  calcium disodium, J0600
  disodium, J3520
Educational Services
  chronic kidney disease, G0420, G0421
Efbemalenograstim, J9361
Efgartigimod, J9332, J9334
Eflapegrastim-xnst, J1449
Eggcrate dry pressure pad/mattress, E0184, E0199
EKG, G0403–G0405
Elbow
  disarticulation, endoskeletal, L6450
  orthosis (EO), E1800, L3700–L3740, L3760, L3671
    dynamic adjustable elbow flexion device, E1800
    elbow arthrosis, L3702–L3766
  protector, E0191
Electric hand, L7007–L7008
Electric, nerve, stimulator, transcutaneous, A4595, E0720–E0749
  conductive garment, E0731
  electric joint stimulation device, E0762
  electrical stimulator supplies, A4595, A4596
  electromagnetic wound treatment device, E0769
  electronic salivary reflex stimulator, E0755
  EMG, biofeedback device, E0746
  functional electrical stimulator, nerve and/or muscle groups, E0770
  functional stimulator sequential muscle groups, E0764
  incontinence treatment system, E0740
  nerve stimulator (FDA), treatment nausea and vomiting, E0765
  osteogenesis stimulator, electrical, surgically implanted, E0749
  osteogenesis stimulator, low-intensity ultrasound, E0760
  osteogenesis stimulator, non-invasive, not spinal, E0747
  osteogenesis stimulator, non-invasive, spinal, E0748
  radiowaves, non-thermal, high frequency, E0761
  stimulator, electrical shock unit, E0745
  stimulator for scoliosis, E0744
  TENS, four or more leads, E0730
  TENS, two lead, E0720
  upper limb, A4540–A4542
Electrical stimulation device used for cancer treatment, E0766, E0767
Electrical work, dialysis equipment, A4870
Electrodes, per pair, A4555, A4556
Electromagnetic, therapy, G0295, G0329
Electronic medication compliance, T1505
Elevating leg rest, K0195

Elliotts B solution, J9175
Elotuzumab, J9176
Elranatamab-bcmm, J1323
Emapalumab injection-lzsg, J9210
Emergency department, visit, G0380–G0384
EMG, E0746
Emtricitabine and tenofovir disoproxil fumarate, J0750
Emtricitabine and tenofovir alafenamide, J0751
Eminase, J0350
Encephalitis, due to vaccine, M1162
Endarterectomy, chemical, M0300
Endoscopy, adapter, UGI, C1606
Endoscope sheath, A4270
Endoscopic
  outlet reduction, C9785
  retrograde cholangiopancreatography, C7541–C7544, C7560
  sleeve gastroplasty, C9784
Endoskeletal system, addition, L5848, L5856–L5857, L5925–L5926, L5961, L5969
Enema, bag, A4458
Enfuvirtide, J1324
Enoxaparin sodium, J1650
Ensifentrine, INH, 3 mg, J7601 ◀
Enteral
  feeding supply kit (syringe) (pump) (gravity), B4034–B4036, B4148
  formulae, B4149–B4156, B4157–B4162
  nutrition infusion pump (with alarm) (without), B9000, B9002
  therapy, supplies, B4000–B9999
    enteral and parenteral pumps, B9002–B9999
    enteral formula/medical supplies, B0434–B4162
    parenteral solutions/supplies, B4164–B5200
Epcoritamab-bysp, J9321
Epinephrine, J0163–J0169 ~~J0171, J0173~~ ◀
Epirubicin HCl, J9178
Epoetin alpha, J0885, Q4081
Epoetin alpha-epbx, Retacrit (for ESRD on dialysis), Q5105
Epoetin alpha-epbx, Retacrit (non-ESRD use), Q5106
Epoetin beta, J0887–J0888
Epoprostenol, J1325
Eptinezumab-jjmr, J3032
Equipment
  decubitus, E0181–E0199
  exercise, A9300, E0935, E0936
  orthopedic, E0910–E0948, E1800–E8002
  oxygen, E0424–E0486, E1353–E1406
  pump, E0781, E0784, E0791
  respiratory, E0424–E0601
  safety, E0700, E0705
  traction, E0830–E0900
  transfer, E0705
  trapeze, E0910–E0912, E0940
  whirlpool, E1300–E1301, E1310
Eravacycline injection, J0122
Erection device, tension ring, L7902
Ergonovine maleate, J1330

Eribulin mesylate, J9179
Ertapenem sodium, J1335
Erythromycin lactobionate, J1364
Erzofri, 1 mg, J2428 ◀
Esketamine, nasal spray, S0013
Esmolol hydrochloride, J1805, J1806
Esomeprazole sodium, J1370 ◀
ESRD (End-Stage Renal Disease); (see also Dialysis)
  diagnosis of, M1187
  machines and accessories, E1500–E1699
    adjustable chair, ESRD, E1570
    centrifuge, dialysis, E1500
    dialysis equipment, NOS, E1699
    hemodialysis, air bubble detector, replacement, E1530
    hemodialysis, bath conductivity meter, E1550
    hemodialysis, blood leak detector, replacement, E1560
    hemodialysis, blood pump, replacement, E1620
    hemodialysis equipment, delivery/installation charges, E1600
    hemodialysis, heparin infusion pump, E1520
    hemodialysis machine, E1590
    hemodialysis, portable travel hemodialyzer system, E1635
    hemodialysis, pressure alarm, E1540
    hemodialysis, reverse osmosis water system, E1615
    hemodialysis, sorbent cartridges, E1636
    hemodialysis, transducer protectors, E1575
    hemodialysis, unipuncture control system, E1580
    hemodialysis, water softening system, E1625
    hemostats, E1637
    peritoneal dialysis, automatic intermittent system, E1592
    peritoneal dialysis clamps, E1634
    peritoneal dialysis, cycler dialysis machine, E1594
    peritoneal dialysis, reciprocating system, E1630
    scale, E1639
    wearable artificial kidney, E1632
  plumbing, A4870
  supplies, A4651–A4929
    acetate concentrate solution, hemodialysis, A4708
    acid concentrate solution, hemodialysis, A4709
    activated carbon filters, hemodialysis, A4680
    ammonia test strip, dialysis, A4774
    automatic blood pressure monitor, A4670
    bicarbonate concentrate, powder, hemodialysis, A4707
    bicarbonate concentrate, solution, A4706
    blood collection tube, vaccum, dialysis, A4770
    blood glucose test strip, dialysis, A4772
    blood pressure cuff only, A4663
    blood tubing, arterial and venous, hemodialysis, A4755
    blood tubing, arterial or venous, hemodialysis, A4750
    chemicals/antiseptics solution, clean dialysis equipment, A4674
    dialysate solution, non-dextrose, A4728
    dialysate solution, peritoneal dialysis, A4720–A4726, A4760–A4766
    dialyzers, hemodialysis, A4690
    disposable catheter tips, peritoneal dialysis, A4860
    disposable cycler set, dialysis machine, A4671
    drainage extension line, dialysis, sterile, A4672

ESRD *(Continued)*
  supplies *(Continued)*
    extension line easy lock connectors, dialysis, A4673
    fistula cannulation set, hemodialysis, A4730
    injectable anesthetic, dialysis, A4737
    occult blood test strips, dialysis, A4773
    peritoneal dialysis, catheter anchoring device, A4653
    protamine sulfate, hemodialysis, A4802
    serum clotting timetube, dialysis, A4771
    shunt accessory, hemodialysis, A4740
    sphygmomanometer, cuff and stethoscope, A4660
    syringes, A4657
    topical anesthetic, dialysis, A4736
    treated water, peritoneal dialysis, A4714
    "Y set" tubing, peritoneal dialysis, A4719
Estrogen conjugated, J1410
Estrone (5, Aqueous), J1435
Etelcalcetide, J0606
Eteplirsen, J1428
Ethacrynate sodium, J1807 ◂
Ethanolamine oleate, J1430
Etidronate disodium, J1436
Etonogestrel implant system, J7307
Etoposide, J9181
  oral, J8560
Etranacogene dezaparvovec-drlb, J1411
Euflexxa, J7323
Evaluation
  conformity, V5020
  contact lens, S0592
  diabetic, G0245, G0246
  footwear, G8410–G8416
  hearing, S0618, V5008, V5010
  hospice, G0337
  multidisciplinary, H2000
  nursing, T1001
  ocularist, S9150
  performance measurement, S3005
  resident, T2011
  speech, S9152
  team, T1024
Everolimus, J7527
Evinacumab-dgnb J1305
Exagamglogene autotem, J3392 ◂
Examination
  gynecological, S0610–S0613
  ophthalmological, S0620, S0621
  pinworm, Q0113
  post operative, unrelated practitioner, G0559 ◂
Excision
  cervical nodes, C7503
  neuroma, C7551
Exercise
  class, S9451
  equipment, A9300
Exoskeletal, addition, L5810–L5966 ◂
External
  ambulatory infusion pump, E0781, E0784
  ambulatory infusion pump continuous glucose sensing, E0787
  ambulatory insulin delivery system, A9274

External *(Continued)*
  power, battery components, L7360–L7368
  power, elbow, L7160–L7191
  urinary supplies, A4356–A4359
Extremity
  belt/harness, E0945
  traction, E0870–E0880
Eye
  case, V2756
  functions, documentation, G8315–G8333
  lens (contact) (spectacle), V2100–V2615
  pad, patch, A6410–A6412
  prosthetic, V2623, V2629
  service (miscellaneous), V2700–V2799
  stent, S1091

F

Face tent, oxygen, A4619
Faceplate, ostomy, A4361
Facility services, dental, G0330
Factor IX, J7193, J7194, J7195, J7200–J7202, J7213
Factor VIIA coagulation factor, recombinant, J7189, J7205, J7212
Factor VIII, anti-hemophilic factor, J7182, J7185, J7190–J7192, J7207–J7209, J7214
Factor X, J7175
Factor XIII, anti-hemophilic factor, J7180, J7188
Factor XIII, A-subunit, J7181
Family Planning Education, H1010
Famotidine, J1308 ◂
Faricimab-svoa, J2777
Fecal microbiota, J1440
Fee
  coordinated care, G9001–G9011
  dispensing, pharmacy, G0333, Q0510–Q0514, S9430
Fentanyl citrate, J3010
  ~~and droperidol, J1810~~
Fern test, Q0114
Ferric citrate, J0609 ◂
Ferric derisomaltose, J1437
Ferric pyrophosphate citrate powder, J1444
Fertility cycle tracking software, A9293
Ferumoxytol, Q0138, Q0139
Fidanacogene elaparvovec-dzkt, J1414 ◂
Filgrastim, J1442, J1447, Q5101, Q5148 ◂
Filler, wound
  alginate dressing, A6199
  foam dressing, A6215
  hydrocolloid dressing, A6240, A6241
  hydrogel dressing, A6248
  not elsewhere classified, A6261, A6262
Film, transparent (for dressing), A6257–A6259
Filter
  aerosol compressor, A7014
  dialysis carbon, A4680
  ostomy, A4368
  tracheostoma, A4481
  ultrasonic generator, A7014
Fistula cannulation set, A4730

◂ New   ↻ Revised   ✓ Reinstated   ~~deleted~~ Deleted

Fitusiran, J7174 ◀
Flebogamma, J1572
Florbetapir F18, A9586
Flortaucipir, A9601
Flotufolastat, C9156
Flowmeter, E0440, E0555, E0580
Floxuridine, J9200
Fluconazole, injection, J1450
Fludeoxyglucose, A9609
Fludarabine phosphate, J8562, J9185
Fluid barrier, dialysis, E1575
Fluid flow, Q4206
Flunisolide inhalation solution, J7641
Fluocinolone, J7311, J7313
   (Yutiq), J7314
Fluorodeoxyglucose F-18 FDG, A9552
Fluorodopa, A9602
Fluoroestradiol F 18, A9591
Fluorouracil, J9190
Fluphenazine decanoate, J2680
Fluphenazine hcl, J2679
Flurpiridaz f18, A9611 ◀
Foam
   dressing, A6209–A6215
   pad adhesive, A5126
Folding walker, E0135, E0143
Foley catheter, A4312–A4316, A4338–A4346
   indwelling catheter, specialty type, A4340–A4342
   indwelling catheter, three-way, continuous irrigation, A4346
   indwelling catheter, two-way, all silicone, A4344
   indwelling catheter, two-way latex, A4338
   insertion tray with drainage bag, A4312
   insertion tray with drainage bag, three-way, continuous irrigation, A4316
   insertion tray with drainage bag, two-way latex, A4314
   insertion tray with drainage bag, two-way, silicone, A4315
   insertion tray without drainage bag, A4313
Folic acid, J1808 ◀
Fomepizole, J1451
Fomivirsen sodium intraocular, J1452
Fondaparinux sodium, J1652
Foot care, G0247
Footdrop splint, L4398
Footplate, E0175, E0970, L3031
Footwear, orthopedic, L3201–L3265
   additional charge for split size, L3257
   Benesch boot, pair, child, L3213
   Benesch boot, pair, infant, L3212
   Benesch boot, pair, junior, L3214
   custom molded shoe, prosthetic shoe, L3250
   custom shoe, depth inlay, L3230
   ladies' shoe, depth inlay, L3216
   ladies' shoe, hightop, L3217
   ladies' shoe, oxford, L3215
   ladies' shoe, oxford/brace, L3224
   men's shoe, depth inlay, L3221
   men's shoe, hightop, L3222
   men's shoe, oxford, L3219
   men's shoe, oxford/brace, L3225

Footwear, orthopedic *(Continued)*
   molded shoe, custom fitted, Plastazote, L3253
   non-standard size or length, L3255
   non-standard size or width, L3254
   Plastazote sandal, L3265
   shoe, hightop, child, L3206
   shoe, hightop, infant, L3204
   shoe, hightop, junior, L3207
   shoe molded/patient model, Plastazote, L3252
   shoe, molded/patient model, silicone, L3251
   shoe, oxford, child, L3202
   shoe, oxford, infant, L3201
   shoe, oxford, junior, L3203
   surgical boot, child, L3209
   surgical boot, infant, L3208
   surgical boot, junior, L3211
   surgical boot/shoe, L3260
Forearm crutches, E0110, E0111
Formoterol, J7640
   fumarate, J7606
Fosaprepitant, J1434, J1453, J1456
Foscarbidopa/Foslevodopa, J7356 ◀
Foscarnet sodium, J1455
Fosdenopterin, J1809 ◀
Fosphenytoin, Q2009
Fracture
   bedpan, E0276
   frame, E0920, E0930, E0946–E0948
      attached to bed/weights, E0920
      attachments for complex cervical traction, E0948
      attachments for complex pelvic traction, E0947
      dual, cross bars, attached to bed, E0946
      free standing/weights, E0930
   orthosis, L2106–L2136, L3980–L3984
      ankle/foot orthosis, fracture, L2106–L2128
      KAFO, fracture orthosis, L2132–L2136
      upper extremity, fracture orthosis, L3980–L3984
   orthotic additions, L2180–L2192, L3995
      addition to upper extremity orthosis, sock, fracture, L3995
      additions lower extremity fracture, L2180–L2192
Fragmin, (see Dalteparin sodium), *J1645*
Frames (spectacles), V2020, V2025
   deluxe frame, V2025
   purchases, V2020
Fremanezumab-vfrm, J3031
Fulvestrant, J9393–J9395
Furosemide, J1938, J̶1̶9̶4̶0̶, J1941 ◀
Fusion
   finger joints, C7506

G

Gadobutrol, A9585
Gadofosveset trisodium, A9583
Gadopiclenol, A9573
Gadoxetate disodium, A9581
Gait trainer, E8000–E8002
Gallium Ga67, A9556
Gallium illuccix, A9596

Gallium locametz, A9800
Gallium nitrate, J1457
Galsulfase, J1458
Gamma globulin, J1460, J1560
  injection, gamma globulin (IM), 1cc, J1460
  injection, gamma globulin (IM), over 10cc, J1560
Gammagard liquid, J1569
Gammaplex, J1557
Gamunex, J1561
Ganciclovir
  implant, J7310
  sodium, J1570, J1574
Garamycin, J1580
Gas system
  compressed, E0424, E0425
  gaseous, E0430, E0431, E0441, E0443
  liquid, E0434–E0440, E0442, E0444
Gastric freezing, hypothermia, M0100
Gatifloxacin, J1590
Gauze
  impregnated, A6222–A6233, A6266
  non-impregnated, A6402–A6404
Gefitinib, J8565
Gel
  conductive, A4558
  pressure pad, E0185, E0196
Gemcitabine HCl, not otherwise specified, J9196, J9201
  Infugem, J9198
Gemtuzumab ozogamicin, J9203
Generator
  neurostimulator (implantable), high frequency, C1822
  neurostimulator (implantable), non-rechargeable, C1827
  neurostimulator (implantable), rechargeable, C1826
  ultrasonic with nebulizer, E0574–E0575
Gentamicin (Sulfate), J1580
Glasses
  air conduction, V5070
  binaural, V5120–V5150
    behind the ear, V5140
    body, V5120
    glasses, V5150
    in the ear, V5130
  bone conduction, V5080
  frames, V2020, V2025
  hearing aid, V5230
Glaucoma
  screening, G0117, G0118
Glofitamab, J9286
Gloves, A4927
Glucagon HCl, J1610–J1612 ◄
Glucose
  monitor with integrated lancing/blood sample collection, E2101
  monitor with integrated voice synthesizer, E2100
  test strips, A4253, A4772
Gluteal pad, L2650
Glycopyrrolate, J1596–J1598
Glycopyrrolate, inhalation solution, concentrated, J7642
Glycopyrrolate, inhalation solution, unit dose, J7643
Gold
  sodium thiomalate, J1600
Golimumab, J1602
Gomco drain bottle, A4912
Gonadorelin HCl, J1620
Goserelin acetate implant; (see also Implant), J9202
Grab bar, trapeze, E0910, E0940
Grade-aid, wheelchair, E0974
Gradient, compression stockings, A6530–A6549
  below knee, 18–30 mmHg, A6530
  below knee, 30–40 mmHg, A6531
  below knee, thigh length, 18–30 mmHg, A6533
  full length/chap style, 18–30 mmHg, A6536
  full length/chap style, 30–40 mmHg, A6537
  full length/chap style, 40–50 mmHg, A6538
  garter belt, A6544
  non-elastic below knee, 30–50 mmhg, A6545
  sleeve, NOS, A6549
  thigh length, 30–40 mmHg, A6534
  thigh length, 40–50 mmHg, A6535
  waist length, 18–30 mmHg, A6539
  waist length, 30–40 mmHg, A6540
  waist length, 40–50 mmHg, A6541
Grafix duo, Q4392 ◄
Granisetron HCl, J1626
  XR, J1627
Gravity traction device, E0941
Gravlee jet washer, A4470
Guidelines, practice, oncology, G9056–G9062

H

Habilitation, prevocational, waiver, T2047
Hair analysis (excluding arsenic), P2031
  Halaven, Injection, eribulin mesylate, 0.1 mg, J9179
Hallus-Valgus dynamic splint, L3100
Hallux prosthetic implant, L8642
Halo procedures, L0810–L0860
  addition HALO procedure, MRI compatible systems, L0859
  addition HALO procedure, replacement liner, L0861
  cervical halo/jacket vest, L0810
  cervical halo/Milwaukee type orthosis, L0830
  cervical halo/plaster body jacket, L0820
Haloperidol, J1630
  decanoate, J1631
Halter, cervical head, E0942
Hand finger orthosis, prefabricated, L3923
Hand restoration, L6900–L6915
  orthosis (WHFO), E1805, E1825, L3800–L3805, L3900–L3954
  partial prosthesis, L6000–L6020
    partial hand, little and/or ring finger remaining, L6010
    partial hand, no finger, L6020
    partial hand, thumb remaining, L6000
    transcarpal/metacarpal or partial hand disarticulation prosthesis, L6025
  rims, wheelchair, E0967

Handgrip (cane, crutch, walker), A4636
Harness, E0942, E0944, E0945
Headgear (for positive airway pressure device), K0185
Hearing
    aid, V5030–V5267, V5298
        aid-body worn, V5100
        assistive listening device, V5268–V5274, V5281–V5290
        battery, use in hearing device, V5266
        contralateral routing, V5171–V5172, V5181, V5211–V5115, V5221
        dispensing fee, binaural, V5160
        dispensing fee, monaural hearing aid, any type, V5241
        dispensing fee, unspecified hearing aid, V5090
        ear impression, each, V5275
        ear mold/insert, disposable, any type, V5265
        ear mold/insert, not disposable, V5264
        glasses, air conduction, V5070
        glasses, bone conduction, V5080
        hearing aid, analog, binaural, CIC, V5248
        hearing aid, analog, binaural, ITC, V5249
        hearing aid, analog, monaural, CIC, V5242
        hearing aid, analog, monaural, ITC, V5243
        hearing aid, BICROS, V5210–V5240
        hearing aid, binaural, V5120–V5150
        hearing aid, CROS, V5170–V5200
        hearing aid, digital, V5254–V5261
        hearing aid, digitally programmable, V5244–V5247, V5250–V5253
        hearing aid, disposable, any type, binaural, V5263
        hearing aid, disposable, any type, monaural, V5262
        hearing aid, monaural, V5030–V5060
        hearing aid, NOC, V5298
        hearing aid or assistive listening device/supplies/accessories, NOS, V5267
        hearing service, miscellaneous, V5299
        semi-implantable, middle ear, V5095
    assessment, S0618, V5008, V5010
    devices, L8614, V5000–V5169, V5171–V5179, V5181–V5209, V5211–V5219, V5221–V5299
    services, V5000–V5999
Heat
    application, E0200–E0239
    infrared heating pad system, A4639, E0221
    lamp, E0200, E0205
    pad, A9273, E0210, E0215, E0237, E0249
Heater (nebulizer), E1372
Heavy duty, wheelchair, E1280–E1298, K0006, K0007, K0801–K0886
    detachable arms, elevating legrests, E1280
    detachable arms, swing away detachable footrest, E1290
    extra heavy duty wheelchair, K0007
    fixed full length arms, elevating legrest, E1295
    fixed full length arms, swing away detachable footrest, E1285
    heavy duty wheelchair, K0006
    power mobility device, not coded by DME PDAC or no criteria, K0900
    power operated vehicle, group 2, K0806–K0808
    power operated vehicle, NOC, K0812
    power wheelchair, group 1, K0813–K0816

Heavy duty, wheelchair (Continued)
    power wheelchair, group 2, K0820–K0843
    power wheelchair, group 3, K0848–K0864
    power wheelchair, group 4, K0868–K0886
    power wheelchair, group 5, pediatric, K0890–K0891
    power wheelchair, NOC, K0898
    power-operated vehicle, group 1, K0800–K0802
    special wheelchair seat depth and/or width, by construction, E1298
    special wheelchair seat depth, by upholstery, E1297
    special wheelchair seat height from floor, E1296
Heel
    elevator, air, E0370
    protector, E0191
    shoe, L3430–L3485
    stabilizer, L3170
Helicopter, ambulance; (see also Ambulance)
Helmet
    cervical, L0100, L0110
    head, A8000–A8004
Hemin, J1640
Hemipelvectomy prosthesis, L5280
Hemi-wheelchair, E1083–E1086
Hemodialysis machine, E1590
Hemodialyzer, portable, E1635
Hemofil M, J7190
Hemophilia clotting factor, J7190–J7198
    anti-inhibitor, per IU, J7198
    anti-thrombin III, human, per IU, J7197
    Factor IX, complex, per IU, J7194
    Factor IX, purified, non-recombinant, per IU, J7193
    Factor IX, recombinant, J7195
    Factor VIII, human, per IU, J7190
    Factor VIII, porcine, per IU, J7191
    Factor VIII, recombinant, per IU, NOS, J7192
    injection, antithrombin recombinant, 50 i.u., J7196
    NOC, J7199
Hemostats, A4850, E1637
Hemostix, A4773
Hepagam B
    IM, J1571
    IV, J1573
Heparin
    infusion pump, dialysis, E1520
    lock flush, J1642
    sodium, J1643, J1644
Hepatitis B, vaccine, administration, G0010
Hep-Lock (U/P), J1642
Hexalite, A4590
High osmolar contrast material, Q9958–Q9964
    HOCM, 400 or greater mg/ml iodine, Q9964
    HOCM, 150–199 mg/ml iodine, Q9959
    HOCM, 200–249 mg/ml iodine, Q9960
    HOCM, 250–299 mg/ml iodine, Q9961
    HOCM, 300–349 mg/ml iodine, Q9962
    HOCM, 350–399 mg/ml iodine, Q9963
    HOCM, up to 149 mg/ml iodine, Q9958
Hip
    disarticulation prosthesis, L5250, L5270
    orthosis (HO), L1600–L1690
Hip-knee-ankle-foot orthosis (HKAFO), L2040–L2090

◄ New   ⟳ Revised   ✓ Reinstated   ~~deleted~~ Deleted

Histrelin
    acetate, J1675
    implant, J9225
HKAFO, L2040–L2090
Home
    certification, home health, G0180
    glucose, monitor, E0607, E2100, E2101, S1030, S1031
    glucose, monitor, lancing/test cartridges, A4271, E2104
    health, aide, G0156, S9122, T1021
    health, aide, in home, per hour, S9122
    health, aide, per visit, T1021
    health, clinical, social worker, G0155
    health, data collection, G0322
    health, hospice, each 15 min, G0156
    health, occupational, therapist, G0152
    health, physical therapist, G0151
    health, physician, certification, G0179–G0182
    health, respiratory therapy, S5180, S5181
    recertification, home health, G0179
    supervision, home health, G0181
    supervision, hospice, G0182
    therapist, speech, S9128
    uterine monitor, S9001
    ventilator, E0458
Home Health Agency Services, T0221, T1022
    care improvement home visit assessment, G9187
Home sleep study test, G0398–G0400
HOPPS, C1000–C9999
Hospice care
    assisted living facility, Q5002
    hospice facility, Q5010
    inpatient hospice facility, Q5006
    inpatient hospital, Q5005
    inpatient psychiatric facility, Q5008
    long-term care facility, Q5007
    nursing long-term facility, Q5003
    patient's home, Q5001
    services, M1159, M1186
    skilled nursing facility, Q5004
Hospice, evaluation, pre-election, G0337
Hospice physician supervision, G0182
Hospital
    bed, E0250–E0304, E0328, E0329
    observation, G0378, G0379
    outpatient clinic visit, assessment, G0463
Hospital Outpatient Payment System, C1000–C9999
Hot water bottle, A9273
Human fibrinogen concentrate, J7178
Humidifier, A7046, E0550–E0563
    durable, diring IPPB treatment, E0560
    durable, extensive, IPPB, E0550
    durable glass bottle type, for regulator, E0555
    heated, used with positive airway pressure device, E0562
    non-heated, used with positive airway pressure, E0561
    water chamber, humidifier, replacement, positive airway device, A7046
Hyalgan, J7321

Hyalomatrix, Q4117
Hyaluronan, J7326, J7327
    derivative, J7332
    durolane, J7318
    gel-Syn, J7328
    genvisc, J7320
    hymovis, J7322
    trivisc, J7329
Hyaluronate, sodium, J7317
Hyaluronidase, J3470, J9316
    ovine, J3471–J3473
Hydralazine HCl, J0360
Hydraulic patient lift, E0630
Hydrocollator, E0225, E0239
Hydrocolloid dressing, A6234–A6241
Hydrocortisone
    acetate, J1700
    sodium phosphate, J1710
    sodium succinate, J1720
Hydrogel dressing, A6231–A6233, A6242–A6248
Hydromorphone, J1171
Hydroxocobalamin, J3424, J3425
Hydroxyprogesterone caproate, J1725–J1726, J1729
Hydroxyzine HCl, J3410
Hygienic item or device, disposable or non-disposable, any type, each, A9286
Hylan G-F 20, J7322
Hyoscyamine Sulfate, J1980
Hyperbaric oxygen chamber, topical, A4575
Hypertonic saline solution, J7130, J7131

I

Ibandronate sodium, J1740
Ibuprofen, J1741
Ibutilide Fumarate, J1742
Icatibant, J1744
Ice
    cap, E0230
    collar, E0230
Idarubicin HCl, J9211
Idursulfase, J1743
Ifosfamide, J9208
Iliac, artery, angiography, G0278
Iloprost, Q4074, J1749
Imaging, PET, G0219, G0235
    any site, NOS, G0235
    whole body, melanoma, non-covered indications, G0219
Imetelstat, J0870 ◄
Imiglucerase, J1786
Immune globulin, J1575
    Alyglo, 500 mg, J1552 ◄
    Bivigam, 500 mg, J1556
    Cuvitru, J1555
    Flebogamma, J1572
    Gammagard liquid, J1569
    Gammaplex, J1557
    Gamunex, J1561

◄ New   ⤺ Revised   ✓ Reinstated   ~~deleted~~ Deleted

Immune globulin (Continued)
    HepaGam B, J1571
    Hizentra, J1559
    Intravenous services, supplies and accessories, Q2052
    NOS, J1566
    Octagam, J1568
    Panzyga, J1576
    Privigen, J1459
    Rho(D), J2788, J2790, *J2791*
    Rhophylac, J2791
    Subcutaneous, J1562
    Xembify, J1558

Immunization counseling, G0310–G0315

Immunosuppressive drug, not otherwise classified, J7599

Implant
    access system, A4301
    aqueous shunt, L8612
    bimatoprost, intracameral implant, J7351
    breast, L8600
    ~~buprenorphine implant, J0570~~
    cochlear, L8614, L8619
    collagen, urinary tract, L8603
    dextranomer/hyaluronic acid copolymer, L8604
    ganciclovir, J7310
    hallux, L8642
    infusion pump, programmable, E0783, E0786
        implantable, programmable, E0783
        implantable, programmable, replacement, E0786
    joint, L8630, L8641, L8658
        interphalangeal joint spacer, silicone or equal, L8658
        metacarpophalangeal joint implant, L8630
        metatarsal joint implant, L8641
    lacrimal duct, A4262, A4263
    metacarpophalangeal joint, L8630
    metatarsal joint, L8641
    neurostimulator pulse generator, L8679, L8681–L8688
    not otherwise specified, L8699
    ocular, L8610
    ossicular, L8613
    osteogenesis stimulator, E0749
    percutaneous access system, A4301
    replacement implantable intraspinal catheter, E0785
    sinuva, J7402
    synthetic, urinary, L8606
    urinary tract, L8603, L8606
    vascular graft, L8670

Implantable radiation dosimeter, A4650

Impregnated gauze dressing, A6222–A6230, *A6231–A6233*

Inclisiran, J1306

Incobotulinumtoxin a, J0588

Incontinence
    appliances and supplies, A4310, A4331, A4332, A4360, A5071–A5075, *A5081–A5093*, A5102–A5114
    garment, A4520, T4521–T4543
        adult sized disposable incontinence product, T4522–T4528

Incontinence (Continued)
    garment (Continued)
        any type, e.g. brief, diaper, A4520
        pediatric sized disposable incontinence product, T4529–T4532
        youth sized disposable incontinence product, T4533–T4534
    supply, A4335, A4356–A4360
        bedside drainage bag, A4357
        disposable external urethral clamp/compression device, A4360
        external urethral clamp or compression device, A4356
        incontinence supply, miscellaneous, A4335
        urinary drainage bag, leg or abdomen, A4358
    treatment system, E0740

Indigotindisulfonate sodium, J9220 ◄

Indium IN-111
    carpromab pendetide, A9507
    ibritumomab tiuxetan, A9542
    labeled autologous platelets, A9571
    labeled autologous white blood cells, A9570
    oxyquinoline, A9547
    pentetate, A9548
    pentetreotide, A9572
    satumomab, A4642

Index visit, M1196, M1204

Inebilizumab-cdon, J1823

Infliximab injection, J1745, J1748

Influenza
    afluria, Q2035
    agriflu, Q2034
    flulaval, Q2036
    fluvirin, Q2037
    fluzone, Q2038
    ~~*immunization, documentation, G8482–G8484*~~
    not otherwise specified, Q2039
    vaccine, administration, G0008
    virus vaccine, Q2034–Q2039

Infusion
    covid, M0249, M0250
    IV, cipaglucosidase, G0138
    pump, ambulatory, with administrative equipment, E0781
    pump, continuous glucose sensing supplies for maintenance, A4226
    pump, heparin, dialysis, E1520
    pump, implantable, E0782, E0783
    pump, implantable, refill kit, A4220
    pump, insulin, E0784
    pump, mechanical, reusable, E0779, E0780
    pump, uninterrupted infusion of Epiprostenol, K0455
    replacement battery, A4602
    saline, J7030–J7060
    supplies, A4219, A4221, A4222, A4225, A4230–A4232, E0776–E0791
    therapy, other than chemotherapeutic drugs, Q0081, Q2054

Inhalation solution; (see also drug name), J7608–J7699, Q4074

◄ New   ↻ Revised   ✓ Reinstated   ~~deleted~~ Deleted

Injection device, needle-free, A4210
Injections; (see also drug name), J0120–J2504,
  J0223, J0224, J0591, J0691, J0693, J0699, J0741,
  J0742, J0791, J0896, J1201, J1303, J1305, J1426,
  J1427, J1429, J1445, J1448, J1554, J1823,
  J1942–J1944, J2406, J2506, J2794, J2798, J3031,
  J3399, J7165–J7169, J7204, J7208, J7311, J7313,
  J7314, J7320, J7321, J7332, J9032, J9036, ~~J9037~~,
  J9039, J9057, J9118, J9153, J9173, J9177, J9199,
  J9201, J9210, J9223, J9229, ~~J9247~~, J9269, J9271,
  J9272, J9299, J9308, J9309, J9313, J9314, J9316,
  J9317, J9348, J9349, J9353, J9355, J9356, Q0244,
  Q0249, Q5112–Q5118, Q5122, Q5123, Q9950,
  Q9991, Q9992
  ado-trastuzumab emtansine, 1 mg, J9354
  aripiprazole, extended release, J0401
  arthrography, sacroiliac, joint, G0259, G0260
  carfilzomib, 1 mg, J9047
  certolizumab pegol, J0717
  dermal filler (LDS), G0429
  filgrastim, J1442
  interferon beta-1a, IM, Q3027
  interferon beta-1a, SC, Q3028
  omacetaxtine mepesuccinate, 0.01 mg, J9262
  pertuzumb, 1 mg, J9306
  sculptra, 0.5 mg, Q2028
  supplies for self-administered, A4211
  ziv-aflibercept, 1 mg, J9400
INR, monitoring, G0248–G0250
  demonstration prior to initiation, home INR, G0248
  physician review and interpretation, home INR, G0250
  provision of test materials, home INR, G0249
Insertion tray, A4310–A4316
Instillation, hexaminolevulinate hydrochloride,
  A9589
Insulin, J1811–J1815, J1817, S5550–S5571
  ambulatory, external, system, A9274
  treatment, outpatient, G9147
Integra flowable wound matrix, Q4114
Interferon
  Alpha, J9212–J9215
  Beta-1a, J1826, Q3027, Q3028
  Beta-1b, J1830
  Gamma, J9216
Intermittent
  assist device with continuous positive airway
    pressure device, E0470–E0472
  limb compression device, E0676
  peritoneal dialysis system, E1592
  positive pressure breathing machine (IPPB),
    E0500
Interphalangeal joint, prosthetic implant,
  L8658, L8659
~~Interprofessional telephone/internet/electronic~~
  ~~medical record,~~ G9037
Interscapular thoracic prosthesis
  endoskeletal, L6570
  upper limb, L6350–L6370
Intervention, alcohol/substance (not tobacco),
  G0396–G0397
Intervention, safety plan, G0560 ◀

Intervention, tobacco, G9016
Intraconazole, J1835
Intraocular
  lenses, V2630–V2632
Intrapulmonary percussive ventilation
  system, E0481
Intrauterine copper contraceptive, J7300
Inversion/eversion correction device, A9285
Iodine I-123
  iobenguane, A9582
  ioflupane, A9584
  sodium iodide, A9509, A9516
Iodine I-125
  serum albumin, A9532
  sodium iodide, A9527
  sodium iothalamate, A9554
Iodine I-131
  iodinated serum albumin, A9524
  sodium iodide capsule, A9517, A9528
  sodium iodide solution, A9529–A9531
Iodine Iobenguane sulfate I-131, A9508
Iodine swabs/wipes, A4247
IPD
  system, E1592
Ipilimumab, J9228
IPPB machine, E0500
Ipratropium bromide, inhalation solution, unit
  dose, J7644, J7645
Irinotecan, J9205, J9206
Iron
  Dextran, J1750
  sucrose, J1756
Irrigation solution for bladder calculi, Q2004
Irrigation supplies, A4320–A4322, A4355,
  A4397–A4400
  irrigation supply, sleeve, each, A4397
  irrigation syringe, bulb, or piston, each, A4320
  irrigation tubing set, bladder irrigation, A4355
  ostomy irrigation set, A4400
  ostomy irrigation supply, bag, A4398
  ostomy irrigation supply, cone/catheter, A4399
Irrigation/evacuation system, bowel
  control unit, E0350
  disposable supplies for, E0352
  manual pump enema, A4459
Isatuximab-irfc, J9227
Isavuconazonium, J1833
Islet, transplant, G0341–G0343, S2102
Isoetharine HCl, inhalation solution
  concentrated, J7647, J7648
  unit dose, J7649, J7650
Isolates, B4150, B4152
Isoniazid, J1834 ◀
Isoproterenol HCl, inhalation solution
  concentrated, J7657, J7658
  unit dose, J7659, J7660
Isosulfan blue, Q9968
Item, non-covered, A9270
IUD, J7300, S4989
IV pole, each, E0776, K0105
Ixabepilone, J9207

◀ New   ⟲ Revised   ✔ Reinstated   ~~deleted~~ Deleted

J

Jacket
  scoliosis, L1300, L1310
Jaw, motion, rehabilitation system, E1700–E1702
Jemperli, J9272
Jenamicin, J1580
Jetria, (ocriplasmin), J7316

K

Kadcyla, ado-trastuzumab emtansine, 1 mg, J9354
Kartop patient lift, toilet or bathroom; (see also Lift), E0625
Keramatrix or kerasorb, J4165
Ketorolac thomethamine, J1885
Kidney
  diagnosis of CKD stage 5, M1188
  ESRD supply, A4650–A4927
  machine, E1500–E1699
  machine, accessories, E1500–E1699
  system, E1510
  wearable artificial, E1632
Kits
  enteral feeding supply (syringe) (pump) (gravity), B4034–B4036
  fistula cannulation (set), A4730
  parenteral nutrition, B4220–B4224
    administration kit, per day, B4224
    supply kit, home mix, per day, B4222
    supply kit, premix, per day, B4220
  surgical dressing (tray), A4550
  tracheostomy, A4625
Knee
  arthroscopy, surgical, G0289, S2112, S2300
    knee, surgical, harvesting cartilage, S2112
    knee, surgical, removal loose body, chondroplasty, different compartment, G0289
    shoulder, surgical, thermally-induced, capsulorraphy, S2300
  disarticulation, prosthesis, L5150, L5160
  joint, miniature, L5826
  orthosis (KO), E1810, L1800–L1885
    dynamic adjustable elbow entension/flexion device, E1800
    dynamic adjustable knee extension/flexion device, E1810
    static-progressive devices, E1801, E1806, E1811, E1816–E1818, E1831, E1841
Knee-ankle-foot device with microprocessor control, L2006
Knee-ankle-foot orthosis (KAFO), K1007, L2000–L2039, L2126–L2136
  addition, high strength, lightweight material, L2755
  base procedure, used with any knee joint, double upright, double bar, L2020
  base procedure, used with any knee joint, full plastic double upright, L2036

Knee-ankle-foot orthosis (KAFO) *(Continued)*
  base procedure, used with any knee joint, single upright, single bar, L2000
  foot orthosis, double upright, double bar, without knee joint, L2030
  foot orthosis, single upright, single bar, without knee joint, L2010
Kovaltry, J7211
Kyphosis pad, L1020, L1025

L

Labetalol hydrochloride, J1920, J1921
Laboratory tests
  chemistry, P2028–P2038
    cephalin flocculation, blood, P2028
    congo red, blood, P2029
    hair analysis, excluding arsenic, P2031
    mucoprotein, blood, P2038
    thymol turbidity, blood, P2033
  microbiology, P7001
  miscellaneous, P9010–P9615, Q0111–Q0115
    blood, split unit, P9011
    blood, whole, transfusion, unit, P9010
    catheterization, collection specimen, multiple patients, P9615
    catheterization, collection specimen, single patient, P9612
    cryoprecipitate, each unit, P9012
    fern test, Q0114
    fresh frozen plasma, donor retested, each unit, P9060
    fresh frozen plasma (single donor), frozen within 8 hours, P9017
    fresh frozen plasma, within 8–24 hours of collection, each unit, P9059
    granulocytes, pheresis, each unit, P9050
    infusion, albumin (human), 25%, 20 ml, P9046
    infusion, albumin (human), 25%, 50 ml, P9047
    infusion, albumin (human), 5%, 250 ml, P9045
    infusion, albumin (human), 5%, 50 ml, P9041
    infusion, plasma protein fraction, human, 5%, 250 ml, P9048
    infusion, plasma protein fraction, human, 5%, 50 ml, P9043
    KOH preparation, Q0112
    pinworm examinations, Q0113
    plasma, cryoprecipitate reduced, each unit, P9044
    plasma, pooled, multiple donor, frozen, P9023
    platelet rich plasma, each unit, P9020
    platelets, each unit, P9019
    platelets, HLA-matched leukocytes reduced, apheresis/pheresis, each unit, P9052
    platelets, irradiated, each unit, P9032
    platelets, leukocytes reduced, CMV-neg, aphresis/pheresis, each unit, P9055
    platelets, leukocytes reduced, each unit, P9031
    platelets, leukocytes reduced, irradiated, each unit, P9033
    platelets, pheresis, each unit, P9034
    platelets, pheresis, irradiated, each unit, P9036

Laboratory tests *(Continued)*
  miscellaneous *(Continued)*
    platelets, pheresis, leukocytes reduced, CMV-neg, irradiated, each unit, P9053
    platelets, pheresis, leukocytes reduced, each unit, P9035
    platelets, pheresis, leukocytes reduced, irradiated, each unit, P9037
    post-coital, direct qualitative, vaginal or cervical mucous, Q0115
    red blood cells, deglycerolized, each unit, P9039
    red blood cells, each unit, P9021
    red blood cells, frozen/deglycerolized/washed, leukocytes reduced, irradiated, each unit, P9057
    red blood cells, irradiated, each unit, P9038
    red blood cells, leukocytes reduced, CMV-neg, irradiated, each unit, P9058
    red blood cells, leukocytes reduced, each unit, P9016
    red blood cells, leukocytes reduced, irradiated, each unit, P9040
    red blood cells, washed, each unit, P9022
    travel allowance, one way, specimen collection, home/nursing home, P9603, P9604
    wet mounts, vaginal, cervical, or skin, Q0111
    whole blood, leukocytes reduced, irradiated, each unit, P9056
    whole blood or red blood cells, leukocytes reduced, CMV-neg, each unit, P9051
    whole blood or red blood cells, leukocytes reduced, frozen, deglycerol, washed, each unit, P9054
  toxicology, P3000–P3001, Q0091

Lacrimal duct, implant
  permanent, A4263
  temporary, A4262

Lactated Ringer's infusion, J7120
Laetrile, J3570
Lanadelumab-flyo, J0593
Lancet, A4258, A4259
Language, screening, V5363
Lanreotide, J1930, J1932
Lanthanum carbonate, J0607–J0608 ◀
Laronidase, J1931
Larynx, artificial, L8500
Laser blood collection device and accessory, A4257, E0620
LASIK, S0800
Lead investigation, T1029
Lead wires, per pair, A4557
Lecanemab-irmb, J0174
Leg
  bag, A4358, A5105, A5112
    leg or abdomen, vinyl, with/without tubes, straps, each, A4358
    urinary drainage bag, leg bag, leg/abdomen, latex, with/without tube, straps, A5112
    urinary suspensory, leg bag, with/without tube, each, A5105
  extensions for walker, E0158
  rest, elevating, K0195
  rest, wheelchair, E0990
  strap, replacement, A5113–A5114

Legg Perthes orthosis, L1700–L1755
  Newington type, L1710
  Patten bottom type, L1755
  Scottish Rite type, L1730
  Tachdjian type, L1720
  Toronto type, L1700
Lenacapavir, J0738, J0752, J1961 ◀
Lens
  aniseikonic, V2118, V2318
  contact, V2500–V2599
    gas permeable, V2510–V2513
    hydrophilic, V2520–V2523
    other type, V2599
    PMMA, V2500–V2503
    scleral, gas, V2530–V2531
  eye, V2100–V2615, V2700–V2799
    bifocal, glass or plastic, V2200–V2299
    contact lenses, V2500–V2599
    low vision aids, V2600–V2615
    miscellaneous, V2700–V2799
    single vision, glass or plastic, V2100–V2199
    trifocal, glass or plastic, V2300–V2399
    variable asphericity, V2410–V2499
  intraocular, V2630–V2632
    anterior chamber, V2630
    iris supported, V2631
    new technology, category 4, IOL, Q1004
    new technology, category 5, IOL, Q1005
    posterior chamber, V2632
    telescopic lens, C1840
  low vision, V2600–V2615
    hand held vision aids, V2600
    single lens spectacle mounted, V2610
    telescopic and other compound lens system, V2615
  progressive, V2781
Lepirudin, J1945
Lesion, destruction, choroid, G0186
Leucovorin calcium, J0640
Leukocyte poor blood, each unit, P9016
Leuprolide acetate, J1950, J1951, J1954, J9217, J9219
Leuprolide injectable, camcevi, J1952
Levalbuterol, all formulations, inhalation solution
  concentrated, J7607, J7612
  unit dose, J7614, J7615
Levetiracetam, J1953
Levocarnitine, J1955
Levofloxacin, J1956
Levoleucovorin injection, J0641
Levoleucovorin injection (khapzory), J0642
Levonorgestrel, (contraceptive), implants and supplies, J7306
Levorphanol tartrate, J1960
Levothyroxine, J0650–J0652
Lexidronam, A9604
Lidocaine, J2002–J2004
Lift
  patient (includes seat lift), E0621–E0635
    bathroom or toilet, E0625
    mechanism incorporated into a combination lift-chair, E0627

◀ New   ↻ Revised   ✓ Reinstated   ~~deleted~~ Deleted

Lightweight, wheelchair (Continued)
  patient (Continued)
    patient lift, electric, E0635
    patient lift, hydraulic or mechanical, E0630
    separate seat lift mechanism, patient owned furniture, non-electric, E0629
    sling or seat, canvas or nylon, E0621
  shoe, L3300–L3334
    lift, elevation, heel, L3334
    lift, elevation, heel and sole, cork, L3320
    lift, elevation, heel and sole, Neoprene, L3310
    lift, elevation, heel, tapered to metatarsals, L3300
    lift, elevation, inside shoe, L3332
    lift, elevation, metal extension, L3330
Lightweight, wheelchair, E1087–E1090, E1240–E1270
  detachable arms, swing away detachable, elevating leg rests, E1240
  detachable arms, swing away detachable footrest, E1260
  fixed full length arms, swing away detachable elevating legrests, E1270
  fixed full length arms, swing away detachable footrest, E1250
  high strength, detachable arms desk, E1088
  high strength, detachable arms desk or full length, E1090
  high strength, fixed full length arms, E1087
  high strength, fixed length arms swing away footrest, E1089
Lincomycin HCl, J2010
Linezolid, J2020, J2021
Liquid barrier, ostomy, A4363
Listening devices, assistive, V5281–V5290
  personal Bluetooth FM/DM, V5286
  personal FM/DM adapter/boot coupling device for receiver, V5289
  personal FM/DM binaural, 2 receivers, V5282
  personal FM/DM, direct audio input, V5285
  personal FM/DM, ear level receiver, V5284
  personal FM/DM monaural, 1 receiver, V5281
  personal FM/DM neck, loop induction receiver, V5283
  personal FM/DM transmitter assistive listening device, V5288
  transmitter microphone, V5290
Lodging, recipient, escort nonemergency transport, A0180, A0200
LOPS, G0245–G0247
  follow-up evaluation and management, G0246
  initial evaluation and management, G0245
  routine foot care, G0247
Lorazepam, J2060
Loss of protective sensation, G0245–G0247
Lovotibeglogene, J3394
Low osmolar contrast material, Q9965–Q9967
Loxapine, for inhalation, J2062
LSO, L0621–L0640
Lubricant, A4332, A4402
Lumbar flexion, L0540
Lumbar-sacral orthosis (LSO), L0621–L0640
Lutetium, A9607
LVRS, services, G0302–G0305
Lymphocyte immune globulin, J7504, J7511

M

Machine
  IPPB, E0500
  kidney, E1500–E1699
Magnesium sulphate, J3475
Maintenance contract, ESRD, A4890
Maintenance, weight, G9888
Mammography, screening, G9899, G9900
Management, patient-caregiver, dementia, G0519–G0528
Mannitol, J2151, ~~J2150~~, J7665 ◀
Marker, tissue, A4648
Marstacimab-hncq, J7172 ◀
Mask
  aerosol, K0180
  oxygen, A4620
Mastectomy
  bra, L8000
  form, L8020
  prosthesis, L8030, L8600
  ~~sleeve, L8010~~
Matristem, Q4118
  micromatrix, 1 mg, Q4118
Mattress
  air pressure, E0186
  alternating pressure, E0277
  dry pressure, E0184
  gel pressure, E0196
  hospital bed, E0271, E0272
  non-powered, pressure reducing, E0373
  overlay, E0371–E0372
  powered, pressure reducing, E0277
  water pressure, E0187
Measurement period
  ace inhibior, M1200, M1203
  ~~anaphylaxis, M1155~~
  dementia, M1164
  herpes zoster, M1174, M1176
  hospice services, M1159, M1165, M1167, M1191
  influenza vaccine, M1168, M1170
  left ventricular function testing, G8682
  pneumococcal conjugate, M1179
  td or tdap vaccine, M1171, M1173
Mecasermin, J2170
Mechlorethamine HCl, J9230
Medicaid, codes, T1000–T9999
Medical and surgical supplies, A4206–A8999
Medical nutritional therapy, G0270, G0271
Medical services, other, M0000–M9999
Medications, high-risk, M1209–M1210
Medroxyprogesterone acetate, J1050
Meloxicam, J1738
Melphalan (apotex), J9249
~~**Melphalan flufenamide** J9247~~
Melphalan (hepzato), J9248
Melphalan NOS, J9245, J9246
Melphalan oral, J8600
Membrane graft/wrap, Q4205, Q4373 ◀
Mental, health, training services, C7900–C7903, G0177

◀ New   ⮂ Revised   ✓ Reinstated   ~~deleted~~ Deleted

Meperidine, J2175
    and promethazine, J2180
Mepivacaine HCl, J0670
Mepolizumab, J2182
Meropenem, J2183–J2185
Mesna, J9209
Metacarpophalangeal joint, prosthetic implant, L8630, L8631
Metaproterenol sulfate, inhalation solution
    concentrated, J7667, J7668
    unit dose, J7669, J7670
Metaraminol bitartrate, J0380
Metatarsal joint, prosthetic implant, L8641
Meter, bath conductivity, dialysis, E1550
Methacholine chloride, J7674
Methadone HCl, J1230
Methergine, J2210
Methocarbamol, J2800
Methotrexate
    (accord), J9252
    oral, J8610–J8612
    sodium, J9260
Methyldopate HCl, J0210
Methylene blue, Q9968
Methylnaltrexone, J2212
Methylprednisolone
    acetate, J1010
    oral, J7509
    sodium succinate, J2919
Metoclopramide HCl, J2765
Metronidazole, J1836
Metoprolol tartrate, J0616 ◄
Micafungin sodium, J2246–J2248
Microbiology test, P7001
Midazolam HCl, J2250–J2253
Miglustat, J1202
Mileage
    ALS, A0390
    ambulance, A0380, A0390
Milrinone lactate, J2260
Mini-bus, nonemergency transportation, A0120
Minocycline hydrochloride, J2265
Mirikizumab, J2267
Mirvetuximab soravtansine-gynx, J9063
Miscellaneous and investigational, A9000–A9999
Mitomycin, J7315, J9280, J9281
Mitoxantrone HCl, J9293
MNT, G0270, G0271
Mobility device, physician, service, G0372
Modalities, with office visit, M0005–M0008
Mogamulizumab injection-kpkc, J9201
Moisture exchanger for use with invasive mechanical ventilation, A4483
Moisturizer, skin, A6250
Molecular diagnostic test reader, K1035
Molecular pathology procedure, G0452
Monitor
    blood glucose, home, E0607
    blood pressure, A4670
    pacemaker, E0610, E0615
Monitoring feature/device, A9279

Monitoring, INR, G0248–G0250
    demonstration prior to initiation, G0248
    physician review and interpretation, G0250
    provision of test materials, G0249
Monoclonal antibodies, J7505, Q0235 ◄
Morphine sulfate, J2270, J2272
    epidural or intrathecal use, J2274
Mosunetuzumab-axgb, J9350
Motion, jaw, rehabilitation system, E1700–E1702
    motion rehabilitation system, E1700
    replacement cushions, E1701
    replacement measuring scales, E1702
Motixafortide, J2277
Mouthpiece (for respiratory equipment), A4617
Moxetumomab pasudotox-tdfx, J9313
Moxifloxacin, J2280, J2281
Mucoprotein, blood, P2038
Multiaxial ankle, L5986
Multidisciplinary services, H2000–H2001, T1023–T1028
Multiple post collar, cervical, L0180–L0200
    occipital/mandibular supports, adjustable, L0180
    occipital/mandibular supports, adjustable cervical bars, L0200
    SQMI, Guilford, Taylor types, L0190
Multi-Podus type AFO, L4396
Muromonab-CD3, J7505
Mycophenolate mofetil, J7514, J7517, J7519 ◄
Mycophenolic acid, J7518
MyOwn skin, Q4226

N

Nabilone, J8650
Nadofaragene firadenovec-vncg, J9029
Natalin, Q4396 ◄
Navigational patient service, G0535 ◄
Nafcillin sodium, J2290–J2291 ◄
Nails, trimming, dystrophic, G0127
Nalbuphine HCl, J2300
Naloxone HCl, J2012–J2313 ~~J2310, J2311~~
Naltrexone, J2315
Nandrolone
    decanoate, J2320
Narrowing device, wheelchair, E0969
Nasal
    application device, K0183
    mechanical allergen barrier/filter, topical, A7023
    pillows/seals (for nasal application device), K0184
    vaccine inhalation, J3530
Nasogastric tubing, B4081, B4082
Natalizumab, J2323, Q5134
Natalin, Q4396 ◄
Navigational patient service, G0535 ◄
Nebulizer, E0570–E0585
    aerosol compressor, E0571, *E0572*
    aerosol mask, A7015
    corrugated tubing, disposable, A7010
    filter, disposable, A7013
    filter, non-disposable, A7014

◄ New   ↻ Revised   ✓ Reinstated   ~~deleted~~ Deleted

Nebulizer *(Continued)*
  heater, E1372
  large volume, disposable, prefilled, A7008
  large volume, disposable, unfilled, A7007
  not used with oxygen, durable, glass, A7017
  pneumatic, administration set, A7003, A7005, A7006
  pneumatic, nonfiltered, A7004
  portable, E0570
  small volume, A7003–A7005
  ultrasonic, E0575
  ultrasonic, dome and mouthpiece, A7016
  ultrasonic, reservoir bottle, non-disposable, A7009
  water collection device, large volume nebulizer, A7012
Necitumumab, J9295
Needle, A4215
  bone marrow biopsy, C1830
  non-coring, A4212
  with syringe, A4206–A4209
Negative pressure wound therapy pump, E2402
  accessories, A6550
Nelarabine, J9261
Neoguard, Q4371 ◀
Neonatal transport, ambulance, base rate, A0225
Neostigmine methylsulfate, J2710
Neothelium, Q4387–Q4389 ◀
Neotrim, Q4265–Q4267
Nerve, conduction, sensory, test, G0255
Nerve stimulator with batteries, E0765
Nesiritide injection, J2324, J2325
Neupogen, injection, filgrastim, 1 mcg, J1442
Neuromodulation stimulator system,
  controller, A4593
  mouth piece, A4594
Neuromuscular stimulator, A4560, E0745
Neurophysiology, intraoperative, monitoring, G0453
Neurostimulator
  battery recharging system, L8695
  external antenna, L8696
  implantable pulse generator, L8679
  pulse generator, L8681–L8688
    dual array, non-rechargeable, with extension, L8688
    dual array, rechargeable, with extension, L8687
    patient programmer (external), replacement only, L8681
    radiofrequency receiver, L8682
    radiofrequency transmitter (external), sacral root receiver, bowel and bladder management, L8684
    radiofrequency transmitter (external), with implantable receiver, L8683
    single array, rechargeable, with extension, L8686
Nicardipine, J2404
Nipocalimab-aahu, 3 mg, C9305 ◀
Nipple prosthesis, custom fabricated, reusable, L8033
Nipple prosthesis, prefabricated, reusable, L8032
Nitrogen N-13 ammonia, A9526
Nivolumab and hyaluronidase, J9289 ◀
Nivol relatlimab, J9298
NMES, E0720–E0749
~~Nogapendekin pmin, C9169~~
Nogapendekin pmin, J9028 ◀

Nonchemotherapy drug, oral, NOS, J8499
Noncovered services, A9270
Nonemergency transportation, A0080–A0210
Nonimpregnated gauze dressing, A6216–A6221, A6402–A6404
Nonprescription drug, A9150
Not otherwise classified drug, J3490, J7599, J7699, J7799, J8499, J8999, J9999, Q0181
Novafix, Q4208
NPH, J1820
NPWT, pump, E2402
NTIOL category 3, Q1003
NTIOL category 4, Q1004
NTIOL category 5, Q1005
Nursing care, T1030–T1031
Nursing service, direct, skilled, outpatient, G0128
Nusinersen, J2326
Nutrition
  enteral infusion pump, B9002
  parenteral infusion pump, B9004, B9006
  parenteral solution, B4164–B5200
  therapy, medical, G0270, G0271

O

O & P supply/accessory/service, L9900
Obecabtagene autoleucel, Q2028 ◀
Observation
  admission, G0379
  hospital, G0378
Occipital/mandibular support, cervical, L0160
Occlusive device, placement, G0269
Occupational, therapy, G0129, S9129
Ocrelizumab, J2350, J2351 ◀
Ocriplasmin, J7316
Octafluoropropane, Q9956
Octagam, J1568
Octreotide acetate, J2353, J2354
Ocular prosthetic implant, L8610
Ofatumumab, J9302
Olanzapine, J2358–J2359
Olaratumab, J9285
Oliceridine, C9101
Olipudase alfa-rpcp, J0218
Omacetaxine Mepesuccinate, J9262
Omadacycline, J0121
Omalizumab, J2357, Q5154 ◀
Omegaven, B4187
OnabotulinumtoxinA, J0585
Oncology
  disease status, G9063–G9139
  practice guidelines, G9056–G9062
  visit, G9050–G9055
Ondansetron HCl, J2405
Ondansetron oral, Q0162
One arm, drive attachment, K0101
Ophthalmological examination, refraction, S0621
Oprelvekin, J2355
Oral device/appliance, E0485–E0486, E0490–E0493
Oral interface, A7047

◀ New   ⮂ Revised   ✓ Reinstated   ~~deleted~~ Deleted

Oral mucoadhesive, A9156
Oral, NOS, drug, J8499
Oral/nasal mask, A7027
   nasal pillows, A7029
   oral cushion, A7028
Oritavancin, J2406, J2407
Oropharyngeal suction catheter, A4628
Orphenadrine, J2360
Orthopedic shoes
   arch support, L3040–L3100
   footwear, *L3000–L3649*, L3201–L3265
   insert, L3000–L3030
   lift, L3300–L3334
   miscellaneous additions, L3500–L3595
   positioning device, L3140–L3170
   transfer, L3600–L3649
   wedge, L3340–L3420
Orthotic additions
   carbon graphite lamination, L2755
   fracture, L2180–L2192, L3995
   halo, L0860
   lower extremity, L2200–L2999, L4320
   ratchet lock, L2430
   scoliosis, L1010–L1120, L1210–L1290, L1320
   shoe, L3300–L3595, L3649
   spinal, L0970–L0984
   upper limb, L3810–L3890, *L3900, L3901,*
      L3970–L3974, *L3975–L3978*, L3995
Orthotic devices
   ankle-foot (AFO); (see also Orthopedic shoes),
      E1815, E1816, E1830, L1900–L1990,
      L2102–L2116, L3160, L4361, *L4397*
   anterior-posterior-lateral, L0700, L0710, L0720 ◀
   cervical, L0100–L0200
   cervical-thoracic-lumbar-sacral (CTLSO), L0700,
      L0710, L0720 ◀
   elbow (EO), E1800, E1801, L3700–L3740,
      L3760–L3761, *L3762*
   fracture, L2102–L2136, L3980–L3986
   halo, L0810–L0830
   hand, (WHFO), E1805, E1825, L3807,
      L3900–L3954, *L3956*
   hand, finger, prefabricated, L3923
   hip (HO), L1600–L1690
   hip-knee-ankle-foot (HKAFO), L2040–L2090
   interface material, E1820
   knee (KO), E1810, E1811, L1800–L1885
   knee-ankle-foot (KAFO); (see also Orthopedic
      shoes), L2000–L2038, L2126–L2136
   Legg Perthes, L1700–L1755
   lumbar, L0625–L0651
   multiple post collar, L0180–L0200
   not otherwise specified, L0999, L1499, L2999,
      L3999, L5999, L7499, L8039, L8239
   pneumatic splint, L4350–L4380
   pronation/supination, E1818
   repair or replacement, L4000–L4210
   replace soft interface material, L4390–L4394
   sacroiliac, L0600–L0620, *L0621–L0624*
   scoliosis, L1000–L1499
   shoe, (see Orthopedic shoes)

Orthotic devices *(Continued)*
   shoulder (SO), L1840, L3650, L3674, *L3678*
   shoulder-elbow-wrist-hand (SEWHO), L3960–L3978
   side bar disconnect, L2768
   spinal, cervical, L0100–L0200
   spinal, DME, K0112–K0116
   thoracic, L0210, *L0220*
   thoracic-hip-knee-ankle (THKO), L1500–L1520
   toe, E1830
   wrist-hand-finger (WHFO), E1805, E1806, E1825,
      L3806–L3809, L3900–L3954, *L3956*
Orthovisc, J7324
Ossicula prosthetic implant, L8613
Osteogenesis stimulator, E0747–E0749, E0760
Ostomy
   accessories, A5093
   belt, A4396
   pouches, A4416–A4435, *A5056, A5057*
   skin barrier, A4401–A4449, *A4462*
   supplies, A4361–A4421, A5051–A5149, *A5200*
Otto Bock, prosthesis, L7007
Outpatient payment system, hospital,
   C1000–C9999
Overdoor, traction, E0860
Oxacillin sodium, J2700
Oxaliplatin, J9263
Oxygen
   ambulance, A0422
   battery charger, E1357
   battery pack/cartridge, E1356
   catheter, transtracheal, A7018
   chamber, hyperbaric, topical, A4575
   concentrator, E1390–E1391
   DC power adapter, E1358
   delivery system (topical), E0446
   equipment, E0424–E0486, *E1353–E1406*
   Liquid oxygen system, E0433
   mask, A4620
   medication supplies, A4611–A4627
   rack/stand, E1355
   regulator, E1352, E1353
   respiratory equipment/supplies, E0424–E0480,
      A4611–A4627, *E0481*
   supplies and equipment, E0425–E0444, E0455
   tent, E0455
   tubing, A4616
   water vapor enriching system, E1405, E1406
   wheeled cart, E1354
Oxymorphone HCl, J2410
Oxytetracycline HCl, J2460
Oxytocin, J2590

P

Pacemaker, duel, C1605
Pacemaker monitor, E0610, E0615
Pacemaker permanent insertion, C7537–C7578
Pacemaker removal, C7540
Paclitaxel, J9267
Paclitaxel protein-bound particles, J9264

Pad
   correction, CTLSO, L1020–L1060
   gel pressure, E0185, E0196
   heat, A9273, E0210, E0215, E0217, E0238, E0249
      electric heat pad, moist, E0215
      electric heat pad, standard, E0210
      hot water bottle, ice cap or collar, heat and/or cold wrap, A9273
      pad for water circulating heat unit, replacement only, E0249
      water circulating heat pad with pump, E0217
   orthotic device interface, E1820
   sheepskin, E0188, E0189
   water circulating cold with pump, E0218
   water circulating heat unit, E0249
   water circulating heat with pump, E0217
Pafolacianine, A9603
Pail, for use with commode chair, E0167
Pain assessment, G8730–G8732
Pain management, chronic, G3002–G3003
Pain measured by the Visual Analog Scale (VAS) or Numeric Pain Scale, G2136–G2141, G2146–G2147
Palate, prosthetic implant, L8618
Palifermin, J2425
Paliperidone palmitate, J2426–J2427
Palonosetron, J2468–J2469, J8655
Pamidronate disodium, J2430
Pan, for use with commode chair, E0167
Panitumumab, J9303
Pantoprazole, J2470–J2472 ◄
Papanicolaou screening smear (Pap), P3000, P3001, Q0091
   cervical or vaginal, up to 3 smears, by technician, P3000
   cervical or vaginal, up to 3 smears, physician interpretation, P3001
   obtaining, preparing and conveyance, Q0091
Papaverine HCl, J2440
Paraffin, A4265
   bath unit, E0235
Parenteral nutrition
   administration kit, B4224
   not otherwise specified, B4185
   pump, B9004, B9006
   solution, B4164, B4184, B4186
      compounded amino acid and carbohydrates, with electrolytes, B4189–B4199, B5000–B5200
      nutrition additives, homemix, B4216
      nutrition administration kit, B4224
      nutrition solution, amino acid, B4168–B4178
      nutrition solution, carbohydrates, B4164, B4180
      nutrition solution, per 10 grams, liquid, B4185
      nutrition supply kit, homemix, B4222
   supply kit, B4220, B4222
Paricalcitol, J2501
Parking fee, nonemergency transport, A0170
Partial Hospitalization, OT, G0129
Pasireotide long acting, J2502
Paste, conductive, A4558
Pathology and laboratory tests, miscellaneous, P9010–P9615
Pathology, surgical, G0416, M1193, M1195

Patient care
   In home, G0529
   Adult daycare center, G0530
   Facility-based, G0531
Patient support system, E0636, M1207–M1208
Patient transfer system, E1035–E1036
Patisiran injection, J0222
Pediculosis (lice) treatment, A9180
PEFR, peak expiratory flow rate meter, A4614
Pegademase bovine, J2504
~~Pegaptanib,~~ ~~J2503~~
Pegaspargase, J9266
Pegcetacoplan, intravitreal, J2781
Pegfilgrastim, J2505, Q5111, Q5122, Q5127, Q5130
Peginesatide, J0890
Pegloticase, J2507
~~Pegulicianine,~~ ~~C9171~~
Pegulicianine, A9615 ◄
Pegunigalsidase, J2508
Pelvic
   belt/harness/boot, E0944
   traction, E0890, E0900, E0947
Pemetrexed, J9292, J9294, J9296–J9297, J9304–J9305, J9322–J9324 ◄
Pemivibart, Q0224
Penicillin
   G benzathine/G benzathine and penicillin G procaine, J0558, J0561
   G potassium, J2540
   G procaine, aqueous, J2510
Penile contracture device, manual, E0201 ◄
Pentamidine isethionate, J2545, J7676
Pentastarch, 10% solution, J2513
Pentazocine HCl, J3070
Pentobarbital sodium, J2515
Pentostatin, J9268
Peramivir, J2547
Percussor, E0480
Percutaneous
   biliary drainage catheter, C7545
   breast biopsies, C7501–C7502
   vertebral augmentations, C7507–C7508
   vertebroplasties, C7504–C7505
Percutaneous access system, A4301
Perflexane lipid microspheres, Q9955
Perflutren lipid microspheres, Q9957
Peroneal strap, L0980
Peroxide, A4244
Perphenazine, J3310
Personal care services, T1019–T1021
   home health aide or CAN, per visit, T1021
   per diem, T1020
   provided by home health aide or CAN, per 15 minutes, T1019
Pertuzumab, J9306, J9316
Pessary, A4561, A4562, A4564
PET, G0219, G0235, G0252
Pharmacologic therapy, G8633
Pharmacy, fee, G0333, Q0521 ~~Q1516–Q0520~~ ◄
Phenobarbital sodium, J2560–J2561
Phentolamine mesylate, J2760

◄ New   ↻ Revised   ✔ Reinstated   ~~deleted~~ Deleted

Phenylephrine hydrochloride, J2371–J2373
Phenylephrine/ketorolac ophthalmic solution, J1097
Phenytoin sodium, J1165
Phisohex solution, A4246
Photofrin, (see Porfimer sodium)
Photorefraction keratectomy, (PRK), S0810
Phototherapeutic keratectomy, (PTK), S0812
Phototherapy light, E0202
Phytonadione, J3430
Pillow, cervical, E0943
Pinworm examination, Q0113
Plasma
   multiple donor, pooled, frozen, P9023, P9070
   single donor, fresh frozen, P9017, P9071
Plasminogen, J2998
Plastazote, L3002, L3252, L3253, L3265, L5654–L5658
   addition to lower extremity socket insert, L5654
   addition to lower extremity socket insert, above knee, L5658
   addition to lower extremity socket insert, below knee, L5655
   addition to lower extremity socket insert, knee disarticulation, L5656, L5657 ◀
   foot insert, removable, plastazote, L3002
   foot, molded shoe, custom fitted, plastazote, L3253
   foot, shoe molded to patient model, plastazote, L3252
   plastazote sandal, L3265
Platelet, P9073, P9100
   concentrate, each unit, P9019
   rich plasma, each unit, P9020
Platelets, P9031–P9037, P9052–P9053, P9055
Platform attachment
   forearm crutch, E0153
   walker, E0154
Plazomicin injection, J0291
Plerixafor, J2562
Plicamycin, J9270
Plumbing, for home ESRD equipment, A4870
Pneumatic
   appliance, E0655–E0673, L4350–L4380
   compressor, E0650–E0652
   splint, L4350–L4380
   ventricular assist device, Q0477, Q0480–Q0505
Pneumatic nebulizer
   administration set, small volume, filtered, A7006
   administration set, small volume, nonfiltered, A7003
   administration set, small volume, nonfiltered, nondisposable, A7005
   small volume, disposable, A7004
Pneumococcal
   vaccine, administration, G0009
Polatuzumab vedotin-piiq, J9309
Porfimer sodium, J9600
Portable
   equipment transfer, R0070–R0076
   gaseous oxygen, K0741, K0742
   hemodialyzer system, E1635
   liquid oxygen system, E0433
   x-ray equipment, Q0092
Positioning seat, T5001

Positive airway pressure device, accessories, A7030–A7039, E0561–E0562
Positive expiratory pressure device, E0484
Post-coital examination, Q0115
Postural drainage board, E0606
Potassium
   chloride, J3480
   hydroxide preparation(KOH), Q0112
Pouch
   fecal collection, A4330
   ostomy, A4375–A4378, A5051–A5054, A5061–A5065
   urinary, A4379–A4383, A5071–A5075
Pozelimab, J9376
Practice, guidelines, oncology, G9056–G9062
Pralatrexate, J9307
Pralidoxime chloride, J2730
Prednisolone
   acetate, J2650
   oral, J7510
Prednisone, J7512
Preparation kits, dialysis, A4914
Preparatory prosthesis, L5510–L5595
   chemotherapy, J8999
   nonchemotherapy, J8499
Prescription digital behavioral therapy, A9291–A9292
Pressure
   alarm, dialysis, E1540
   pad, A4640, E0180–E0199
Privigen, J1459
Procainamide HCl, J2690
Procedure
   HALO, L0810–L0861
   noncovered, G0293, G0294
   scoliosis, L1000–L1499
Prochlorperazine, J0780
Progenamatrix, Q4222
Programmer/Programable, A9268–A9269
Prolonged Service
   home or residence, G0318
   hospital inpatient/observation, G0316
   nursing facility, G0317
Prolotherapy, M0076
Promazine HCl, J2950
Promethazine
   and meperdine, J2180
   HCl, J2550
~~Prophylaxis, Q0516–Q0518~~
Propranolol HCl, J1800
Prostate, cancer, screening, G0102, G0103
Prosthesis
   artificial larynx battery/accessory, L8505
   breast, L8000–L8035, L8600
   eye, L8610, L8611, V2623–V2629
   fitting, L5400–L5460, L6380–L6388
   foot/ankle one piece system, L5979
   hand, L6000–L6020, L6026
   implants, L8600–L8690
   larynx, L8500
   lower extremity, L5700–L5999, L8640–L8642, L8720, L8721
   mandible, L8617
   maxilla, L8616

◀ New   ⮐ Revised   ✓ Reinstated   ~~deleted~~ Deleted

Prosthesis (Continued)
   maxillofacial, provided by a non-physician,
      L8040–L8048
   miscellaneous service, L8499
   ocular, V2623–V2629
   repair of, L7520, L8049
   socks (shrinker, sheath, stump sock), L8400–L8485
   taxes, orthotic/prosthetic/other, L9999
   tracheo-esophageal, L8507–L8509
   upper extremity, L6000–L7406 ◄
   vacuum erection system, L7900

Prosthetic additions
   lower extremity, L5610–L5999
   powered upper extremity range of motion assist
      device, L8701–L8702
   upper extremity, L6600–L7406 ◄

Prosthetic, eye, V2623
Protamine sulfate, J2720
Protectant, skin, A6250
Protector, heel or elbow, E0191
Protein C Concentrate, J2724
Protirelin, J2725
Psychotherapy, crisis, G0017–G0018
Psychotherapy, group, partial hospitalization,
   G0410–G0411
Pulse generator, E2120
Pump
   alternating pressure pad, E0182
   ambulatory infusion, E0781, E0787
   ambulatory insulin, E0784
   blood, dialysis, E1620
   breast, E0602–E0604
   enteral infusion, B9000, B9002
   external infusion, E0779
   heparin infusion, E1520
   implantable infusion, E0782, E0783
   implantable infusion, refill kit, A4220
   infusion, supplies, A4226, A4230, A4232
   negative pressure wound therapy, E2402
   parenteral infusion, B9004, B9006
   suction, portable, E0600
   water circulating pad, E0236
   wound, negative, pressure, E2402
Purification system, E1610, E1615
Pyridoxine HCl, J3415

Q

Quad cane, E0105
Quinupristin/dalfopristin, J2770

R

Rack/stand, oxygen, E1355
Radiation therapy, Stereotactic, G0563 ◄
Radiesse, Q2026
Radioelements for brachytherapy, Q3001
Radiological, supplies, A4641, A4642

Radiology service, R0070–R0076
**Radiopharmaceutical diagnostic and therapeutic
   imaging agent,** A4641, A4642, A9500–A9699
Radiosurgery, robotic, G0339–G0340
Radiosurgery, stereotactic, G0339, G0340
Rail
   bathtub, E0241, E0242, E0246
   bed, E0305, E0310
   toilet, E0243
Ranibizumab, J2778, Q5128
Rasburicase, J2783
Ravulizumab injection-cwvz, J1303
Reaching/grabbing device, A9281
Reagent strip, A4252
Reciprocating peritoneal dialysis system, E1630
Reclast, J3488, J3489
Reclining, wheelchair, E1014, E1050–E1070,
   E1100–E1110
Reconstruction, angiography, G0288
Rectal Control System for Vaginal insertion, A4563
Red blood cells, P9021, P9022, P9027
Regadenoson, J2785
Regular insulin, *J1815,* J1820
Regulator, oxygen, E1353
Rehabilitation
   cardiac, S9472
   program, H2001
   psychosocial, H2017, H2018
   pulmonary, S9473
   system, jaw, motion, E1700–E1702
   vestibular, S9476
Releuko, Q5125
Remdesivir, J0248
Remestemcel-l-rknd, J3402 ◄
Remimazolam, J2249
Removal, cerumen, G0268
Renew matrix, Q4378 ◄
Repair
   contract, ESRD, A4890
   durable medical equipment, E1340
   maxillofacial prosthesis, L8049
   orthosis, L4000–L4130
   prosthetic, L7500, L7510
Repair of
   enterocutaneous fistula, C9796
Replacement
   battery, A4630
   electronic system, G0555 ◄
   pad (alternating pressure), A4640
   tanks, dialysis, A4880
   tip for cane, crutches, walker, A4637
   underarm pad for crutches, A4635
Reslizumab, J2786
Respiratory
   DME, A7000–A7527
   equipment, E0424–E0601
   function, therapeutic, procedure, G0237–G0239,
      S5180–S5181
   supplies, A4604–A4629, A7049
Restraint/Enclosures; Pelvic Device, E0710–E0716
Restrata minimatrix, A2026

◄ New   ⮂ Revised   ✓ Reinstated   ~~deleted~~ Deleted

Reteplase, J2993
Retifanlimab-dlwr, J9345
Revakinagene taroretcel-lwey, J3403 ◀
Revascularization, C9603–C9608
Revefenacin inhalation solution, J7677
Rezafungin, J0349
Rho(D) immune globulin, human, J2788, J2790, J2792
Rib belt, thoracic, A4572, L0220
Rifampin, 1 mg, J2804 ◀
sRilanocept, J2793
RimabotulinumtoxinB, J0587
Ring, ostomy, A4404
Ringers lactate infusion, J7120
Risankizumab, J2327
Risk-adjusted functional status
   elbow, wrist or hand, G8667–G8670
   hip, G8651–G8654
   lower leg, foot or ankle, G8655–G8658
   lumbar spine, G8659–G8662
   neck, cranium, mandible, thoracic spine, ribs, or other, G8671–G8674
   shoulder, G8663–G8666
Risk management, ASCVD, G0537–G0538 ◀
Risperidone (risperdal consta), J2794
   (perseris), J2798
   (rykindo), J2801
   (uzedy), J2799
Rituximab, J9312
   abbs (Truxina), Q5115
Robin-Aids, L6000, L6010, L6020, L6855, L6860
Rocking bed, E0462
Rolapitant, J8670
Rollabout chair, E1031
Romidepsin, J9315
~~Romiplostim, J2796~~
Romiplostim, J2802 ◀
Romosozumab injection-aqqg, J3111
Ropivacaine HCl, J2795
Rozanolixizumab-noli, J9333
Rubidium Rb-82, A9555
Rybrevant, J9061
Rylaze, J9021

S

Sacituzumab govitecan-hziy, J9317
Sacral nerve stimulation test lead, A4290
Safety equipment, E0700
   vest, wheelchair, E0980
Saline
   hypertonic, J7130, *J7131*
   infusion, *J7030–J7060*
   solution, A4216–A4218, J7030–J7050
~~Saliva~~
   ~~artificial, A9155~~
Samarium SM 153 Lexidronamm, A9605
Sargramostim (GM-CSF), J2820
Scale, E1639

Scoliosis, L1000–L1499
   additions, L1010–L1120, L1210–L1290
Screening
   alcohol misuse, G0442
   cancer, cervical or vaginal, G0101
   colorectal, cancer, G0104–G0105, G0120–G0122, G0328 ↩
   cytopathology cervical or vaginal, G0123, G0124, G0141–G0148
   depression, G0444
   dysphagia, documentation, V5364
   enzyme immunoassay, G0432
   glaucoma, G0117, G0118
   infectious agent antibody detection, G0433, G0435
   language, V5363
   mammography, digital image, G9899, G9900
   prostate, cancer, G0102, G0103
   speech, V5362
   TB, M1003
Sculptra, Q2028
Sealant
   skin, A6250
Seat
   attachment, walker, E0156
   insert, wheelchair, E0992
   lift (patient), E0621, E0627–E0629
   upholstery, wheelchair, E0975, *E0981*
Sebelipase alfa , J2840
Secretin, J2850
Secukinumab, J3247
Semen analysis, G0027
Semi-reclining, wheelchair, E1100, *E1110*
Sensitivity study, P7001
Sensory nerve conduction test, G0255
Sermorelin acetate, Q0515
Serum clotting time tube, A4771
Service
   Advanced primary care management, G0556–G0558 ◀
   Allied Health, home health, hospice, G0151–G0161
   behavioral health and/or substance abuse, H0001–H9999
   ~~co-management, G9038~~
   doula birth worker, T1032–T1033
   integration, G0019–G0022
   healing, traditional, H0051
   hearing, V5000–V5999
   laboratory, P0000–P9999
   mental, health, training, G0177
   navigation, G0023–G0024, G0140, G0146
   non-covered, A9270
   oncology, M0010
   outpatient, intensive, G0137
   physician, for mobility device, G0372
   pulmonary, for LVRS, G0302–G0305
   recovery support, G0535 ◀
   skilled, RN/LPN, home health, hospice, G0162
   social, psychological, G0409–G0411
   speech-language, V5336–V5364
   ~~therapeutic, C9784–C9795~~
   vision, V2020–V2799

Sevelamer carbonate, J0601 ◀
Sevelamer PDR carbonate, J0602 ◀
Sevelamer hydrochloride, J0603 ◀
SEWHO, L3960–L3974, *L3975–L3978*
SEXA, *G0130*
Sheepskin pad, E0188, E0189
Shoes
    arch support, L3040–L3100
    for diabetics, A5500–A5514
    insert, L3000–L3030, *L3031*
    lift, L3300–L3334
    miscellaneous additions, L3500–L3595
    orthopedic, L3201–L3265
    positioning device, L3140–L3170
    transfer, L3600–L3649
    wedge, L3340–L3485
Shoulder
    disarticulation, prosthetic, L6300–L6320, L6550
    orthosis (SO), L3650–L3674
    spinal, cervical, L0100–L0200
Shoulder sling, A4566
Shoulder-elbow-wrist-hand orthosis (SEWHO),
    L3960–L3969, *L3971–L3978*
Shunt accessory for dialysis, A4740
    aqueous, L8612
Sigmoidoscopy, cancer screening, G0104, ~~G0106~~
Siltuximab, J2860
Simulation, complex, with PET/CT, G0562 ◀
Sincalide, J2805–~~J2806~~
Sipuleucel-T, Q2043
Sirolimus, J7520, J9331
Sitz bath, E0160–E0162
Skin
    barrier, ostomy, A4362, A4363, A4369–A4373,
        A4385, A5120
    bond or cement, ostomy, A4364
    sealant, protectant, moisturizer, A6250
    substitute, Q4100–Q4258, Q4265–Q4345
Sling, A4565
    patient lift, E0621, E0630, E0635
Smear, Papanicolaou, screening, P3000, *P3001,* Q0091
SNCT, G0255
Social worker, clinical, home, health, G0155
Social worker, nonemergency transport, A0160
Social work/psychological services, CORF, G0409
Sock
    body sock, L0984
    prosthetic sock, *L8417,* L8420–L8435, L8470,
        L8480, L8485
    stump sock, L8470–L8485
Sodium
    chloride injection, J2912
    ferric gluconate complex in sucrose, J2916
    fluoride F-18, A9580
    hyaluronate
        Euflexxa, J7323
        GELSYN-3, J7328
        Hyalgan, J7321
        Orthovisc, J7324
        Supartz, J7321
        Synvisc and Synvisc-One, J7325
        Visco-3, J7321

Sodium (*Continued*)
    nithlodote, J0211
    phosphate P32, A9563
    pyrophosphate, J1443
    succinate, J1720
    thiosulfate, J0208–J0209, J0211
Solution
    calibrator, A4256
    dialysate, A4760
    elliotts b, J9175
    enteral formulae, B4149–B4156, *B4157–B4162*
    parenteral nutrition, B4164–B5200
Solvent, adhesive remover, A4455
Somatrem, J2940
Somatropin, J2941
Sorbent cartridge, ESRD, E1636
Special size, wheelchair, E1220–E1239
Specialty absorptive dressing, A6251–A6256
Specialty care, H2040–H2041
Spectacle lenses, V2100–V2199
Spectinomycin HCl, J3320
Speech assessment, V5362–V5364
Speech generating device, E2500–E2599
Speech, pathologist, G0153
Speech-Language pathology, services, V5336–V5364
Speech Volume System, E3000, 32000
Spesolimab-sbzo, J1747
Spherocylinder, single vision, V2100–V2114
    bifocal, *V2203–V2214*
    trifocal, *V2303–V2314*
Spinal orthosis
    cervical, L0100–L0200
    cervical-thoracic-lumbar-sacral (CTLSO), L0700,
        L0710, L0720 ◀
    DME, K0112–K0116
    halo, L0810–L0830
    multiple post collar, L0180–L0200
    scoliosis, L1000–L1499
    torso supports, L0960
Splint, A4570, L3100, L4350–L4380
    ankle, L4390–L4398
    dynamic, E1800, E1805, E1810, E1815, E1825,
        E1830, E1840
    footdrop, L4398
    supplies, miscellaneous, Q4051
Standard, wheelchair, E1130, K0001
Static progressive stretch, E1801, E1806, E1811,
    E1816, E1818, E1821
Status
    disease, oncology, G9063–G9139
STELARA, ustekinumab, 1 mg, J3357
Stent, transcatheter, placement, C9600, C9601
Stereotactic, radiosurgery, G0339, G0340
Sterile cefuroxime sodium, J0697
Sterile water, A4216–A4217
Stimulation, electrical, non-attended, G0281–G0283
Stimulators
    neuromuscular, E0743–E0745
    osteogenesis, electrical, E0747–E0749
    salivary reflex, E0755
    stoma absorptive cover, A5083

◀ New   ↻ Revised   ✓ Reinstated   ~~deleted~~ Deleted

Stimulators *(Continued)*
   transcutaneous, electric, nerve, A4595–A4596, E0720–E0749
   ultrasound, E0760
Stockings
   gradient, compression, A6530–A6549
   surgical, A4490–A4510
Stoma, plug or seal, A5081
Stomach tube, B4083
Streptokinase, J2995
Streptomycin, J3000
Streptozocin, J9320
Strip, blood glucose test, A4253–A4772
   urine reagent, A4250
Strontium-89 chloride, supply of, A9600
Study, bone density, G0130
Stump sock, L8470–L8485
Stylet, A4212
Substance/Alcohol, assessment, G0396, G0397, H0001, H0003, H0049
Succinylcholine chloride, J0330
Sucroferric oxyhydroxide, J0605 ◀
Suction pump
   gastric, home model, E2000
   portable, E0600
   respiratory, home model, E0600
   urine and/or fecal system, home model, E2001
Sulfameth/trimethoprim, 5mg/1mg, J2865 ◀
Sumatriptan succinate, J3030
Summit aaa, Q4397 ◀
Supartz, J7321
Supplies
   battery, A4233–A4236, A4601, A4611–A4613, A4638
   cast, A4580, A4590, Q4001–Q4051
   catheters, A4300–A4306
   continuous glucose monitor, A4238, A4239
   contraceptive, A4267–A4269
   diabetic shoes, A5500–A5513
   dialysis, A4653–A4928
   digital device, G0552 ◀
   DME, other, A4630–A4640
   docking station, oral, K1037
   dressings, A6000–A6513
   electrical stimulator (external), A4438, L8678
   enteral, therapy, B4000–B9999
   hip orthosis, L1681
   home, nasal spray, G0532 ◀
   incontinence, A4310–A4355, A5102–A5200
   infusion, A4221, A4222, A4230–A4232, E0776–E0791
   lung expansion, A7021
   needle, A4212, A4215
   needle-free device, A4210
   nerve stimulator, A4543–A4545
   ostomy, A4361–A4434, A5051–A5093, A5120–A5200
   parenteral, therapy, B4000–B9999
   radiological, A4641, A4642
   refill kit, infusion pump, A4220
   respiratory, A4604–A4629
   self-administered injections, A4211
   splint, Q4051

Supplies *(Continued)*
   sterile water/saline and/or dextrose, A4216–A4218
   surgical, miscellaneous, A4649
   syringe, A4206–A4209, A4213, A4232
   syringe with needle, A4206–A4209
   ultrasonic diathermy treatment, K1036
   urinary, external, A4356–A4360
Supply/accessory/service, A9900
Support
   arch, L3040–L3090
   cervical, L0100–L0200
   spinal, L0960
   stockings, L8100–L8239
Surederm, Q4220
Surgical
   arthroscopy, knee, G0289, S2112
   boot, L3208–L3211
   dressing, A6196–A6406
   procedure, noncovered, G0293, G0294
   stocking, A4490–A4510
   supplies, A4649
   tray, A4550
Surgicord, Q4218–Q4219
Surgraft, Q4209, Q4263, Q4268–Q4269, Q4393–Q9394 ◀
Susvimo, J2779
Sutimlimab-jome, J1302
Swabs, betadine or iodine, A4247
Synojoynt, J7331
Synvisc and Synvisc-One, J7325
Syringe, A4213
   with needle, A4206–A4209
System
   external, ambulatory insulin, A9274
   rehabilitation, jaw, motion, E1700–E1702
   transport, E1035–E1039

T

Tables, bed, E0274, E0315
Tacrolimus
   oral, J7503, J7507, J7508, J7521 ◀
   parenteral, J7525
Tagraxofusp injections-erzs, J9269
Taliglucerase, J3060
Talimogene laheroareovec, J9325
Talquetamab-tgvs, J3055
Tape, A4450–A4452
~~**Tarlatamab,** C9170~~
Tarlatamab, J9026 ◀
Taurolidine, J0911
Taxi, non-emergency transportation, A0100
Team, conference, G0175, G9007, S0220, S0221
Tebentafusp-tebn, J9274
Technetium TC 99M
   Arcitumomab, A9568
   Bicisate, A9557
   Depreotide, A9536
   Disofenin, A9510
   Exametazine, A9521

Technetium TC 99M (Continued)
   Exametazine labeled autologous white blood cells, A9569
   Fanolesomab, A9566
   Glucepatate, A9550
   Labeled red blood cells, A9560
   Macroaggregated albumin, A9540
   Mebrofenin, A9537
   Mertiatide, A9562
   Oxidronate, A9561
   Pentetate, A9539, A9567
   Pertechnetate, A9512
   Pyrophosphate, A9538
   Sestamibi, A9500
   Succimer, A9551
   Sulfur colloid, A9541
   Teboroxime, A9501
   Tetrofosmin, A9502
   Tilmanocept, A9520

Teclistamab-cqyv, J9380
Tedizolid phosphate, J3090
TEEV, J0900
Telavancin, J3095
Telehealth, Q3014, G0320–G0321, G0544–G0551 ◄
Telehealth transmission, T1014
Telisotuzumab vedotin-tilv, 1 mg, C9306 ◄
Temozolomide
   injection, J9328
   oral, J8700
Temporary codes, Q0000–Q9999, S0009–S9999
Temsirolimus, J9330
Tenecteplase, J3101
Teniposide, Q2017
TENS, A4595–A4596, E0720–E0749
Tent, oxygen, E0455
Teplizumab-mzwv, J9381
Teprotumumab-trbw, J3241
Terbutaline sulfate, J3105
   inhalation solution, concentrated, J7680
   inhalation solution, unit dose, J7681
Teriparatide, J3110
Terminal devices, L6700–L6895
Test
   sensory, nerve, conduction, G0255
Testosterone
   cypionate and estradiol cypionate, J1071, J1072 ◄
   enanthate, J3121
   undecanoate, J3145
Tetanus immune globulin, human, J1670
Tetracycline, J0120
Tezepelumab, J2356
Thallous Chloride TL 201, A9505
Theophylline, J2810
Therapeutic lightbox, A4634, E0203
Therapy
   activity, G0176
   electromagnetic, G0295, G0329
   enteral, supplies, B4000–B9999
   immune checkpoint inhibitor, M1180
   medical, nutritional, G0270, G0271

Therapy (Continued)
   occupational, G0129, H5300, S9129
   occupational, health, G0152
   parenteral, supplies, B4000–B9999
   respiratory, function, procedure, G0237–S0239, S5180, S5181
   speech, home, G0153, S9128
   wound, negative, pressure, pump, E2402
Theraskin, Q4121
Thermometer, A4931–A4932
   dialysis, A4910
Thiamine HCl, J3411
Thiethylperazine maleate, J3280
Thiotepa, J9341, J9342 ~~J9340~~ ◄
Thoracic orthosis, L0210
Thoracic-hip-knee-ankle (THKAO), L1500–L1520
Thoracic-lumbar-sacral orthosis (TLSO)
   scoliosis, L1200–L1290
   spinal, L0450–L0492
Thymol turbidity, blood, P2033
Thyroidectomy, C7555
Thyrotropin Alfa, J3240
Tigecycline, J3243, J3244
Tinzarparin sodium, J1655
Tip (cane, crutch, walker) replacement, A4637
Tire, wheelchair, E2211–E2225, E2381–E2395
Tirofiban, J3246
Tisagenlecleucel, Q2040
Tislelizumab, J9329
Tisotumab vedotin-TFTV, J9273
Tissue marker, A4648
~~Tixagev and cilgav,~~ ~~Q0221~~
TLSO, L0450–L0492, L1200–L1290
Tobacco
   intervention, G9016, G0029–G0030
Tobramycin
   inhalation solution, unit dose, J7682, J7685
   sulfate, J3260
Tocilizumab, J2362, Q0237, Q5133, Q5135, Q5156 ◄
Toe device, E1831
Tofersen, J1304
Toilet accessories, E0167–E0179, E0243, E0244, E0625
Tolazoline HCl, J2670
Toll, non emergency transport, A0170
Topical hyperbaric oxygen chamber, A4575
Topotecan, J8705, J9351
Toripalimab, J3263
Torsemide, J3265
Trabectedin, J9352
Tracheostoma heat moisture exchange system, A7501–A7509
Tracheostomy
   care kit, A4629
   filter, A4481
   speaking valve, L8501
   supplies, A4623, A4629, A7523–A7524
   tube, A7520–A7522
Tracheotomy mask or collar, A7525–A7526
Traction
   cervical, E0855, E0856
   device, ambulatory, E0830

◄ New   ⤺ Revised   ✓ Reinstated   ~~deleted~~ Deleted

HCPCS 2026 INDEX / Truss

Traction *(Continued)*
  equipment, E0840–E0948
  extremity, E0870–E0880
  pelvic, E0890, E0900, E0947
Training
  caregiver, G0539–G0543 ◄
  diabetes, outpatient, G0108, G0109
  home health or hospice, G0162
  services, mental, health, G0177
Tranexamic acid, J3290 ◄
Transcutaneous electrical nerve stimulator (TENS), E0720–E0770
Transducer protector, dialysis, E1575
Transfer (shoe orthosis), L3600–L3640
Transfer system with seat, E1035
Transparent film (for dressing), A6257–A6259
Transplant
  heart (history of), M1151–M1152
  islet, G0341–G0343, S2102
Transport
  chair, E1035–E1039
  system, E1035–E1039
  x-ray, R0070–R0076
Transportation
  ambulance, A0021–A0999, Q3019, Q3020
  corneal tissue, V2785
  EKG (portable), R0076
  handicapped, A0130
  non-emergency, A0080–A0210, T2001–T2005
  service, including ambulance, A0021, A0999, T2006
  taxi, non-emergency, A0100
  toll, non-emergency, A0170
  volunteer, non-emergency, A0080, A0090
  x-ray (portable), R0070, R0075, R0076
Transportation services
  air services, A0430, A0431, A0435, A0436
  ALS disposable supplies, A0398
  ALS mileage, A0390
  ALS specialized service, A0392, A0394, A0396
  ambulance, ALS, A0426, A0427, A0433
  ambulance, outside state, Medicaid, A0021
  ambulance oxygen, A0422
  ambulance, waiting time, A0420
  ancillary, lodging, escort, A0200
  ancillary, lodging, recipient, A0180
  ancillary, meals, escort, A0210
  ancillary, meals, recipient, A0190
  ancillary, parking fees, tolls, A0170
  BLS disposable supplies, A0382
  BLS mileage, A0380
  BLS specialized service, A0384
  emergency, neonatal, one-way, A0225
  extra ambulance attendant, A0424
  ground mileage, A0425
  non-emergency, air travel, A0140
  non-emergency, bus, A0110
  non-emergency, case worker, A0160
  non-emergency, mini-bus, A0120
  non-emergency, no vested interest, A0080
  non-emergency, taxi, A0100
  non-emergency, wheelchair van, A0130

Transportation services *(Continued)*
  non-emergency, with vested interest, A0090
  paramedic intercept, A0432
  response and treat, no transport, A0998
  specialty transport, A0434
Transtracheal oxygen catheter, A7018
Trapeze bar, E0910–E0912, E0940
Trauma, response, team, G0390
Tray
  insertion, A4310–A4316
  irrigation, A4320
  surgical; (see also kits), A4550
  wheelchair, E0950
Trastuzumab injection excludes biosimilar, J9316, J9355
  anns (kanjinti), Q5117
  dkst (Ogivri), Q5114
  dttb (Ontruzant), Q5112
  fam-trastuzumab deruxtecan-nxki, J9358
  hercessi, Q5146 ◄
  pkrb (Herzuma), Q5113
  qyyp (trazimera), Q5116
Trastuzumab and Hyaluronidase-oysk, J9356
Travoprost intracameral implant, J7355
Treatment
  bone, G0412–G0415
  electronic positional OSA, E0530
  pediculosis (lice), A9180
  services, behavioral health, H0002–H2037
  therapeutic, monthly, G0553–G0554 ◄
Tremelimumab-actl, J9347
Treosulfan, J0614 ◄
Treprostinil, J3285
Triamcinolone, J3301–J3303
  acetonide, J3300, J3301
  diacetate, J3302
  hexacetonide, J3303
  inhalation solution, concentrated, J7683
  inhalation solution, unit dose, J7684
Triferic avnu J1445
Triflupromazine HCl, J3400
Trifocal, glass or plastic, V2300–V2399
  aniseikonic, V2318
  lenticular, V2315, V2321
  specialty trifocal, by report, V2399
  sphere, plus or minus, V2300–V2302
  spherocylinder, V2303–V2314
  trifocal add-over 3.25d, V2320
  trifocal, seg width over 28 mm, V2319
Trigraft, Q4377 ◄
Trilaciclib J1448
Triluron intraarticular injection, J7332
Trimethobenzamide HCl, J3250
Trimetrexate glucuoronate, J3305
Trimming, nails, dystrophic, G0127
Triptorelin pamoate, J3315
Truss, L8300–L8330
  addition to standard pad, scrotal pad, L8330
  addition to standard pad, water pad, L8320
  double, standard pads, L8310
  single, standard pad, L8300

 New   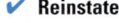 Revised   ✔ Reinstated   ~~deleted~~ Deleted

39

Tube/Tubing
   anchoring device, A5200
   blood, A4750, A4755
   corrugated tubing, non-disposable, used with large volume nebulizer,10 feet, A4337
   drainage extension, A4331
   enema, A4457
   gastrostomy, B4087, B4088
   irrigation, A4355
   larynectomy, A4622
   nasogastric, B4081, B4082
   oxygen, A4616
   serum clotting time, A4771
   stomach, B4083
   suction pump, each, A7002
   tire, K0091, K0093, K0095, K0097
   tracheostomy, A4622
   urinary drainage, K0280
Tympanostomy, with tube delivery device, G0561 ◀

U

Ublituximab-xiiy, J2329
Ultrasonic nebulizer, E0575
Ultrasound, S8055, S9024
   paranasal sinus ultrasound, S9024
   ultrasound guidance, multifetal pregnancy reduction, technical component, S8055
Ultraviolet, cabinet/system, E0691, E0694
Ultraviolet light therapy system, A4633, E0691–E0694
   light therapy system in 6 foot cabinet, E0694
   replacement bulb/lamp, A4633
   therapy system panel, 4 foot, E0692
   therapy system panel, 6 foot, E0693
   treatment area 2 sq feet or less, E0691
Unclassified drug, J3490
Underpads, disposable, A4554
Unipuncture control system, dialysis, E1580
Upper extremity addition, locking elbow, L6693
Upper extremity fracture orthosis, L3980–L3999
Upper limb prosthesis, L6000–L7499
Urea, J3350
Ureterostomy supplies, A4454–A4590
Urethral suppository, Alprostadil, J0275
Urinal, E0325, E0326
Urinary
   catheter, A4338–A4346, A4351–A4353
      indwelling catheter, A4338–A4346
      intermittent urinary catheter, A4351–A4353
      male external catheter, A4349
   collection and retention (supplies), A4310–A4360
      bedside drainage bag, A4357
      disposable external urethral clamp, A4360
      external urethral clamp, A4356
      female external urinary collection device, A4328
      insertion trays, A4310–A4316, A4354–A4355
      irrigation syringe, A4322
      irrigation tray, A4320
      male external catheter/integral collection chamber, A4326

Urinary *(Continued)*
      perianal fecal collection pouch, A4330
      therapeutic agent urinary catheter irrigation, A4321
      urinary drainage bag, leg/abdomen, A4358
   supplies, external, A4335, A4356–A4358
      bedside drainage bag, A4357
      external urethral clamp/compression device, A4356
      incontinence supply, A4335
      urinary drainage bag, leg or abdomen, A4358
   tract endoscope, C1747
   tract implant, collagen, L8603
   tract implant, synthetic, L8606
Urine
   sensitivity study, P7001
   tests, A4250
Urofollitropin, J3355
Urokinase, J3364, J3365
Ustekinumab, J3357, J3758, Q5098–Q5100, Q5137–Q5138, Q9996–Q9999 ◀
U-V lens, V2755

V

Vabra aspirator, A4480
Vaccination, administration
   flublok, Q2033
   hepatitis B, G0010
   HIV prevention, G0012
   influenza virus, G0008
   pneumococcal, G0009
Vaccine
   administration, influenza, G0008
   administration, pneumococcal, G0009
   counseling, G0011, G0013
   hepatitis B, administration, G0010
Vadadustat, J0901 ◀
Vaginal
   cancer, screening, G0101
   cytopathologist, G0123
   cytopathology, G0123, G0124, G0141–G0148
   screening, cervical/vaginal, thin-layer, cytopathologist, G0123
   screening, cervical/vaginal, thin-layer, physician interpretation, G0124
   screening cytopathology smears, automated, G0141–G0148
Valoctocogene, J1412
Vancomycin HCl, J3373–J3375 ~~J3370–J3372~~ ◀
Vaporizer, E0605
Vascular
   catheter (appliances and supplies), A4300–A4306
      disposable drug delivery system, >50 ml/hr, A4305
      disposable drug delivery system, <50 ml/hr, A4306
      implantable access catheter, external, A4300
      implantable access total, catheter, A4301
   graft material, synthetic, L8670
      embolization or occlusion procedure, C9797
Vasopressin, J2598–J2599, J2601
Vasoxyl, J3390

◀ New   ↻ Revised   ✔ Reinstated   ~~deleted~~ Deleted

Ventricular assist device (Continued)
Vedolizumab, J3380
Vehicle, power-operated, K0800–K0899
Velaglucerase alfa, J3385
Velmanase, J0217
Venous pressure clamp, dialysis, A4918
Ventilator
   battery, A4611–A4613
   home ventilator, any type, E0465–E0469
     used with invasive interface (e.g., tracheostomy tube), E0465
     used with non-invasive interface (e.g., mask, chest shell), E0466
   moisture exchanger, disposable, A4483
Ventricular assist device, Q0478–Q0504, Q0506–Q0509
   battery clips, electric or electric/pneumatic, replacement, Q0497
   battery, lithium-ion, electric or electric/pneumatic, replacement, Q0506
   battery, other than lithium-ion, electric or electric/pneumatic, replacement, Q0496
   battery, pneumatic, replacement, Q0503
   battery/power-pack charger, electric or electric/pneumatic, replacement, Q0495
   belt/vest/bag, carry external components, replacement, Q0499
   driver, replacement, Q0480
   ejection, fraction, left, M1150
   emergency hand pump, electric or electric/pneumatic, replacement, Q0494
   emergency power source, electric, replacement, Q0490
   emergency power source, electric/pneumatic, replacement, Q0491
   emergency power supply cable, electric, replacement, Q0492
   emergency power supply cable, electric/pneumatic, replacement, Q0493
   filters, electric or electric/pneumatic, replacement, Q0500
   holster, electric or electric/pneumatic, replacement, Q0498
   leads (pneumatic/electrical), replacement, Q0487
   microprocessor control unit, electric/pneumatic combination, replacement, Q0482
   microprocessor control unit, pneumatic, replacement, Q0481
   miscellaneous supply, external VAD, Q0507
   miscellaneous supply, implanted device, Q0508
   miscellaneous supply, implanted device, payment not made under Medicare Part A, Q0509
   mobility cart, replacement, Q0502
   monitor control cable, electric, replacement, Q0485
   monitor control cable, electric/pneumatic, replacement, Q0486
   monitor/display module, electric, replacement, Q0483
   monitor/display module, electric/electric pneumatic, replacement, Q0484
   power adapter, pneumatic, replacement, vehicle type, Q0504

Waiver (Continued)
   power adapter, vehicle type, Q0478
   power module, replacement, Q0479
   power-pack base, electric, replacement, Q0488
   power-pack base, electric/pneumatic, replacement, Q0489
   shower cover, electric or electric/pneumatic, replacement, Q0501
Verteporfin, J3396
Vest, safety, wheelchair, E0980
Vinblastine sulfate, J9360
Vincristine sulfate, J9370
Vinorelbine tartrate, J9390
Vision service, V2020–V2799
   bifocal, glass or plastic, V2200–V2299
   contact lenses, V2500–V2599
   frames, V2020–V2025
   intraocular lenses, V2630–V2632
   low-vision aids, V2600–V2615
   miscellaneous, V2700–V2799
   prosthetic eye, V2623–V2629
   spectacle lenses, V2100–V2199
   trifocal, glass or plastic, V2300–V2399
   variable asphericity, V2410–V2499
Visit, emergency department, G0380–G0384
Visual, function, postoperative cataract surgery, G0915–G0918
Vitamin B-12 cyanocobalamin, J3420
Vitamin K, J3430
Voice
   amplifier, L8510
   prosthesis, L8511–L8514
Von Willebrand Factor Complex, human, J7179, J7183, J7187
Voriconazole, J3465
Vutrisiran, J0225

W

Waiver, T2012–T2050
   assessment/plan of care development, T2024
   case management, per month, T2022
   day habilitation, per 15 minutes, T2021
   day habilitation, per diem, T2020
   habilitation, educational, per diem, T2012
   habilitation, educational, per hour, T2013
   habilitation, prevocational, per diem, T2014
   habilitation, prevocational, per hour, T2015
   habilitation, residential, 15 minutes, T2017
   habilitation, residential, per diem, T2016
   habilitation, supported employment, 15 minutes, T2019
   habilitation, supported employment, per diem, T2018
   targeted case management, per month, T2023
   waiver services NOS, T2025
Walker, E0130–E0149
   accessories, A4636, A4637
   attachments, E0153–E0159
   enclosed, four-sided frame, E0144
   folding (pickup), E0135

Walker (Continued)
   folding, wheeled, E0143, E0152
   heavy duty, multiple braking system, E0147
   heavy duty, wheeled, rigid or folding, E0149
   heavy duty, without wheels, E0148
   rigid (pickup), E0130
   rigid, wheeled, E0141
   with trunk support, E0140
Walking splint, L4386
Washer, Gravlee jet, A4470
Water
   dextrose, J7042, J7060, J7070
   distilled (for nebulizer), A7018
   pressure pad/mattress, E0187, E0198
   purification system (ESRD), E1610, E1615
   softening system (ESRD), E1625
   sterile, A4714
WBC/CBC, G0306
Wedges, shoe, L3340–L3420
Wellness, promoting, M0005
Wellness visit; annual, G0438, G0439
Wet mount, Q0111
Wheel attachment, rigid pickup walker, E0155
Wheelchair, E0950–E1298, K0001–K0108, K0801–K0899
   accessories, E0192, E0950–E1034, E1065–E1069, E2211–E2231, E2291–E2298, E2301–E2399, E2626–E2633 ◀
   amputee, E1170–E1200
   back, fully reclining, manual, E1226
   component or accessory, not otherwise specified, K0108
   cushions, E2601–E2625
   custom manual wheelchair base, K0008
   custom motorized/power base, K0013
   dynamic positioning hardware for back, E2398
   foot box, E0954
   heavy duty, E1280–E1298, K0006, K0007, K0801–K0886
   lateral thigh or knee support, E0953
   lightweight, E1087–E1090, E1240–E1270
   narrowing device, E0969
   power add-on, E0983–E0984
   reclining, fully, E1014, E1050–E1070, E1100–E1110
   semi-reclining, E1100–E1110
   shock absorber, E1015–E1018
   specially sized, E1220, E1230
   standard, E1130, K0001
   stump support system, K0551
   tire, E0999
   transfer board or device, E0705
   tray, K0107
   van, non-emergency, A0130
   youth, E1091
WHFO with inflatable air chamber, L3807
Whirlpool equipment, E1300–E1310
WHO, wrist extension, L3914
Wig, A9282
Wipes, A4245, A4247

Wound
   cleanser, A6260
   closure, adhesive, G0168
   cover, Q4354–Q4367 ◀
      alginate dressing, A6196–A6198
      collagen dressing, A6020–A6024
      foam dressing, A6209–A6214
      hydrocolloid dressing, A6234–A6239
      hydrogel dressing, A6242–A6247
      non-contact wound warming cover, and accessory, E0231–E0232
      specialty absorptive dressing, A2001–A2010, A2015–A2039, A6251–A6256 ◀
   filler
      alginate dressing, A6199
      collagen based, A6010
      foam dressing, A6215
      hydrocolloid dressing, A6240–A6241
      hydrogel dressing, A6248
      not elsewhere classified, A6261–A6262
Woundfix, Woundfix Plus, Q4217
   matrix, Q4114, Q4346–Q4353 ◀
   pouch, A6154
   therapy, negative, pressure, pump, E2402
   wound suction, A9272, K0743
Wrapping, fabric, abdominal aneurysm, M0301
Wrist
   disarticulation prosthesis, L6050, L6055
   electronic wrist rotator, L7259
   hand/finger orthosis (WHFO), E1805, E1825, L3800–L3954

X

Xenon Xe 133, A9558
Xenon Xe 129, A9610
Xipere, J3299
X-ray
   equipment, portable, Q0092, R0070, R0075
   single, energy, absorptiometry (SEXA), G0130
   transport, R0070–R0076
Xylocaine HCl, J2000

Y

Yttrium Y-90 ibritumomab, A9543

Z

Zanidatamab-hrii, J9276 ◀
Zenocutuzumab-zbco, J9382 ◀
Ziconotide, J2278
Zidovudine, J3485
Ziprasidone mesylate, J3486
Zolbetuximab-clzb, J1326 ◀
Zoledronic acid, J3489
Zynlonta, J9359

2026
TABLE OF DRUGS

IA	Intra-arterial administration
IU	International unit
IV	Intravenous administration
IM	Intramuscular administration
IT	Intrathecal
SC	Subcutaneous administration
INH	Administration by inhaled solution
VAR	Various routes of administration
OTH	Other routes of administration
ORAL	Administered orally

Intravenous administration includes all methods, such as gravity infusion, injections, and timed pushes. The "VAR" posting denotes various routes of administration and is used for drugs that are commonly administered into joints, cavities, tissues, or topical applications, in addition to other parenteral administrations. Listings posted with "OTH" indicate other administration methods, such as suppositories or catheter injections.

Blue typeface terms are added by publisher.

DRUG NAME	DOSAGE	METHOD OF ADMINISTRATION	HCPCS CODE
A			
Abatacept	10 mg	IV	J0129
Abbokinase	5,000 IU vial	IV	J3364
	250,000 IU vial	IV	J3365
Abbokinase, Open Cath	5,000 IU vial	IV	J3364
Abciximab	10 mg	IV	J0130
Abelcet	10 mg	IV	J0289
Abilify Maintena	1 mg		J0401
ABLC	50 mg	IV	J0285
AbobotulinumtoxinA	5 units	IM	J0586
Abraxane	1 mg		J9264
Accuneb	1 mg		J7613
Acetadote	100 mg		J0132
Acetaminophen	10 mg	IM, IV	J0131, J0136-J0138
Acetazolamide sodium	up to 500 mg	IM, IV	J1120
Acetylcysteine			
injection	100 mg	IV	J0132
unit dose form	per gram	INH	J7604, J7608
Achromycin	up to 250 mg	IM, IV	J0120
Actemra	1 mg		J3262
Acthib			J3490
Acthrel	1 mcg		J0795
Actimmune	3 million units	SC	J9216
Activase	1 mg	IV	J2997
Acyclovir	5 mg		J0133
			J8499
Adagen	25 IU		J2504
~~Adalimumab~~	~~20 mg~~	~~SC, IM~~	~~J0135, Q5131~~
Adcetris	1 mg	IV	J9042
Adenosine	1 mg	IV	J0153
Ado-trastuzumab Emtansine	1 mg	IV	J9354
~~Adrenalin Chloride~~	~~up to 1 ml ampule~~	~~SC, IM~~	~~J0171~~
~~Adrenalin, epinephrine~~	~~0.1 mg~~	~~SC, IM~~	~~J0171~~

◀ New   ⮌ Revised   ✔ Reinstated   ~~deleted~~ Deleted

DRUG NAME	DOSAGE	METHOD OF ADMINISTRATION	HCPCS CODE
Adriamycin, PFS, RDF	10 mg	IV	J9000
Adrucil	500 mg	IV	J9190
Aduhelm	2 mg	IV	J0172
Advate	per IU		J7192
Adzynma	10 iu		J7171
Afamelanotide implant	1 mg	IV	J7352
Aflibercept	1 mg	OTH	J0177- J0178
Agalsidase beta	1 mg	IV	J0180
Aggrastat	0.25 mg	IM, IV	J3246
A-hydrocort	up to 50 mg	IV, IM, SC	J1710
	up to 100 mg		J1720
Akineton	per 5 mg	IM, IV	J0190
Akynzeo	300 mg and 0.5 mg		J8655
Alatrofloxacin mesylate, injection	100 mg	IV	J0200
Albumin			P9041, P9045, P9046, P9047
Albuterol	0.5 mg	INH	J7620
concentrated form	1 mg	INH	J7610, J7611
unit dose form	1 mg	INH	J7609, J7613
Aldesleukin	per single use vial	IM, IV	J9015
Aldomet	up to 250 mg	IV	J0210
Aldurazyme	0.1 mg		J1931
Alefacept	0.5 mg	IM, IV	J0215
Alemtuzumab	1 mg		J0202
Alfentanil hydrochloride	500 mcg	IM	J0216
Alferon N	250,000 IU	IM	J9215
Alglucerase	per 10 units	IV	J0205
Alglucosidase alfa	10 mg	IV	J0220, J0221
Alimta	10 mg		J9305
Alkaban-AQ	1 mg	IV	J9360
Alkeran	2 mg	ORAL	J8600
	50 mg	IV	J9245
AlloDerm	per square centimeter		Q4116
AlloSkin	per square centimeter		Q4115
Allopurinol sodium	1 mg	IM	J0206
Aloxi	25 mcg		J2469
Alpha 1-proteinase inhibitor, human	10 mg	IV	J0256, J0257
Alphanate			J7186
AlphaNine SD	per IU		J7193
Alprolix	per IU		J7201
Alprostadil			
injection	1.25 mcg	OTH	J0270
urethral suppository	each	OTH	J0275
Alteplase recombinant	1 mg	IV	J2997
Alupent	per 10 mg	INH	J7667, J7668
noncompounded, unit dose	10 mg	INH	J7669
unit dose	10 mg	INH	J7670
AmBisome	10 mg	IV	J0289

◀ New   ↻ Revised   ✔ Reinstated   ~~deleted~~ Deleted

2026 TABLE OF DRUGS / Amcort

DRUG NAME	DOSAGE	METHOD OF ADMINISTRATION	HCPCS CODE
Amcort	per 5 mg	IM	J3302
Amgen	1 mcg	SC	J9212
Amifostine	500 mg	IV	J0207
Amikacin sulfate	100 mg	IM, IV	J0278
Aminocaproic Acid			J0281, J3490 ◀
Aminolevulinic acid HCl	unit dose (354 mg)	OTH	J7308
Aminolevulinic acid HCl 10% Gel	10 mg	OTH	J7345
Aminolevulinate	1 g	OTH	J7309
Aminophylline/Aminophyllin	up to 250 mg	IV	J0280
Amiodarone HCl	30 mg	IV	J0282-J0283
Amisulpride	1 mg	IM	J0184
Amitriptyline HCl	up to 20 mg	IM	J1320
Amobarbital	up to 125 mg	IM, IV	J0300
Amphadase	1 ml		J3470
Amphocin	50 mg	IV	J0285
Amphotericin B	50 mg	IV	J0285
Amphotericin B, lipid complex	10 mg	IV	J0287-J0289
Ampicillin			
sodium	up to 500 mg	IM, IV	J0290
sodium/sulbactam sodium	per 1.5 g	IM, IV	J0295
Amvuttra	1 mg	IM	J0225
Amygdalin			J3570
Amytal	up to 125 mg	IM, IV	J0300
Anabolin LA 100	up to 50 mg	IM	J2320
Anadulafungin	1 mg	IV	J0348
Anascorp	up to 120 mg	IV	J0716
Anastrozole	1 mg		J8999
Ancef	500 mg	IV, IM	J0690
Andrest 90-4	1 mg	IM	J3121
Andro-Cyp	1 mg		J1071
Andro-Cyp 200	1 mg		J1071
Andro L.A. 200	1 mg	IM	J3121
Andro-Estro 90-4	1 mg	IM	J3121
Andro/Fem	1 mg		J1071
Androgyn L.A.	1 mcg	IM	J3121
Androlone-50	up to 50 mg		J2320
Androlone-D 100	up to 50 mg	IM	J2320
Andronaq-50	up to 50 mg	IM	J3140
Andronaq-LA	1 mg		J1071
Andronate-100	1 mg		J1071
Andronate-200	1 mg		J1071
Andropository 100	1 mg	IM	J3121
Andryl 200	1 mg	IM	J3121
Anectine	up to 20 mg	IM, IV	J0330
Anergan 25	up to 50 mg	IM, IV	J2550
	12.5 mg	ORAL	Q0169
Anergan 50	up to 50 mg	IM, IV	J2550
	12.5 mg	ORAL	Q0169

◀ New   ↺ Revised   ✔ Reinstated   ~~deleted~~ Deleted

DRUG NAME	DOSAGE	METHOD OF ADMINISTRATION	HCPCS CODE
Angiomax	1 mg		J0583
Anidulafungin	1 mg	IV	J0348
Anistreplase	30 units	IV	J0350
Antiflex	up to 60 mg	IM, IV	J2360
Anti-Inhibitor	per IU	IV	J7198
Antispas	up to 20 mg	IM	J0500
Antithrombin III (human)	per IU	IV	J7197
Antithrombin recombinant	50 IU	IV	J7196
Anzemet	10 mg	IV	J1260
	50 mg	ORAL	S0174
	100 mg	ORAL	Q0180
Apidra Solostar	per 50 units		J1817
A.P.L.	per 1,000 USP units	IM	J0725
Apligraf	per square centimeter		Q4101
Apomorphine Hydrochloride	1 mg	SC	J0364
Aprepitant	1 mg	IV	J0185
Aprepitant	5 mg	ORAL	J8501
Apresoline	up to 20 mg	IV, IM	J0360
Aprotinin	10,000 kiu		J0365
AquaMEPHYTON	per 1 mg	IM, SC, IV	J3430
Aralast	10 mg	IV	J0256
Aralen	up to 250 mg	IM	J0390
Aramine	per 10 mg	IV, IM, SC	J0380
Aranesp			
ESRD use	1 mcg		J0882
Non-ESRD use	1 mcg		J0881
Arbutamine	1 mg	IV	J0395
Arcalyst	1 mg		J2793
Aredia	per 30 mg	IV	J2430
Arfonad, see Trimethaphan camsylate			
Arformoterol tartrate	15 mcg	INH	J7605
Argatroban			
(for ESRD use)	1 mg	IV	J0884, J0892, J0899
(for non-ESRD use)	1 mg	IV	J0883, J0891, J0898
Aridol	~~25% in 50 ml~~	~~IV~~	~~J2150~~
	5 mg	INH	J7665
Arimidex			J8999
Aripiprazole	0.25 mg	IM	J0400
Aripiprazole (abilify asimtufii)	1 mg	IM	J0402
Aripiprazole, extended release	1 mg	IV	J0401
Aripiprazole lauroxil	1 mg	IV	J1942
Aripiprazole lauroxil (aristada)	1 mg	IV	J1944
Aripiprazole lauroxil (aristada initio)	1 mg	IV	J1943
Aristocort Forte	per 5 mg	IM	J3302
Aristocort Intralesional	per 5 mg	IM	J3302
Aristospan Intra-Articular	per 5 mg	VAR	J3303

◄ New   ↻ Revised   ✔ Reinstated   ~~deleted~~ Deleted

DRUG NAME	DOSAGE	METHOD OF ADMINISTRATION	HCPCS CODE
Aristospan Intralesional	per 5 mg	VAR	J3303
Arixtra	per 0.5 m		J1652
Aromasin			J8999
Arranon	50 mg		J9261
Arrestin	up to 200 mg	IM	J3250
	250 mg	ORAL	Q0173
Arsenic trioxide	1 mg	IV	J9017
Artesunate	1 mg	IM	J0391
Arzerra	10 mg		J9302
Asparaginase	1,000 units	IV, IM	J9019
	10,000 units	IV, IM	J9020
Astagraf XL	0.1 mg		J7508
Astramorph PF	up to 10 mg	IM, IV, SC	J2270
Atezolizumab	10 mg	IV	J9022, J9024 ◀
Atgam	250 mg	IV	J7504
Atidarsagene autotemcel			J3391 ◀
Ativan	2 mg	IM, IV	J2060
Atropine			
concentrated form	per mg	INH	J7635
unit dose form	per mg	INH	J7636
sulfate	0.01 mg	IV, IM, SC	J0461, J0462, J7636 ◀
Atrovent, unit dose form	per mg	INH	J7644, J7645
ATryn	50 IU	IV	J7196
Aurothioglucose	up to 50 mg	IM	J2910
Autologous cultured chondrocytes implant		OTH	J7330
Autoplex T	per IU	IV	J7198, J7199
~~AUVI-Q~~	~~0.15 mg~~		~~J0171~~
Avastin	10 mg		J9035
Avelox	100 mg		J2280
Avacincaptad pegol	0.1 mg	IM	J2782
Avelumab	10 mg	IV	J9023
Avonex	30 mcg	IM	J1826
	1 mcg	IM	Q3027
	1 mcg	SC	Q3028
Axatilimab-csfr	0.1 mg	IM	J9038 ◀
Azacitidine	1 mg	SC	J9025
Azasan	50 mg		J7500
Azathioprine	50 mg	ORAL	J7500
Azathioprine, parenteral	100 mg	IV	J7501
Azithromycin, dihydrate	1 gram	ORAL	Q0144
Azithromycin, injection	500 mg	IV	J0456
Azmiro	1 mg	IM	J1072 ◀
Aztreonam	100 mg	IM	J0457
Aztreonam/Avibactam	7.5 mg/2.5 mg	IM	J0458 ◀
B			
Baciim			J3490
Bacitracin			J3490

◀ New   ↻ Revised   ✔ Reinstated   ~~deleted~~ Deleted

DRUG NAME	DOSAGE	METHOD OF ADMINISTRATION	HCPCS CODE
Baclofen	10 mg	IT	J0475
Baclofen for intrathecal trial	50 mcg	OTH	J0476
Bactocill	up to 250 mg	IM, IV	J2700
BAL in oil	per 100 mg	IM	J0470
Bamlan and etesev		IV	M0245
Bamlanivimab and etesevima	2100 mg	IV	Q0245
Banflex	up to 60 mg	IV, IM	J2360
Basiliximab	20 mg		J0480
BCG live intravesical instillation	1 mg	OTH	J9030
Bebulin	per IU		J7194
Beclomethasone inhalation solution, unit dose form	per mg	INH	J7622
~~Belantamab mafodotin-blmf~~	~~0.5 mg~~	~~IV~~	~~J9037~~
Belatacept	1 mg	IV	J0485
Beleodaq	10 mg		J9032
Belimumab	10 mg	IV	J0490
Belinostat	10 mg	IV	J9032
Bena-D 10	up to 50 mg	IV, IM	J1200
Bena-D 50	up to 50 mg	IV, IM	J1200
Benadryl	up to 50 mg	IV, IM	J1200
Benahist 10	up to 50 mg	IV, IM	J1200
Benahist 50	up to 50 mg	IV, IM	J1200
Ben-Allergin-50	up to 50 mg	IV, IM	J1200
	50 mg	ORAL	Q0163
Bendamustine HCl			
~~Apotex~~	~~1 mg~~	~~IV~~	~~J9058~~
~~Baxter~~	~~1 mg~~	~~IV~~	~~J9059~~
Bendeka	1 mg	IV	J9034
Hydrochloride	1 mg	IV	J9033
Vivimusta	1 mg	IV	J9056
Bendamustine HCl (Belrapzo/bendamustine)	1 mg	IV	J9036
Benefix	per IU	IV	J7195
Benlysta	10 mg		J0490
Benoject-10	up to 50 mg	IV, IM	J1200
Benoject-50	up to 50 mg	IV, IM	J1200
Benralizumab	1 mg	IV	J0517
Bentyl	up to 20 mg	IM	J0500
Benzocaine			J3490
Benztropine mesylate	per 1 mg	IM, IV	J0515
Beremagene	per 0.1 ml		J3401
Berinert	10 units		J0597

DRUG NAME	DOSAGE	METHOD OF ADMINISTRATION	HCPCS CODE
Berubigen	up to 1,000 mcg	IM, SC	J3420
Beta amyloid	per study dose	OTH	A9599
Betalin 12	up to 1,000 mcg	IM, SC	J3420
Betameth	per 3 mg	IM, IV	J0702
Betamethasone Acetate			J3490
Betamethasone Acetate & Betamethasone Sodium Phosphate	per 3 mg	IM	J0702
Betamethasone inhalation solution, unit dose form	per mg	INH	J7624
Betaseron	0.25 mg	SC	J1830
Bethanechol chloride	up to 5 mg	SC	J0520
Bethkis	300 mg		J7682
Betibeglogene autotemce		IM	J3393
Bevacizumab	10 mg	IV	J9035
Bevacizumab-adcd	10 mg	IM	Q5129
Bevacizumab-awwb	10 mg	IV	Q5107
Bevacizumab-bvzr (Zirabev)	10 mg	IV	Q5118
Bezlotoxumab	10 mg	IV	J0565
Bicillin C-R	100,000 units		J0558
Bicillin C-R 900/300	100,000 units	IM	J0558, J0561
Bicillin L-A	100,000 units	IM	J0561
BiCNU	100 mg	IV	J9050
Biperiden lactate	per 5 mg	IM, IV	J0190
Bitolterol mesylate			
concentrated form	per mg	INH	J7628
unit dose form	per mg	INH	J7629
Bivalirudin	1 mg	IV	J0582, J0583 ◀
Blenoxane	15 units	IM, IV, SC	J9040
Bleomycin sulfate	15 units	IM, IV, SC	J9040
Blinatumomab	1 mcg	IV	J9039
Blincyto	1 mcg		J9039
Boniva	1 mg		J1740
Bortezomib	0.1 mg	IV	J9041
Bortezomib	0.1 mg		J9046, J9049, J9051, J9054 ◀
Botox	1 unit		J0585
Bravelle	75 IU		J3355
Brentuximab Vedotin	1 mg	IV	J9042
Brethine			
concentrated form	per 1 mg	INH	J7680
unit dose	per 1 mg	INH	J7681
	up to 1 mg	SC, IV	J3105

◀ New   ↪ Revised   ✔ Reinstated   ~~deleted~~ Deleted

DRUG NAME	DOSAGE	METHOD OF ADMINISTRATION	HCPCS CODE	
Bricanyl Subcutaneous	up to 1 mg	SC, IV	J3105	
Brompheniramine maleate	per 10 mg	IM, SC, IV	J0945	
Bronkephrine, *see* Ethylnorepinephrine HCl				
Bronkosol				
concentrated form	per mg	INH	J7647, J7648	
unit dose form	per mg	INH	J7649, J7650	
Brovana			J7605	
Budesonide inhalation solution				
concentrated form	0.25 mg	INH	J7633, J7634	
unit dose form	0.5 mg	INH	J7626, J7627	
Bumetanide	0.5 mg	IM, IV, ORAL	J1939, J3490	
Bupivacaine	0.5 mg	IM	J0665, J0666 J3490	◀
Bupivacaine and meloxicam	1 mg/0.03 mg	OTH	J0668	◀
Buprenex	0.3 mg		J0592	
Buprenorphine Hydrochloride	0.1 mg	IM	J0592	
Buprenorphine/Naloxone	1 mg	ORAL	J0571	
	< 3 mg	ORAL	J0572	
	> 3 mg but < 6 mg	ORAL	J0573	
	> 6 mg but < 10 mg	ORAL	J0574	
	> 10 mg	ORAL	J0575	
Buprenorphine extended release	< 100 mg	ORAL	Q9991	
	> 100 mg	ORAL	Q9992	
		IM	J0577, J0578	
Burosumab-twza	1 mg	IV	J05894	
Busulfan	1 mg	IV	J0594	
	2 mg	ORAL	J8510	
Butorphanol tartrate	1 mg		J0595	
C				
C1 Esterase Inhibitor	10 units	IV	J0596-J0599	
Cabazitaxel	1 mg	IV	J9043, J9064	
Cabergoline	0.25 mg	ORAL	J8515	
Cabote Rilpivir	2 mg/3 mg	IV	J0741	
Cabotegravir	1 mg	IM	J0739	
Cafcit	5 mg	IV	J0706	
Caffeine citrate	5 mg	IV	J0706	
Calaspargase pegol-mknl	10 units	IV	J9118	
Calcijex	0.1 mcg	IM	J0636	
Calcimar	up to 400 units	SC, IM	J0630	
Calcitonin-salmon	up to 400 units	SC, IM	J0630	

◀ New   ↻ Revised   ✔ Reinstated   ~~deleted~~ Deleted

DRUG NAME	DOSAGE	METHOD OF ADMINISTRATION	HCPCS CODE
Calcitriol	0.1 mcg	IM	J0636
Calcitrol			J8499
Calcium acetate	23 mg	ORAL	J0615
Calcium chloride	2 mg	IM	J1618
Calcium gluconate	10 mg	IM	J0611-J0613
Calcium glycerophosphate and calcium lactate	per 10 ml	IM, SC	J0620
Caldolor	100 mg	IV	J1741
Calphosan	per 10 ml	IM, SC	J0620
Camcevi	1 mg	IV	J1952
Camptosar	20 mg	IV	J9206
Canakinumab	1 mg	SC	J0638
Cancidas	5 mg		J0637
Cantharidin	3.2 mg	Topical	J7354
Capecitabine	50 mg	Oral	J8522
Capsaicin patch	per sq cm	OTH	J7336
Carbidopa 5 mg/levodopa 20 mg enteral suspension		IV	J7340
Carbocaine	per 10 ml	VAR	J0670
Carbocaine with Neo-Cobefrin	per 10 ml	VAR	J0670
Carboplatin	50 mg	IV	J9045
Carboprost tromethamine	0.1 mg	IM	J0675
Carfilzomib	1 mg	IV	J9047
Carimune	500 mg		J1566
Carmustine	100 mg	IV	J9050, J9052
Carnitor	per 1 g	IV	J1955
Carticel			J7330
Casimersen	10 mg	IV	J1426
Caspofungin acetate	5 mg	IV	J0637
Cathflo Activase	1 mg		J2997
Caverject	per 1.25 mcg		J0270
Cefadyl	up to 1 g	IV, IM	J0710
Cefazolin sodium	500 mg	IV, IM	J0688-J0690
Cefepime hydrochloride	500 mg	IV	J0692, J0701, J0703
Cefiderocol	10 mg	IV	J0699
Cefizox	per 500 mg	IM, IV	J0715
Cefotaxime sodium	per 1 g	IV, IM	J0698
Cefotetan			J3490
Cefotetan disodium	10 mg	IV, IM	J0525
Cefoxitin sodium	1 g/500 mg	IV, IM	J0687-J0690, J0694
Ceftaroline fosamil	1 mg	IV	J0712

◄ New ⮂ Revised ✔ Reinstated ~~deleted~~ Deleted

DRUG NAME	DOSAGE	METHOD OF ADMINISTRATION	HCPCS CODE
Ceftazidime	per 500 mg	IM, IV	J0713
Ceftazidime and avibactam	0.5 g/0.125 g	IV	J0714
Ceftizoxime sodium	per 500 mg	IV, IM	J0715
Ceftobiprole medocaril sodium	3 mg	IM	J0681 ◄
Ceftolozane 50 mg and Tazobactam 25 mg		IV	J0695
Ceftriaxone sodium	per 250 mg	IV, IM	J0696
Cefuroxime sodium, sterile	per 750 mg	IM, IV	J0697
Celestone Soluspan	per 3 mg	IM	J0702
CellCept	250 mg	ORAL	J7517
Cel-U-Jec	per 4 mg	IM, IV	Q0511
Cenacort A-40	1 mg		J3300
	per 10 mg	IM	J3301
Cenacort Forte	per 5 mg	IM	J3302
Centruroides Immune F(ab)	up to 120 mg	IV	J0716
~~Cephalothin sodium~~	~~up to 1 g~~	~~IM, IV~~	~~J1890~~
Cephapirin sodium	up to 1 g	IV, IM	J0710
Ceprotin	10 IU		J2724
Ceredase	per 10 units	IV	J0205
Cerezyme	10 units		J1786
Cerliponase alfa	1 mg	IV	J0567
Certolizumab pegol	1 mg	SC	J0717
Cerubidine	10 mg	IV	J9150
Cetirizine hydrochloride	0.5 mg	IM	J1201
Cetuximab	10 mg	IV	J9055
Chealamide	per 150 mg	IV	J3520
Chirhostim	1 mcg	IV	J2850
Chloramphenicol Sodium Succinate	up to 1 g	IV	J0720
Chlordiazepoxide HCl	up to 100 mg	IM, IV	J1990
Chloromycetin Sodium Succinate	up to 1 g	IV	J0720
Chloroprocaine	1 mg		J2401-J2403
Chloroquine HCl	up to 250 mg	IM	J0390
Chlorothiazide sodium	per 500 mg	IV	J1205
Chlorpromazine	5 mg	ORAL	Q0161
Chlorpromazine HCl	up to 50 mg	IM, IV	J3230
Cholografin Meglumine	per ml		Q9961
Chorex-5	per 1,000 USP units	IM	J0725
Chorex-10	per 1,000 USP units	IM	J0725
Chorignon	per 1,000 USP units	IM	J0725
Chorionic Gonadotropin	per 1,000 USP units	IM	J0725
Choron 10	per 1,000 USP units	IM	J0725

◄ New   ↻ Revised   ✔ Reinstated   ~~deleted~~ Deleted

2026 TABLE OF DRUGS / Cidofovir

DRUG NAME	DOSAGE	METHOD OF ADMINISTRATION	HCPCS CODE
Cidofovir	375 mg	IV	J0740
Cilastatin sodium, imipenem	per 250 mg	IV, IM	J0743
Cimzia	1 mg	SC	J0717
Cinacalcet	1 mg	ORAL	J0604
Cinryze	10 units		J0598
Cipaglucosidase alfa-atga	5 mg	IM	J1203
Cipro IV	200 mg	IV	J0706
Ciprofloxacin	200 mg	IV	J0706
otic suspension	6 mg	OTH	J7342
			J3490
Cisplatin, powder or solution	per 10 mg	IV	J9060
Cladribine	per mg	IV	J9065
Claforan	per 1 gm	IM, IV	J0698
Cleocin Phosphate			J3490
Clevidipine butyrate	1 mg	IM	J0759
Clindamycin			J3490
Clindamycin phosphate	300 mg	IM	J0736, J0737
Clofarabine	1 mg	IV	J9027
Clolar	1 mg		J9027
Clonidine Hydrochloride	1 mg	Epidural	J0735
Coagulation factor Xa (recombinant), inactivated-zhzo (Andexxa)	10 mg		J7169
Cobex	up to 1,000 mcg	IM, SC	J3420
Codeine phosphate	per 30 mg	IM, IV, SC	J0745
Codimal-A	per 10 mg	IM, SC, IV	J0945
Cogentin	per 1 mg	IM, IV	J0515
Colistimethate sodium	up to 150 mg	IM, IV	J0770
Collagenase, Clostridium Histolyticum	0.01 mg	OTH	J0775
Coly-Mycin M	up to 150 mg	IM, IV	J0770
Compa-Z	up to 10 mg	IM, IV	J0780
Copanlisib	1 mg	IV	J9057
Compazine	up to 10 mg	IM, IV	J0780
	5 mg	ORAL	Q0164
			J8498
Compounded drug, not otherwise classified			J7999
Compro			J8498
Concizumab-mtci	0.5 mg	IM	J7173
Conray	per ml		Q9961
Conray 30	per ml		Q9958
Conray 43	per ml		Q9960
Copaxone	20 mg		J1595

◀ New   ↻ Revised   ✔ Reinstated   ~~deleted~~ Deleted

DRUG NAME	DOSAGE	METHOD OF ADMINISTRATION	HCPCS CODE
Cophene-B	per 10 mg	IM, SC, IV	J0945
Copper contraceptive, intrauterine		OTH	J7300
Cordarone	30 mg	IV	J0282
Corgonject-5	per 1,000 USP units	IM	J0725
Corifact	1 IU		J7180
Corticorelin ovine triflutate	1 mcg		J0795
Corticotropin	up to 40 units	IV, IM, SC	J0801-J0802
Cortisone Acetate Micronized			J3490
Cortrosyn	per 0.25 mg	IM, IV	J0835
Corvert	1 mg		J1742
Cosibelimab-ipdl	2 mg	IM	J9275 ◀
Cosmegen	0.5 mg	IV	J9120
Cosyntropin	per 0.25 mg	IM, IV	J0833, J0834
Cotranzine	up to 10 mg	IM, IV	J0780
Crizanlizumab-tmca		IV	J0791
Crofab	up to 1 gram		J0840
Cromolyn Sodium			J8499
Cromolyn sodium, unit dose form	per 10 mg	INH	J7631, J7632
Crotalidae immune f(ab')2 (equine)	120 mg	IV	J0841
Crotalidae Polyvalent Immune Fab	up to 1 gram	IV	J0840
Crovalimab-akkz	10 mg	IM	J1307 ◀
Crysticillin 600 A.S.	up to 600,000 units	IM, IV	J2510
Cubicin	1 mg		J0878
Cutaquig	100 mg	IM	J1551
Cuvitru			J7799
Cyclophosphamide	100 mg	IM, IV	J9072-J9076 ◀
oral	25 mg	ORAL	J8530
Cyclosporine	25 mg	ORAL	J7515
	100 mg	ORAL	J7502
parenteral	250 mg	IV	J7516
Cymetra	1 cc		Q4112
Cyramza	5 mg		J9308
Cysto-Conray II	per ml		Q9958
Cystografin	per ml		Q9958
Cytarabine	100 mg	SC, IV	J9100
Cytarabine liposome	10 mg	IT	J9098
CytoGam	per vial		J0850
Cytomegalovirus immune globulin intravenous (human)	per vial	IV	J0850
Cytosar-U	100 mg	SC, IV	J9100
Cytovene	500 mg	IV	J1570

◀ New   ⇄ Revised   ✓ Reinstated   ~~deleted~~ Deleted

2026 TABLE OF DRUGS / Cytoxan

DRUG NAME	DOSAGE	METHOD OF ADMINISTRATION	HCPCS CODE
Cytoxan	100 mg	IV	J8530
D			
D-5-W, infusion	1000 cc	IV	J7070
Dacarbazine	100 mg	IV	J9130
Daclizumab	25 mg	IV	J7513
Dacogen	1 mg		J0894
Dactinomycin	0.5 mg	IV	J9120
Dalalone	1 mg	IM, IV, OTH	J1100
~~Dalalone L.A.~~	~~1 mg~~	~~IM~~	~~J1094~~
Dalbavancin	5 mg	IV	J0875
Dalteparin sodium	per 2500 IU	SC	J1645
Daprodustat	1 mg	oral	J0889
Daptomycin	1 mg	IV	J0782-J0874, J0877, J0878
Daptomycin (xellia)	1 mg	IM, IV	J0873
Datopotamab deruxtecan-dlnk	1 mg	IV	J9011
Daratumumab	10 mg	IV	J9145
Darbepoetin Alfa	1 mcg	IV, SC	J0881, J0882
Darzalex	10 mg		J9145
Daunorubicin citrate, liposomal formulation	10 mg	IV	J9151
Daunorubicin HCl	10 mg	IV	J9150
Daunoxome	10 mg	IV	J9151
Daxibotulinumtoxina-lanm	1 unit	IM	J0589
DDAVP	1 mcg	IV, SC	J2597
Decadron	1 mg	IM, IV, OTH	J1100
	0.25 mg		J8540
Decadron Phosphate	1 mg	IM, IV, OTH	J1100
~~Decadron-LA~~	~~1 mg~~	~~IM~~	~~J1094~~
Deca-Durabolin	up to 50 mg	IM	J2320
Decaject	1 mg	IM, IV, OTH	J1100
~~Decaject-L.A.~~	~~1 mg~~	~~IM~~	~~J1094~~
Decitabine	1 mg	IV	J0893, J0894
Decolone-50	up to 50 mg	IM	J2320
Decolone-100	up to 50 mg	IM	J2320
De-Comberol	1 mg		J1071
Deferoxamine mesylate	500 mg	IM, SC, IV	J0895
Definity	per ml		J3490, Q9957
Degarelix	1 mg	SC	J9155
Dehist	per 10 mg	IM, SC, IV	J0945
Deladumone	1 mg	IM	J3121
Deladumone OB	1 mg	IM	J3121
Delandistrogene moxeparvovec-rokl	per dose	IV	J1413

◀ New ↻ Revised ✔ Reinstated ~~deleted~~ Deleted

DRUG NAME	DOSAGE	METHOD OF ADMINISTRATION	HCPCS CODE
Delatest	1 mg	IM	J3121
Delatestadiol	1 mg	IM	J3121
Delatestryl	1 mg	IM	J3121
Delestrogen	up to 10 mg	IM	J1380
Delta-Cortef	5 mg	ORAL	J7510
Demadex	10 mg/ml	IV	J3265
Demerol HCl	per 100 mg	IM, IV, SC	J2175
Denileukin diftitox-cxdl	1 mcg	IV	J9161 ◄
Denosumab	1 mg	SC	J0897
Deoxycholic acid	1 mg	IM	J0591
DepAndro 100	1 mg		J1071
DepAndro 200	1 mg		J1071
DepAndrogyn	1 mg		J1071
DepGynogen	up to 5 mg	IM	J1000
DepoCyt	10 mg		J9098
Depo-estradiol cypionate	up to 5 mg	IM	J1000
Depogen	up to 5 mg	IM	J1000
Depo-Provera Contraceptive	1 mg		J1050
Depotest	1 mg		J1071
Depo-Testadiol	1 mg		J1071
Depo-Testosterone	1 mg		J1071
Depotestrogen	1 mg		J1071
Dermagraft	per square centimeter		Q4106
Desferal Mesylate	500 mg	IM, SC, IV	J0895
Desmopressin acetate	1 mcg	IV, SC	J2597
Dexacen-4	1 mg	IM, IV, OTH	J1100
~~Dexacen LA-8~~	~~1 mg~~	~~IM~~	~~J1094~~
Dexamethasone			
concentrated form	per mg	INH	J7637
intravitreal implant	0.1 mg	OTH	J7312
lacrimal ophthalmic insert	0.1 mg	OTH	J1096
unit form	per mg	INH	J7638
oral	0.25 mg	ORAL	J8540, J8541
~~acetate~~	~~1 mg~~	~~IM~~	~~J1094~~
sodium phosphate	1 mg	IM, IV, OTH	J1100
Dexasone	1 mg	IM, IV, OTH	J1100
~~Dexasone L.A.~~	~~1 mg~~	~~IM~~	~~J1094~~
Dexferrum	50 mg		J1750
Dexmedetomidine	1 mcg	ORAL	J1105
Dexone	0.25 mg	ORAL	J8540
	1 mg	IM, IV, OTH	J1100

◄ New   ↻ Revised   ✔ Reinstated   ~~deleted~~ Deleted

2026 TABLE OF DRUGS / Dexpak

DRUG NAME	DOSAGE	METHOD OF ADMINISTRATION	HCPCS CODE
~~Dexone LA~~	~~1 mg~~	~~IM~~	~~J1094~~
Dexpak	0.25 mg	ORAL	J8540
Dexrazoxane hydrochloride	250 mg	IV	J1190
Dextran 40	500 ml	IV	J7100
Dextran 75	500 ml	IV	J7110
Dextrose 5%/normal saline solution	500 ml = 1 unit	IV	J7042
Dextrose/water (5%)	500 ml = 1 unit	IV	J7060
D.H.E. 45	per 1 mg		J1110
Diamox	up to 500 mg	IM, IV	J1120
Diazepam	up to 5 mg	IM, IV	J3360
Diazoxide	up to 300 mg	IV	J1730
Dibent	up to 20 mg	IM	J0500
Diclofenac sodium	37.5	IV	J1130
Dicyclomine HCl	up to 20 mg	IM	J0500
Didronel	per 300 mg	IV	J1436
Diethylstilbestrol diphosphate	250 mg	IV	J9165
Diflucan	200 mg	IV	J1450
DigiFab	per vial		J1162
Digoxin	up to 0.5 mg	IM, IV	J1160
Digoxin immune fab (ovine)	per vial		J1162
Dihydrex	up to 50 mg	IV, IM	J1200
	50 mg	ORAL	Q0163
Dihydroergotamine mesylate	per 1 mg	IM, IV	J1110
Dilantin	per 50 mg	IM, IV	J1165
Dilaudid	250 mg	OTH	S0092
Dilomine	up to 20 mg	IM	J0500
Dilor	up to 500 mg	IM	J1180
Diltiazem hydrochloride	0.5 mg	IM	J1163 ◀
Dimenhydrinate	up to 50 mg	IM, IV	J1240
Dimercaprol	per 100 mg	IM	J0470
Dimethyl sulfoxide	50%, 50 ml	OTH	J1212
Dinate	up to 50 mg	IM, IV	J1240
Dioval	up to 10 mg	IM	J1380
Dioval 40	up to 10 mg	IM	J1380
Dioval XX	up to 10 mg	IM	J1380
Diphenacen-50	up to 50 mg	IV, IM	J1200
	50 mg	ORAL	Q0163
Diphenhydramine HCl			
IV	up to 50 mg	IV, IM	J1200
oral	50 mg	ORAL	Q0163

◀ New ↪ Revised ✔ Reinstated ~~deleted~~ Deleted

2026 TABLE OF DRUGS / Droperidol

DRUG NAME	DOSAGE	METHOD OF ADMINISTRATION	HCPCS CODE
Diprivan	10 mg		J2704
			J3490
Dipyridamole	per 10 mg	IV	J1245
Disotate	per 150 mg	IV	J3520
Di-Spaz	up to 20 mg	IM	J0500
Ditate-DS	1 mg	IM	J3121
Diuril Sodium	per 500 mg	IV	J1205
DMSO, Dimethyl sulfoxide 50%	50 ml	OTH	J1212
Dobutamine HCl	per 250 mg	IV	J1250
Dobutrex	per 250 mg	IV	J1250
Docefrez	1 mg		J9171
Docetaxel	20 mg	IV	J9170
Docetaxel (docivyx)	1 mg	IV	J9172
Docetaxel (beizray)	1 mg	1 mg	J9174 ◄
Dolasetron mesylate			
injection	10 mg	IV	J1260
tablets	100 mg	ORAL	Q0180
Dolophine HCl	up to 10 mg	IM, SC	J1230
Dommanate	up to 50 mg	IM, IV	J1240
Donanemab-azbt	2 mg	IM	J0175
Donbax	10 mg		J1267
Dopamine	40 mg		J1265
Dopamine HCl	40 mg		J1265
Doribax	10 mg		J1267
Doripenem	10 mg	IV	J1267
Dornase alpha, unit dose form	per mg	INH	J7639
Dotarem	0.1 ml		A9575
Doxercalciferol	1 mcg	IV	J1270
Doxil	10 mg	IV	J9000, Q2050
Doxorubicin HCL	10 mg	IV	J9000
Doxy	100 mg		J3490
Doxycycline hyclate	1 mg	IM	J1271 ◄
Dramamine	up to 50 mg	IM, IV	J1240
Dramanate	up to 50 mg	IM, IV	J1240
Dramilin	up to 50 mg	IM, IV	J1240
Dramocen	up to 50 mg	IM, IV	J1240
Dramoject	up to 50 mg	IM, IV	J1240
Dronabinol	2.5 mg	ORAL	Q0167
Droperidol	up to 5 mg	IM, IV	J1790
~~Droperidol and fentanyl citrate~~	~~up to 2 ml ampule~~	~~IM, IV~~	~~J1810~~

◄ New   ⇄ Revised   ✔ Reinstated   ~~deleted~~ Deleted

2026 TABLE OF DRUGS / Droxia

DRUG NAME	DOSAGE	METHOD OF ADMINISTRATION	HCPCS CODE
Droxia		ORAL	J8999
Drug administered through a metered dose inhaler		INH	J3535
DTIC-Dome	100 mg	IV	J9130
Dua-Gen L.A.	1 mg	IM	J3121
DuoNeb	up to 2.5 mg		J7620
Duopa	20 ml		J7340
Duoval P.A.	1 mg	IM	J3121
Durabolin	up to 50 mg	IM	J2320
Duracillin A.S.	up to 600,000 units	IM, IV	J2510
Duraclon	1 mg	Epidural	J0735
Dura-Estrin	up to 5 mg	IM	J1000
Duragen-10	up to 10 mg	IM	J1380
Duragen-20	up to 10 mg	IM	J1380
Duragen-40	up to 10 mg	IM	J1380
Duralutin, see Hydroxyprogesterone Caproate			
Duramorph	up to 10 mg	IM, IV, SC	J2270, J2274
Duratest-100	1 mg		J1071
Duratest-200	1 mg		J1071
Duratestrin	1 mg		J1071
Durathate-200	1 mg	IM	J3121
Durvalumab	10 mg	IV	J9173
Dymenate	up to 50 mg	IM, IV	J1240
Dyphylline	up to 500 mg	IM	J1180
Dysport	5 units		J0586
Dalvance	5 mg		J0875
E			
Ecallantide	1 mg	SC	J1290
~~Eculizumab~~	~~10 mg~~	~~IV~~	~~J1300~~
Eculizumab	2 mg	IV	J1299 ◀
Edaravone	1 mg	IV	J1301
Edetate calcium disodium	up to 1,000 mg	IV, SC, IM	J0600
Edetate disodium	per 150 mg	IV	J3520
Efbemalenograstim alfa-vuxw	0.5 mg	IM	J9361
Efgartigimod	2 mg	IM	J9332, J9334
Eflapegrastim-xnst	0.1 mg	IM	J1449
Elaprase	1 mg		J1743
Elavil	up to 20 mg	IM	J1320
Elelyso	10 units		J3060
Eligard	7.5 mg		J9217
Elitek	0.5 mg		J2783

◀ New ↩ Revised ✔ Reinstated ~~deleted~~ Deleted

2026 TABLE OF DRUGS / Epogen

DRUG NAME	DOSAGE	METHOD OF ADMINISTRATION	HCPCS CODE
Ellence	2 mg		J9178
Elliotts B solution	1 ml	OTH	J9175
Eloctate	per IU		J7205
Elosulfase alfa	1 mg	IV	J1322
Elotuzumab	1 mg	IV	J9176
Eloxatin	0.5 mg		J9263
Elranatamab-bcmm	1 mg		J1323
Elspar	10,000 units	IV, IM	J9020
Emapalunab-lzsg	1 mg	IV	J9210
Emend			J1453, J8501
Emete-Con, see Benzquinamide			
Eminase	30 units	IV	J0350
Empliciti	1 mg		J9176
Emtricitabine and tenofovir disoproxil fumarate	200 mg	ORAL	J0750
	300 mg	ORAL	
Emtricitabine and tenofovir alafenamide	200 mg	ORAL	J0751
	25 mg	ORAL	
Enbrel	25 mg	IM, IV	J1438
Endrate ethylenediamine-tetra-acetic acid	per 150 mg	IV	J3520
Enfortumab vedotin-ejfv	0.25 mg	IM	J9177
Enfuvirtide	1 mg	SC	J1324
Engerix-B			J3490
Enovil	up to 20 mg	IM	J1320
Enoxaparin sodium	10 mg	SC	J1650
Ensifentrine	3 mg	INH	J7601 ◀
Entyvio			J3380
Eovist	1 ml		A9581
Epcoritamab-bysp	0.16 mg	SC	J9321
Epinephrine			~~J0173~~, J7799
Epinephrine, adrenalin	~~0.1 mg~~	SC, IM	J0163-J0169 ◀
			~~J0171~~
Epirubicin hydrochloride	2 mg		J9178
Epoetin alfa, ESRD use	100 units	IV, SC	Q4081
Epoetin alfa, non-ESRD use	1000 units	IV	J0885
Epoetin alfa-epbx (Retacrit) ESRD use	100 units	IV	Q5105
Epoetin alfa-epbx (Retacrit) non-ESRD use	1000 units	IV	Q5106
Epoetin beta, ESRD use	1 mcg	IV	J0887
Epoetin beta, non-ESRD use	1 mcg	IV	J0888
Epogen	1,000 units		J0885
			Q4081

◀ New　↻ Revised　✓ Reinstated　~~deleted~~ Deleted

2026 TABLE OF DRUGS / Epoprostenol

DRUG NAME	DOSAGE	METHOD OF ADMINISTRATION	HCPCS CODE	
Epoprostenol	0.5 mg	IV	J1325	
Eptifibatide, injection	5 mg	IM, IV	J1327	
Eravacycline	1 mg	IV	J0122	
Eraxis	1 mg	IV	J0348	
Erbitux	10 mg		J9055	
Ergonovine maleate	up to 0.2 mg	IM, IV	J1330	
Eribulin mesylate	0.1 mg	IV	J9179	
Erivedge	150 mg		J8999	
Ertapenem sodium	500 mg	IM, IV	J1335	
Erwinase	1,000 units	IV, IM	J9019	
	10,000 units	IV, IM	J9020	
Erythromycin lactobionate	500 mg	IV	J1364	
Erzofri	1 mg	IM	J2428	◀
Esmolol hydrochloride	10 mg	IM	J1805, J1806	
Esomeprazole sodium	1 mg	IV	J1370	◀
Estra-D	up to 5 mg	IM	J1000	
Estradiol				
L.A.	up to 10 mg	IM	J1380	
L.A. 20	up to 10 mg	IM	J1380	
L.A. 40	up to 10 mg	IM	J1380	
Estradiol cypionate	up to 5 mg	IM	J1000	
Estradiol valerate	up to 10 mg	IM	J1380	
Estra-L 20	up to 10 mg	IM	J1380	
Estra-L 40	up to 10 mg	IM	J1380	
Estra-Testrin	1 mg	IM	J3121	
Estro-Cyp	up to 5 mg	IM	J1000	
Estrogen, conjugated	per 25 mg	IV, IM	J1410	
Estroject L.A.	up to 5 mg	IM	J1000	
Estrone	per 1 mg	IM	J1435	
Estrone 5	per 1 mg	IM	J1435	
Estrone Aqueous	per 1 mg	IM	J1435	
Estronol	per 1 mg	IM	J1435	
Estronol-L.A.	up to 5 mg	IM	J1000	
Etanercept, injection	25 mg	IM, IV	J1438	
Etelcalcetide	0.1 mg	IV	Q4078	
Eteplirsen	10 mg	IV	J1428	
Ethcrynate sodium	1 mg	IV	J1807	◀
Ethamolin	100 mg		J1430	
Ethanolamine	100 mg		J1430, J3490	
Ethyol	500 mg	IV	J0207	

◀ New   ↩ Revised   ✔ Reinstated   ~~deleted~~ Deleted

DRUG NAME	DOSAGE	METHOD OF ADMINISTRATION	HCPCS CODE
Etidronate disodium	per 300 mg	IV	J1436
Etonogestrel implant			J7307
Etopophos	10 mg	IV	J9181
Etoposide	10 mg	IV	J9181
oral	50 mg	ORAL	J8560
Etranacogene dezaparvovec-drlb	per dose	IM	J1411
Euflexxa	per dose	OTH	J7323
Everolimus	0.25 mg	ORAL	J7527
Everone	1 mg	IM	J3121
Evinacumab-dgnb	5 mg	IV	J1305
Evomela	50 mg		J9245
Exagamglogen autotemcel	per dose	IM	J3392 ◀
Eylea	1 mg	OTH	J0178
F			
Fabrazyme	1 mg	IV	J0180
Factor IX			
anti-hemophilic factor, purified, non-recombinant	per IU	IV	J7193
anti-hemophilic factor, recombinant	per IU	IV	J7195, J7200-J7202
complex	per IU	IV	J7194
coagulation (recombinant)	1 IU	IV	J7213
Factor VIIa (coagulation factor, recombinant)	1 mcg	IV	J7189
Factor VIII (anti-hemophilic factor)	per IU	IV	J7208
human	per IU	IV	J7190
porcine	per IU	IV	J7191
recombinant	per IU	IV	J7182, J7185, J7192, J7188
Factor VIII (anti-hemophilic factor, recombinant)			
(Afstyla)	per IU	IV	J7210
Esperoct	per IU	IV	J7204
Jivi	per IU	IV	J7208
(Kovaltry)	per IU	IV	J7211
Novoeight	per IU	IV	J7182
Obizur	per IU	IV	J7188
Xyntha	per IU	IV	J7185
Factor VIII, anti-hemophilic factor (recombinant)(esperoct)	per IU	IV	J7204
Factor VIII (recombinant)	per IU	IV	J7205, J7207, J7209, J7214
Factor X (human)	per IU	IV	J7175
Factor XIII A-subunit (recombinant)	per IU	IV	J7181
Factors, other hemophilia clotting	per IU	IV	J7196

◀ New   ⮂ Revised   ✓ Reinstated   ~~deleted~~ Deleted

2026 TABLE OF DRUGS / Factrel

DRUG NAME	DOSAGE	METHOD OF ADMINISTRATION	HCPCS CODE	
Factrel	per 100 mcg	SC, IV	J1620	
Fam-trastuzumab deruxtecan-nxki	1 mg	IM	J9358	
Famotidine			J3490	
Famotidine	0.25 mg	IM	J1308	◄
Faricimab-svoa	0.1 mg	IM	J2777	
Faslodex	25 mg		J9395	
Fecal microbiota	1 ml		J1440	
Feiba NF			J7198	
Feiba VH Immuno	per IU	IV	J7196	
Fentanyl citrate	0.1 mg	IM, IV	J3010	
Feraheme	1 mg		Q0138, Q0139	
Ferric carboxymaltose	1 mg	IV	J1439	
Ferric citrate	3 mg	ORAL	J0609	◄
Ferric pyrophosphate citrate powder	0.1 mg of iron	IV	J1444	
Ferric pyrophosphate citrate solution (triferic)	0.1 mg of iron	IV	J1443	
Ferric pyrophosphate citrate solution (triferic avnu)	0.1 mg of iron	IV	J1445	
Ferrlecit	12.5 mg		J2916	
Ferumoxytol	1 mg		Q0138, Q0139	
Fidanacogene elaparvovec-dzkt	per therapeutic dose	IM	J1414	◄
Filgrastim-aafi	1 mcg	IV	Q5110	
Filgrastim				
(G-CSF)	1 mcg	SC, IV	J1442, Q5101	
(TBO)	1 mcg	IV	J1447	
Firazyr	1 mg	SC	J1744	
Firmagon	1 mg		J9155	
Fitusiran	0.04 mg	IM	J7174	◄
Flebogamma	500 mg	IV	J1572	
	1 cc		J1460	
Flexoject	up to 60 mg	IV, IM	J2360	
Flexon	up to 60 mg	IV, IM	J2360	
Flolan	0.5 mg	IV	J1325	
Flo-Pred	5 mg		J7510	
Florbetaben f18, diagnostic	per study dose	IV	Q9983	
Floxuridine	500 mg	IV	J9200	
Fluconazole	200 mg	IV	J1450	
Fludara	1 mg	ORAL	J8562	
	50 mg	IV	J9185	
Fludarabine phosphate	1 mg	ORAL	J8562	
	50 mg	IV	J9185	
Flunisolide inhalation solution, unit dose form	per mg	INH	J7641	
Fluocinolone		OTH	J7311, J7313	

◄ New   ↻ Revised   ✓ Reinstated   ~~deleted~~ Deleted

DRUG NAME	DOSAGE	METHOD OF ADMINISTRATION	HCPCS CODE	
Fluocinolone acetonide (Yutiq)	0.01 mg	OTH	J7314	
Fluorouracil	500 mg	IV	J9190	
Fluphenazine decanoate	up to 25 mg		J2680	
Fluphenazine HCL	1.25 mg	ORAL	J2679	
Flutamide			J8999	
Flutemetamol f18, diagnostic	per study dose	IV	Q9982	
Folex	50 mg	IA, IM, IT, IV	J9260	
Folex PFS	50 mg	IA, IM, IT, IV	J9260	
Folic acid	0.1 mg	IM	J1808	◄
Follutein	per 1,000 USP units	IM	J0725	
Folotyn	1 mg		J9307	
Fomepizole	15 mg		J1451	
Fomivirsen sodium	1.65 mg	Intraocular	J1452	
Fondaparinux sodium	0.5 mg	SC	J1652	
Formoterol	12 mcg	INH	J7640	
Formoterol fumarate	20 mcg	INH	J7606	
Fortaz	per 500 mg	IM, IV	J0713	
Fosaprepitant	1 mg	IV	J1434, J1453, J1456	
Foscarnet sodium	per 1,000 mg	IV	J1455	
Foscarbidopa/Foslevodopa	0.25 mg/5 mg	SC	J7356	◄
Foscavir	per 1,000 mg	IV	J1455	
Fosdenopterin	0.1 mg	IV	J1809	◄
Fosnetupitant 235 mg and palonosetron 0.25 mg		IV	J1454	
Fosphenytoin	50 mg	IV	Q2009	
Fragmin	per 2,500 IU		J1645	
Fremanezumab-vfrm	1 mg	IV	J3031	
FUDR	500 mg	IV	J9200	
Fulvestrant	25 mg	IM	J9393, J9394, J9395	
Fungizone intravenous	50 mg	IV	J0285	
~~Furomide M.D.~~	~~up to 20 mg~~	~~IM, IV~~	~~J1940~~	
Furosemide	up to 20 mg	IM, IV	J1938 ~~J1940~~, J1941	◄
G				
Gablofen	10 mg		J0475	
	50 mcg		J0476	
Gadavist	0.1 ml		A9585	
Gadopiclenol	1 ml	IM	A9573	
Gadoxetate disodium	1 ml	IV	A9581	
Gallium nitrate	1 mg	IV	J1457	

◄ New   ↻ Revised   ✔ Reinstated   ~~deleted~~ Deleted

2026 TABLE OF DRUGS / Galsulfase

DRUG NAME	DOSAGE	METHOD OF ADMINISTRATION	HCPCS CODE
Galsulfase	1 mg	IV	J1458
Gamastan	1 cc	IM	J1460
	over 10 cc	IM	J1560
Gamma globulin	1 cc	IM	J1460
	over 10 cc	IM	J1560
Gammagard Liquid	500 mg	IV	J1569
Gammagard S/D			J1566
GammaGraft	per square centimeter		Q4111
Gammaplex	500 mg	IV	J1557
Gammar	1 cc	IM	J1460
	over 10 cc	IM	J1560
Gammar-IV, see Immune globin intravenous (human)			
Gamulin RH			
immune globulin, human	100 IU		J2791
	1 dose package, 300 mcg	IM	J2790
immune globulin, human, solvent detergent	100 IU	IV	J2792
Gamunex	500 mg	IV	J1561
Ganciclovir, implant	4.5 mg	OTH	J7310
Ganciclovir sodium	500 mg	IV	J1570, J1574
Ganirelix			J3490
Garamycin, gentamicin	up to 80 mg	IM, IV	J1580
Gastrografin	per ml		Q9963
Gatifloxacin	10 mg	IV	J1590
Gazyva	10 mg		J9301
Gefitinib	250 mg	ORAL	J8565
Gel-One	per dose	OTH	J7326
Gemcitabine HCl	200 mg	IV	J9201, J9196
Gemcitabine HCl, not otherwise specified	200 mg	IV	J9201
Gemcitabine HCl (Infugem)	100 mg	IV	J9198
Gemsar	200 mg	IV	J9201
Gemtuzumab ozogamicin	5 mg	IV	J9300
Gengraf	100 mg		J7502
	25 mg	ORAL	J7515
Genotropin	1 mg		J2941
Gentamicin Sulfate	up to 80 mg	IM, IV	J1580, J7699
Gentran	500 ml	IV	J7100
Gentran 75	500 ml	IV	J7110
Geodon	10 mg		J3486
Gesterol 50	per 50 mg		J2675

◀ New   ↪ Revised   ✔ Reinstated   ~~deleted~~ Deleted

2026 TABLE OF DRUGS / Hemophilia clotting factors

DRUG NAME	DOSAGE	METHOD OF ADMINISTRATION	HCPCS CODE
Givosiran	0.5 mg	IM	J0223
Glassia	10 mg	IV	J0257
Glatiramer Acetate	20 mg	SC	J1595
Gleevec (Film-Coated)	400 mg		J8999
Glofitamab	2.5 mg	IV	J9286
GlucaGen	per 1 mg		J1610
Glucagon (gvoke)	0.01 mg	SC, IM, IV	J1620 ◄
Glucagon HCl	per 1 mg	SC, IM, IV	J1610, J1611
Glukor	per 1,000 USP units	IM	J0725
Glycopyrrolate	0.1 mg	IM, IV, ORAL	J1596-J1598
concentrated form	per 1 mg	INH	J7642
unit dose form	per 1 mg	INH	J7643
Gold sodium thiomalate	up to 50 mg	IM	J1600
Golimumab	1 mg	IV	J1602
Golodirsen	10 mg	IM	J1429
Gonadorelin HCl	per 100 mcg	SC, IV	J1620
Gonal-F			J3490
Gonic	per 1,000 USP units	IM	J0725
Goserelin acetate implant	per 3.6 mg	SC	J9202
Graftjacket	per square centimeter		Q4107
Graftjacket Xpress	1 cc		Q4113
Granisetron HCl			
extended release	0.1 mg	IV	J1627
injection	100 mcg	IV	J1626
oral	1 mg	ORAL	Q0166
Guselkumab	1 mg	IV	J1628
Gynogen L.A. A10	up to 10 mg	IM	J1380
Gynogen L.A. A20	up to 10 mg	IM	J1380
Gynogen L.A. A40	up to 10 mg	IM	J1380
H			
Halaven	0.1 mg		J9179
Haldol	up to 5 mg	IM, IV	J1630
Haloperidol	up to 5 mg	IM, IV	J1630
Haloperidol decanoate	per 50 mg	IM	J1631
Haloperidol Lactate	up to 5 mg		J1630
Hectoral	1 mcg	IV	J1270
Helixate FS	per IU		J7192
Hemin	1 mg		J1640
Hemofil M	per IU	IV	J7190
Hemophilia clotting factors (e.g., anti-inhibitors)	per IU	IV	J7198
NOC	per IU	IV	J7199

◄ New   ↻ Revised   ✓ Reinstated   ~~deleted~~ Deleted

DRUG NAME	DOSAGE	METHOD OF ADMINISTRATION	HCPCS CODE
Hepagam B	0.5 ml	IM	J1571
	0.5 ml	IV	J1573
Heparin sodium	1,000 units	IV, SC	J1643, J1644
Heparin sodium (heparin lock flush)	10 units	IV	J1642
Heparin Sodium (Procine)	per 1,000 units		J1644
Hep-Lock	10 units	IV	J1642
Hep-Lock U/P	10 units	IV	J1642
Herceptin	10 mg	IV	J9355
Hexabrix 320	per ml		Q9967
Hexadrol Phosphate	1 mg	IM, IV, OTH	J1100
Hexaminolevulinate hydrochloride	100 mg	IV	A9589
Histaject	per 10 mg	IM, SC, IV	J0945
Histerone 50	up to 50 mg	IM	J3140
Histerone 100	up to 50 mg	IM	J3140
Histrelin			
acetate	10 mcg		J1675
implant	50 mg	OTH	J9225, J9226
Hizentra, see Immune globulin			
Humalog	per 5 units		J1815
	per 50 units		J1817
Human fibrinogen concentrate	100 mg	IV	J7178
Human fibrinogen concentrate (fibryga)	1 mg	IV	J7177
Humate-P	per IU		J7187
Humatrope	1 mg		J2941
~~Humira~~	~~20 mg~~		~~J0135~~
Humulin	per 5 units		J1815
	per 50 units		J1817
Hyalgan, Spurtaz or VISCO-3	per dose	IA	J7321
Hyaluronan or derivative	per dose	IV	J7327
Durolane	1 mg	IA	J7318
Gel-Syn	0.1 mg	IA	J7328
Gelsyn-3	0.1 mg	IV	J7328
Gen Visc 850	1 mg	IA	J7320
Hyalgan or supartz	per dose	IA	J7321
Hymovis	1 mg	IA	J7322
Synojoynt	1 mg	VAR	J7331
Triluron	1 mg	IV	J7332
Trivisc	1 mg	IV	J7329
Hyaluronic Acid			J3490
Hyaluronidase	up to 150 units	SC, IV	J3470

◀ New   ↻ Revised   ✓ Reinstated   ~~deleted~~ Deleted

2026 TABLE OF DRUGS / Ibandronate sodium

DRUG NAME	DOSAGE	METHOD OF ADMINISTRATION	HCPCS CODE
Hyaluronidase			
ovine	up to 999 units	VAR	J3471
ovine	per 1000 units	VAR	J3472
recombinant	1 usp	SC	J3473
Hyate:C	per IU	IV	J7191
Hybolin Decanoate	up to 50 mg	IM	J2320
Hycamtin	0.25 mg	ORAL	J8705
	4 mg	IV	J9351
Hydralazine HCl	up to 20 mg	IV, IM	J0360
Hydrate	up to 50 mg	IM, IV	J1240
Hydrea			J8999
Hydrocortisone acetate	up to 25 mg	IV, IM, SC	J1700
Hydrocortisone sodium phosphate	up to 50 mg	IV, IM, SC	J1710
Hydrocortisone succinate sodium	up to 100 mg	IV, IM, SC	J1720
Hydrocortone Acetate	up to 25 mg	IV, IM, SC	J1700
Hydrocortone Phosphate	up to 50 mg	IM, IV, SC	J1710
Hydromorphone	0.1 mg	Oral	J1171
Hydroxocobalamin	10 mcg	IM	J3425
Hydroxocobalamin	25 mg	IV	J3424
Hydroxyprogesterone Caproate	1 mg	IM	J1725
(Makena)	10 mg	IV	J1726
NOS	10 mg	IV	J1729
Hydroxyurea			J8999
Hydroxyzine HCl	up to 25 mg	IM	J3410
Hydroxyzine Pamoate	25 mg	ORAL	Q0177
Hylan G-F 20		OTH	J7322
Hylenex	1 USP unit		J3473
Hyoscyamine sulfate	up to 0.25 mg	SC, IM, IV	J1980
Hyperrho S/D	300 mcg		J2790
	100 IU		J2792
Hyperstat IV	up to 300 mg	IV	J1730
Hyper-Tet	up to 250 units	IM	J1670
HypRho-D	300 mcg	IM	J2790
			J2791
	50 mcg		J2788
Hyrexin-50	up to 50 mg	IV, IM	J1200
Hyzine-50	up to 25 mg	IM	J3410
I			
Ibalizumab-uiyk	10 mg	IV	J1746
Ibandronate sodium	1 mg	IV	J1740

◀ New   ↻ Revised   ✔ Reinstated   ~~deleted~~ Deleted

2026 TABLE OF DRUGS / Ibuprofen

DRUG NAME	DOSAGE	METHOD OF ADMINISTRATION	HCPCS CODE	
Ibuprofen	100 mg	IV	J1741	
Ibutilide fumarate	1 mg	IV	J1742	
Icatibant	1 mg	SC	J1744	
Idamycin	5 mg	IV	J9211	
Idarubicin HCl	5 mg	IV	J9211	
Idursulfase	1 mg	IV	J1743	
Ifex	1 g	IV	J9208	
Ifosfamide	1 g	IV	J9208	
Ilaris	1 mg		J0638	
Iloprost	20 mcg, 0.1 mcg	INH, IM	Q4074, J1749	
Ilotycin, see Erythromycin lactobionate				
Iluvien	0.01 mg		J7313	
Imetelstat	1 mg	IM	J0870	◀
Imferon	50 mg		J1750	
Imiglucerase	10 units	IV	J1786	
Imipenem 4 mg, cilistatin 4 mg, relebactam 2 mg			J0742	
Imitrex	6 mg	SC	J3030	
Imlygic	per 1 million plaque forming units		J9325, J9999	
Immune globulin				
Alyglo	500 mg	IM, IV	J1552	◀
Asceniv	500 mg	IV	J1554	
Bivigam	500 mg	IV	J1556	
Cuvitru	100 mg	IV	J1555	
Flebogamma	500 mg	IV	J1572	
Gammagard Liquid	500 mg	IV	J1569	
Gammaplex	500 mg	IV	J1557	
Gamunex	500 mg	IV	J1561	
HepaGam B	0.5 ml	IM	J1571	
	0.5 ml	IV	J1573	
Hizentra	100 mg	SC	J1559	
Hyaluronidase, (HYQVIA)	100 mg	IV	J1575	
NOS	500 mg	IV	J1566, J1599	
Octagam	500 mg	IV	J1568	
Panzyga	500 mg	IV	J1576	
Privigen	500 mg	IV	J1459	
Rhophylac	100 IU	IM	J2791	
Subcutaneous	100 mg	SC	J1562	
Xembify	100 mg	IM	J1558	
Immunosuppressive drug, not otherwise classified			J7599	

◀ New   ⮌ Revised   ✔ Reinstated   ~~deleted~~ Deleted

DRUG NAME	DOSAGE	METHOD OF ADMINISTRATION	HCPCS CODE
Imuran	50 mg	ORAL	J7500
	100 mg	IV	J7501
Inapsine	up to 5 mg	IM, IV	J1790
Inclisiran	1 mg	IM	J1306
Incobotulinumtoxin type A	1 unit	IM	J0588
Increlex	1 mg		J2170
Inderal	up to 1 mg	IV	J1800
Indigotindisulfonate sodium	1 mg	IM	J9220 ◄
Inebilizumab-cdon	1 mg	IV	J1823
Infed	50 mg		J1750
Infergen	1 mcg	SC	J9212
Inflectra			Q5102
Infliximab			
dyyb	10 mg	IM, IV	Q5103, J1748
abda	10 mg	IM, IV	Q5104
axxq, biosimilar, (AVSOLA)	10 mg	IM, IV	Q5121
qbtx	10 mg	IM, IV	Q5109
Infumorph	10 mg		J2274
Injectafer	1 mg		J1439
Injection factor XL, glycopegylated	1 IU	IV	J7203
Injection sulfur hexafluoride lipid microspheres	per ml	IV	Q9950
Innohep	1,000 iu	SC	J1655
~~Innovar~~	~~up to 2 ml ampule~~	~~IM, IV~~	~~J1810~~
Inotuzumab orogamicin	0.1 mg	IV	J9229
Isoniazid	1 mg	ORAL, IM	J1834 ◄
Insulin	5 units, 50 units	SC	J1811-J1815
Insulin-Humalog	per 50 units		J1817
Insulin lispro	50 units	SC	J1817
Intal, unit dose form	per 10 mg	INH	J7631, J7632
Integra			
Bilayer Matrix Wound Dressing (BMWD)	per square centimeter		Q4104
Dermal Regeneration Template (DRT)	per square centimeter		Q4105
Flowable Wound Matrix	1 cc		Q4114
Matrix	per square centimeter		Q4108
Integrilin IV injection	5 mg	IM, IV	J1327
Interferon alfa-2a, recombinant	3 million units	SC, IM	J9213
Interferon alfa-2b, recombinant	1 million units	SC, IM	J9214
Interferon alfa-n3 (human leukocyte derived)	250,000 IU	IM	J9215
Interferon alphacon-1, recombinant	1 mcg	SC	J9212

◄ New   ⮂ Revised   ✔ Reinstated   ~~deleted~~ Deleted

DRUG NAME	DOSAGE	METHOD OF ADMINISTRATION	HCPCS CODE
Interferon beta-1a	30 mcg	IM	J1826
	1 mcg	IM	Q3027
	1 mcg	SC	Q3028
Interferon beta-1b	0.25 mg	SC	J1830
Interferon gamma-1b	3 million units	SC	J9216
Intrauterine copper contraceptive		OTH	J7300
Intron-A	1 million units		J9214
Invanz	500 mg		J1335
Invega Sustenna	1 mg		J2426
Ipilimumab	1 mg	IV	J9228
Ipratropium bromide, unit dose form	per mg	INH	J3535, J7620, J7644, J7645
Irinotecan	20 mg	IV	J9206, J9205
Iron dextran	50 mg	IV, IM	J1750
Iron oxide, superparamagnetic	per study dose		A9697
Iron sucrose	1 mg	IV	J1756
Irrigation solution for Tx of bladder calculi	per 50 ml	OTH	Q2004
Isatuximab-irfc	10 mg	IV	J9227
Isavuconazonium	1 mg	IV	J1833
Isocaine HCl	per 10 ml	VAR	J0670
Isoetharine HCl			
concentrated form	per mg	INH	J7647, J7648
unit dose form	per mg	INH	J7649, J7650
Isoproterenol HCl			
concentrated form	per mg	INH	J7657, J7658
unit dose form	per mg	INH	J7659, J7660
Isovue	per ml		Q9966, Q9967
Isuprel			
concentrated form	per mg	INH	J7657, J7658
unit dose form	per mg	INH	J7659, J7660
Itraconazole	50 mg	IV	J1835
Ixabepilone	1 mg	IV	J9207
Ixempra	1 mg		J9207
J			
Jemperli	10 mg	IV	J9272
Jenamicin	up to 80 mg	IM, IV	J1580
Jetrea	0.125 mg		J7316
Jevtana	1 mg		J9043
K			
Kabikinase	per 250,000 IU	IV	J2995

DRUG NAME	DOSAGE	METHOD OF ADMINISTRATION	HCPCS CODE
Kadcyla	1 mg		J9354
Kalbitor	1 mg		J1290
~~Keflin~~	~~up to 1 g~~	~~IM, IV~~	~~J1890~~
Kefurox	per 750 mg		J0697
Kefzol	500 mg	IV, IM	J0690
Kenaject-40	1 mg		J3300
	per 10 mg	IM	J3301
Kenalog-10	1 mg		J3300
	per 10 mg	IM	J3301
Kenalog-40	1 mg		J3300
	per 10 mg	IM	J3301
Kepivance	50 mcg		J2425
Keppra	10 mg		J1953
Keroxx	1 cc	IV	Q4202
Kestrone 5	per 1 mg	IM	J1435
Ketorolac tromethamine	per 15 mg	IM, IV	J1885
Key-Pred 25	up to 1 ml	IM	J2650
Key-Pred 50	up to 1 ml	IM	J2650
Key-Pred-SP, see Prednisolone sodium phosphate			
Keytruda	1 mg		J9271
K-Flex	up to 60 mg	IV, IM	J2360
Khapzory	0.5 mg	IV	J0642
Kinevac	5 mcg	IV	J2805
Kitabis PAK	per 300 mg		J7682
Koate-HP (anti-hemophilic factor)			
human	per IU	IV	J7190
porcine	per IU	IV	J7191
recombinant	per IU	IV	J7192
Kogenate			
human	per IU	IV	J7190
porcine	per IU	IV	J7191
recombinant	per IU	IV	J7192
Konakion	per 1 mg	IM, SC, IV	J3430
Konyne-80	per IU	IV	J7194
Krystexxa	1 mg		J2507
Kyleena	19.5 mg	OTH	J7296
Kyprolis	1 mg		J9047
Kytril	1 mg	ORAL	Q0166
	1 mg	IV	S0091
	100 mcg	IV	J1626

◄ New   ↻ Revised   ✔ Reinstated   ~~deleted~~ Deleted

DRUG NAME	DOSAGE	METHOD OF ADMINISTRATION	HCPCS CODE
L			
L.A.E. 20	up to 10 mg	IM	J1380
Labetalol hydrochloride	5 mg	IM	J1920, J1921
Laetrile, Amygdalin, vitamin B-17			J3570
Lanadelumab-flyo	1 mg	IV	J0593
Lanoxin	up to 0.5 mg	IM, IV	J1160
Lanreotide	1 mg	SC	J1930, J1932
Lanthanum carbonate	5 mg	ORAL	J0607-J0608 ◀
Lantus	per 5 units		J1815
Largon, *see* Propiomazine HCl			
Laronidase	0.1 mg	IV	J1931
~~Lasix~~	~~up to 20 mg~~	~~IM, IV~~	~~J1940~~
Lecanemab-irmb	1 mg	IM	J0174
Lefamulin	1 mg		J0691
Lemtrada	1 mg		J0202
Lenacapavir	1 mg	IM	J0738, J0759, J1961 ◀
Lepirudin	50 mg		J1945
Leucovorin calcium	per 50 mg	IM, IV	J0640
Leukeran			J8999
Leukine	50 mcg	IV	J2820
Leuprolide acetate	per 1 mg	IM	J9218
Leuprolide acetate (for depot suspension)	per 3.75 mg	IM	J1950
	7.5 mg	IM	J1954, J9217
Leuprolide acetate (for depot suspension) (fensolvi)	0.25 mg	IV	J1951
Leuprolide acetate implant	65 mg	OTH	J9219
Leustatin	per mg	IV	J9065
Levalbuterol HCl			
concentrated form	0.5 mg	INH	J7607, J7612
unit dose form	0.5 mg	INH	J7614, J7615
Levaquin I.U.	250 mg	IV	J1956
Levetiracetam	10 mg	IV	J1953
Levocarnitine	per 1 gm	IV	J1955
Levo-Dromoran	up to 2 mg	SC, IV	J1960
Levofloxacin	250 mg	IV	J1956
Levoleucovorin NOS	0.5 mg	IV	J0641
Levonorgestrel implant		OTH	J7306
Levonorgestrel-releasing intrauterine contraceptive system	52 mg	OTH	J7297, J7298
Kyleena	19.5 mg	OTH	J7296
Levorphanol tartrate	up to 2 mg	SC, IV	J1960

◀ New   ↪ Revised   ✔ Reinstated   ~~deleted~~ Deleted

DRUG NAME	DOSAGE	METHOD OF ADMINISTRATION	HCPCS CODE
Levothyroxine	10 mcg	IM	J0650-J0652
Levsin	up to 0.25 mg	SC, IM, IV	J1980
Levulan Kerastick	unit dose (354 mg)	OTH	J7308
Lexiscan	0.1 mg		J2785
Librium	up to 100 mg	IM, IV	J1990
Lidocaine	0.1 mg, 1 mg	IM	J2002-J2004
Liletta	52 mg	OTH	J7297
Lincocin	up to 300 mg	IV	J2010
Lincomycin HCl	up to 300 mg	IV	J2010
Linezolid	200 mg	IV	J2020, J2021
Lioresal	10 mg	IT	J0475
			J0476
Liposomal			
Cytarabine	2.27 mg	IV	J9153
Daunorubicin	1 mg	IV	J9153
Liquaemin Sodium	1,000 units	IV, SC	J1644
LMD (10%)	500 ml	IV	J7100
Locort	1.5 mg		J8540
Lorazepam	2 mg	IM, IV	J2060
Lovenox	10 mg	SC	J1650
Lovotibeglogene autotemcel		IM	J3394
Loxapine	1 mg	OTH	J2062
Lucentis	0.1 mg		J2778
Lufyllin	up to 500 mg	IM	J1180
Lumasiran	0.5 mg	IV	J0224
Lumason	per ml		Q9950
Luminal Sodium	up to 120 mg	IM, IV	J2560
Lumizyme	10 mg		J0221
Lupon Depot	7.5 mg		J9217
	3.75 mg		J1950
Lupron	per 1 mg	IM	J9218
	per 3.75 mg	IM	J1950
	7.5 mg	IM	J9217
Lurbinectedin	0.1 mg	IV	J9223
Luspatercept-aamt	0.25 mg	IM	J0896
Lyophilized, see Cyclophosphamide, lyophilized			
M			
~~Macugen~~	~~0.3 mg~~		~~J2503~~
Magnesium sulfate	500 mg		J3475
Magnevist	per ml		A9579

◀ New   ⤺ Revised   ✔ Reinstated   ~~deleted~~ Deleted

2026 TABLE OF DRUGS / Makena

DRUG NAME	DOSAGE	METHOD OF ADMINISTRATION	HCPCS CODE
Makena	1 mg		J1725
Mannitol	250 mg 25% in 50 ml	IV	J2151 J2150 ◄
	5 mg	INH	J7665
Marcaine			J3490
Margetuximab-cmkb	5 mg	IV	J9353
Marinol	2.5 mg	ORAL	Q0167
Marmine	up to 50 mg	IM, IV	J1240
Marstacimab-hncq	0.5 mg	SC	J7172 ◄
Matulane	50 mg		J8999
Maxipime	500 mg	IV	J0692
MD-76R	per ml		Q9963
MD Gastroview	per ml		Q9963
Mecasermin	1 mg	SC	J2170
Mechlorethamine HCl (nitrogen mustard), HN2	10 mg	IV	J9230
Medrol	per 4 mg	ORAL	J7509
Medroxyprogesterone acetate	1 mg	IM	J1050
Mefoxin	1 g	IV, IM	J0694
Megestrol Acetate			J8999
Meloxicam	1 mg	IV	J1738
Melphalan (evomela)	1 mg	IV	J9246
Melphalan (hepzato)	1 mg	IV	J9248
Melphalan (apotex)	1 mg	IV	J9249
Melphanlan flufenamide	1 mg	IV	J9247
Melphalan HCl	50 mg	IV	J9245
Melphalan, oral	2 mg	ORAL	J8600
Menoject LA	1 mg		J1071
Mepergan injection	up to 50 mg	IM, IV	J2180
Meperidine and promethazine HCl	up to 50 mg	IM, IV	J2180
Meperidine HCl	per 100 mg	IM, IV, SC	J2175
Mepivacaine HCl	per 10 ml	VAR	J0670
Mepolizumab	1 mg	IV	J2182
Mercaptopurine			J8999
Meropenem	100 mg	IV	J2183-J2185
Merrem	100 mg		J2185
Mesna	200 mg	IV	J9209
Mesnex	200 mg	IV	J9209
Metaprel			
concentrated form	per 10 mg	INH	J7667, J7668
unit dose form	per 10 mg	INH	J7669, J7670

◄ New   ↻ Revised   ✓ Reinstated   deleted Deleted

DRUG NAME	DOSAGE	METHOD OF ADMINISTRATION	HCPCS CODE
Metaproterenol sulfate			
concentrated form	per 10 mg	INH	J7667, J7668
unit dose form	per 10 mg	INH	J7669, J7670
Metaraminol bitartrate	per 10 mg	IV, IM, SC	J0380
Metastron	per millicurie		A9600
Methacholine chloride	1 mg	INH	J7674
Methadone HCl	up to 10 mg	IM, SC	J1230
Methergine	up to 0.2 mg		J2210
Methocarbamol	up to 10 ml	IV, IM	J2800
Methotrexate LPF	50 mg	IV, IM, IT, IA	J9260
Methotrexate (accord)	50 mg	IV, IM, IT, IA	J9252
Methotrexate, oral	2.5 mg	ORAL	J8610-J8612
Methotrexate sodium	50 mg	IV, IM, IT, IA	J9260
Methyldopate HCl	up to 250 mg	IV	J0210
Methylergonovine maleate	up to 0.2 mg		J2210
Methylnaltrexone	0.1 mg	SC	J2212
Methylprednisolone acetate	1 mg	IM	J1010
Methylprednisolone, oral	per 4 mg	ORAL	J7509
Methylprednisolone sodium succinate	5 mg	IM	J2919
Metoclopramide HCl	up to 10 mg	IV	J2765
Metoprolol tartrate	1 mg	IM	J0616 ◀
Metrodin	75 IU		J3355
Metronidazole	10 mg	IM	J1836, J3490
Metvixia	1 g	OTH	J7309
Miacalcin	up to 400 units	SC, IM	J0630
Micafungin sodium	1 mg		J2246-J2248
MicRhoGAM	50 mcg		J2788
Midazolam HCl	per 1 mg	IM, IV	J2250-J2253
Miglustat	65 mg	Oral	J1202
Milrinone lactate	5 mg	IV	J2260
Minocine	1 mg		J2265
Minocycline Hydrochloride	1 mg	IV	J2265
Mircera	1 mcg		J0887, J0888
Mirena	52 mg	OTH	J7297, J7298
Mirikizumab-mrkz	1 mg	IM	J2267
Mirvetuximab soravtansine-gynx	1 mg	IM	J9063
Mithracin	2,500 mcg	IV	J9270
Mitomycin	0.2 mg	Ophthalmic	J7315
	5 mg	IV	J9280

◀ New   ⟲ Revised   ✓ Reinstated   ~~deleted~~ Deleted

2026 TABLE OF DRUGS / Mitosol

DRUG NAME	DOSAGE	METHOD OF ADMINISTRATION	HCPCS CODE
Mitosol	0.2 mg	Ophthalmic	J7315
	5 mg	IV	J9280
Mitoxantrone HCl	per 5 mg	IV	J9293
Mogamulizumab-kpkc	1 mg	IV	J9204
Mometasone furoate sinus implant, (sinuva)	10 mcg	OTH	J7402
Monocid, see Cefonicic sodium			
Monoclate-P			
human	per IU	IV	J7190
porcine	per IU	IV	J7191
Monoclonal antibodies, parenteral	5 mg	IV	J7505
Mononine	per IU	IV	J7193
Monovisc			J7327
Morphine sulfate	up to 10 mg	IM, IV, SC	J2270, J2272
preservative-free	10 mg	SC, IM, IV	J2274
Mosunetuzumab-axgb	1 mg	IM	J9350
Motixafortide	0.25 mg	SC	J2277
Moxetumomab Pasudotox-tdfk	0.01 mg	IV	J9313
Moxifloxacin	100 mg	IV	J2280, J2281
Mozobil	1 mg		J2562
Mucomyst			
unit dose form	per gram	INH	J7604, J7608
Mucosol			
injection	100 mg	IV	J0132
unit dose	per gram	INH	J7604, J7608
MultiHance	per ml		A9577
MultiHance Multipack	per ml		A9578
Muromonab-CD3	5 mg	IV	J7505
Muse		OTH	J0275
	1.25 mcg	OTH	J0270
Mustargen	10 mg	IV	J9230
Mutamycin			
	0.2 mg	Ophthalmic	J7315
	5 mg	IV	J9280
Mycamine	1 mg		J2248
Mycophenolate Mofetil	250 mg	ORAL	J7514, J7517, J7519 ◀
Mycophenolic acid	180 mg	ORAL	J7518
Myfortic	180 mg		J7518
Myleran	1 mg		J0594
	2 mg	ORAL	J8510

◀ New   ⤺ Revised   ✔ Reinstated   ~~deleted~~ Deleted

DRUG NAME	DOSAGE	METHOD OF ADMINISTRATION	HCPCS CODE
Mylotarg	5 mg	IV	J9300
Myobloc	per 100 units	IM	J0587
Myochrysine	up to 50 mg	IM	J1600
Myolin	up to 60 mg	IV, IM	J2360
N			
Nabilone	1 mg	ORAL	J8650
Nadofaragene firadenovec-vncg	per therapeutic dose	IM	J9029
Nafcillin			J3490
Nafcillin sodium	20 mg	IM	J2290-J2291 ◄
Naglazyme	1 mg		J1458
Nalbuphine HCl	per 10 mg	IM, IV, SC	J2300
Naloxone HCl	0.1 mg/per 1 mg	IM, IV, SC	J2312-J2313 ◄ ~~J2310, J2311,~~ ~~J3490~~
Naltrexone			J3490
Naltrexone, depot form	1 mg	IM	J2315
Nandrobolic L.A.	up to 50 mg	IM	J2320
Nandrolone decanoate	up to 50 mg	IM	J2320
~~Narcan~~	~~1 mg~~	~~IM, IV, SC~~	~~J2310~~
Naropin	1 mg		J2795
Nasahist B	per 10 mg	IM, SC, IV	J0945
Nasal vaccine inhalation		INH	J3530
Natalizumab	1 mg	IV	J2323
Natrecor	0.1 mg		J2325
Navane, *see* Thiothixene			
Navelbine	per 10 mg	IV	J9390
Naxitamab-gqgk	1 mg	IV	J9348
ND Stat	per 10 mg	IM, SC, IV	J0945
Nebcin	up to 80 mg	IM, IV	J3260
NebuPent	per 300 mg	INH	J2545, J7676
Necitumumab	1 mg	IV	J9295
Nelarabine	50 mg	IV	J9261
Nembutal Sodium Solution	per 50 mg	IM, IV, OTH	J2515
Neocyten	up to 60 mg	IV, IM	J2360
Neo-Durabolic	up to 50 mg	IM	J2320
Neoquess	up to 20 mg	IM	J0500
Neoral	100 mg		J7502
	25 mg		J7515
Neostigmine methylsulfate	up to 0.5 mg	IM, IV, SC	J2710
Nesiritide	0.1 mg	IV	J2325
Netupitant 300 mg and palonosetron 0.5 mg		ORAL	J8655

◄ New   ⤺ Revised   ✓ Reinstated   ~~deleted~~ Deleted

DRUG NAME	DOSAGE	METHOD OF ADMINISTRATION	HCPCS CODE
Neumega	5 mg	SC	J2355
Neupogen			
(G-CSF)	1 mcg	SC, IV	J1442
Neutrexin	per 25 mg	IV	J3305
Nicardipine	0.1 mg	IV	J2404
Nipent	per 10 mg	IV	J9268
Nithlodote			
Sodium nitrate and sodium thiosulfate	3 mg/125 mg	IM	J0211
Nitroglycerin	5 mg	IM	J2305
Nivol relatlimab	3 mg/1 mg	IM	J9298
Nivolumab	1 mg	IV	J9299
Nivolumab and hyaluronidase	2 mg	IV	J9289 ◄
Nogapendekin pmin	1 mcg	OTH	J9028 ◄
Nolvadex			J8999
Nordryl	up to 50 mg	IV, IM	J1200
	50 mg	ORAL	Q0163
Norflex	up to 60 mg	IV, IM	J2360
Norzine	up to 10 mg	IM	J3280
Not otherwise classified drugs			J3490
other than inhalation solution administered through DME			J7799
inhalation solution administered through DME			J7699
anti-neoplastic			J9999
chemotherapeutic		ORAL	J8999
immunosuppressive			J7599
nonchemotherapeutic		ORAL	J8499
Novantrone	per 5 mg	IV	J9293
Novarel	per 1,000 USP Units		J0725
Novolin	per 5 units		J1815
	per 50 units		J1817
Novolog	per 5 units		J1815
	per 50 units		J1817
Novo Seven	1 mcg	IV	J7189
Novoeight			J7182
NPH	5 units	SC	J1815
Nplate	100 units		J0587
	~~10 mcg~~		~~J2796~~
Nubain	per 10 mg	IM, IV, SC	J2300
Nulecit	12.5 mg		J2916
Nulojix	1 mg	IV	J0485
Numorphan	up to 1 mg	IV, SC, IM	J2410

◄ New   ↻ Revised   ✓ Reinstated   ~~deleted~~ Deleted

DRUG NAME	DOSAGE	METHOD OF ADMINISTRATION	HCPCS CODE
Numorphan H.P.	up to 1 mg	IV, SC, IM	J2410
Nusinersen	0.1 mg	IV	J2326
Nutropin	1 mg		J2941
O			
Oasis Burn Matrix	per square centimeter		Q4103
Oasis Wound Matrix	per square centimeter		Q4102
Obinutuzumab	10 mg		J9301
Ocriplasmin	0.125 mg	IV	J7316
Ocrelizumab	1 mg	IV	J2350
Ocrelizumab and hyaluronidase-ocsq	1 mg	IM	J2351 ◄
Octagam	500 mg	IV	J1568
Octreotide Acetate, ~~injection~~	1 mg	IM	J2353
	25 mcg	IV, SQ	J2354
Oculinum	per unit	IM	J0585
Ofatumumab	10 mg	IV	J9302
Ofev			J8499
Ofirmev	10 mg	IV	J0131
O-Flex	up to 60 mg	IV, IM	J2360
Oforta	10 mg		J8562
Olanzapine	1 mg, 0.5 mg	IM	J2358-J2359
Olaratumab	10 mg	IV	J9285
Olipudase alfa-rpcp	1 mg	IM	J0218
Omadacycline	1 mg	IV	J0121
Omacetaxine Mepesuccinate	0.01 mg	IV	J9262
Omalizumab	5 mg	SC	J2357
Omnipaque	per ml		Q9965, Q9966, Q9967
Omnipen-N	up to 500 mg	IM, IV	J0290
	per 1.5 gm	IM, IV	J0295
Omniscan	per ml		A9579
Omnitrope	1 mg		J2941
Omontys	0.1 mg	IV, SC	J0890
OnabotulinumtoxinA	1 unit	IM	J0585
Onasemnogene abeparvovec-xioi, per treatment, vector genomes	up to 5x10 15	IM	J3399
Oncaspar	per single dose vial	IM, IV	J9266
Oncovin	1 mg	IV	J9370
Ondansetron HCl	1 mg	IV	J2405
	1 mg	ORAL	Q0162
Onivyde	1 mg		J9205
Opana	up to 1 mg		J2410
Opdivo	1 mg		J9299

◄ New   ↻ Revised   ✔ Reinstated   ~~deleted~~ Deleted

2026 TABLE OF DRUGS / Oprelvekin

DRUG NAME	DOSAGE	METHOD OF ADMINISTRATION	HCPCS CODE
Oprelvekin	5 mg	SC	J2355
Optimark	per ml		A9579
Optiray	per ml		Q9966, Q9967
Optison	per ml		Q9956
Oraminic II	per 10 mg	IM, SC, IV	J0945
Orapred	per 5 mg	ORAL	J7510
Orbactiv	10 mg		J2407
Orencia	10 mg		J0129
Oritavancin (kimyrsa)	10 mg	IV	J2406
Oritavancin (orbactiv)	10 mg	IV	J2407
Ormazine	up to 50 mg	IM, IV	J3230
Orphenadrine citrate	up to 60 mg	IV, IM	J2360
Orphenate	up to 60 mg	IV, IM	J2360
Orthovisc		OTH	J7324
Or-Tyl	up to 20 mg	IM	J0500
Osmitrol			J7799
Ovidrel			J3490
Oxacillin sodium	up to 250 mg	IM, IV	J2700
Oxaliplatin	0.5 mg	IV	J9263
Oxilan	per ml		Q9967
Oxlumo	0.5 mg	IV	J0224
Oxymorphone HCl	up to 1 mg	IV, SC, IM	J2410
Oxytetracycline HCl	up to 50 mg	IM	J2460
Oxytocin	up to 10 units	IV, IM	J2590
Ozurdex	0.1 mg		J7312
P			
Paclitaxel	1 mg	IV	J9267
Paclitaxel protein-bound particles	1 mg	IV	J9259, J9264
Pafolacianine	0.1 mg	IM	J9603
Palifermin	50 mcg	IV	J2425
Paliperidone palmitate	1 mg	IM	J2426-J2427
Palonosetron HCl	25 mcg	IV	J2468-J2469
Netupitant 300 mg and palonosetron 0.5 mg		ORAL	J8655
Pamidronate disodium	per 30 mg	IV	J2430
Panhematin	1 mg		J1640
Panitumumab	10 mg	IV	J9303
Pantoprazole	40 mg	IM	J2470-J2472 ◄ J2470, J2471
Papaverine HCl	up to 60 mg	IV, IM	J2440
Paragard T 380 A		OTH	J7300

◄ New   ⮂ Revised   ✔ Reinstated   deleted Deleted

DRUG NAME	DOSAGE	METHOD OF ADMINISTRATION	HCPCS CODE
Paraplatin	50 mg	IV	J9045
Paricalcitol, injection	1 mcg	IV, IM	J2501
Pasireotide, long acting	1 mg	IV	J2502
Pathogen(s) test for platelets		OTH	P9100
Patisiran	0.1 mg	IV	J0222
Peforomist	20 mcg		J7606
Pegademase bovine	25 IU		J2504
~~Pegaptinib~~	~~0.3 mg~~	~~OTH~~	~~J2503~~
Pegaspargase	per single dose vial	IM, IV	J9266
Pegasys			J3490
Pegcetacoplan	1 mg	IVT	J2781
Pegfilgrastim-bmez, biosimilar, (ziextenzo)	0.5 mg	IM	Q5120
Pegfilgrastim-cbqv	0.5 mg	IM	Q5111
Pegfilgrastim-fpgk	0.5 mg	IM	Q5127
Pegfilgrastim-jmdb	0.5 mg	SC	Q5108
Pegfilgrastim-pbbk	0.5 mg	IM	Q5130
Peginesatide	0.1 mg	IV, SC	J0890
Peg-Intron			J3490
Pegloticase	1 mg	IV	J2507
Pegunigalsidase	1 mg	IV	J2508
Pembrolizumab	1 mg	IV	J9271
Pemetrexed	10 mg	IV	J9292, J9294, J9296-J9297, J9305, J9314, J9322-J9324 ◀
Pemetrexed (Pemfexy)	10 mg	IV	J9304
Penicillin G Benzathine	100,000 units	IM	J0561
Penicillin G Benzathine and Penicillin G Procaine	100,000 units	IM	J0558
Penicillin G potassium	up to 600,000 units	IM, IV	J2540
Penicillin G procaine, aqueous	up to 600,000 units	IM, IV	J2510
Penicillin G Sodium			J3490
Pentam	per 300 mg		J7676
Pentamidine isethionate	per 300 mg	INH, IM	J2545, J7676
Pentastarch, 10%	100 ml		J2513
Pentazocine HCl	30 mg	IM, SC, IV	J3070
Pentobarbital sodium	per 50 mg	IM, IV, OTH	J2515
Pentostatin	per 10 mg	IV	J9268
Peramivir	1 mg	IV	J2547
Perjeta	1 mg		J9306
Permapen	up to 600,000	IM	J0561

◀ New ↻ Revised ✔ Reinstated ~~deleted~~ Deleted

2026 TABLE OF DRUGS / Perphenazine

DRUG NAME	DOSAGE	METHOD OF ADMINISTRATION	HCPCS CODE
Perphenazine			
injection	up to 5 mg	IM, IV	J3310
tablets	4 mg	ORAL	Q0175
Persantine IV	per 10 mg	IV	J1245
Pertuzumab	1 mg	IV	J9306
Pet Imaging			
Fluciclovine F-18, diagnostic	1 millicurie	IV	A9588
Gallium Ga-68, dotatate, diagnostic	0.1 millicurie	IV	A9587
Gallium ga-68, psma-11, (ucla)	1 millicurie	IV	A9594
Gallium ga-68, psma-11, (ucsf)	1 millicurie	IV	A9593
Pfizerpen	up to 600,000 units	IM, IV	J2540
Pfizerpen A.S.	up to 600,000 units	IM, IV	J2510
Phenadoz			J8498
Phenazine 25	up to 50 mg	IM, IV	J2550
	12.5 mg	ORAL	Q0169
Phenazine 50	up to 50 mg	IM, IV	J2550
	12.5 mg	ORAL	Q0169
Phenergan	12.5 mg	ORAL	Q0169
	up to 50 mg	IM, IV	J2550
			J8498
Phenobarbital sodium	up to 120 mg	IM, IV	J2560-J2561
Phentolamine mesylate	up to 5 mg	IM, IV	J2760
Phenylephrine hydrochloride (biorphen)	20 mcg	IM	J2371-J2373
Phenylephrine 10.16 mg/Ketorolac 2.88	1 ml	VAR	J1097
Phenytoin sodium	per 50 mg	IM, IV	J1165
Photofrin	75 mg	IV	J9600
Phytonadione (Vitamin K)	per 1 mg	IM, SC, IV	J3430
Piperacillin/Tazobactam Sodium, injection	1.125 g	IV	J2543
Pitocin	up to 10 units	IV, IM	J2590
Plantinol AQ	10 mg	IV	J9060
Plasma			
cryoprecipitate reduced	each unit	IV	P9044
pooled multiple donor, frozen	each unit	IV	P9023, P9070
(single donor), pathogen reduced, frozen	each unit	IV	P9071
Plasminogen TVMH	1 mg		J2998
Plas+SD	each unit	IV	P9023
Platelets, pheresis, pathogen reduced	each unit	IV	P9073
Pathogen(s) test for platelets		OTH	P9100
Platinol	10 mg	IV, IM	J9060

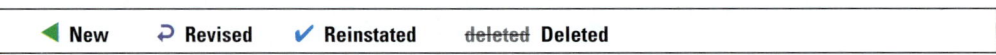
◀ New   ⤾ Revised   ✓ Reinstated   ~~deleted~~ Deleted

2026 TABLE OF DRUGS / Prochlorperazine

DRUG NAME	DOSAGE	METHOD OF ADMINISTRATION	HCPCS CODE
Plazomicin	5 mg	IV	J0291
Plerixafor	1 mg	SC	J2562
Plicamycin	2,500 mcg	IV	J9270
Polatuzumab vedotin	1 mg	IV	J9309
Polocaine	per 10 ml	VAR	J0670
Polycillin-N	up to 500 mg	IM, IV	J0290
	per 1.5 gm	IM, IV	J0295
Polygam	500 mg		J1566
Porfimer Sodium	75 mg	IV	J9600
Portrazza	1 mg		J9295
Positron emission tomography radiopharmaceutical, diagnostic			
for non-tumor identification, NOC		IV	A9598
for tumor identification, NOC		IV	A9597
Potassium chloride	per 2 mEq	IV	J3480
Potassium Chloride	up to 1,000 cc		J7120
Pozelimab	1 mg	IM	J9376
Pralatrexate	1 mg	IV	J9307
Pralidoxime chloride	up to 1 g	IV, IM, SC	J2730
Predalone-50	up to 1 ml	IM	J2650
Predcor-25	up to 1 ml	IM	J2650
Predcor-50	up to 1 ml	IM	J2650
Predicort-50	up to 1 ml	IM	J2650
Prednisolone acetate	up to 1 ml	IM	J2650
Prednisolone, oral	5 mg	ORAL	J7510
Prednisone, immediate release or delayed release	1 mg	ORAL	J7512
Predoject-50	up to 1 ml	IM	J2650
Pregnyl	per 1,000 USP units	IM	J0725
Premarin Intravenous	per 25 mg	IV, IM	J1410
Prescription, chemotherapeutic, not otherwise specified		ORAL	J8999
Prescription, nonchemotherapeutic, not otherwise specified		ORAL	J8499
Prialt	1 mcg		J2278
Primacor	5 mg	IV	J2260
Primatrix	per square centimeter		Q4110
Primaxin	per 250 mg	IV, IM	J0743
Priscoline HCl	up to 25 mg	IV	J2670
Privigen	500 mg	IV	J1459
~~Probuphine System Kit~~			~~J0570~~
Procainamide HCl	up to 1 g	IM, IV	J2690
Prochlorperazine	up to 10 mg	IM, IV	J0780
			J8498

◀ New   ↻ Revised   ✔ Reinstated   ~~deleted~~ Deleted

2026 TABLE OF DRUGS / Prochlorperazine maleate

DRUG NAME	DOSAGE	METHOD OF ADMINISTRATION	HCPCS CODE
Prochlorperazine maleate	5 mg	ORAL	Q0164
	5 mg		S0183
Procrit			J0885
			Q4081
Pro-Depo, see Hydroxyprogesterone Caproate			
Profasi HP	per 1,000 USP units	IM	J0725
Profilnine Heat-Treated			
non-recombinant	per IU	IV	J7193
recombinant	per IU	IU	J7195, J7200-J7202
complex	per IU	IV	J7194
Profonol	10 mg/ml		J3490
Progestaject	per 50 mg		J2675
Progesterone	per 50 mg	IM	J2675
Prograf			
oral	1 mg	ORAL	J7507
parenteral	5 mg		J7525
Prohance Multipack	per ml		A9576, A9579
Prokine	50 mcg	IV	J2820
Proleukin	per single use vial	IM, IV	J9015
Prolia	1 mg		J0897
Prolixin Decanoate	up to 25 mg	IM, SC	J2680
Promazine HCl	up to 25 mg	IM	J2950
Promethazine			J8498
Promethazine HCl			
injection	up to 50 mg	IM, IV	J2550
oral	12.5 mg	ORAL	Q0169
Promethegan			J8498
Pronestyl	up to 1 g	IM, IV	J2690
Proplex SX-T			
non-recombinant	per IU	IV	J7193
recombinant	per IU		J7195, J7200-J7202
complex	per IU	IV	J7194
Proplex T			
non-recombinant	per IU	IV	J7193
recombinant	per IU		J7195, J7200-J7202
complex	per IU	IV	J7194
Propofol	10 mg	IV	J2704
Propranolol HCl	up to 1 mg	IV	J1800

◀ New　⤺ Revised　✔ Reinstated　~~deleted~~ Deleted

DRUG NAME	DOSAGE	METHOD OF ADMINISTRATION	HCPCS CODE
Prorex-25			
	up to 50 mg	IM, IV	J2550
	12.5 mg	ORAL	Q0169
Prorex-50	up to 50 mg	IM, IV	J2550
	12.5 mg	ORAL	Q0169
Prostaglandin E1	per 1.25 mcg		J0270
Prostaphlin	up to 1 g	IM, IV	J2690
Prostigmin	up to 0.5 mg	IM, IV, SC	J2710
Prostin VR Pediatric	0.5 mg		J0270
Protamine sulfate	per 10 mg	IV	J2720
Protein C Concentrate	10 IU	IV	J2724
Prothazine	up to 50 mg	IM, IV	J2550
	12.5 mg	ORAL	Q0169
Prothrombin complex concentrate (human), kcentra	per i.u. of factor ix activity	OTH	J7165, J7168
Protirelin	per 250 mcg	IV	J2725
Protonix			J3490
Protopam Chloride	up to 1 g	IV, IM, SC	J2730
Provenge			Q2043
Proventil			
concentrated form	1 mg	INH	J7610, J7611
unit dose form	1 mg	INH	J7609, J7613
Provocholine	per 1 mg		J7674
Prozine-50	up to 25 mg	IM	J2950
Pulmicort Respules			
concentrated form	0.25 mg	INH	J7633, J7634
unit dose	0.5 mg	INH	J7626, J7627
Pulmozyme	per mg		J7639
Pyridoxine HCl	100 mg		J3415
Q			
Quelicin	up to 20 mg	IV, IM	J0330
Quinupristin/dalfopristin	500 mg (150/350)	IV	J2770
Qutenza	per square cm		J7336
R			
Ramucirumab	5 mg	IV	J9308
Ranibizumab	0.1 mg	OTH, IM	J2778, Q5128
Rapamune	1 mg	ORAL	J7520
Rasburicase	0.5 mg	IV	J2783
Ravulizumab-cwvz	10 mg	IV	J1303
Rebif	11 mcg		Q3026
Reclast	1 mg		J3489

◀ New   ⮂ Revised   ✔ Reinstated   ~~deleted~~ Deleted

DRUG NAME	DOSAGE	METHOD OF ADMINISTRATION	HCPCS CODE
Recombinate			
human	per IU	IV	J7190
porcine	per IU	IV	J7191
recombinant	per IU	IV	J7192
Recombivax			J3490
Redisol	up to 1,000 mcg	IM, SC	J3420
Regadenoson	0.1 mg	IV	J2785
Regitine	up to 5 mg	IM, IV	J2760
Reglan	up to 10 mg	IV	J2765
Regular	5 units	SC	J1815
Relefact TRH	per 250 mcg	IV	J2725
Relistor	0.1 mg	SC	J2212
Remestemcel-l-rknd	per therapeutic dose		J3402 ◄
Remicade	10 mg	IM, IV	J1745
Remimazolam	1 mg	IM	J2249
Remodulin	1 mg		J3285
Renflexis			Q5102
ReoPro	10 mg	IV	J0130
Resectisol			J7799
Reslizumab	1 mg	IV	J2786
Retavase	18.1 mg	IV	J2993
Reteplase	18.8 mg	IV	J2993
Retifanlimab-dlwr	1 mg	IM	J9345
Retisert			J7311
Retrovir	10 mg	IV	J3485
Revakinagene taroretcel-lwey	per implant		J3403 ◄
Revefenacin inhalation solution	—	INH	J7677
Rezafungin	1 mg	IM	J0349
Rheomacrodex	500 ml	IV	J7100
Rhesonativ	300 mcg	IM	J2790
	50 mg		J2788
Rheumatrex Dose Pack	2.5 mg	ORAL	J8610
Rho(D)			
immune globulin		IM, IV	J2791
immune globulin, human	1 dose package/ 300 mcg	IM	J2790
	50 mg	IM	J2788
immune globulin, human, solvent detergent	100	IV, IU	J2792
RhoGAM	300 mcg	IM	J2790
	50 mg		J2788
Rhophylac	100 IU	IM, IV	J2791

◄ New   ⮂ Revised   ✔ Reinstated   ~~deleted~~ Deleted

2026 TABLE OF DRUGS / Saline solution

DRUG NAME	DOSAGE	METHOD OF ADMINISTRATION	HCPCS CODE	
Riastap	100 mg		J7178	
Rifadin			J3490	
Rifampin	1 mg	IM	J2804, J3490	◀
Rilonacept	1 mg	SC	J2793	
RimabotulinumtoxinB	100 units	IM	J0587	
Rimso-50	50 ml		J1212	
Ringers lactate infusion	up to 1,000 cc	IV	J7120, J7121	
Risankizumab	1 mg	IV	J2327	
Risperdal Consta	0.5 mg		J2794	
Risperidone	0.5 mg	IM	J2794	
Risperidone (perseris)	0.5 mg	IV	J2798	
Risperidone (rykindo)	0.5 mg	IV	J2801	
Risperidone (uzedy)	1 mg	IV	J2799	
Rituxan	100 mg	IV	J9312	
Rituximab	100 mg	IV	J9312	
Rituximab-abbs	10 mg	IV	Q5115	
Rituximab-arrx, biosimilar, (riabni)	10 mg	IV	Q5123	
Rituximab-pvvr, biosimilar, (Ruxience)	10 mg	IV	Q5119	
Rixubis			J7200	
Robaxin	up to 10 ml	IV, IM	J2800	
Rocephin	per 250 mg	IV, IM	J0696	
Roferon-A	3 million units	SC, IM	J9213	
Rolapitant	0.5 mg	IV	J2797	
Rolapitant, oral, 1 mg	1 mg	ORAL	J8670	
Romidepsin lyophilized	1 mg	IV	J9319	
Romidepsin, non-lyophilized	0.1 mg	IV	J9318	
~~Romiplostim~~	~~10 mcg~~	~~SC~~	~~J2796~~	
Romiplostim	10 mcg	SC	J2802	◀
Romosozumab-aqqg	1 mg	IV	J3111	
Ropivacaine Hydrochloride	1 mg	OTH	J2795	
Rozanolixizumab-noli	1 mg	IV	J9333	
Rubex	10 mg	IV	J9000	
Rubramin PC	up to 1,000 mcg	IM, SC	J3420	
S				
Saizen	1 mg		J2941	
Saline solution	10 ml		A4216	
5% dextrose	500 ml	IV	J7042	
infusion	250 cc	IV	J7050	
	1,000 cc	IV	J7030	
sterile	500 ml = 1 unit	IV, OTH	J7040	

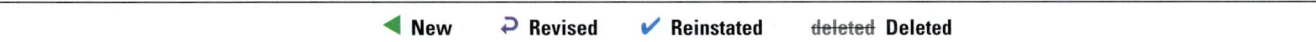

◀ New   ⤺ Revised   ✔ Reinstated   ~~deleted~~ Deleted

2026 TABLE OF DRUGS / Sandimmune

DRUG NAME	DOSAGE	METHOD OF ADMINISTRATION	HCPCS CODE
Sandimmune	25 mg	ORAL	J7515
	100 mg	ORAL	J7502
	250 mg	OTH	J7516
Sandoglobulin, see Immune globulin intravenous (human)			
Sandostatin, Lar Depot	25 mcg		J2354
	1 mg	IM	J2353
Sargramostim (GM-CSF)	50 mcg	IV	J2820
Sculptra	0.5 mg	IV	Q2028
Sebelelipase alfa	1 mg	IV	J2840
Secukinumab	1 mg	IV	J3247
Selestoject	per 4 mg	IM, IV	J0702
Sermorelin acetate	1 mcg	SC	Q0515
Serostim	1 mg		J2941
Sevelamer carbonate	20 mg	ORAL	J0601 ◄
Sevelamer PDR carbonate	20 mg	ORAL	J0602 ◄
Sevelamer hydrochloride	20 mg	ORAL	J0603 ◄
Signifor LAR	20 ml		J2502
Siltuximab	10 mg	IV	J2860
Simponi Aria	1 mg		J1602
Simulect	20 mg		J0480
Sincalide	5 mcg	IV, IM	J2805 ~~J2806~~
Sinografin	per ml		Q9963
Sinusol-B	per 10 mg	IM, SC, IV	J0945
Sirolimus	1 mg	ORAL	J7520
Sirolimus protien-bound	1 mg	IM	J9331
Sivextro	1 mg		J3090
Skyla	13.5 mg	OTH	J7301
Smz-TMP			J3490
Sodium Chloride	1,000 cc		J7030
	500 ml = 1 unit		J7040
	500 ml		A4217
	250 cc		J7050
Bacteriostatic	10 ml		A4216
Sodium Chloride Concentrate			J7799
Sodium ferricgluconate in sucrose	12.5 mg		J2916
Sodium Hyaluronate			J3490
Euflexxa			J7323
Hyalgan			J7321
Orthovisc			J7324
Sodium Thiosulfate	100 mg	IM	J0208-J0209

◄ New ⇌ Revised ✓ Reinstated ~~deleted~~ Deleted

2026 TABLE OF DRUGS / Synribo

DRUG NAME	DOSAGE	METHOD OF ADMINISTRATION	HCPCS CODE	
Solganal	up to 50 mg	IM	J2910	
~~Soliris~~	~~10 mg~~		~~J1300~~	
Solu-Cortef	up to 50 mg	IV, IM, SC	J1710	
	100 mg		J1720	
Solurex	1 mg	IM, IV, OTH	J1100	
~~Solurex LA~~	~~1 mg~~	~~IM~~	~~J1094~~	
Somatrem	1 mg	SC	J2940	
Somatropin	1 mg	SC	J2941	
Somatulin Depot	1 mg		J1930	
Sparine	up to 25 mg	IM	J2950	
Spasmoject	up to 20 mg	IM	J0500	
Spectinomycin HCl	up to 2 g	IM	J3320	
Spesolimab-sbzo	1 mg	IM	J1747	
Sporanox	50 mg	IV	J1835	
Staphcillin, *see* Methicillin sodium				
Stelara	1 mg		J3357	
Stilphostrol	250 mg	IV	J9165	
Streptase	250,000 IU	IV	J2995	
Streptokinase	per 250,000	IU, IV	J2995	
Streptomycin	up to 1 g	IM	J3000	
Streptomycin Sulfate	up to 1 g	IM	J3000	
Streptozocin	1 gm	IV	J9320	
Strontium-89 chloride	per millicurie		A9600	
Sublimaze	0.1 mg	IM, IV	J3010	
Succinylcholine chloride	up to 20 mg	IV, IM	J0330	
Sucroferric oxyhydroxide	5 mg	ORAL	J0605	◀
Sufentanil Citrate			J3490	
Sulfameth/trimethoprim	5 mg/1 mg	IM	J2865	◀
Sumarel Dosepro	6 mg		J3030	
Sumatriptan succinate	6 mg	SC	J3030	
Supartz		OTH	J7321	
Supprelin LA	50 mg		J9226	
Surostrin	up to 20 mg	IV, IM	J0330	
~~Sus-Phrine~~	~~up to 1 ml ampule~~	~~SC, IM~~	~~J0171~~	
Sutimlimab-jome	10 mg	IM	J1302	
Susvimo	0.1 mg		J2779	
Synercid	500 mg (150/350)	IV	J2770	
Synkavite	per 1 mg	IM, SC, IV	J3430	
Synribo	0.01 mg		J9262	

◀ New   ⮂ Revised   ✔ Reinstated   ~~deleted~~ Deleted

2026 TABLE OF DRUGS / Syntocinon

DRUG NAME	DOSAGE	METHOD OF ADMINISTRATION	HCPCS CODE
Syntocinon	up to 10 units	IV, IM	J2590
Synvisc and Synvisc-One	1 mg	OTH	J7325
Syrex	10 ml		A4216
Sytobex	1,000 mcg	IM, SC	J3420
T			
Tacrolimus			
(Envarsus XR)	0.25 mg	ORAL	J7503
oral, extended release	0.1 mg	ORAL	J7508
oral, immediate release	1 mg	ORAL	J7507
oral, suspension	0.1 mg	ORAL	J7521 ◄
parenteral	5 mg	IV	J7525
Tafasitamab	2 mg	IV	J9349
Tagraxofusp-erzs	10 mcg	IV	J9269
Taliglucerase Alfa	10 units	IV	J3060
Talimogene laherparepvec	per 1 million plaque forming units	IV	J9325
Talquetamab-tgvs	0.25 mg	SC	J3055
Talwin	30 mg	IM, SC, IV	J3070
Tamoxifen Citrate			J8999
Taractan, see Chlorprothixene			
Tarlatamab-dlle	1 mg	IM	J9026 ◄
Taurolidine (heparin sodium 100 units)	1.35 mg		J0911
Taxol	1 mg	IV	J9267
Taxotere	20 mg	IV	J9171
Tazicef	per 500 mg		J0713
Tazidime, see Ceftazidime Technetium TC Sestambi	per dose		A9500
			J0713
Tebentafusp-tebn	1 mcg	IM	J9274
Teclistamab-cqyv	0.5 mg	IM	J9380
Tedizolid phosphate	1 mg	IV	J3090
TEEV	1 mg	IM	J3121
Teflaro	1 mg		J0712
Telavancin	10 mg	IV	J3095
Temodar	5 mg	ORAL	J8700, J9328
Temozolomide	1 mg	IV	J9328
	5 mg	ORAL	J8700
Temsirolimus	1 mg	IV	J9330
Tenecteplase	1 mg	IV	J3101
Teniposide	50 mg		Q2017
~~Tepadina~~	~~15 mg~~		~~J9340~~
Teplizumab-mzwv	5 mcg	IM	J9381

◄ New   ⇌ Revised   ✔ Reinstated   ~~deleted~~ Deleted

DRUG NAME	DOSAGE	METHOD OF ADMINISTRATION	HCPCS CODE
Teprotumumab-trbw	10 mg	IV	J3241
Tequin	10 mg	IV	J1590
Terbutaline sulfate	up to 1 mg	SC, IV	J3105
concentrated form	per 1 mg	INH	J7680
unit dose form	per 1 mg	INH	J7681
Teriparatide	10 mcg	SC	J3110
Terramycin IM	up to 50 mg	IM	J2460
Testa-C	1 mg		J1071
Testadiate	1 mg	IM	J3121
Testadiate-Depo	1 mg		J1071
Testaject-LA	1 mg		J1071
Testaqua	up to 50 mg	IM	J3140
Test-Estro Cypionates	1 mg		J1071
Test-Estro-C	1 mg		J1071
Testex	up to 100 mg	IM	J3150
Testo AQ	up to 50 mg		J3140
Testoject-50	up to 50 mg	IM	J3140
Testoject-LA	1 mg		J1071
Testone			
LA 100	1 mg	IM	J3121
LA 200	1 mg	IM	J3121
Testopel Pellets			J3490
Testosterone Aqueous	up to 50 mg	IM	J3140
Testosterone cypionate	1 mg	IM	J1071, J1072 ◀
Testosterone enanthate	1 mg	IM	J3121
Testosterone undecanoate	1 mg	IM	J3145
Testradiol 90/4	1 mg	IM	J3121
Testrin PA	1 mg	IM	J3121
Testro AQ	up to 50 mg		J3140
Tetanus immune globulin, human	up to 250 units	IM	J1670
Tetracycline	up to 250 mg	IM, IV	J0120
Tezepelumab-ekko	1 mg		J2356
Thallous Chloride TI-201	per MCI		A9505
Theelin Aqueous	per 1 mg	IM	J1435
Theophylline	per 40 mg	IV	J2810
Thiamine HCl	100 mg		J3411
Thiethylperazine maleate			
injection	up to 10 mg	IM	J3280
oral	10 mg	ORAL	Q0174
Thiotepa (tepylute)	1 mg ~~15 mg~~	IV	J9341 ~~J9340~~ ◀
not otherwise specified	1 mg	IV	J9342 ◀

◀ New   ↻ Revised   ✓ Reinstated   ~~deleted~~ Deleted

2026 TABLE OF DRUGS / Thorazine

DRUG NAME	DOSAGE	METHOD OF ADMINISTRATION	HCPCS CODE
Thorazine	up to 50 mg	IM, IV	J3230
Thrombate III	per IU		J7197
Thymoglobulin (see also Immune globulin)			
anti-thymocyte globulin, equine	250 mg	IV	J7504
anti-thymocyte globulin, rabbit	25 mg	IV	J7511
Thypinone	per 250 mcg	IV	J2725
Thyrogen	0.9 mg	IM, SC	J3240
Thyrotropin Alfa, injection	0.9 mg	IM, SC	J3240
Ticon			
injection	up to 200 mg	IM	J3250
oral	250 mg	ORAL	Q0173
Tigan			
injection	up to 200 mg	IM	J3250
oral	250 mg	ORAL	Q0173
Tigecycline	1 mg	IV	J3243, J3244
Tiject-20			
injection	up to 200 mg	IM	J3250
oral	250 mg	ORAL	Q0173
Tinzaparin	1,000 IU	SC	J1655
Tirofiban Hydrochloride, injection	0.25 mg	IM, IV	J3246
Tislelizumab-jsgr	1 mg	IM	J9329
TNKase	1 mg	IV	J3101
Tobi	300 mg	INH	J7682, J7685
Tobramycin, inhalation solution	300 mg	INH	J7682, J7685
Tobramycin sulfate	up to 80 mg	IM, IV	J3260
Tocilizumab	1 mg	IV	J3262
Tofersen	1 mg	IM, IV	J1304
Tofranil, see Imipramine HCl			
Tolazoline HCl	up to 25 mg	IV	J2670
Toposar	10 mg		J9181
Topotecan	0.25 mg	ORAL	J8705
	0.1 mg	IV	J9351
Toradol	per 15 mg	IM, IV	J1885
Torecan			
injection	up to 10 mg	IM	J3280
oral	10 mg	ORAL	Q0174
Toripalimab	1 mg	IM	J3263
Torisel	1 mg		J9330

◀ New   ⇄ Revised   ✔ Reinstated   deleted Deleted

2026 TABLE OF DRUGS / Trilaciclib

DRUG NAME	DOSAGE	METHOD OF ADMINISTRATION	HCPCS CODE	
Tornalate				
concentrated form	per mg	INH	J7628	
unit dose	per mg	INH	J7629	
Torsemide	10 mg/ml	IV	J3265	
Totacillin-N	up to 500 mg	IM, IV	J0290	
	per 1.5 gm	IM, IV	J0295	
Trabectedin	0.1 mg	IV	J9352	
Tranexamic acid	5 mg	IV	J3290	◄
Trastuzumab	10 mg	IV	J9355	
Trastuzumab-anns (kanjinti)	10 mg	IV	Q5117	
Trastuzumab-dkst	10 mg	IV	Q5114	
Trastuzumab-dttb	10 mg	IV	Q5112	
Trastuzumab-pkrb	10 mg	IV	Q5113	
Trastuzumab-qyyp (trazimera)	10 mg	IV	Q5116	
Trastuzumab and Hyaluronidase	10 mg	IV	J9356	
Travoprost intracameral implant	1 mcg		J7355	
Treanda	1 mg	IV	J3490	↩
Trelstar	3.75 mg		J3315	
Tremelimumab-actl	1 mg	IM	J9347	
Treosulfan	50 mg	IM	J0614	◄
Treprostinil	1 mg		J3285, J7686	
Trexall	2.5 mg	ORAL	J8610	
Triam-A	1 mg		J3300	
	per 10 mg	IM	J3301	
Triamcinolone				
concentrated form	per 1 mg	INH	J7683	
unit dose	per 1 mg	INH	J7684	
Triamcinolone acetonide	1 mg		J3300	
	per 10 mg	IM	J3301	
Triamcinolone acetonide XR	1 mg	IM	J3304	
Triamcinolone diacetate	per 5 mg	IM	J3302	
Triamcinolone hexacetonide	per 5 mg	VAR	J3303	
Triesence	1 mg		J3300	
	per 10 mg	IM	J3301	
~~Triethylene thio-Phosphoramide/T~~	~~15 mg~~		~~J9340~~	
Triflupromazine HCl	up to 20 mg	IM, IV	J3400	
Tri-Kort	1 mg		J3300	
	per 10 mg	IM	J3301	
Trilaciclib	1 mg	IV	J1448	

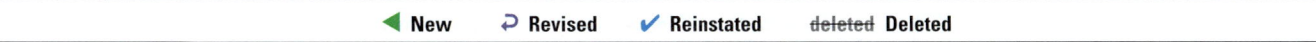

◄ New   ↩ Revised   ✔ Reinstated   ~~deleted~~ Deleted

DRUG NAME	DOSAGE	METHOD OF ADMINISTRATION	HCPCS CODE
Trilafon	4 mg	ORAL	Q0175
	up to 5 mg	IM, IV	J3310
Trilog	1 mg		J3300
	per 10 mg	IM	J3301
Trilone	per 5 mg		J3302
Trimethobenzamide HCl			
injection	up to 200 mg	IM	J3250
oral	250 mg	ORAL	Q0173
Trimetrexate glucuronate	per 25 mg	IV	J3305
Triptorelin Pamoate	3.75 mg	SC	J3315
Triptorelin XR	3.75 mg	SC	J3316
Trisenox	1 mg	IV	J9017
Trobicin	up to 2 g	IM	J3320
Trovan	100 mg	IV	J0200
Tysabri	1 mg		J2323
Tyvaso	1.74 mg		J7686
U			
Ublituximab-xiiy	1 mg	IM	J2329
Ultravist 240	per ml		Q9966
Ultravist 300	per ml		Q9967
Ultravist 370	per ml		Q9967
Ultrazine-10	up to 10 mg	IM, IV	J0780
Unasyn	per 1.5 gm	IM, IV	J0295
Unclassified drugs (*see also* Not elsewhere classified)			J3490
Unclassified drugs or biological used for ESRD on dialysis		IV	J3591
Unspecified oral antiemetic			Q0181
Urea	up to 40 g	IV	J3350
Ureaphil	up to 40 g	IV	J3350
Urecholine	up to 5 mg	SC	J0520
Urofollitropin	75 IU		J3355
Urokinase	5,000 IU vial	IV	J3364
	250,000 IU vial	IV	J3365
Ustekinumab	1 mg	SC	J3357
	1 mg	IV	J3358
V			
Vadadustat	1 mg	ORAL	J0901 ◄
Valcyte			J3490
Valergen 10	10 mg	IM	J1380
Valergen 20	10 mg	IM	J1380
Valergen 40	up to 10 mg	IM	J1380

◄ New   ⮌ Revised   ✔ Reinstated   ~~deleted~~ Deleted

DRUG NAME	DOSAGE	METHOD OF ADMINISTRATION	HCPCS CODE
Valertest No. 1	1 mg	IM	J3121
Valertest No. 2	1 mg	IM	J3121
Valganciclovir HCL			J8499
Valium	up to 5 mg	IM, IV	J3360
Valoctocogene roxaparvovec-rvox	per ml	IV	J1412
Valrubicin, intravesical	200 mg	OTH	J9357
Valstar	200 mg	OTH	J9357
~~Vancocin~~	~~500 mg~~	~~IV, IM~~	~~J3370~~
~~Vancoled~~	~~500 mg~~	~~IV, IM~~	~~J3370~~
Vancomycin HCl	10 mg ~~500 mg~~	IV, IM	J3373-J3375 ~~J3370, J3371, J3372~~
Vantas	50 mg		J9226, J9225
Varubi	90 mg		J8670
Vasceze	per 10 mg		J1642
Vasopressin	1 unit	IM	J2598-J2599, J2601
Vasoxyl, see Methoxamine HCl			
Vectibix	10 mg		J9303
Vedolizumab	1 mg	IV	J3380
Velaglucerase alfa	100 units	IV	J3385
Velban	1 mg	IV	J9360
Velcade	0.1 mg		J9041
Veletri	0.5 mg		J1325
Velmanase	1 mg	IM	J0217
Velsar	1 mg	IV	J9360
Venofer	1 mg	IV	J1756
Ventavis	20 mcg		Q4074
Ventolin	0.5 mg	INH	J7620
concentrated form	1 mg	INH	J7610, J7611
unit dose form	1 mg	INH	J7609, J7613
VePesid	50 mg	ORAL	J8560
Veritas Collagen Matrix			J3490
Versed	per 1 mg	IM, IV	J2250
Verteporfin	0.1 mg	IV	J3396
Vesprin	up to 20 mg	IM, IV	J3400
Vestronidase alfa-vjbk	1 mg	IV	J3397
VFEND IV	10 mg	IV	J3465
V-Gan 25	up to 50 mg	IM, IV	J2550
	12.5 mg	ORAL	Q0169

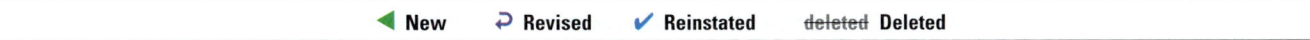

◀ New   ⤺ Revised   ✔ Reinstated   ~~deleted~~ Deleted

DRUG NAME	DOSAGE	METHOD OF ADMINISTRATION	HCPCS CODE
V-Gan 50	up to 50 mg	IM, IV	J2550
	12.5 mg	ORAL	Q0169
Viadur	65 mg	OTH	J9219
Vibativ	10 mg		J3095
Viltolarsen	10 mg	IV	J1427
Vinblastine sulfate	1 mg	IV	J9360
Vincasar PFS	1 mg	IV	J9370
Vincristine sulfate	1 mg	IV	J9370
Vinorelbine tartrate	per 10 mg	IV	J9390
Vispaque	per ml		Q9966, Q9967
Vistaject-25	up to 25 mg	IM	J3410
Vistaril	up to 25 mg	IM	J3410
	25 mg	ORAL	Q0177
Vistide	375 mg	IV	J0740
Visudyne	0.1 mg	IV	J3396
Vitamin B-12 cyanocobalamin	up to 1,000 mcg	IM, SC	J3420
Vitamin K, phytonadione, menadione, menadiol sodium diphosphate	per 1 mg	IM, SC, IV	J3430
Vitrase	per 1 USP unit		J3471
Vivaglobin	100 mg		J1562
Vivitrol	1 mg		J2315
Von Willebrand Factor Complex, human	per IU VWF:RCo	IV	J7187
Wilate	per IU VWF	IV	J7183
Vonvendi	per IU VWF	IV	J7179
Voretigene neparvovec-rzyl	1 billion vector genomes	IV	J3398
Voriconazole	10 mg	IV	J3465
Vpriv	100 units		J3385
Vutrisiran	1 mg	IM	J0225
W			
Wehamine	up to 50 mg	IM, IV	J1240
Wehdryl	up to 50 mg	IM, IV	J1200
	50 mg	ORAL	Q0163
Wellcovorin	per 50 mg	IM, IV	J0640
Wilate	per IU	IV	J7183
Win Rho SD	100 IU	IV	J2792
Wyamine Sulfate, see Mephentermine sulfate			
Wycillin	up to 600,000 units	IM, IV	J2510
Wydase	up to 150 units	SC, IV	J3470
X			
Xeomin	1 unit		J0588
Xgera	1 mg		J0987

◀ New   ⮂ Revised   ✓ Reinstated   ~~deleted~~ Deleted

DRUG NAME	DOSAGE	METHOD OF ADMINISTRATION	HCPCS CODE
Xgeva	1 mg		J0897
Xiaflex	0.01 mg		J0775
Xipere	1 mg		J3299
Xolair	5 mg		J2357
Xopenex	0.5 mg	INH	J7620
concentrated form	1 mg	INH	J7610, J7611, J7612
unit dose form	1 mg	INH	J7609, J7613, J7614
Xyntha	per IU	IV	J7185, J7192, J7182, J7188
Y			
Yervoy, see Ipilimumab			
Yondelis	0.1 mg		J9352, J9999
Z			
Zaltrap	1 mg		J9400
Zanidatamab-hrii	2 mg	IM	J9276 ◄
Zanosar	1 g	IV	J9320
Zantac	25 mg	IV, IM	J2780
Zarxio	1 mcg		Q5101
Zemaira	10 mg	IV	J0256
Zemdri	5 mg	IV	J0291
Zemplar	1 mcg	IM, IV	J2501
Zenapax	25 mg	IV	J7513
Zenocutuzumab-zbco	1 mg	IV	J9382 ◄
Zerbaxa	1 gm		J0695
Zetran	up to 5 mg	IM, IV	J3360
Ziconotide	1 mcg	OTH	J2278
Zidovudine	10 mg	IV	J3485
Zinacef	per 750 mg	IM, IV	J0697
Zinecard	per 250 mg		J1190
Ziprasidone Mesylate	10 mg	IM	J3486
Zithromax	1 gm	ORAL	Q0144
injection	500 mg	IV	J0456
Ziv-Aflibercept	1 mg	IV	J9400
Zmax	1 g		Q0144
Zofran	1 mg	IV	J2405
	1 mg	ORAL	Q0162
Zoladex	per 3.6 mg	SC	J9202
Zolbetuximab-clzb	2 mg	IM	J1326 ◄
Zoledronic Acid	1 mg	IV	J3489

◄ New　⇄ Revised　✔ Reinstated　deleted Deleted

2026 TABLE OF DRUGS / Zolicef

DRUG NAME	DOSAGE	METHOD OF ADMINISTRATION	HCPCS CODE
Zolicef	500 mg	IV, IM	J0690
Zometra	1 mg		J3489
Zorbtive	1 mg		J2941
Zortress	0.25 mg	ORAL	J7527
Zosyn	1.125 g	IV	J2543
Zovirax	5 mg		J8499
Zymfentra	10 mg	IM	**J1748**
Zyprexa Relprevv	1 mg		J2358
Zyvox	200 mg	IV	J2020

◄ New   ⇌ Revised   ✔ Reinstated   deleted Deleted

HCPCS 2026

LEVEL II NATIONAL CODES

2026 HCPCS quarterly updates available on the companion website at: http://www.codingupdates.com

DISCLAIMER

Every effort has been made to make this text complete and accurate, but no guarantee, warranty, or representation is made for its accuracy or completeness. This text is based on the Centers for Medicare and Medicaid Services Healthcare Common Procedure Coding System (HCPCS).

2026 HCPCS LEVEL II NATIONAL CODES

Do not report HCPCS modifiers with MIPS CPT Category II codes, rather, use Performance Measurement Modifiers 1P, 2P, 3P, and 8P, as instructed in the CPT guidelines for Category II codes under 'Modifiers'.

LEVEL II NATIONAL MODIFIERS

*	A1	Dressing for one wound
*	A2	Dressing for two wounds
*	A3	Dressing for three wounds
*	A4	Dressing for four wounds
*	A5	Dressing for five wounds
*	A6	Dressing for six wounds
*	A7	Dressing for seven wounds
*	A8	Dressing for eight wounds
*	A9	Dressing for nine or more wounds
⊛	AA	Anesthesia services performed personally by anesthesiologist
		IOM: 100-04, 12, 90.4
	AB	Audiology service furnished personally by an audiologist without a physician/npp order for non-acute hearing assessment unrelated to disequilibrium, or hearing aids, or examinations for the purpose of prescribing, fitting, or changing hearing aids; service may be performed once every 12 months, per beneficiary
⊛	AD	Medical supervision by a physician: more than four concurrent anesthesia procedures
		IOM: 100-04, 12, 90.4
*	AE	Registered dietician
*	AF	Specialty physician
*	AG	Primary physician
⊛	AH	Clinical psychologist
		IOM: 100-04, 12, 170
*	AI	Principal physician of record
⊛	AJ	Clinical social worker
		IOM: 100-04, 12, 170; 100-04, 12, 150
*	AK	Nonparticipating physician
⊛	AM	Physician, team member service
		Not assigned for Medicare
		Cross Reference QM
*	AO	Alternate payment method declined by provider of service
*	AP	Determination of refractive state was not performed in the course of diagnostic ophthalmological examination
*	AQ	Physician providing a service in an unlisted health professional shortage area (HPSA)
*	AR	Physician provider services in a physician scarcity area
*	AS	Physician assistant, nurse practitioner, or clinical nurse specialist services for assistant at surgery
*	AT	Acute treatment (this modifier should be used when reporting service 98940, 98941, 98942)
*	AU	Item furnished in conjunction with a urological, ostomy, or tracheostomy supply
*	AV	Item furnished in conjunction with a prosthetic device, prosthetic or orthotic
*	AW	Item furnished in conjunction with a surgical dressing
*	AX	Item furnished in conjunction with dialysis services
*	AY	Item or service furnished to an ESRD patient that is not for the treatment of ESRD
⊘	AZ	Physician providing a service in a dental health professional shortage area for the purpose of an electronic health record incentive payment
*	BA	Item furnished in conjunction with parenteral enteral nutrition (PEN) services
*	BL	Special acquisition of blood and blood products
*	BO	Orally administered nutrition, not by feeding tube
*	BP	The beneficiary has been informed of the purchase and rental options and has elected to purchase the item
*	BR	The beneficiary has been informed of the purchase and rental options and has elected to rent the item
*	BU	The beneficiary has been informed of the purchase and rental options and after 30 days has not informed the supplier of his/her decision
*	CA	Procedure payable only in the inpatient setting when performed emergently on an outpatient who expires prior to admission
*	CB	Service ordered by a renal dialysis facility (RDF) physician as part of the ESRD beneficiary's dialysis benefit, is not part of the composite rate, and is separately reimbursable

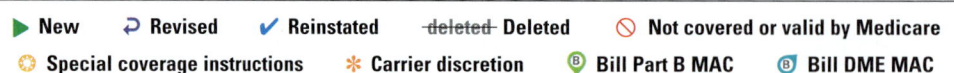

▶ New   ⤺ Revised   ✓ Reinstated   ̶d̶e̶l̶e̶t̶e̶d̶ Deleted   ⊘ Not covered or valid by Medicare   ⊛ Special coverage instructions   * Carrier discretion   Ⓑ Bill Part B MAC   Ⓑ Bill DME MAC

LEVEL II NATIONAL MODIFIERS

* **CC** — Procedure code change (Use CC when the procedure code submitted was changed either for administrative reasons or because an incorrect code was filed)
* **CD** — AMCC test has been ordered by an ESRD facility or MCP physician that is part of the composite rate and is not separately billable
* **CE** — AMCC test has been ordered by an ESRD facility or MCP physician that is a composite rate test but is beyond the normal frequency covered under the rate and is separately reimbursable based on medical necessity
* **CF** — AMCC test has been ordered by an ESRD facility or MCP physician that is not part of the composite rate and is separately billable
* **CG** — Policy criteria applied
* **CH** — 0 percent impaired, limited or restricted
* **CI** — At least 1 percent but less than 20 percent impaired, limited or restricted
* **CJ** — At least 20 percent but less than 40 percent impaired, limited or restricted
* **CK** — At least 40 percent but less than 60 percent impaired, limited or restricted
* **CL** — At least 60 percent but less than 80 percent impaired, limited or restricted
* **CM** — At least 80 percent but less than 100 percent impaired, limited or restricted
* **CN** — 100 percent impaired, limited or restricted
* **CO** — Outpatient occupational therapy services furnished in whole or in part by an occupational therapy assistant
* **CR** — Catastrophe/Disaster related
* **CS** — Cost-sharing waived for specified covid-19 testing-related services that result in and order for or administration of a covid-19 test and/or used for cost-sharing waived preventive services furnished via telehealth in rural health clinics and federally qualified health centers during the covid-19 public health emergency
* **CT** — Computed tomography services furnished using equipment that does not meet each of the attributes of the national electrical manufacturers association (NEMA) XR-29-2013 standard

    Coding Clinic: 2017, Q1, P6

* **CQ** — Outpatient physical therapy services furnished in whole or in part by a physical therapist assistant
* **DA** — Oral health assessment by a licensed health professional other than a dentist
* **E1** — Upper left, eyelid

    Coding Clinic: 2016, Q3, P3

* **E2** — Lower left, eyelid

    Coding Clinic: 2016, Q3, P3

* **E3** — Upper right, eyelid

    Coding Clinic: 2011, Q3, P6

* **E4** — Lower right, eyelid
* **EA** — Erythropoetic stimulating agent (ESA) administered to treat anemia due to anti-cancer chemotherapy

    CMS requires claims for non-ESRD ESAs (J0881 and J0885) to include one of three modifiers: EA, EB, EC.

* **EB** — Erythropoetic stimulating agent (ESA) administered to treat anemia due to anti-cancer radiotherapy

    CMS requires claims for non-ESRD ESAs (J0881 and J0885) to include one of three modifiers: EA, EB, EC.

* **EC** — Erythropoetic stimulating agent (ESA) administered to treat anemia not due to anti-cancer radiotherapy or anti-cancer chemotherapy

    CMS requires claims for non-ESRD ESAs (J0881 and J0885) to include one of three modifiers: EA, EB, EC.

* **ED** — Hematocrit level has exceeded 39% (or hemoglobin level has exceeded 13.0 g/dl) for 3 or more consecutive billing cycles immediately prior to and including the current cycle
* **EE** — Hematocrit level has not exceeded 39% (or hemoglobin level has not exceeded 13.0 g/dl) for 3 or more consecutive billing cycles immediately prior to and including the current cycle
* **EJ** — Subsequent claims for a defined course of therapy, e.g., EPO, sodium hyaluronate, infliximab
* **EM** — Emergency reserve supply (for ESRD benefit only)
* **EP** — Service provided as part of Medicaid early periodic screening diagnosis and treatment (EPSDT) program
* **ER** — Items and services furnished by a provider-based, off-campus emergency department
* **ET** — Emergency services
* **EX** — Expatriate beneficiary

MIPS | Quantity Physician | Quantity Hospital | Female only | Male only | Age | DMEPOS | A2-Z3 ASC Payment Indicator | A-Y ASC Status Indicator | Coding Clinic

* EY	No physician or other licensed health care provider order for this item or service		* G2	Most recent URR reading of 60 to 64.9
				IOM: 100-04, 8, 50.9
	Items billed before a signed and dated order has been received by the supplier must be submitted with an EY modifier added to each related HCPCS code.		* G3	Most recent URR reading of 65 to 69.9
				IOM: 100-04, 8, 50.9
			* G4	Most recent URR reading of 70 to 74.9
				IOM: 100-04, 8, 50.9
* F1	Left hand, second digit		* G5	Most recent URR reading of 75 or greater
* F2	Left hand, third digit			
* F3	Left hand, fourth digit			*IOM: 100-04, 8, 50.9*
* F4	Left hand, fifth digit		* G6	ESRD patient for whom less than six dialysis sessions have been provided in a month
* F5	Right hand, thumb			
* F6	Right hand, second digit			
* F7	Right hand, third digit			*IOM: 100-04, 8, 50.9*
* F8	Right hand, fourth digit		◎ G7	Pregnancy resulted from rape or incest or pregnancy certified by physician as life threatening
* F9	Right hand, fifth digit			
* FA	Left hand, thumb			
⊘ FB	Item provided without cost to provider, supplier or practitioner, or full credit received for replaced device (examples, but not limited to, covered under warranty, replaced due to defect, free samples)			*IOM: 100-02, 15, 20.1; 100-03, 3, 170.3*
			* G8	Monitored anesthesia care (MAC) for deep complex, complicated, or markedly invasive surgical procedure
			* G9	Monitored anesthesia care for patient who has history of severe cardiopulmonary condition
◎ FC	Partial credit received for replaced device			
			* GA	Waiver of liability statement issued as required by payer policy, individual case
* FP	Service provided as part of family planning program			
				An item/service is expected to be denied as not reasonable and necessary and an ABN is on file. Modifier GA can be used on either a specific or a miscellaneous HCPCS code. Modifiers GA and GY should never be reported together on the same line for the same HCPCS code.
* FQ	The service was furnished using audio-only communication technology			
* FR	The supervising practitioner was present through two-way, audio/video communication technology			
* FS	Split (or shared) evaluation and management visit			
			* GB	Claim being resubmitted for payment because it is no longer covered under a global payment demonstration
* FT	Unrelated evaluation and management (e/m) visit during a postoperative period, or on the same day as a procedure or another E/M visit. (report when an e/m visit is furnished within the global period but is unrelated, or when one or more additional E/M visits furnished on the same day are unrelated)			
			◎ GC	This service has been performed in part by a resident under the direction of a teaching physician
				IOM: 100-04, 12, 90.4, 100
			◎ GE	This service has been performed by a resident without the presence of a teaching physician under the primary care exception
* FX	X-ray taken using film			
	Coding Clinic: 2017, Q1, P6		* GF	Non-physician (e.g., nurse practitioner (NP), certified registered nurse anesthetist (CRNA), certified registered nurse (CRN), clinical nurse specialist (CNS), physician assistant (PA)) services in a critical access hospital
* FY	X-ray taken using computed radiography technology/cassette-based imaging			
* G0	Telehealth services for diagnosis, evaluation, or treatment, of symptoms of an acute stroke			
			* GG	Performance and payment of a screening mammogram and diagnostic mammogram on the same patient, same day
* G1	Most recent URR reading of less than 60			
	IOM: 100-04, 8, 50.9			

▶ New   ⤴ Revised   ✓ Reinstated   ~~deleted~~ Deleted   ⊘ Not covered or valid by Medicare
◎ Special coverage instructions   * Carrier discretion   Ⓑ Bill Part B MAC   Ⓑ Bill DME MAC

LEVEL II NATIONAL MODIFIERS

✱	**GH**	Diagnostic mammogram converted from screening mammogram on same day
✱	**GJ**	"Opt out" physician or practitioner emergency or urgent service
✱	**GK**	Reasonable and necessary item/service associated with a GA or GZ modifier
		An upgrade is defined as an item that goes beyond what is medically necessary under Medicare's coverage requirements. An item can be considered an upgrade even if the physician has signed an order for it. When suppliers know that an item will not be paid in full because it does not meet the coverage criteria stated in the LCD, the supplier can still obtain partial payment at the time of initial determination if the claim is billed using one of the upgrade modifiers (GK or GL). (https://www.cms.gov/manuals/downloads/clm104c01.pdf)
✱	**GL**	Medically unnecessary upgrade provided instead of non-upgraded item, no charge, no Advance Beneficiary Notice (ABN)
✱	**GM**	Multiple patients on one ambulance trip
✱	**GN**	Services delivered under an outpatient speech language pathology plan of care
✱	**GO**	Services delivered under an outpatient occupational therapy plan of care
✱	**GP**	Services delivered under an outpatient physical therapy plan of care
✱	**GQ**	Via asynchronous telecommunications system
✱	**GR**	This service was performed in whole or in part by a resident in a Department of Veterans Affairs medical center or clinic, supervised in accordance with VA policy
✺	**GS**	Dosage of erythropoietin-stimulating agent has been reduced and maintained in response to hematocrit or hemoglobin level
✺	**GT**	Via interactive audio and video telecommunication systems
✱	**GU**	Waiver of liability statement issued as required by payer policy, routine notice
✺	**GV**	Attending physician not employed or paid under arrangement by the patient's hospice provider
✺	**GW**	Service not related to the hospice patient's terminal condition
✱	**GX**	Notice of liability issued, voluntary under payer policy
		GX modifier must be submitted with non-covered charges only. This modifier differentiates from the required uses in conjunction with ABN. (https://www.cms.gov/manuals/downloads/clm104c01.pdf)
⊘	**GY**	Item or service statutorily excluded, does not meet the definition of any Medicare benefit or, for non-Medicare insurers, is not a contract benefit
		Examples of "statutorily excluded" include: Infusion drug not administered using a durable infusion pump, a wheelchair that is for use for mobility outside the home or hearing aids. GA and GY should never be coded together on the same line for the same HCPCS code. (https://www.cms.gov/manuals/downloads/clm104c01.pdf)
⊘	**GZ**	Item or service expected to be denied as not reasonable or necessary
		Used when an ABN is not on file and can be used on either a specific or a miscellaneous HCPCS code. It would never be correct to place any combination of GY, GZ or GA modifiers on the same claim line and will result in rejected or denied claim for invalid coding. (https://www.cms.gov/manuals/downloads/clm104c01.pdf)
⊘	**H9**	Court-ordered
⊘	**HA**	Child/adolescent program
⊘	**HB**	Adult program, nongeriatric
⊘	**HC**	Adult program, geriatric
⊘	**HD**	Pregnant/parenting women's program
⊘	**HE**	Mental health program
⊘	**HF**	Substance abuse program
⊘	**HG**	Opioid addiction treatment program
⊘	**HH**	Integrated mental health/substance abuse program
⊘	**HI**	Integrated mental health and intellectual disability/developmental disabilities program
⊘	**HJ**	Employee assistance program
⊘	**HK**	Specialized mental health programs for high-risk populations
⊘	**HL**	Intern
⊘	**HM**	Less than bachelors degree level
⊘	**HN**	Bachelors degree level
⊘	**HO**	Masters degree level
⊘	**HP**	Doctoral level
⊘	**HQ**	Group setting
⊘	**HR**	Family/couple with client present

🏷 MIPS	Qp Quantity Physician	Qh Quantity Hospital	♀ Female only	
♂ Male only	A Age	♿ DMEPOS	A2-Z3 ASC Payment Indicator	A-Y ASC Status Indicator	Coding Clinic

⊘	HS	Family/couple without client present		* JW	Drug amount discarded/not administered to any patient
⊘	HT	Multi-disciplinary team			
⊘	HU	Funded by child welfare agency			Use JW to identify unused drugs or biologicals from single use vial/package that are appropriately discarded. Bill on separate line for payment of discarded drug/biological.
⊘	HV	Funded by state addictions agency			
⊘	HW	Funded by state mental health agency			
⊘	HX	Funded by county/local agency			
⊘	HY	Funded by juvenile justice agency			*IOM: 100-4, 17, 40*
⊘	HZ	Funded by criminal justice agency			Coding Clinic: 2023, Q3, P14-19; 2016, Q4, P4-7; 2010, Q3, P10

* **J1** — Competitive acquisition program no-pay submission for a prescription number

JZ — Zero drug amount discarded/not administered to any patient

Coding Clinic: 2023, Q3, P14-19

* **J2** — Competitive acquisition program, restocking of emergency drugs after emergency administration

* **K0** — Lower extremity prosthesis functional Level 0 - does not have the ability or potential to ambulate or transfer safely with or without assistance and a prosthesis does not enhance their quality of life or mobility.

* **J3** — Competitive acquisition program (CAP), drug not available through CAP as written, reimbursed under average sales price methodology

* **K1** — Lower extremity prosthesis functional Level 1 - has the ability or potential to use a prosthesis for transfers or ambulation on level surfaces at fixed cadence. Typical of the limited and unlimited household ambulator.

* **J4** — DMEPOS item subject to DMEPOS competitive bidding program that is furnished by a hospital upon discharge

* **J5** — Off-the-shelf orthotic subject to dmepos competitive bidding program that is furnished as part of a physical therapist or occupational therapist professional service

* **K2** — Lower extremity prosthesis functional Level 2 - has the ability or potential for ambulation with the ability to traverse low level environmental barriers such as curbs, stairs or uneven surfaces. Typical of the limited community ambulator.

* **JA** — Administered intravenously

This modifier is informational only (not a payment modifier) and may be submitted with all injection codes. According to Medicare, reporting this modifier is voluntary. (CMS Pub. 100-04, chapter 8, section 60.2.3.1 and Pub. 100-04, chapter 17, section 80.11)

* **K3** — Lower extremity prosthesis functional Level 3 - has the ability or potential for ambulation with variable cadence. Typical of the community ambulator who has the ability to traverse most environmental barriers and may have vocational, therapeutic, or exercise activity that demands prosthetic utilization beyond simple locomotion.

* **JB** — Administered subcutaneously
* **JC** — Skin substitute used as a graft
* **JD** — Skin substitute not used as a graft
* **JE** — Administered via dialysate

~~JG~~ — ~~Drug or biological acquired with 340B drug pricing program discount, reported for informational purposes~~

* **K4** — Lower extremity prosthesis functional Level 4 - has the ability or potential for prosthetic ambulation that exceeds the basic ambulation skills, exhibiting high impact, stress, or energy levels, typical of the prosthetic demands of the child, active adult, or athlete.

JK — One month supply or less of drug or biological

JL — Three month supply of drug or biological

* **KA** — Add on option/accessory for wheelchair
* **KB** — Beneficiary requested upgrade for ABN, more than 4 modifiers identified on claim
* **KC** — Replacement of special power wheelchair interface
* **KD** — Drug or biological infused through DME
* **KE** — Bid under round one of the DMEPOS competitive bidding program for use with non-competitive bid base equipment

---

▶ New ↻ Revised ✓ Reinstated ~~deleted~~ Deleted ⊘ Not covered or valid by Medicare
✱ Special coverage instructions * Carrier discretion Ⓑ Bill Part B MAC Ⓑ Bill DME MAC

LEVEL II NATIONAL MODIFIERS

* **KF** — Item designated by FDA as Class III device
* **KG** — DMEPOS item subject to DMEPOS competitive bidding program number 1
* **KH** — DMEPOS item, initial claim, purchase or first month rental
* **KI** — DMEPOS item, second or third month rental
* **KJ** — DMEPOS item, parenteral enteral nutrition (PEN) pump or capped rental, months four to fifteen
* **KK** — DMEPOS item subject to DMEPOS competitive bidding program number 2
* **KL** — DMEPOS item delivered via mail
* **KM** — Replacement of facial prosthesis including new impression/moulage
* **KN** — Replacement of facial prosthesis using previous master model
* **KO** — Single drug unit dose formulation
* **KP** — First drug of a multiple drug unit dose formulation
* **KQ** — Second or subsequent drug of a multiple drug unit dose formulation
* **KR** — Rental item, billing for partial month
* **KS** — Glucose monitor supply for diabetic beneficiary not treated with insulin
* **KT** — Beneficiary resides in a competitive bidding area and travels outside that competitive bidding area and receives a competitive bid item
* **KU** — DMEPOS item subject to DMEPOS competitive bidding program number 3
* **KV** — DMEPOS item subject to DMEPOS competitive bidding program that is furnished as part of a professional service
* **KW** — DMEPOS item subject to DMEPOS competitive bidding program number 4
* **KX** — Requirements specified in the medical policy have been met

  Used for physical, occupational, or speech-language therapy to request an exception to therapy payment caps and indicate the services are reasonable and necessary and that there is documentation of medical necessity in the patient's medical record. (Pub 100-04 Attachment - Business Requirements Centers for Medicare and Medicaid Services, Transmittal 2457, April 27, 2012)

  Medicare requires modifier KX for implanted permanent cardiac pacemakers, single chamber or duel chamber, for one of the following CPT codes: 33206, 33207, 33208.

* **KY** — DMEPOS item subject to DMEPOS competitive bidding program number 5
* **KZ** — New coverage not implemented by managed care
* **LC** — Left circumflex coronary artery
* **LD** — Left anterior descending coronary artery
* **LL** — Lease/rental (use the LL modifier when DME equipment rental is to be applied against the purchase price)
* **LM** — Left main coronary artery
* **LR** — Laboratory round trip
* **LS** — FDA-monitored intraocular lens implant
* **LT** — Left side (used to identify procedures performed on the left side of the body)

  Modifiers LT and RT identify procedures which can be performed on paired organs. Used for procedures performed on one side only. Should also be used when the procedures are similar but not identical and are performed on paired body parts.

  Coding Clinic: 2016, Q3, P5

* **LU** — Fractionated payment
* **M2** — Medicare secondary payer (MSP)
* ~~MA~~ — ~~Ordering professional is not required to consult a clinical decision support mechanism due to service being rendered to a patient with a suspected or confirmed emergency medical condition~~
* ~~MB~~ — ~~Ordering professional is not required to consult a clinical decision support mechanism due to the significant hardship exception of insufficient internet access~~
* ~~MC~~ — ~~Ordering professional is not required to consult a clinical decision support mechanism due to the significant hardship exception of electronic health record or clinical decision support mechanism vendor issues~~
* ~~MD~~ — ~~Ordering professional is not required to consult a clinical decision support mechanism due to the significant hardship exception of extreme and uncontrollable circumstances~~
* ~~ME~~ — ~~The order for this service adheres to appropriate use criteria in the clinical decision support mechanism consulted by the ordering professional~~

| MIPS | Qp Quantity Physician | Qh Quantity Hospital | ♀ Female only |
| ♂ Male only | Age | DMEPOS | A2-Z3 ASC Payment Indicator | A-Y ASC Status Indicator | Coding Clinic |

	~~MF~~	~~The order for this service does not adhere to the appropriate use criteria in the clinical decision support mechanism consulted by the ordering professional~~
	~~MG~~	~~The order for this service does not have applicable appropriate use criteria in the qualified clinical decision support mechanism consulted by the ordering professional~~
	~~MH~~	~~Unknown if ordering professional consulted a clinical decision support mechanism for this service, related information was not provided to the furnishing professional or provider~~
*	MS	Six month maintenance and servicing fee for reasonable and necessary parts and labor which are not covered under any manufacturer or supplier warranty
	N1	Group 1 oxygen coverage criteria met
	N2	Group 2 oxygen coverage criteria met
	N3	Group 3 oxygen coverage criteria met
*	NB	Nebulizer system, any type, FDA-cleared for use with specific drug
*	NR	New when rented (use the NR modifier when DME which was new at the time of rental is subsequently purchased)
*	NU	New equipment
*	P1	A normal healthy patient
*	P2	A patient with mild systemic disease
*	P3	A patient with severe systemic disease
*	P4	A patient with severe systemic disease that is a constant threat to life
*	P5	A moribund patient who is not expected to survive without the operation
*	P6	A declared brain-dead patient whose organs are being removed for donor purposes
⊘	PA	Surgical or other invasive procedure on wrong body part
⊘	PB	Surgical or other invasive procedure on wrong patient
⊘	PC	Wrong surgery or other invasive procedure on patient
*	PD	Diagnostic or related non diagnostic item or service provided in a wholly owned or operated entity to a patient who is admitted as an inpatient within 3 days
*	PI	Positron emission tomography (PET) or PET/computed tomography (CT) to inform the initial treatment strategy of tumors that are biopsy proven or strongly suspected of being cancerous based on other diagnostic testing
*	PL	Progressive addition lenses
*	PM	Post mortem
*	PN	Non-excepted service provided at an off-campus, outpatient, provider-based department of a hospital
*	PO	Expected services provided at off-campus, outpatient, provider-based department of a hospital
*	PS	Positron emission tomography (PET) or PET/computed tomography (CT) to inform the subsequent treatment strategy of cancerous tumors when the beneficiary's treating physician determines that the PET study is needed to inform subsequent anti-tumor strategy
*	PT	Colorectal cancer screening test; converted to diagnostic text or other procedure

Assign this modifier with the appropriate CPT procedure code for colonoscopy, flexible sigmoidoscopy, or barium enema when the service is initiated as a colorectal cancer screening service but then becomes a diagnostic service. MLN Matters article MM7012 (PDF, 75 KB) Reference Medicare Transmittal 3232 April 3, 2015.

Coding Clinic: 2011, Q1, P10

⊙	Q0	Investigational clinical service provided in a clinical research study that is in an approved clinical research study
⊙	Q1	Routine clinical service provided in a clinical research study that is in an approved clinical research study
*	Q2	Demonstration procedure/service
*	Q3	Live kidney donor surgery and related services
*	Q4	Service for ordering/referring physician qualifies as a service exemption
⊙	Q5	Service furnished under a reciprocal billing arrangement by a substitute physician or by a substitute physical therapist furnishing outpatient physical therapy services in a health professional shortage area, a medically underserved area, or a rural area

IOM: 100-04, 1, 30.2.10

▶ New   ↻ Revised   ✓ Reinstated   ~~deleted~~ Deleted   ⊘ Not covered or valid by Medicare
⊙ Special coverage instructions   * Carrier discretion   Ⓑ Bill Part B MAC   Ⓑ Bill DME MAC

LEVEL II NATIONAL MODIFIERS

◉ **Q6**	Service furnished under a fee-for-time compensation arrangement by a substitute physician or by a substitute physical therapist furnishing outpatient physical therapy services in a health professional shortage area, a medically underserved area, or a rural area *IOM: 100-04, 1, 30.2.11*		◉ **QP**	Documentation is on file showing that the laboratory test(s) was ordered individually or ordered as a CPT-recognized panel other than automated profile codes 80002-80019, G0058, G0059, and G0060
✱ **Q7**	One Class A finding		~~QQ~~	~~Ordering professional consulted a qualified clinical decision support mechanism for this service and the related data was provided to the furnishing professional~~
✱ **Q8**	Two Class B findings			
✱ **Q9**	One Class B and two Class C findings			
✱ **QA**	Prescribed amounts of stationary oxygen for daytime use while at rest and nighttime use differ and the average of the two amounts is less than 1 liter per minute (lpm)		✱ **QR**	Prescribed amounts of stationary oxygen for daytime use while at rest and nighttime use differ and the average of the two amounts is greater than 4 liters per minute (lpm)
✱ **QB**	Prescribed amounts of stationary oxygen for daytime use while at rest and nighttime use differ and the average of the two amounts exceeds 4 liters per minute (lpm) and portable oxygen is prescribed		◉ **QS**	Monitored anesthesia care service *IOM: 100-04, 12, 30.6, 501*
			✱ **QT**	Recording and storage on tape by an analog tape recorder
✱ **QC**	Single channel monitoring		✱ **QW**	CLIA-waived test
✱ **QD**	Recording and storage in solid state memory by a digital recorder		✱ **QX**	CRNA service: with medical direction by a physician
✱ **QE**	Prescribed amount of stationary oxygen while at rest is less than 1 liter per minute (LPM)		◉ **QY**	Medical direction of one certified registered nurse anesthetist (CRNA) by an anesthesiologist *IOM: 100-04, 12, 50K, 90*
✱ **QF**	Prescribed amount of stationary oxygen while at rest exceeds 4 liters per minute (LPM) and portable oxygen is prescribed		✱ **QZ**	CRNA service: without medical direction by a physician
			✱ **RA**	Replacement of a DME, orthotic or prosthetic item
✱ **QG**	Prescribed amount of stationary oxygen while at rest is greater than 4 liters per minute (LPM)			Contractors will deny claims for replacement parts when furnished in conjunction with the repair of a capped rental item and billed with modifier RB, including claims for parts submitted using code E1399, that are billed during the capped rental period (i.e., the last day of the 13th month of continuous use or before). Repair includes all maintenance, servicing, and repair of capped rental DME because it is included in the allowed rental payment amounts. (Pub 100-20 One-Time Notification Centers for Medicare & Medicaid Services, Transmittal: 901, May 13, 2011)
✱ **QH**	Oxygen conserving device is being used with an oxygen delivery system			
◉ **QJ**	Services/items provided to a prisoner or patient in state or local custody, however, the state or local government, as applicable, meets the requirements in 42 CFR 411.4 (B)			
◉ **QK**	Medical direction of two, three, or four concurrent anesthesia procedures involving qualified individuals *IOM: 100-04, 12, 50K, 90*			
✱ **QL**	Patient pronounced dead after ambulance called		✱ **RB**	Replacement of a part of a DME, orthotic or prosthetic item furnished as part of a repair
✱ **QM**	Ambulance service provided under arrangement by a provider of services		✱ **RC**	Right coronary artery
✱ **QN**	Ambulance service furnished directly by a provider of services		✱ **RD**	Drug provided to beneficiary, but not administered "incident-to"

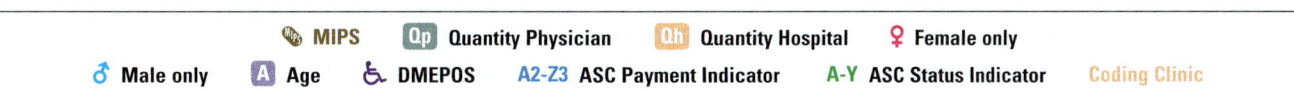

* RE	Furnished in full compliance with FDA-mandated risk evaluation and mitigation strategy (REMS)	⊘ SV	Pharmaceuticals delivered to patient's home but not utilized
* RI	Ramus intermedius coronary artery	* SW	Services provided by a certified diabetic educator
* RR	Rental (use the 'RR' modifier when DME is to be rented)	⊘ SY	Persons who are in close contact with member of high-risk population (use only with codes for immunization)
* RT	Right side (used to identify procedures performed on the right side of the body)	* T1	Left foot, second digit
		* T2	Left foot, third digit
		* T3	Left foot, fourth digit
		* T4	Left foot, fifth digit
		* T5	Right foot, great toe
		* T6	Right foot, second digit
		* T7	Right foot, third digit
		* T8	Right foot, fourth digit
		* T9	Right foot, fifth digit
		* TA	Left foot, great toe

Modifiers LT and RT identify procedures which can be performed on paired organs. Used for procedures performed on one side only. Should also be used when the procedures are similar but not identical and are performed on paired body parts.

Coding Clinic: 2016, Q3, P5

⊘ SA	Nurse practitioner rendering service in collaboration with a physician	↪ * TB	Drug or biological acquired with 340B drug pricing program discount, reported for informational purposes
⊘ SB	Nurse midwife	* TC	Technical component; under certain circumstances, a charge may be made for the technical component alone; under those circumstances the technical component charge is identified by adding modifier TC to the usual procedure number; technical component charges are institutional charges and not billed separately by physicians; however, portable x-ray suppliers only bill for technical component and should utilize modifier TC; the charge data from portable x-ray suppliers will then be used to build customary and prevailing profiles.
* SC	Medically necessary service or supply		
⊘ SD	Services provided by registered nurse with specialized, highly technical home infusion training		
⊘ SE	State and/or federally funded programs/services		
* SF	Second opinion ordered by a professional review organization (PRO) per Section 9401, P.L. 99-272 (100% reimbursement – no Medicare deductible or coinsurance)		
* SG	Ambulatory surgical center (ASC) facility service		

Only valid for surgical codes. After 1/1/08 not required for ASC facility charges.

⊘ SH	Second concurrently administered infusion therapy	⊘ TD	RN
		⊘ TE	LPN/LVN
⊘ SJ	Third or more concurrently administered infusion therapy	⊘ TF	Intermediate level of care
		⊘ TG	Complex/high tech level of care
⊘ SK	Member of high risk population (use only with codes for immunization)	⊘ TH	Obstetrical treatment/services, prenatal or postpartum
⊘ SL	State supplied vaccine	⊘ TJ	Program group, child and/or adolescent
⊘ SM	Second surgical opinion	⊘ TK	Extra patient or passenger, non-ambulance
⊘ SN	Third surgical opinion		
⊘ SQ	Item ordered by home health	⊘ TL	Early intervention/individualized family service plan (IFSP)
⊘ SS	Home infusion services provided in the infusion suite of the IV therapy provider	⊘ TM	Individualized education program (IEP)
		⊘ TN	Rural/outside providers' customary service area
⊘ ST	Related to trauma or injury	⊘ TP	Medical transport, unloaded vehicle
⊘ SU	Procedure performed in physician's office (to denote use of facility and equipment)	⊘ TQ	Basic life support transport by a volunteer ambulance provider

▶ New ↪ Revised ✓ Reinstated ~~deleted~~ Deleted ⊘ Not covered or valid by Medicare ● Special coverage instructions * Carrier discretion ⒷBill Part B MAC ⒷBill DME MAC

LEVEL II NATIONAL MODIFIERS

⊘	**TR**	School-based individual education program (IEP) services provided outside the public school district responsible for the student
✱	**TS**	Follow-up service
⊘	**TT**	Individualized service provided to more than one patient in same setting
⊘	**TU**	Special payment rate, overtime
⊘	**TV**	Special payment rates, holidays/weekends
⊘	**TW**	Back-up equipment
⊘	**U1**	Medicaid Level of Care 1, as defined by each State
⊘	**U2**	Medicaid Level of Care 2, as defined by each State
⊘	**U3**	Medicaid Level of Care 3, as defined by each State
⊘	**U4**	Medicaid Level of Care 4, as defined by each State
⊘	**U5**	Medicaid Level of Care 5, as defined by each State
⊘	**U6**	Medicaid Level of Care 6, as defined by each State
⊘	**U7**	Medicaid Level of Care 7, as defined by each State
⊘	**U8**	Medicaid Level of Care 8, as defined by each State
⊘	**U9**	Medicaid Level of Care 9, as defined by each State
⊘	**UA**	Medicaid Level of Care 10, as defined by each State
⊘	**UB**	Medicaid Level of Care 11, as defined by each State
⊘	**UC**	Medicaid Level of Care 12, as defined by each State
⊘	**UD**	Medicaid Level of Care 13, as defined by each State
✱	**UE**	Used durable medical equipment
⊘	**UF**	Services provided in the morning
⊘	**UG**	Services provided in the afternoon
⊘	**UH**	Services provided in the evening
✱	**UJ**	Services provided at night
⊘	**UK**	Services provided on behalf of the client to someone other than the client (collateral relationship)
✱	**UN**	Two patients served
✱	**UP**	Three patients served
✱	**UQ**	Four patients served
✱	**UR**	Five patients served
✱	**US**	Six or more patients served
✱	**V1**	Demonstration Modifier 1
✱	**V2**	Demonstration Modifier 2
✱	**V3**	Demonstration Modifier 3
✱	**V4**	Demonstration modifier 4
✱	**V5**	Vascular catheter (alone or with any other vascular access)
✱	**V6**	Arteriovenous graft (or other vascular access not including a vascular catheter)
✱	**V7**	Arteriovenous fistula only (in use with two needles)
✱	**VM**	Medicare diabetes prevention program (MDPP) virtual make-up session
✱	**VP**	Aphakic patient
✱	**X1**	Continuous/broad services: for reporting services by clinicians, who provide the principal care for a patient, with no planned endpoint of the relationship; services in this category represent comprehensive care, dealing with the entire scope of patient problems, either directly or in a care coordination role; reporting clinician service examples include, but are not limited to: primary care, and clinicians providing comprehensive care to patients in addition to specialty care
✱	**X2**	Continuous/focused services: for reporting services by clinicians whose expertise is needed for the ongoing management of a chronic disease or a condition that needs to be managed and followed with no planned endpoint to the relationship; reporting clinician service examples include but are not limited to: a rheumatologist taking care of the patient's rheumatoid arthritis longitudinally but not providing general primary care services
✱	**X3**	Episodic/broad services: for reporting services by clinicians who have broad responsibility for the comprehensive needs of the patient that is limited to a defined period and circumstance such as a hospitalization; reporting clinician service examples include but are not limited to the hospitalist's services rendered providing comprehensive and general care to a patient while admitted to the hospital

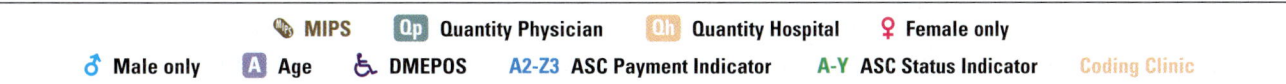

* X4	Episodic/focused services: for reporting services by clinicians who provide focused care on particular types of treatment limited to a defined period and circumstance; the patient has a problem, acute or chronic, that will be treated with surgery, radiation, or some other type of generally time-limited intervention; reporting clinician service examples include but are not limited to, the orthopedic surgeon performing a knee replacement and seeing the patient through the postoperative period
* X5	Diagnostic services requested by another clinician: for reporting services by a clinician who furnishes care to the patient only as requested by another clinician or subsequent and related services requested by another clinician; this modifier is reported for patient relationships that may not be adequately captured by the above alternative categories; reporting clinician service examples include but are not limited to, the radiologist's interpretation of an imaging study requested by another clinician
* XE	Separate encounter, a service that is distinct because it occurred during a separate encounter
* XP	Separate practitioner, a service that is distinct because it was performed by a different practitioner
* XS	Separate structure, a service that is distinct because it was performed on a separate organ/structure
* XU	Unusual non-overlapping service, the use of a service that is distinct because it does not overlap usual components of the main service

Ambulance Modifiers

Modifiers that are used on claims for ambulance services are created by combining two alpha characters. Each alpha character, with the exception of X, represents an origin (source) code or a destination code. The pair of alpha codes creates one modifier. The first position alpha-code = origin; the second position alpha-code = destination. On form CMS-1491, used to report ambulance services, Item 12 should contain the origin code and Item 13 should contain the destination code. Origin and destination codes and their descriptions are as follows:

D	Diagnostic or therapeutic site other than P or H when these are used as origin codes
E	Residential, domiciliary, custodial facility (other than an 1819 facility)
G	Hospital-based ESRD facility
H	Hospital
I	Site of transfer (e.g., airport or helicopter pad) between modes of ambulance transport
J	Freestanding ESRD facility
N	Skilled nursing facility
P	Physician's office
R	Residence
S	Scene of accident or acute event
X	Intermediate stop at physician's office on way to hospital (destination code only)

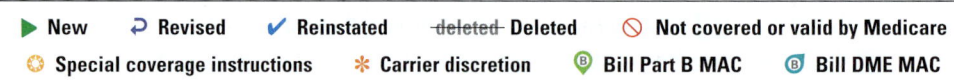

TRANSPORT SERVICES INCLUDING AMBULANCE (A0000-A0999)

- ⊘ **A0021** Ambulance service, outside state per mile, transport (Medicaid only) B Qp Qh E1
  Cross Reference A0030
- ⊘ **A0080** Non-emergency transportation, per mile - vehicle provided by volunteer (individual or organization), with no vested interest B Qp Qh E1
- ⊘ **A0090** Non-emergency transportation, per mile - vehicle provided by individual (family member, self, neighbor) with vested interest B Qp Qh E1
- ⊘ **A0100** Non-emergency transportation; taxi B Qp Qh E1
- ⊘ **A0110** Non-emergency transportation and bus, intra- or interstate carrier B Qp Qh E1
- ⊘ **A0120** Non-emergency transportation: mini-bus, mountain area transports, or other transportation systems B Qp Qh E1
- ⊘ **A0130** Non-emergency transportation: wheelchair van B Qp Qh E1
- ⊘ **A0140** Non-emergency transportation and air travel (private or commercial), intra- or interstate B Qp Qh E1
- ⊘ **A0160** Non-emergency transportation: per mile - caseworker or social worker B Qp Qh E1
- ⊘ **A0170** Transportation: ancillary: parking fees, tolls, other B Qp Qh E1
- ⊘ **A0180** Non-emergency transportation: ancillary: lodging - recipient B Qp Qh E1
- ⊘ **A0190** Non-emergency transportation: ancillary: meals - recipient B Qp Qh E1
- ⊘ **A0200** Non-emergency transportation: ancillary: lodging - escort B Qp Qh E1
- ⊘ **A0210** Non-emergency transportation: ancillary: meals - escort B Qp Qh E1
- ⊘ **A0225** Ambulance service, neonatal transport, base rate, emergency transport, one way B Qp Qh E1
- ⊘ **A0380** BLS mileage (per mile) B Qp Qh E1
  Cross Reference A0425
- ⊘ **A0382** BLS routine disposable supplies B Qp Qh E1
- ⊘ **A0384** BLS specialized service disposable supplies; defibrillation (used by ALS ambulances and BLS ambulances in jurisdictions where defibrillation is permitted in BLS ambulances) B Qp Qh E1
- ⊘ **A0390** ALS mileage (per mile) B Qp Qh E1
  Cross Reference A0425
- ⊘ **A0392** ALS specialized service disposable supplies; defibrillation (to be used only in jurisdictions where defibrillation cannot be performed in BLS ambulances) B Qp Qh E1
- ⊘ **A0394** ALS specialized service disposable supplies; IV drug therapy B Qp Qh E1
- ⊘ **A0396** ALS specialized service disposable supplies; esophageal intubation B Qp Qh E1
- ⊘ **A0398** ALS routine disposable supplies B Qp Qh E1
- ⊘ **A0420** Ambulance waiting time (ALS or BLS), one half (½) hour increments B Qp Qh E1

Waiting Time Table			
UNITS	TIME	UNITS	TIME
1	½ to 1 hr.	6	3 to 3½ hrs.
2	1 to 1½ hrs.	7	3½ to 4 hrs.
3	1½ to 2 hrs.	8	4 to 4½ hrs.
4	2 to 2½ hrs.	9	4½ to 5 hrs.
5	2½ to 3 hrs.	10	5 to 5½ hrs.

- ⊘ **A0422** Ambulance (ALS or BLS) oxygen and oxygen supplies, life sustaining situation B Qp Qh E1
- ⊘ **A0424** Extra ambulance attendant, ground (ALS or BLS) or air (fixed or rotary winged); (requires medical review) B Qp Qh E1
- ✶ **A0425** Ground mileage, per statute mile B Qp Qh A
- ✶ **A0426** Ambulance service, advanced life support, non-emergency transport, Level 1 (ALS 1) B Qp Qh A
- ✶ **A0427** Ambulance service, advanced life support, emergency transport, Level 1 (ALS 1-Emergency) B Qp Qh A
- ✶ **A0428** Ambulance service, basic life support, non-emergency transport (BLS) B Qp Qh A
- ✶ **A0429** Ambulance service, basic life support, emergency transport (BLS-Emergency) B Qp Qh A
- ✶ **A0430** Ambulance service, conventional air services, transport, one way (fixed wing) B Qp Qh A
- ✶ **A0431** Ambulance service, conventional air services, transport, one way (rotary wing) B Qp Qh A

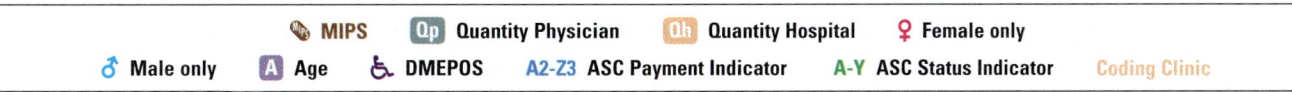

🖐 MIPS   Qp Quantity Physician   Qh Quantity Hospital   ♀ Female only
♂ Male only   A Age   ♿ DMEPOS   A2-Z3 ASC Payment Indicator   A-Y ASC Status Indicator   Coding Clinic

* A0432	Paramedic intercept (PI), rural area, transport furnished by a volunteer ambulance company, which is prohibited by state law from billing third party payers Ⓑ Qp Qh	A	* A2016	Permeaderm B, per square centimeter	N1	N
* A0433	Advanced life support, Level 2 (ALS2) Ⓑ Qp Qh	A	* A2017	Permeaderm glove, each	N1	N
* A0434	Specialty care transport (SCT) Ⓑ Qp Qh	A	* A2018	Permeaderm C, per square centimeter	N1	N

* A0432 — Paramedic intercept (PI), rural area, transport furnished by a volunteer ambulance company, which is prohibited by state law from billing third party payers Ⓑ Qp Qh — A

* A0433 — Advanced life support, Level 2 (ALS2) Ⓑ Qp Qh — A

* A0434 — Specialty care transport (SCT) Ⓑ Qp Qh — A

* A0435 — Fixed wing air mileage, per statute mile Ⓑ Qp Qh — A

* A0436 — Rotary wing air mileage, per statute mile Ⓑ Qp Qh — A

⊘ A0888 — Noncovered ambulance mileage, per mile (e.g., for miles traveled beyond closest appropriate facility) Ⓑ Qp Qh — E1
MCM: 2125

⊘ A0998 — Ambulance response and treatment, no transport Ⓑ Qp Qh — E1
IOM: 100-02, 10, 20

◉ A0999 — Unlisted ambulance service Ⓑ — A
IOM: 100-02, 10, 20

MEDICAL AND SURGICAL SUPPLIES
(A2001-A8004)

Wound Supplies

* A2001 — Innovamatrix ac, per square centimeter — N1 N
* A2002 — Mirragen advanced wound matrix, per square centimeter — N1 N
* A2004 — Xcellistem, 1 mg — N1 N
* A2005 — Microlyte matrix, per square centimeter — N1 N
* A2006 — Novosorb synpath dermal matrix, per square centimeter — N1 N
* A2007 — Restrata, per square centimeter — N1 N
* A2008 — Theragenesis, per square centimeter — N1 N
* A2009 — Symphony, per square centimeter — N1 N
* A2010 — Apis, per square centimeter — N1 N
* A2011 — Supra sdrm, per square centimeter — N1 N
* A2012 — Suprathel, per square centimeter — N1 N
* A2013 — Innovamatrix fs, per square centimeter — N1 N
* A2014 — Omeza collagen matrix, per 100 mg — N1 N
* A2015 — Phoenix wound matrix, per square centimeter — N1 N
* A2016 — Permeaderm B, per square centimeter — N1 N
* A2017 — Permeaderm glove, each — N1 N
* A2018 — Permeaderm C, per square centimeter — N1 N
* A2019 — Kerecis omega3 marigen shield, per square centimeter — N1 N
* A2020 — Ac5 advanced wound system (ac5) — N1 N
* A2021 — Neomatrix, per square centimeter — N1 N
* A2022 — Innovaburn or innovamatrix xl, per square centimeter — N1 N
* A2023 — Innovamatrix pd, 1 mg — N1 N
* A2024 — Resolve matrix or xenopatch, per square centimeter — N1 N
* A2025 — Miro3d, per cubic centimeter — N1 N
* A2026 — Restrata minimatrix, 5 mg — N1 N
* A2027 — Matriderm, per square centimeter — N1 N
* A2028 — Micromatrix flex, per mg — N1 N
* A2029 — Mirotract wound matrix sheet, per cubic centimeter — N1 N
▶ * A2030 — Miro3d fibers, per mg — N1 N
▶ * A2031 — Mirodry wound matrix, per square centimeter — N1 N
▶ * A2032 — Myriad matrix, per square centimeter — N1 N
▶ * A2033 — Myriad morcells, 4 mg — N1 N
▶ * A2034 — Foundation drs solo, per square centimeter — N1 N
▶ * A2035 — Corplex p or theracor p or allacor p, per mg — N1 N
▶ * A2036 — Cohealyx collagen dermal matrix, per square centimeter — N1 N
▶ * A2037 — G4derm plus, per milliliter — N1 N
▶ * A2038 — Marigen pacto, per square centimeter — N1 N
▶ * A2039 — Innovamatrix fd, per square centimeter — N1 N
* A4100 — Skin substitute, FDA cleared as a device, not otherwise specified — N1 N

Injection and Infusion

* A4206 — Syringe with needle, sterile 1 cc or less, each Ⓑ Ⓑ — N
* A4207 — Syringe with needle, sterile 2 cc, each Ⓑ Ⓑ — N
* A4208 — Syringe with needle, sterile 3 cc, each Ⓑ Ⓑ — N
* A4209 — Syringe with needle, sterile 5 cc or greater, each Ⓑ Ⓑ — N
⊘ A4210 — Needle-free injection device, each Ⓑ Qp Qh — E1
IOM: 100-03, 4, 280.1

▶ New ⇆ Revised ✓ Reinstated ~~deleted~~ Deleted ⊘ Not covered or valid by Medicare ◉ Special coverage instructions * Carrier discretion Ⓑ Bill Part B MAC Ⓑ Bill DME MAC

MEDICAL AND SURGICAL SUPPLIES

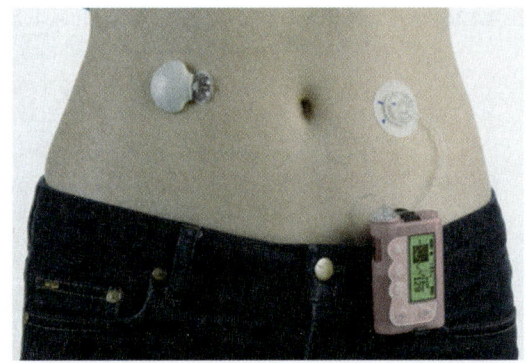

Figure 1 Insulin pump.

○ **A4211** Supplies for self-administered injections ⒷⒷ Qp Qh N
IOM: 100-02, 15, 50

∗ **A4212** Non-coring needle or stylet with or without catheter Ⓑ Qp Qh N

∗ **A4213** Syringe, sterile, 20 cc or greater, each ⒷⒷ N

∗ **A4215** Needle, sterile, any size, each ⒷⒷ N

○ **A4216** Sterile water, saline and/or dextrose diluent/flush, 10 ml ⒷⒷ ♿ N
Other: Sodium Chloride, Bacteriostatic, Syrex
IOM: 100-02, 15, 50

○ **A4217** Sterile water/saline, 500 ml ⒷⒷ ♿ N
Other: Sodium Chloride
IOM: 100-02, 15, 50

○ **A4218** Sterile saline or water, metered dose dispenser, 10 ml Ⓑ Ⓑ N
Other: Sodium Chloride

○ **A4220** Refill kit for implantable infusion pump Ⓑ Qp Qh N
Do not report with 95990 or 95991 since Medicare payment for these codes includes the refill kit.
IOM: 100-03, 4, 280.1

∗ **A4221** Supplies for maintenance of non-insulin drug infusion catheter, per week (list drugs separately) Ⓑ Ⓑ Qp Qh ♿ N
Includes dressings for catheter site and flush solutions not directly related to drug infusion.

∗ **A4222** Infusion supplies for external drug infusion pump, per cassette or bag (list drug separately) Ⓑ Qp Qh ♿ N
Includes cassette or bag, diluting solutions, tubing and/or administration supplies, port cap changes, compounding charges, and preparation charges.

∗ **A4223** Infusion supplies not used with external infusion pump, per cassette or bag (list drugs separately) Ⓑ N
IOM: 100-03, 4, 280.1

∗ **A4224** Supplies for maintenance of insulin infusion catheter, per week Ⓑ Qp Qh ♿ N

○ **A4225** Supplies for external insulin infusion pump, syringe type cartridge, sterile, each Ⓑ Qp Qh ♿ N
IOM: 100-03, 1, 50.3

∗ **A4226** Supplies for maintenance of insulin infusion pump with dosage rate adjustment using therapeutic continuous glucose sensing, per week E1

○ **A4230** Infusion set for external insulin pump, non-needle cannula type Ⓑ N
Requires prior authorization and copy of invoice.
IOM: 100-03, 4, 280.1

○ **A4231** Infusion set for external insulin pump, needle type Ⓑ N
Requires prior authorization and copy of invoice.
IOM: 100-03, 4, 280.1

⊘ **A4232** Syringe with needle for external insulin pump, sterile, 3 cc Ⓑ Qp Qh E1
Reports insulin reservoir for use with external insulin infusion pump (E0784); may be glass or plastic; includes needle for drawing up insulin. Does not include insulin for use in reservoir.
IOM: 100-03, 4, 280.1

Replacement Batteries

∗ **A4233** Replacement battery, alkaline (other than J cell), for use with medically necessary home blood glucose monitor owned by patient, each Ⓑ Qh ♿ E1

∗ **A4234** Replacement battery, alkaline, J cell, for use with medically necessary home blood glucose monitor owned by patient, each Ⓑ Qh ♿ E1

∗ **A4235** Replacement battery, lithium, for use with medically necessary home blood glucose monitor owned by patient, each Ⓑ Qp Qh ♿ E1

∗ **A4236** Replacement battery, silver oxide, for use with medically necessary home blood glucose monitor owned by patient, each Ⓑ Qh ♿ E1

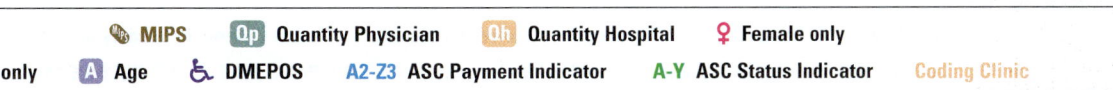

Miscellaneous Supplies

* **A4238** Supply allowance for adjunctive, non-implanted continuous glucose monitor (cgm), includes all supplies and accessories, 1 month supply = 1 unit of service ⓑ ♿ Y

* **A4239** Supply allowance for non-adjunctive, non-implanted continuous glucose monitor (cgm), includes all supplies and accessories, 1 month supply = 1 unit of service ⓑ ♿ Y

* **A4244** Alcohol or peroxide, per pint ⓑ ⓑ N

* **A4245** Alcohol wipes, per box ⓑ ⓑ N

* **A4246** Betadine or Phisohex solution, per pint ⓑ ⓑ N

* **A4247** Betadine or iodine swabs/wipes, per box ⓑ ⓑ N

* **A4248** Chlorhexidine containing antiseptic, 1 ml ⓑ ⓑ N

⊘ **A4250** Urine test or reagent strips or tablets (100 tablets or strips) ⓑ ⓑ Qp Qh E1

IOM: 100-02, 15, 110

⊘ **A4252** Blood ketone test or reagent strip, each ⓑ Qp Qh E1

Medicare Statute 1861(n)

✹ **A4253** Blood glucose test or reagent strips for home blood glucose monitor, per 50 strips ⓑ Qp Qh ♿ N

Test strips (1 unit = 50 strips); non-insulin treated (every 3 months) 100 test strips (1×/day testing), 100 lancets (1×/day testing); modifier KS

IOM: 100-03, 1, 40.2

✹ **A4255** Platforms for home blood glucose monitor, 50 per box ⓑ Qp Qh ♿ N

IOM: 100-03, 1, 40.2

✹ **A4256** Normal, low and high calibrator solution/chips ⓑ Qp Qh ♿ N

IOM: 100-03, 1, 40.2

* **A4257** Replacement lens shield cartridge for use with laser skin piercing device, each ⓑ Qp Qh ♿ E1

✹ **A4258** Spring-powered device for lancet, each ⓑ Qp Qh ♿ N

IOM: 100-03, 1, 40.2

✹ **A4259** Lancets, per box of 100 ⓑ Qp Qh ♿ N

IOM: 100-03, 1, 40.2

⊘ **A4261** Cervical cap for contraceptive use ⓑ Qp Qh ♀ E1

Medicare Statute 1862A1

✹ **A4262** Temporary, absorbable lacrimal duct implant, each ⓑ Qp Qh N

IOM: 100-04, 12, 20.3, 30.4

✹ **A4263** Permanent, long term, non-dissolvable lacrimal duct implant, each ⓑ Qp Qh N

Bundled with insertion if performed in physician office.

IOM: 100-04, 12, 30.4

⊘ **A4264** Permanent implantable contraceptive intratubal occlusion device(s) and delivery system ⓑ Qp Qh ♀ E1

Reports the Essure device.

✹ **A4265** Paraffin, per pound ⓑ ⓑ Qp Qh ♿ N

IOM: 100-03, 4, 280.1

⊘ **A4266** Diaphragm for contraceptive use ⓑ Qp Qh ♀ E1

⊘ **A4267** Contraceptive supply, condom, male, each ⓑ Qp Qh ♂ E1

⊘ **A4268** Contraceptive supply, condom, female, each ⓑ Qp Qh ♀ E1

⊘ **A4269** Contraceptive supply, spermicide (e.g., foam, gel), each ⓑ Qp Qh E1

* **A4270** Disposable endoscope sheath, each ⓑ Qp Qh N

A4271 Integrated lancing and blood sample testing cartridges for home blood glucose monitor, per 50 tests ⓑ A

* **A4280** Adhesive skin support attachment for use with external breast prosthesis, each ⓑ Qh ♀ ♿ N

* **A4281** Tubing for breast pump, replacement ⓑ ♀ E1

* **A4282** Adapter for breast pump, replacement ⓑ ♀ E1

* **A4283** Cap for breast pump bottle, replacement ⓑ ♀ E1

* **A4284** Breast shield and splash protector for use with breast pump, replacement ⓑ ♀ E1

* **A4285** Polycarbonate bottle for use with breast pump, replacement ⓑ ♀ E1

* **A4286** Locking ring for breast pump, replacement ⓑ ♀ E1

* **A4287** Disposable collection and storage bag for breast milk, any size, any type, each ⓑ ⓑ ♀ Y

▶ * **A4288** Valve for breast pump, replacement ⓑ ♀ Y

* **A4290** Sacral nerve stimulation test lead, each ⓑ N

Service not separately priced by Part B (e.g., services not covered, bundled, used by Part A only)

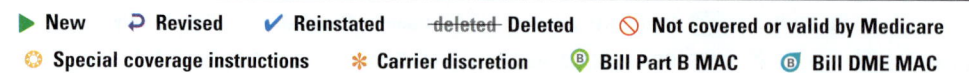

▶ New ⮂ Revised ✓ Reinstated ~~deleted~~ Deleted ⊘ Not covered or valid by Medicare
✹ Special coverage instructions * Carrier discretion ⓑ Bill Part B MAC ⓑ Bill DME MAC

MEDICAL AND SURGICAL SUPPLIES

Implantable Catheters

- **A4300** Implantable access catheter, (e.g., venous, arterial, epidural subarachnoid, or peritoneal, etc.) external access ⓑ Qp Qh N
  IOM: 100-02, 15, 120

- **A4301** Implantable access total; catheter, port/reservoir (e.g., venous, arterial, epidural, subarachnoid, peritoneal, etc.) ⓑ Qp Qh N

Disposable Drug Delivery System

- **A4305** Disposable drug delivery system, flow rate of 50 ml or greater per hour ⓑ ⓑ Qp Qh N

- **A4306** Disposable drug delivery system, flow rate of less than 50 ml per hour ⓑ ⓑ Qp Qh N

Incontinence Appliances and Care Supplies

- **A4310** Insertion tray without drainage bag and without catheter (accessories only) ⓑ Qp Qh ♿ N
  IOM: 100-02, 15, 120

- **A4311** Insertion tray without drainage bag with indwelling catheter, Foley type, two-way latex with coating (Teflon, silicone, silicone elastomer, or hydrophilic, etc.) ⓑ ⓑ Qp Qh ♿ N
  IOM: 100-02, 15, 120

- **A4312** Insertion tray without drainage bag with indwelling catheter, Foley type, two-way, all silicone ⓑ ⓑ Qp Qh ♿ N

  Must meet criteria for indwelling catheter and medical record must justify need for:
  - Recurrent encrustation
  - Inability to pass a straight catheter
  - Sensitivity to latex

  Must be medically necessary.
  IOM: 100-02, 15, 120

- **A4313** Insertion tray without drainage bag with indwelling catheter, Foley type, three-way, for continuous irrigation ⓑ ⓑ Qp Qh ♿ N

  Must meet criteria for indwelling catheter and medical record must justify need for:
  - Recurrent encrustation
  - Inability to pass a straight catheter
  - Sensitivity to latex

  Must be medically necessary.
  IOM: 100-02, 15, 120

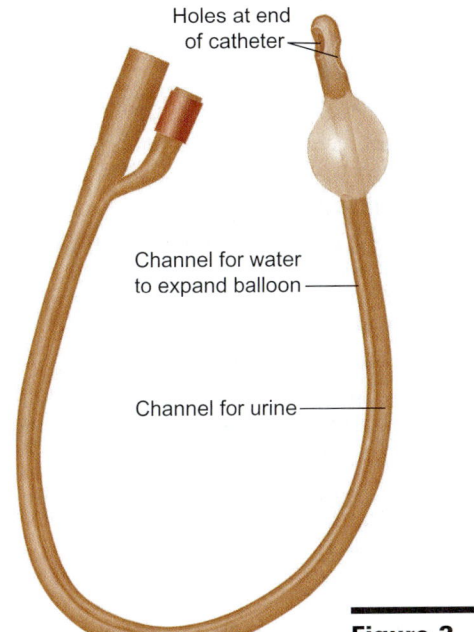

Figure 2 Foley catheter.

- **A4314** Insertion tray with drainage bag with indwelling catheter, Foley type, two-way latex with coating (Teflon, silicone, silicone elastomer or hydrophilic, etc.) ⓑ ⓑ Qp Qh ♿ N
  IOM: 100-02, 15, 120

- **A4315** Insertion tray with drainage bag with indwelling catheter, Foley type, two-way, all silicone ⓑ ⓑ Qp Qh ♿ N
  IOM: 100-02, 15, 120

- **A4316** Insertion tray with drainage bag with indwelling catheter, Foley type, three-way, for continuous irrigation ⓑ ⓑ Qp Qh ♿ N
  IOM: 100-02, 15, 120

- **A4320** Irrigation tray with bulb or piston syringe, any purpose ⓑ ⓑ Qp Qh ♿ N
  IOM: 100-02, 15, 120

- **A4321** Therapeutic agent for urinary catheter irrigation ⓑ ⓑ ♿ N
  IOM: 100-02, 15, 120

- **A4322** Irrigation syringe, bulb, or piston, each ⓑ ⓑ Qp Qh ♿ N
  IOM: 100-02, 15, 120

- **A4326** Male external catheter with integral collection chamber, any type, each ⓑ ⓑ Qp Qh ♂ ♿ N
  IOM: 100-02, 15, 120

- **A4327** Female external urinary collection device; meatal cup, each ⓑ ⓑ Qp Qh ♀ ♿ N
  IOM: 100-02, 15, 120

| 🌐 MIPS | Qp Quantity Physician | Qh Quantity Hospital | ♀ Female only |
| ♂ Male only | A Age | ♿ DMEPOS | A2-Z3 ASC Payment Indicator | A-Y ASC Status Indicator | Coding Clinic |

117

A4328 Female external urinary collection device; pouch, each ⓑ Ⓑ Qp Qh ♀ ♿ N
IOM: 100-02, 15, 120

A4330 Perianal fecal collection pouch with adhesive, each ⓑ Ⓑ Qp Qh ♿ N
IOM: 100-02, 15, 120

A4331 Extension drainage tubing, any type, any length, with connector/adaptor, for use with urinary leg bag or urostomy pouch, each ⓑ Ⓑ Qh ♿ N
IOM: 100-02, 15, 120

A4332 Lubricant, individual sterile packet, each ⓑ Ⓑ Qp Qh ♿ N
IOM: 100-02, 15, 120

A4333 Urinary catheter anchoring device, adhesive skin attachment, each ⓑ Ⓑ ♿ N
IOM: 100-02, 15, 120

A4334 Urinary catheter anchoring device, leg strap, each ⓑ Ⓑ ♿ N
IOM: 100-02, 15, 120

A4335 Incontinence supply; miscellaneous ⓑ Ⓑ Qp Qh N
IOM: 100-02, 15, 120

A4336 Incontinence supply, urethral insert, any type, each ⓑ Ⓑ ♿ N
IOM: 100-02, 15, 120

A4337 Incontinence supply, rectal insert, any type, each ⓑ Ⓑ Qp Qh N
IOM: 100-02, 15, 120

A4338 Indwelling catheter; Foley type, two-way latex with coating (Teflon, silicone, silicone elastomer, or hydrophilic, etc.), each ⓑ Ⓑ Qp Qh ♿ N
IOM: 100-02, 15, 120

A4340 Indwelling catheter; specialty type (e.g., coude, mushroom, wing, etc.), each ⓑ Ⓑ Qp Qh ♿ N

Must meet criteria for indwelling catheter and medical record must justify need for:
• Recurrent encrustation
• Inability to pass a straight catheter
• Sensitivity to latex
Must be medically necessary.

IOM: 100-02, 15, 120

A4341 Indwelling intraurethral drainage device with valve, patient inserted, replacement only, each Ⓑ Qp Qh N

A4342 Accessories for patient inserted indwelling intraurethral drainage device with valve, replacement only, each Ⓑ Qp Qh ♿ N

A4344 Indwelling catheter, Foley type, two-way, all silicone, or polyurethane each ⓑ Ⓑ Qp Qh ♿ N1 N

Must meet criteria for indwelling catheter and medical record must justify need for:
• Recurrent encrustation
• Inability to pass a straight catheter
• Sensitivity to latex
Must be medically necessary.

IOM: 100-02, 15, 120

A4346 Indwelling catheter; Foley type, three way for continuous irrigation, each ⓑ Ⓑ Qp Qh ♿ N
IOM: 100-02, 15, 120

A4349 Male external catheter, with or without adhesive, disposable, each ⓑ Ⓑ ♂ ♿ N
IOM: 100-02, 15, 120

A4351 Intermittent urinary catheter; straight tip, with or without coating (Teflon, silicone, silicone elastomer, or hydrophilic, etc.), each ⓑ Ⓑ Qp Qh ♿ N
IOM: 100-02, 15, 120

A4352 Intermittent urinary catheter; coude (curved) tip, with or without coating (Teflon, silicone, silicone elastomeric, or hydrophilic, etc.), each ⓑ Ⓑ Qp Qh ♿ N
IOM: 100-02, 15, 120

A4353 Intermittent urinary catheter, with insertion supplies ⓑ Ⓑ Qh ♿ N
IOM: 100-02, 15, 120

A4354 Insertion tray with drainage bag but without catheter ⓑ Ⓑ Qp Qh ♿ N
IOM: 100-02, 15, 120

A4355 Irrigation tubing set for continuous bladder irrigation through a three-way indwelling Foley catheter, each ⓑ Ⓑ Qp Qh ♿ N
IOM: 100-02, 15, 120

External Urinary Supplies

A4356 External urethral clamp or compression device (not to be used for catheter clamp), each ⓑ Ⓑ Qp Qh ♿ N
IOM: 100-02, 15, 120

▶ New ↻ Revised ✓ Reinstated ~~deleted~~ Deleted ⊘ Not covered or valid by Medicare
※ Special coverage instructions ✱ Carrier discretion Ⓑ Bill Part B MAC Ⓑ Bill DME MAC

MEDICAL AND SURGICAL SUPPLIES

- **A4357** Bedside drainage bag, day or night, with or without anti-reflux device, with or without tube, each ⓑ ⓑ Qp Qh ♿ N
  IOM: 100-02, 15, 120
- **A4358** Urinary drainage bag, leg or abdomen, vinyl, with or without tube, with straps, each ⓑ ⓑ Qp ♿ N
  IOM: 100-02, 15, 120
- **A4360** Disposable external urethral clamp or compression device, with pad and/or pouch, each ⓑ ⓑ ♿ N

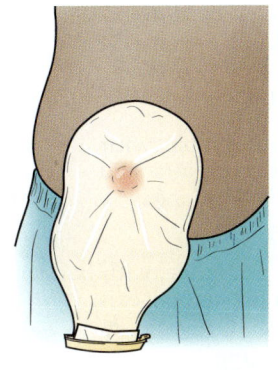

Figure 3 Ostomy pouch.

Ostomy Supplies

- **A4361** Ostomy faceplate, each ⓑ ⓑ Qp Qh ♿ N
  IOM: 100-02, 15, 120
- **A4362** Skin barrier; solid, 4 × 4 or equivalent; each ⓑ ⓑ Qp Qh ♿ N
  IOM: 100-02, 15, 120
- **A4363** Ostomy clamp, any type, replacement only, each ⓑ ⓑ Qp Qh ♿ E1
- **A4364** Adhesive, liquid or equal, any type, per oz ⓑ ⓑ Qp Qh ♿ N
  Fee schedule category: Ostomy, tracheostomy, and urologicals items.
  IOM: 100-02, 15, 120
- **A4366** Ostomy vent, any type, each ⓑ ⓑ Qh ♿ N
- **A4367** Ostomy belt, each ⓑ ⓑ Qp Qh ♿ N
  IOM: 100-02, 15, 120
- **A4368** Ostomy filter, any type, each ⓑ ⓑ Qp Qh ♿ N
- **A4369** Ostomy skin barrier, liquid (spray, brush, etc.), per oz ⓑ ⓑ ♿ N
  IOM: 100-02, 15, 120
- **A4371** Ostomy skin barrier, powder, per oz ⓑ ⓑ ♿ N
  IOM: 100-02, 15, 120
- **A4372** Ostomy skin barrier, solid 4 × 4 or equivalent, standard wear, with built-in convexity, each ⓑ ⓑ Qh ♿ N
  IOM: 100-02, 15, 120
- **A4373** Ostomy skin barrier, with flange (solid, flexible, or accordion), with built-in convexity, any size, each ⓑ ⓑ Qh ♿ N
  IOM: 100-02, 15, 120
- **A4375** Ostomy pouch, drainable, with faceplate attached, plastic, each ⓑ ⓑ Qp Qh ♿ N
  IOM: 100-02, 15, 120
- **A4376** Ostomy pouch, drainable, with faceplate attached, rubber, each ⓑ ⓑ Qp Qh ♿ N
  IOM: 100-02, 15, 120
- **A4377** Ostomy pouch, drainable, for use on faceplate, plastic, each ⓑ ⓑ Qp Qh ♿ N
  IOM: 100-02, 15, 120
- **A4378** Ostomy pouch, drainable, for use on faceplate, rubber, each ⓑ ⓑ Qp Qh ♿ N
  IOM: 100-02, 15, 120
- **A4379** Ostomy pouch, urinary, with faceplate attached, plastic, each ⓑ ⓑ Qp Qh ♿ N
  IOM: 100-02, 15, 120
- **A4380** Ostomy pouch, urinary, with faceplate attached, rubber, each ⓑ ⓑ Qp Qh ♿ N
  IOM: 100-02, 15, 120
- **A4381** Ostomy pouch, urinary, for use on faceplate, plastic, each ⓑ ⓑ Qp Qh ♿ N
  IOM: 100-02, 15, 120
- **A4382** Ostomy pouch, urinary, for use on faceplate, heavy plastic, each ⓑ ⓑ Qp Qh ♿ N
  IOM: 100-02, 15, 120
- **A4383** Ostomy pouch, urinary, for use on faceplate, rubber, each ⓑ ⓑ Qp Qh ♿ N
  IOM: 100-02, 15, 120
- **A4384** Ostomy faceplate equivalent, silicone ring, each ⓑ ⓑ Qp Qh ♿ N
  IOM: 100-02, 15, 120
- **A4385** Ostomy skin barrier, solid 4 × 4 or equivalent, extended wear, without built-in convexity, each ⓑ ⓑ Qp Qh ♿ N
  IOM: 100-02, 15, 120

MIPS | Qp Quantity Physician | Qh Quantity Hospital | ♀ Female only
♂ Male only | A Age | ♿ DMEPOS | A2-Z3 ASC Payment Indicator | A-Y ASC Status Indicator | Coding Clinic

2026 HCPCS LEVEL II NATIONAL CODES

⊛ **A4387** Ostomy pouch closed, with barrier attached, with built-in convexity (1 piece), each ⓑ Ⓑ Qh ♿   N
IOM: 100-02, 15, 120

⊛ **A4388** Ostomy pouch, drainable, with extended wear barrier attached (1 piece), each ⓑ Ⓑ Qh ♿   N
IOM: 100-02, 15, 120

⊛ **A4389** Ostomy pouch, drainable, with barrier attached, with built-in convexity (1 piece), each ⓑ Ⓑ Qp Qh ♿   N
IOM: 100-02, 15, 120

⊛ **A4390** Ostomy pouch, drainable, with extended wear barrier attached, with built-in convexity (1 piece), each ⓑ Ⓑ Qh ♿   N
IOM: 100-02, 15, 120

⊛ **A4391** Ostomy pouch, urinary, with extended wear barrier attached (1 piece), each ⓑ Ⓑ Qh ♿   N
IOM: 100-02, 15, 120

⊛ **A4392** Ostomy pouch, urinary, with standard wear barrier attached, with built-in convexity (1 piece), each ⓑ Ⓑ Qp Qh ♿   N
IOM: 100-02, 15, 120

⊛ **A4393** Ostomy pouch, urinary, with extended wear barrier attached, with built-in convexity (1 piece), each ⓑ Ⓑ Qh ♿   N
IOM: 100-02, 15, 120

⊛ **A4394** Ostomy deodorant, with or without lubricant, for use in ostomy pouch, per fluid ounce ⓑ Ⓑ ♿   N
IOM: 100-02, 15, 20

⊛ **A4395** Ostomy deodorant for use in ostomy pouch, solid, per tablet ⓑ Ⓑ ♿   N
IOM: 100-02, 15, 20

⊛ **A4396** Ostomy belt with peristomal hernia support ⓑ Ⓑ Qh ♿   N
IOM: 100-02, 15, 120

⊛ **A4398** Ostomy irrigation supply; bag, each ⓑ Ⓑ Qp Qh ♿   N
IOM: 100-02, 15, 120

⊛ **A4399** Ostomy irrigation supply; cone/catheter, with or without brush ⓑ Ⓑ Qp Qh ♿   N
IOM: 100-02, 15, 120

⊛ **A4400** Ostomy irrigation set ⓑ Ⓑ Qp Qh ♿   N
IOM: 100-02, 15, 120

⊛ **A4402** Lubricant, per ounce ⓑ Ⓑ Qp Qh ♿   N
IOM: 100-02, 15, 120

⊛ **A4404** Ostomy ring, each ⓑ Ⓑ Qp Qh   N
IOM: 100-02, 15, 120

⊛ **A4405** Ostomy skin barrier, non-pectin based, paste, per ounce ⓑ Ⓑ ♿   N
IOM: 100-02, 15, 120

⊛ **A4406** Ostomy skin barrier, pectin-based, paste, per ounce ⓑ Ⓑ ♿   N
IOM: 100-02, 15, 120

⊛ **A4407** Ostomy skin barrier, with flange (solid, flexible, or accordion), extended wear, with built-in convexity, 4 × 4 inches or smaller, each ⓑ Ⓑ Qp Qh ♿   N
IOM: 100-02, 15, 120

⊛ **A4408** Ostomy skin barrier, with flange (solid, flexible, or accordion), extended wear, with built-in convexity, larger than 4 × 4 inches, each ⓑ Qh ♿   N
IOM: 100-02, 15, 120

⊛ **A4409** Ostomy skin barrier, with flange (solid, flexible, or accordion), extended wear, without built-in convexity, 4 × 4 inches or smaller, each ⓑ Ⓑ Qh ♿   N
IOM: 100-02, 15, 120

⊛ **A4410** Ostomy skin barrier, with flange (solid, flexible, or accordion), extended wear, without built-in convexity, larger than 4 × 4 inches, each ⓑ Ⓑ Qp Qh ♿   N
IOM: 100-02, 15, 120

⊛ **A4411** Ostomy skin barrier, solid 4 × 4 or equivalent, extended wear, with built-in convexity, each ⓑ Ⓑ Qh ♿   N

⊛ **A4412** Ostomy pouch, drainable, high output, for use on a barrier with flange (2 piece system), without filter, each ⓑ Ⓑ Qh ♿   N
IOM: 100-02, 15, 120

⊛ **A4413** Ostomy pouch, drainable, high output, for use on a barrier with flange (2 piece system), with filter, each ⓑ Ⓑ Qp Qh ♿   N
IOM: 100-02, 15, 120

⊛ **A4414** Ostomy skin barrier, with flange (solid, flexible, or accordion), without built-in convexity, 4 × 4 inches or smaller, each ⓑ Ⓑ Qh ♿   N
IOM: 100-02, 15, 120

⊛ **A4415** Ostomy skin barrier, with flange (solid, flexible, or accordion), without built-in convexity, larger than 4 × 4 inches, each ⓑ Ⓑ Qh ♿   N
IOM: 100-02, 15, 120

✱ **A4416** Ostomy pouch, closed, with barrier attached, with filter (1 piece), each ⓑ Ⓑ Qp Qh ♿   N

✱ **A4417** Ostomy pouch, closed, with barrier attached, with built-in convexity, with filter (1 piece), each ⓑ Ⓑ Qh ♿   N

▶ New ↻ Revised ✓ Reinstated ~~deleted~~ Deleted ⊘ Not covered or valid by Medicare
⊛ Special coverage instructions ✱ Carrier discretion ⓑ Bill Part B MAC Ⓑ Bill DME MAC

MEDICAL AND SURGICAL SUPPLIES

* **A4418** Ostomy pouch, closed; without barrier attached, with filter (1 piece), each ⓑ ⓑ Qh ♿ N

* **A4419** Ostomy pouch, closed; for use on barrier with non-locking flange, with filter (2 piece), each ⓑ ⓑ Qp Qh ♿ N

* **A4420** Ostomy pouch, closed; for use on barrier with locking flange (2 piece), each ⓑ ⓑ Qh ♿ N

* **A4421** Ostomy supply; miscellaneous ⓑ ⓑ N

⊛ **A4422** Ostomy absorbent material (sheet/pad/crystal packet) for use in ostomy pouch to thicken liquid stomal output, each ⓑ ⓑ ♿ N

   IOM: 100-02, 15, 120

* **A4423** Ostomy pouch, closed; for use on barrier with locking flange, with filter (2 piece), each ⓑ ⓑ Qp Qh ♿ N

* **A4424** Ostomy pouch, drainable, with barrier attached, with filter (1 piece), each ⓑ ⓑ Qh ♿ N

* **A4425** Ostomy pouch, drainable; for use on barrier with non-locking flange, with filter (2 piece system), each ⓑ ⓑ Qh ♿ N

* **A4426** Ostomy pouch, drainable; for use on barrier with locking flange (2 piece system), each ⓑ ⓑ Qp Qh ♿ N

* **A4427** Ostomy pouch, drainable; for use on barrier with locking flange, with filter (2 piece system), each ⓑ ⓑ Qh ♿ N

* **A4428** Ostomy pouch, urinary, with extended wear barrier attached, with faucet-type tap with valve (1 piece), each ⓑ ⓑ Qh ♿ N

* **A4429** Ostomy pouch, urinary, with barrier attached, with built-in convexity, with faucet-type tap with valve (1 piece), each ⓑ ⓑ Qp Qh ♿ N

* **A4430** Ostomy pouch, urinary, with extended wear barrier attached, with built-in convexity, with faucet-type tap with valve (1 piece), each ⓑ ⓑ Qh ♿ N

* **A4431** Ostomy pouch, urinary; with barrier attached, with faucet-type tap with valve (1 piece), each ⓑ ⓑ Qh ♿ N

* **A4432** Ostomy pouch, urinary; for use on barrier with non-locking flange, with faucet-type tap with valve (2 piece), each ⓑ ⓑ Qp Qh ♿ N

* **A4433** Ostomy pouch, urinary; for use on barrier with locking flange (2 piece), each ⓑ ⓑ Qh ♿ N

* **A4434** Ostomy pouch, urinary; for use on barrier with locking flange, with faucet-type tap with valve (2 piece), each ⓑ ⓑ Qh ♿ N

* **A4435** Ostomy pouch, drainable, high output, with extended wear barrier (one-piece system), with or without filter, each ⓑ ⓑ Qp Qh ♿ N

* **A4436** Irrigation supply; sleeve, reusable, per month ♿ N

* **A4437** Irrigation supply; sleeve, disposable, per month ♿ N

* **A4438** Adhesive clip applied to the skin to secure external electrical nerve stimulator controller, each A

Miscellaneous Supplies

⊛ **A4450** Tape, non-waterproof, per 18 square inches ⓑ ⓑ ♿ N

   If used with surgical dressings, billed with AW modifier (in addition to appropriate A1-A9 modifier).

   IOM: 100-02, 15, 120

⊛ **A4452** Tape, waterproof, per 18 square inches ⓑ ⓑ ♿ N

   If used with surgical dressings, billed with AW modifier (in addition to appropriate A1-A9 modifier).

   IOM: 100-02, 15, 120

↻ ⊛ **A4453** Rectal catheter with or without balloon, for use with any type transanal irrigation system, each ⓑ N

   If used with surgical dressings, billed with AW modifier (in addition to appropriate A1-A9 modifier).

⊛ **A4455** Adhesive remover or solvent (for tape, cement or other adhesive), per ounce ⓑ ⓑ Qp Qh ♿ N

   IOM: 100-02, 15, 120

⊛ **A4456** Adhesive remover, wipes, any type, each ⓑ ⓑ ♿ N

   May be reimbursed for male or female clients to home health DME providers and DME medical suppliers in the home setting.

   IOM: 100-02, 15, 120

   A4457 Enema tube, with or without adapter, any type, replacement only, each ⓑ ⓑ E1

* **A4458** Enema bag with tubing, reusable ⓑ N

↻ * **A4459** Manual transanal irrigation system, includes water reservoir, pump, tubing, and accessories, without catheter, any type ⓑ Qp Qh N

* **A4461** Surgical dressing holder, non-reusable, each ⓑ ⓑ Qp Qh ♿ N

* **A4463** Surgical dressing holder, reusable, each ⓑ ⓑ Qh ♿ N

* **A4465** Non-elastic binder for extremity ⓑ Qp Qh N

⊘ **A4467** Belt, strap, sleeve, garment, or covering, any type ⓑ Qp Qh E1

| 🍁 MIPS | Qp Quantity Physician | Qh Quantity Hospital | ♀ Female only |
| ♂ Male only | A Age | ♿ DMEPOS | A2-Z3 ASC Payment Indicator | A-Y ASC Status Indicator | Coding Clinic |

2026 HCPCS LEVEL II NATIONAL CODES

A4468	Exsufflation belt, includes all supplies and accessories E1
✱ A4470	Gravlee jet washer N
	Symptoms suggestive of endometrial disease must be present for this disposable diagnostic tool to be covered.
	IOM: 100-02, 16, 90; 100-03, 4, 230.5
✱ A4480	VABRA aspirator N
	Symptoms suggestive of endometrial disease must be present for this disposable diagnostic tool to be covered.
	IOM: 100-02, 16, 90; 100-03, 4, 230.6
✱ A4481	Tracheostoma filter, any type, any size, each N
	IOM: 100-02, 15, 120
✱ A4483	Moisture exchanger, disposable, for use with invasive mechanical ventilation N
	IOM: 100-02, 15, 120
⊘ A4490	Surgical stockings above knee length, each E1
	IOM: 100-02, 15, 100; 100-02, 15, 110; 100-03, 4, 280.1
⊘ A4495	Surgical stockings thigh length, each E1
	IOM: 100-02, 15, 100; 100-02, 15, 110; 100-03, 4, 280.1
⊘ A4500	Surgical stockings below knee length, each E1
	IOM: 100-02, 15, 100; 100-02, 15, 110; 100-03, 4, 280.1
⊘ A4510	Surgical stockings full length, each E1
	IOM: 100-02, 15, 100; 100-02, 15, 110; 100-03, 4, 280.1
A4520	Incontinence garment, any type (e.g., brief, diaper), each E1
	IOM: 100-03, 4, 280.1
A4540	Distal transcutaneous electrical nerve stimulator, stimulates peripheral nerves of the upper arm E1
A4541	Monthly supplies for use of device coded at E0733 Y
A4542	Supplies and accessories for external upper limb tremor stimulator of the peripheral nerves of the wrist Y
⊘ A4543	Supplies for transcutaneous electrical nerve stimulator, for nerves in the auricular region, per month Y
⊘ A4544	Electrode for external lower extremity nerve stimulator for restless legs syndrome Y
⊘ A4545	Supplies and accessories for external tibial nerve stimulator (e.g., socks, gel pads, electrodes, etc.), needed for one month Y
✱ A4550	Surgical trays B
	No longer payable by Medicare; included in practice expense for procedures. Some private payers may pay, most private payers follow Medicare guidelines.
	IOM: 100-04, 12, 20.3, 30.4
⊘ A4553	Non-disposable underpads, all sizes E1
	IOM: 100-03, 4, 280.1
⊘ A4554	Disposable underpads, all sizes E1
	IOM: 100-03, 4, 280.1
⊘ A4555	Electrode/transducer for use with electrical stimulation device used for cancer treatment, replacement only E1
* A4556	Electrodes (e.g., apnea monitor), per pair N
* A4557	Lead wires (e.g., apnea monitor), per pair N
* A4558	Conductive gel or paste, for use with electrical device (e.g., TENS, NMES), per oz N
* A4559	Coupling gel or paste, for use with ultrasound device, per oz N
A4560	Neuromuscular electrical stimulator (NMES), disposable, replacement only E1
* A4561	Pessary, reusable, rubber, any type N
* A4562	Pessary, reusable, non-rubber, any type N
* A4563	Rectal control system for vaginal insertion, for long term use, includes pump and all supplies and accessories, any type each A
* A4564	Pessary, disposable, any type A
* A4565	Slings N
⊘ A4566	Shoulder sling or vest design, abduction restrainer, with or without swathe control, prefabricated, includes fitting and adjustment E1

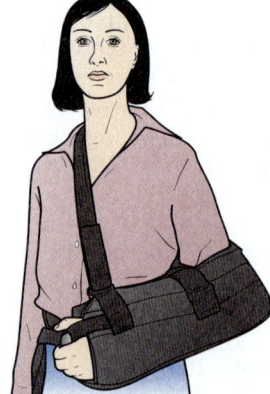

Figure 4 Arm sling.

▶ New   ⤺ Revised   ✓ Reinstated   ~~deleted~~ Deleted   ⊘ Not covered or valid by Medicare
✱ Special coverage instructions   * Carrier discretion   🅑 Bill Part B MAC   🅑 Bill DME MAC

MEDICAL AND SURGICAL SUPPLIES

⊘ **A4570** Splint ⓑ Qp Qh   E1
     IOM: 100-02, 6, 10; 100-02, 15, 100; 100-04, 4, 240

✱ **A4575** Topical hyperbaric oxygen chamber, disposable ⓑ Qp Qh   A

⊘ **A4580** Cast supplies (e.g., plaster) ⓑ Qp Qh   E1
     IOM: 100-02, 6, 10; 100-02, 15, 100; 100-04, 4, 240

⊘ **A4590** Special casting material (e.g., fiberglass) ⓑ Qp Qh   E1
     IOM: 100-02, 6, 10; 100-02, 15, 100; 100-04, 4, 240

   A4593 Neuromodulation stimulator system, adjunct to rehabilitation therapy regime, controller ⓑ   E1

   A4594 Neuromodulation stimulator system, adjunct to rehabilitation therapy regime, mouthpiece each ⓑ   E1

✵ **A4595** Electrical stimulator supplies, 2 lead, per month (e.g., TENS, NMES) ⓠ ⓑ Qp Qh ♿   N
     IOM: 100-03, 2, 160.13

   A4596 Cranial electrotherapy stimulation (CES) system supplies and accessories, per month ⓑ ♿   N

✱ **A4600** Sleeve for intermittent limb compression device, replacement only, each ⓑ   E1

✱ **A4601** Lithium ion battery, rechargeable, for non-prosthetic use, replacement ⓑ   E1

✱ **A4602** Replacement battery for external infusion pump owned by patient, lithium, 1.5 volt, each ⓑ Qp Qh ♿   N

✱ **A4604** Tubing with integrated heating element for use with positive airway pressure device ⓑ Qh ♿   N

✱ **A4605** Tracheal suction catheter, closed system, each ⓑ Qh ♿   N

✱ **A4606** Oxygen probe for use with oximeter device, replacement ⓑ Qp Qh   N

✱ **A4608** Transtracheal oxygen catheter, each ⓑ ♿   N

Supplies for Respiratory and Oxygen Equipment

⊘ **A4611** Battery, heavy duty; replacement for patient owned ventilator ⓑ Qp Qh   E1
     Medicare Statute 1834(a)(3)(a)

⊘ **A4612** Battery cables; replacement for patient-owned ventilator ⓑ Qh   E1
     Medicare Statute 1834(a)(3)(a)

⊘ **A4613** Battery charger; replacement for patient-owned ventilator ⓑ Qh   E1
     Medicare Statute 1834(a)(3)(a)

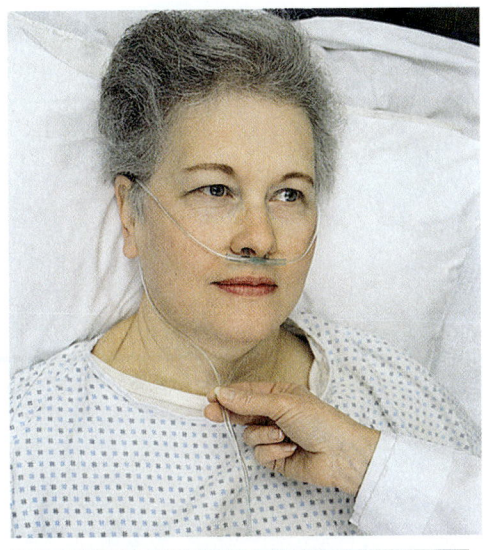

Figure 5   Nasal cannula.

✱ **A4614** Peak expiratory flow rate meter, hand held ⓑ ⓑ Qp Qh ♿   N

✵ **A4615** Cannula, nasal ⓠ ⓑ ♿   N
     IOM: 100-03, 2, 160.6; 100-04, 20, 100.2

✵ **A4616** Tubing (oxygen), per foot ⓠ ⓑ ♿   N
     IOM: 100-03, 2, 160.6; 100-04, 20, 100.2

✵ **A4617** Mouth piece ⓠ ⓑ ♿   N
     IOM: 100-03, 2, 160.6; 100-04, 20, 100.2

✵ **A4618** Breathing circuits ⓠ ⓑ Qp Qh ♿   N
     IOM: 100-03, 2, 160.6; 100-04, 20, 100.2

✵ **A4619** Face tent ⓠ ⓑ ♿   N
     IOM: 100-03, 2, 160.6; 100-04, 20, 100.2

✵ **A4620** Variable concentration mask ⓠ ⓑ ♿   N
     IOM: 100-03, 2, 160.6; 100-04, 20, 100.2

✵ **A4623** Tracheostomy, inner cannula ⓠ ⓑ Qh ♿   N
     IOM: 100-02, 15, 120; 100-03, 1, 20.9

✱ **A4624** Tracheal suction catheter, any type, other than closed system, each ⓠ ⓑ Qh ♿   N

     Sterile suction catheters are medically necessary only for tracheostomy suctioning. Limitations include three suction catheters per day when covered for medically necessary tracheostomy suctioning. Assign DX V44.0 or V55.0 on the claim form. (CMS Manual System, Pub. 100-3, NCD manual, Chapter 1, Section 280-1)

👆 MIPS	Qp Quantity Physician	Qh Quantity Hospital	♀ Female only	
♂ Male only	A Age	♿ DMEPOS	A2-Z3 ASC Payment Indicator	A-Y ASC Status Indicator Coding Clinic

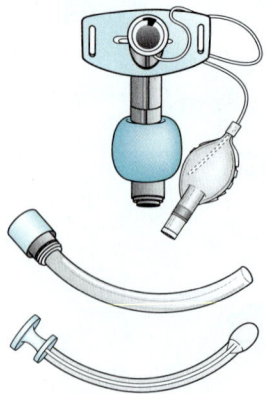

Figure 6 Tracheostomy cannula.

○ **A4625** Tracheostomy care kit for new tracheostomy Ⓑ Ⓑ Qp Qh ♿ N

Dressings used with tracheostomies are included in the allowance for the code. This starter kit is covered after a surgical tracheostomy. (https://www.noridianmedicare.com/dme/coverage/docs/lcds/current_lcds/tracheostomy_care_supplies.htm)

IOM: 100-02, 15, 120

○ **A4626** Tracheostomy cleaning brush, each Ⓑ Ⓑ ♿ N

IOM: 100-02, 15, 120

⊘ **A4627** Spacer, bag, or reservoir, with or without mask, for use with metered dose inhaler Ⓑ Ⓑ Qp Qh E1

IOM: 100-02, 15, 110

✱ **A4628** Oral and/or oropharyngeal suction catheter, each Ⓑ Qh ♿ N

No more than three catheters per week are covered for medically necessary oropharyngeal suctioning because the catheters can be reused if cleansed and disinfected. (MS Manual System, Pub. 100-3, NCD manual, Chapter 1, Section 280-1)

○ **A4629** Tracheostomy care kit for established tracheostomy Ⓑ Ⓑ Qh ♿ N

IOM: 100-02, 15, 120

Replacement Parts

○ **A4630** Replacement batteries, medically necessary, transcutaneous electrical stimulator, owned by patient Ⓑ ♿ E1

IOM: 100-03, 3, 160.7

✱ **A4633** Replacement bulb/lamp for ultraviolet light therapy system, each Ⓑ Qp Qh ♿ E1

✱ **A4634** Replacement bulb for therapeutic light box, tabletop model Ⓑ N

○ **A4635** Underarm pad, crutch, replacement, each Ⓑ Qp Qh ♿ E1

IOM: 100-03, 4, 280.1

○ **A4636** Replacement, handgrip, cane, crutch, or walker, each Ⓑ Qh ♿ E1

IOM: 100-03, 4, 280.1

○ **A4637** Replacement, tip, cane, crutch, walker, each Ⓑ Qh ♿ E1

IOM: 100-03, 4, 280.1

✱ **A4638** Replacement battery for patient-owned ear pulse generator, each Ⓑ Qp Qh ♿ E1

✱ **A4639** Replacement pad for infrared heating pad system, each Ⓑ ♿ E1

○ **A4640** Replacement pad for use with medically necessary alternating pressure pad owned by patient Ⓑ Qp Qh ♿ E1

IOM: 100-03, 4, 280.1; 100-08, 5, 5.2.3

Supplies for Radiological Procedures

✱ **A4641** Radiopharmaceutical, diagnostic, not otherwise classified Ⓖ N

Is not an applicable tracer for PET scans

✱ **A4642** Indium In-111 satumomab pendetide, diagnostic, per study dose, up to 6 millicuries Ⓑ Qp Qh N

Miscellaneous Supplies

✱ **A4648** Tissue marker, implantable, any type, each Ⓑ Qp Qh N

Coding Clinic: 2024, Q3, P20; 2018, Q2, P4,5; 2013, Q3, P9

✱ **A4649** Surgical supply miscellaneous Ⓑ Ⓑ Qp N

✱ **A4650** Implantable radiation dosimeter, each Ⓑ Qp Qh N

○ **A4651** Calibrated microcapillary tube, each Ⓑ N

IOM: 100-04, 3, 40.3

○ **A4652** Microcapillary tube sealant Ⓑ N

IOM: 100-04, 3, 40.3

Supplies for Dialysis

✱ **A4653** Peritoneal dialysis catheter anchoring device, belt, each Ⓑ Qp Qh N

○ **A4657** Syringe, with or without needle, each Ⓑ Qp Qh N

IOM: 100-04, 8, 90.3.2

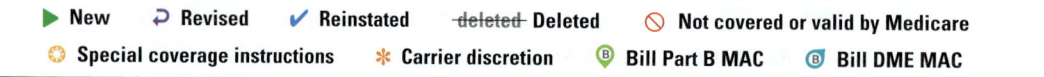

MEDICAL AND SURGICAL SUPPLIES

- **A4660** Sphygmomanometer/blood pressure apparatus with cuff and stethoscope ⓑ Qp Qh N
  IOM: 100-04, 8, 90.3.2

- **A4663** Blood pressure cuff only ⓑ Qp Qh N
  IOM: 100-04, 8, 90.3.2

- ⊘ **A4670** Automatic blood pressure monitor ⓑ Qp Qh E1
  IOM: 100-04, 8, 90.3.2

- **A4671** Disposable cycler set used with cycler dialysis machine, each ⓑ Qp Qh B
  IOM: 100-04, 8, 90.3.2

- **A4672** Drainage extension line, sterile, for dialysis, each ⓑ Qp Qh B
  IOM: 100-04, 8, 90.3.2

- **A4673** Extension line with easy lock connectors, used with dialysis ⓑ Qp Qh B
  IOM: 100-04, 8, 90.3.2

- **A4674** Chemicals/antiseptics solution used to clean/sterilize dialysis equipment, per 8 oz ⓑ Qp Qh B
  IOM: 100-04, 8, 90.3.2

- **A4680** Activated carbon filters for hemodialysis, each ⓑ Qp Qh N
  IOM: 100-04, 8, 90.3.2

- **A4690** Dialyzers (artificial kidneys), all types, all sizes, for hemodialysis, each ⓑ Qp Qh N
  IOM: 100-04, 8, 90.3.2

- **A4706** Bicarbonate concentrate, solution, for hemodialysis, per gallon ⓑ Qp Qh N
  IOM: 100-04, 8, 90.3.2

- **A4707** Bicarbonate concentrate, powder, for hemodialysis, per packet ⓑ Qp Qh N
  IOM: 100-04, 8, 90.3.2

- **A4708** Acetate concentrate solution, for hemodialysis, per gallon ⓑ Qp Qh N
  IOM: 100-04, 8, 90.3.2

- **A4709** Acid concentrate, solution, for hemodialysis, per gallon ⓑ Qp Qh N
  IOM: 100-04, 8, 90.3.2

- **A4714** Treated water (deionized, distilled, or reverse osmosis) for peritoneal dialysis, per gallon ⓑ Qp Qh N
  IOM: 100-03, 4, 230.7; 100-04, 3, 40.3

- **A4719** "Y set" tubing for peritoneal dialysis ⓑ Qp Qh N
  IOM: 100-04, 8, 90.3.2

- **A4720** Dialysate solution, any concentration of dextrose, fluid volume greater than 249 cc, but less than or equal to 999 cc, for peritoneal dialysis ⓑ Qp Qh N
  Do not use AX modifier.
  IOM: 100-04, 8, 90.3.2

- **A4721** Dialysate solution, any concentration of dextrose, fluid volume greater than 999 cc but less than or equal to 1999 cc, for peritoneal dialysis ⓑ Qp Qh N
  IOM: 100-04, 8, 90.3.2

- **A4722** Dialysate solution, any concentration of dextrose, fluid volume greater than 1999 cc but less than or equal to 2999 cc, for peritoneal dialysis ⓑ Qp Qh N
  IOM: 100-04, 8, 90.3.2

- **A4723** Dialysate solution, any concentration of dextrose, fluid volume greater than 2999 cc but less than or equal to 3999 cc, for peritoneal dialysis ⓑ Qp Qh N
  IOM: 100-04, 8, 90.3.2

- **A4724** Dialysate solution, any concentration of dextrose, fluid volume greater than 3999 cc but less than or equal to 4999 cc for peritoneal dialysis ⓑ Qp Qh N
  IOM: 100-04, 8, 90.3.2

- **A4725** Dialysate solution, any concentration of dextrose, fluid volume greater than 4999 cc but less than or equal to 5999 cc, for peritoneal dialysis ⓑ Qp Qh N
  IOM: 100-04, 8, 90.3.2

- **A4726** Dialysate solution, any concentration of dextrose, fluid volume greater than 5999 cc, for peritoneal dialysis ⓑ Qp Qh N
  IOM: 100-04, 8, 90.3.2

- ✱ **A4728** Dialysate solution, non-dextrose containing, 500 ml ⓑ Qp Qh B

- **A4730** Fistula cannulation set for hemodialysis, each ⓑ Qp Qh N
  IOM: 100-04, 8, 90.3.2

- **A4736** Topical anesthetic, for dialysis, per gram ⓑ Qp Qh N
  IOM: 100-04, 8, 90.3.2

- **A4737** Injectable anesthetic, for dialysis, per 10 ml ⓑ Qp Qh N
  IOM: 100-04, 8, 90.3.2

- **A4740** Shunt accessory, for hemodialysis, any type, each ⓑ Qp Qh N
  IOM: 100-04, 8, 90.3.2

- **A4750** Blood tubing, arterial or venous, for hemodialysis, each ⓑ Qp Qh N
  IOM: 100-04, 8, 90.3.2

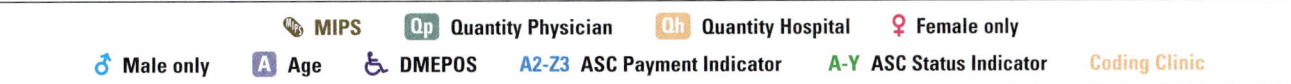

✺ A4755	Blood tubing, arterial and venous combined, for hemodialysis, each Ⓑ Qp Qh	N
	IOM: 100-04, 8, 90.3.2	
✺ A4760	Dialysate solution test kit, for peritoneal dialysis, any type, each Ⓑ Qp Qh	N
	IOM: 100-04, 8, 90.3.2	
✺ A4765	Dialysate concentrate, powder, additive for peritoneal dialysis, per packet Ⓑ Qp Qh	N
	IOM: 100-04, 8, 90.3.2	
✺ A4766	Dialysate concentrate, solution, additive for peritoneal dialysis, per 10 ml Ⓑ Qp Qh	N
	IOM: 100-04, 8, 90.3.2	
✺ A4770	Blood collection tube, vacuum, for dialysis, per 50 Ⓑ Qp Qh	N
	IOM: 100-04, 8, 90.3.2	
✺ A4771	Serum clotting time tube, for dialysis, per 50 Ⓑ Qp Qh	N
	IOM: 100-04, 8, 90.3.2	
✺ A4772	Blood glucose test strips, for dialysis, per 50 Ⓑ Qp Qh	N
	IOM: 100-04, 8, 90.3.2	
✺ A4773	Occult blood test strips, for dialysis, per 50 Ⓑ Qp Qh	N
	IOM: 100-04, 8, 90.3.2	
✺ A4774	Ammonia test strips, for dialysis, per 50 Ⓑ Qp Qh	N
	IOM: 100-04, 8, 90.3.2	
✺ A4802	Protamine sulfate, for hemodialysis, per 50 mg Ⓑ Qp Qh	N
	IOM: 100-04, 8, 90.3.2	
✺ A4860	Disposable catheter tips for peritoneal dialysis, per 10 Ⓑ Qp Qh	N
	IOM: 100-04, 8, 90.3.2	
✺ A4870	Plumbing and/or electrical work for home hemodialysis equipment Ⓑ Qp Qh	N
	IOM: 100-04, 8, 90.3.2	
✺ A4890	Contracts, repair and maintenance, for hemodialysis equipment Ⓑ Qp Qh	N
	IOM: 100-02, 15, 110.2	
✺ A4911	Drain bag/bottle, for dialysis, each Ⓑ Qp Qh	N
✺ A4913	Miscellaneous dialysis supplies, not otherwise specified Ⓑ Qp Qh	N
	Items not related to dialysis must not be billed with the miscellaneous codes A4913 or E1699.	
✺ A4918	Venous pressure clamp, for hemodialysis, each Ⓑ Qp Qh	N
✺ A4927	Gloves, non-sterile, per 100 Ⓑ Qp Qh	N
✺ A4928	Surgical mask, per 20 Ⓑ Qp Qh	N
✺ A4929	Tourniquet for dialysis, each Ⓑ Qp Qh	N
✺ A4930	Gloves, sterile, per pair Ⓑ Qp Qh	N
* A4931	Oral thermometer, reusable, any type, each Ⓑ Qp Qh	N
* A4932	Rectal thermometer, reusable, any type, each Ⓑ Qp Qh	N

Additional Ostomy Supplies

✺ A5051	Ostomy pouch, closed; with barrier attached (1 piece), each ⓞ Ⓑ Qp Qh ♿	N
	IOM: 100-02, 15, 120	
✺ A5052	Ostomy pouch, closed; without barrier attached (1 piece), each ⓞ Ⓑ Qp Qh ♿	N
	IOM: 100-02, 15, 120	
✺ A5053	Ostomy pouch, closed; for use on faceplate, each ⓞ Ⓑ Qp Qh ♿	N
	IOM: 100-02, 15, 120	
✺ A5054	Ostomy pouch, closed; for use on barrier with flange (2 piece), each ⓞ Ⓑ Qp ♿	N
	IOM: 100-02, 15, 120	
✺ A5055	Stoma cap ⓞ Ⓑ Qp Qh ♿	N
	IOM: 100-02, 15, 120	
✺ A5056	Ostomy pouch, drainable, with extended wear barrier attached, with filter (1 piece), each ⓞ Ⓑ Qp Qh ♿	N
	IOM: 100-02, 15, 120	
✺ A5057	Ostomy pouch, drainable, with extended wear barrier attached, with built in convexity, with filter (1 piece), each ⓞ Ⓑ Qp Qh ♿	N
	IOM: 100-02, 15, 120	
* A5061	Ostomy pouch, drainable; with barrier attached (1 piece), each ⓞ Ⓑ Qp Qh ♿	N
	IOM: 100-02, 15, 120	
✺ A5062	Ostomy pouch, drainable; without barrier attached (1 piece), each ⓞ Ⓑ Qp Qh ♿	N
	IOM: 100-02, 15, 120	
✺ A5063	Ostomy pouch, drainable; for use on barrier with flange (2 piece system), each ⓞ Ⓑ Qp Qh ♿	N
	IOM: 100-02, 15, 120	

▶ New ⤺ Revised ✓ Reinstated ~~deleted~~ Deleted 🚫 Not covered or valid by Medicare
✺ Special coverage instructions * Carrier discretion Ⓑ Bill Part B MAC Ⓑ Bill DME MAC

MEDICAL AND SURGICAL SUPPLIES

- **A5071** Ostomy pouch, urinary; with barrier attached (1 piece), each   N
  IOM: 100-02, 15, 120

- **A5072** Ostomy pouch, urinary; without barrier attached (1 piece), each   N
  IOM: 100-02, 15, 120

- **A5073** Ostomy pouch, urinary; for use on barrier with flange (2 piece), each   N
  IOM: 100-02, 15, 120

- **A5081** Stoma plug or seal, any type   N
  IOM: 100-02, 15, 120

- **A5082** Continent device; catheter for continent stoma   N
  IOM: 100-02, 15, 120

- *** A5083** Continent device, stoma absorptive cover for continent stoma   N

- **A5093** Ostomy accessory; convex insert   N
  IOM: 100-02, 15, 120

Additional Incontinence and Ostomy Supplies

- **A5102** Bedside drainage bottle with or without tubing, rigid or expandable, each   N
  IOM: 100-02, 15, 120

- **A5105** Urinary suspensory, with leg bag, with or without tube, each   N
  IOM: 100-02, 15, 120

- **A5112** Urinary drainage bag, leg bag, leg or abdomen, latex, with or without tube, with straps, each   N
  IOM: 100-02, 15, 120

- **A5113** Leg strap; latex, replacement only, per set   E1
  IOM: 100-02, 15, 120

- **A5114** Leg strap; foam or fabric, replacement only, per set   E1
  IOM: 100-02, 15, 120

- **A5120** Skin barrier, wipes or swabs, each   N
  IOM: 100-02, 15, 120

- **A5121** Skin barrier; solid, 6 × 6 or equivalent, each   N
  IOM: 100-02, 15, 120

- **A5122** Skin barrier; solid, 8 × 8 or equivalent, each   N
  IOM: 100-02, 15, 120

- **A5126** Adhesive or non-adhesive; disk or foam pad   N
  IOM: 100-02, 15, 120

- **A5131** Appliance cleaner, incontinence and ostomy appliances, per 16 oz   N
  IOM: 100-02, 15, 120

- **A5200** Percutaneous catheter/tube anchoring device, adhesive skin attachment   N
  IOM: 100-02, 15, 120

Diabetic Shoes, Fitting, and Modifications

- **A5500** For diabetics only, fitting (including follow-up), custom preparation and supply of off-the-shelf depth-inlay shoe manufactured to accommodate multi-density insert(s), per shoe   Y
  IOM: 100-02, 15, 140

- **A5501** For diabetics only, fitting (including follow-up), custom preparation and supply of shoe molded from cast(s) of patient's foot (custom-molded shoe), per shoe   Y

  The diabetic patient must have at least one of the following conditions: peripheral neuropathy with evidence of callus formation, pre-ulcerative calluses, previous ulceration, foot deformity, previous amputation or poor circulation.

  IOM: 100-02, 15, 140

- **A5503** For diabetics only, modification (including fitting) of off-the-shelf depth-inlay shoe or custom-molded shoe with roller or rigid rocker bottom, per shoe   Y
  IOM: 100-02, 15, 140

- **A5504** For diabetics only, modification (including fitting) of off-the-shelf depth-inlay shoe or custom-molded shoe with wedge(s), per shoe   Y
  IOM: 100-02, 15, 140

- **A5505** For diabetics only, modification (including fitting) of off-the-shelf depth-inlay shoe or custom-molded shoe with metatarsal bar, per shoe   Y
  IOM: 100-02, 15, 140

- **A5506** For diabetics only, modification (including fitting) of off-the-shelf depth-inlay shoe or custom-molded shoe with off-set heel(s), per shoe   Y
  IOM: 100-02, 15, 140

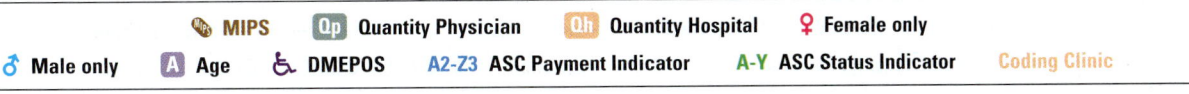

MIPS   Qp Quantity Physician   Qh Quantity Hospital   ♀ Female only   ♂ Male only   A Age   DMEPOS   A2-Z3 ASC Payment Indicator   A-Y ASC Status Indicator   Coding Clinic

A5507 — For diabetics only, not otherwise specified modification (including fitting) of off-the-shelf depth-inlay shoe or custom-molded shoe, per shoe Ⓑ Qp Qh ♿ Y

Only used for not otherwise specified therapeutic modifications to shoe or for repairs to a diabetic shoe(s)

IOM: 100-02, 15, 140

A5508 — For diabetics only, deluxe feature of off-the-shelf depth-inlay shoe or custom-molded shoe, per shoe Ⓑ Qp Qh Y

IOM: 100-02, 15, 40

A5510 — For diabetics only, direct formed, compression molded to patient's foot without external heat source, multiple-density insert(s) prefabricated, per shoe Ⓑ Qp Qh N

IOM: 100-02, 15, 140

A5512 — For diabetics only, multiple density insert, direct formed, molded to foot after external heat source of 230 degrees Fahrenheit or higher, total contact with patient's foot, including arch, base layer minimum of 1/4 inch material of shore a 35 durometer or 3/16 inch material of shore a 40 durometer (or higher), prefabricated, each Ⓑ Qp Qh ♿ Y

A5513 — For diabetics only, multiple density insert, custom molded from model of patient's foot, total contact with patient's foot, including arch, base layer minimum of 3/16 inch material of shore a 35 durometer (or higher), includes arch filler and other shaping material, custom fabricated, each Ⓑ Qp Qh ♿ Y

A5514 — For diabetics only, multiple density insert, made by direct carving with cam technology from a rectified CAD model created from a digitized scan of the patient, total contact with patient's foot, including arch, base layer minimum of 3/16 inch material of shore a 35 durometer (or higher), includes arch filler and other shaping material, custom fabricated, each Ⓑ ♿ Y

Dressings

A6000 — Non-contact wound warming wound cover for use with the non-contact wound warming device and warming card Ⓑ Qp Qh E1

IOM: 100-02, 16, 20

A6010 — Collagen based wound filler, dry form, sterile, per gram of collagen Ⓑ Ⓑ ♿ N

IOM: 100-02, 15, 100

A6011 — Collagen based wound filler, gel/paste, per gram of collagen Ⓑ ♿ N

IOM: 100-02, 15, 100

A6021 — Collagen dressing, sterile, size 16 sq. in. or less, each Ⓑ ♿ N

IOM: 100-02, 15, 100

A6022 — Collagen dressing, sterile, size more than 16 sq. in. but less than or equal to 48 sq. in., each Ⓑ Qp ♿ N

IOM: 100-02, 15, 100

A6023 — Collagen dressing, sterile, size more than 48 sq. in., each Ⓑ ♿ N

IOM: 100-02, 15, 100

A6024 — Collagen dressing wound filler, sterile, per 6 inches Ⓑ Ⓑ ♿ N

IOM: 100-02, 15, 100

A6025 — Gel sheet for dermal or epidermal application (e.g., silicone, hydrogel, other), each Ⓑ Ⓑ N

If used for the treatment of keloids or other scars, a silicone gel sheet will not meet the definition of the surgical dressing benefit and will be denied as noncovered.

A6154 — Wound pouch, each Ⓑ Ⓑ Qp Qh ♿ N

Waterproof collection device with drainable port that adheres to skin around wound. Usual dressing change is up to 3 times per week.

IOM: 100-02, 15, 100

A6196 — Alginate or other fiber gelling dressing, wound cover, sterile, pad size 16 sq. in. or less, each dressing Ⓑ Ⓑ Qp ♿ N

IOM: 100-02, 15, 100

A6197 — Alginate or other fiber gelling dressing, wound cover, sterile, pad size more than 16 sq. in., but less than or equal to 48 sq. in., each dressing Ⓑ Ⓑ Qp ♿ N

IOM: 100-02, 15, 100

A6198 — Alginate or other fiber gelling dressing, wound cover, sterile, pad size more than 48 sq. in., each dressing Ⓑ Ⓑ Qp N

IOM: 100-02, 15, 100

A6199 — Alginate or other fiber gelling dressing, wound filler, sterile, per 6 inches Ⓑ Ⓑ Qp ♿ N

IOM: 100-02, 15, 100

A6203 — Composite dressing, sterile, pad size 16 sq. in. or less, with any size adhesive border, each dressing Ⓑ Ⓑ Qp N

Usual composite dressing change is up to 3 times per week, one wound cover per dressing change.

IOM: 100-02, 15, 100

▶ New   ⟲ Revised   ✓ Reinstated   ~~deleted~~ Deleted   ⊘ Not covered or valid by Medicare
✺ Special coverage instructions   ✱ Carrier discretion   Ⓑ Bill Part B MAC   Ⓑ Bill DME MAC

MEDICAL AND SURGICAL SUPPLIES

A6204 Composite dressing, sterile, pad size more than 16 sq. in. but less than or equal to 48 sq. in., with any size adhesive border, each dressing ⓑ Ⓑ Qp ♿ N

Usual composite dressing change is up to 3 times per week, one wound cover per dressing change.

IOM: 100-02, 15, 100

A6205 Composite dressing, sterile, pad size more than 48 sq. in., with any size adhesive border, each dressing ⓑ Ⓑ Qp Qh N

Usual composite dressing change is up to 3 times per week, one wound cover per dressing change.

IOM: 100-02, 15, 100

A6206 Contact layer, sterile, 16 sq. in. or less, each dressing ⓑ Ⓑ Qp N

Contact layers are porous to allow wound fluid to pass through for absorption by separate overlying dressing and are not intended to be changed with each dressing change. Usual dressing change is up to once per week.

IOM: 100-02, 15, 100

A6207 Contact layer, sterile, more than 16 sq. in. but less than or equal to 48 sq. in., each dressing ⓑ Ⓑ Qp ♿ N

Contact layer dressings are used to line the entire wound; they are not intended to be changed with each dressing change. Usual dressing change is up to once per week.

IOM: 100-02, 15, 100

A6208 Contact layer, sterile, more than 48 sq. in., each dressing ⓑ Ⓑ Qp N

Contact layer dressings are used to line the entire wound; they are not intended to be changed with each dressing change. Usual dressing change is up to once per week.

IOM: 100-02, 15, 100

A6209 Foam dressing, wound cover, sterile, pad size 16 sq. in. or less, without adhesive border, each dressing ⓑ Ⓑ Qp ♿ N

Made of open cell, medical grade expanded polymer; with nonadherent property over wound site.

IOM: 100-02, 15, 100

A6210 Foam dressing, wound cover, sterile, pad size more than 16 sq. in. but less than or equal to 48 sq. in., without adhesive border, each dressing ⓑ Ⓑ Qp ♿ N

Foam dressings are covered items when used on full thickness wounds (e.g., stage III or IV ulcers) with moderate to heavy exudates. Usual dressing change for a foam wound cover when used as primary dressing is up to 3 times per week. When foam wound cover is used as a secondary dressing for wounds with very heavy exudates, dressing change may be up to 3 times per week. Usual dressing change for foam wound fillers is up to once per day (A6209-A6215).

IOM: 100-02, 15, 100

A6211 Foam dressing, wound cover, sterile, pad size more than 48 sq. in., without adhesive border, each dressing ⓑ Ⓑ Qp ♿ N

IOM: 100-02, 15, 100

A6212 Foam dressing, wound cover, sterile, pad size 16 sq. in. or less, with any size adhesive border, each dressing ⓑ Ⓑ Qp ♿ N

IOM: 100-02, 15, 100

A6213 Foam dressing, wound cover, sterile, pad size more than 16 sq. in. but less than or equal to 48 sq. in., with any size adhesive border, each dressing ⓑ Ⓑ Qp N

IOM: 100-02, 15, 100

A6214 Foam dressing, wound cover, sterile, pad size more than 48 sq. in., with any size adhesive border, each dressing ⓑ Ⓑ Qp ♿ N

IOM: 100-02, 15, 100

A6215 Foam dressing, wound filler, sterile, per gram ⓑ Ⓑ Qp N

IOM: 100-02, 15, 100

A6216 Gauze, non-impregnated, non-sterile, pad size 16 sq. in. or less, without adhesive border, each dressing ⓑ Ⓑ Qp ♿ N

IOM: 100-02, 15, 100

A6217 Gauze, non-impregnated, non-sterile, pad size more than 16 sq. in. but less than or equal to 48 sq. in., without adhesive border, each dressing ⓑ Ⓑ Qp ♿ N

IOM: 100-02, 15, 100

| 🏷 MIPS | Qp Quantity Physician | Qh Quantity Hospital | ♀ Female only |
| ♂ Male only | A Age | ♿ DMEPOS | A2-Z3 ASC Payment Indicator | A-Y ASC Status Indicator | Coding Clinic |

A6218	Gauze, non-impregnated, non-sterile, pad size more than 48 sq. in., without adhesive border, each dressing N
	IOM: 100-02, 15, 100
A6219	Gauze, non-impregnated, sterile, pad size 16 sq. in. or less, with any size adhesive border, each dressing N
	IOM: 100-02, 15, 100
A6220	Gauze, non-impregnated, sterile, pad size more than 16 sq. in. but less than or equal to 48 sq. in., with any size adhesive border, each dressing N
	IOM: 100-02, 15, 100
A6221	Gauze, non-impregnated, sterile, pad size more than 48 sq. in., with any size adhesive border, each dressing N
	IOM: 100-02, 15, 100
A6222	Gauze, impregnated with other than water, normal saline, or hydrogel, sterile, pad size 16 sq. in. or less, without adhesive border, each dressing N
	Substances may have been incorporated into dressing material (i.e., iodinated agents, petrolatum, zinc paste, crystalline sodium chloride, chlorhexadine gluconate [CHG], bismuth tribromophenate [BTP], water, aqueous saline, hydrogel, or agents).
	IOM: 100-02, 15, 100
A6223	Gauze, impregnated with other than water, normal saline, or hydrogel, sterile, pad size more than 16 sq. in. but less than or equal to 48 sq. in., without adhesive border, each dressing N
	IOM: 100-02, 15, 100
A6224	Gauze, impregnated with other than water, normal saline, or hydrogel, sterile, pad size more than 48 sq. in., without adhesive border, each dressing N
	IOM: 100-02, 15, 100
A6228	Gauze, impregnated, water or normal saline, sterile, pad size 16 sq. in. or less, without adhesive border, each dressing N
	IOM: 100-02, 15, 100
A6229	Gauze, impregnated, water or normal saline, sterile, pad size more than 16 sq. in. but less than or equal to 48 sq. in., without adhesive border, each dressing N
	IOM: 100-02, 15, 100
A6230	Gauze, impregnated, water or normal saline, sterile, pad size more than 48 sq. in., without adhesive border, each dressing N
	IOM: 100-02, 15, 100
A6231	Gauze, impregnated, hydrogel, for direct wound contact, sterile, pad size 16 sq. in. or less, each dressing N
	IOM: 100-02, 15, 100
A6232	Gauze, impregnated, hydrogel, for direct wound contact, sterile, pad size greater than 16 sq. in., but less than or equal to 48 sq. in., each dressing N
	IOM: 100-02, 15, 100
A6233	Gauze, impregnated, hydrogel, for direct wound contact, sterile, pad size more than 48 sq. in., each dressing N
	IOM: 100-02, 15, 100
A6234	Hydrocolloid dressing, wound cover, sterile, pad size 16 sq. in. or less, without adhesive border, each dressing N
	This type of dressing is usually used on wounds with light to moderate exudate with an average of three dressing changes per week.
	IOM: 100-02, 15, 100
A6235	Hydrocolloid dressing, wound cover, sterile, pad size more than 16 sq. in. but less than or equal to 48 sq. in., without adhesive border, each dressing N
	IOM: 100-02, 15, 100
A6236	Hydrocolloid dressing, wound cover, sterile, pad size more than 48 sq. in., without adhesive border, each dressing N
	IOM: 100-02, 15, 100
A6237	Hydrocolloid dressing, wound cover, sterile, pad size 16 sq. in. or less, with any size adhesive border, each dressing N
	IOM: 100-02, 15, 100

▶ New   ↻ Revised   ✓ Reinstated   ~~deleted~~ Deleted   ⊘ Not covered or valid by Medicare
✺ Special coverage instructions   ✱ Carrier discretion   Ⓑ Bill Part B MAC   Ⓓ Bill DME MAC

MEDICAL AND SURGICAL SUPPLIES

A6238 Hydrocolloid dressing, wound cover, sterile, pad size more than 16 sq. in. but less than or equal to 48 sq. in., with any size adhesive border, each dressing ⓑ Ⓑ Qp Qh ♿ N

IOM: 100-02, 15, 100

A6239 Hydrocolloid dressing, wound cover, sterile, pad size more than 48 sq. in., with any size adhesive border, each dressing ⓑ Ⓑ Qp Qh N

IOM: 100-02, 15, 100

A6240 Hydrocolloid dressing, wound filler, paste, sterile, per ounce ⓑ Ⓑ Qp Qh ♿ N

IOM: 100-02, 15, 100

A6241 Hydrocolloid dressing, wound filler, dry form, sterile, per gram ⓑ Ⓑ Qp Qh ♿ N

IOM: 100-02, 15, 100

A6242 Hydrogel dressing, wound cover, sterile, pad size 16 sq. in. or less, without adhesive border, each dressing ⓑ Ⓑ Qp ♿ N

Considered medically necessary when used on full thickness wounds with minimal or no exudate (e.g., stage III or IV ulcers).

Usually up to one dressing change per day is considered medically necessary, but if well documented and medically necessary, the payer may allow more frequent dressing changes.

IOM: 100-02, 15, 100

A6243 Hydrogel dressing, wound cover, sterile, pad size more than 16 sq. in. but less than or equal to 48 sq. in., without adhesive border, each dressing ⓑ Ⓑ Qp ♿ N

IOM: 100-02, 15, 100

A6244 Hydrogel dressing, wound cover, sterile, pad size more than 48 sq. in., without adhesive border, each dressing ⓑ Ⓑ Qp Qh ♿ N

IOM: 100-02, 15, 100

A6245 Hydrogel dressing, wound cover, sterile, pad size 16 sq. in. or less, with any size adhesive border, each dressing ⓑ Ⓑ Qp ♿ N

Coverage of a non-elastic gradient compression wrap is limited to one per 6 months per leg.

IOM: 100-02, 15, 100

A6246 Hydrogel dressing, wound cover, sterile, pad size more than 16 sq. in. but less than or equal to 48 sq. in., with any size adhesive border, each dressing ⓑ Ⓑ Qp Qh ♿ N

IOM: 100-02, 15, 100

A6247 Hydrogel dressing, wound cover, sterile, pad size more than 48 sq. in., with any size adhesive border, each dressing ⓑ Ⓑ Qp Qh ♿ N

IOM: 100-02, 15, 100

A6248 Hydrogel dressing, wound filler, gel, per fluid ounce ⓑ Ⓑ Qp ♿ N

IOM: 100-02, 15, 100

A6250 Skin sealants, protectants, moisturizers, ointments, any type, any size ⓑ Ⓑ Qp Qh N

IOM: 100-02, 15, 100

A6251 Specialty absorptive dressing, wound cover, sterile, pad size 16 sq. in. or less, without adhesive border, each dressing ⓑ Ⓑ Qp ♿ N

IOM: 100-02, 15, 100

A6252 Specialty absorptive dressing, wound cover, sterile, pad size more than 16 sq. in. but less than or equal to 48 sq. in., without adhesive border, each dressing ⓑ Ⓑ Qp ♿ N

IOM: 100-02, 15, 100

A6253 Specialty absorptive dressing, wound cover, sterile, pad size more than 48 sq. in., without adhesive border, each dressing ⓑ Ⓑ Qp ♿ N

IOM: 100-02, 15, 100

A6254 Specialty absorptive dressing, wound cover, sterile, pad size 16 sq. in. or less, with any size adhesive border, each dressing ⓑ Ⓑ Qp ♿ N

IOM: 100-02, 15, 100

A6255 Specialty absorptive dressing, wound cover, sterile, pad size more than 16 sq. in. but less than or equal to 48 sq. in., with any size adhesive border, each dressing ⓑ Ⓑ Qp ♿ N

IOM: 100-02, 15, 100

A6256 Specialty absorptive dressing, wound cover, sterile, pad size more than 48 sq. in., with any size adhesive border, each dressing ⓑ Ⓑ Qp Qh N

Considered medically necessary when used for moderately or highly exudative wounds (e.g., stage III or IV ulcers).

IOM: 100-02, 15, 100

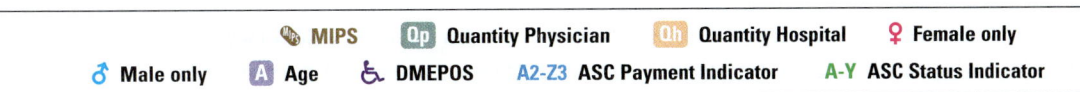

⊛ **A6257**	Transparent film, sterile, 16 sq. in. or less, each dressing ⓑ Ⓑ Qp ♿	N

Considered medically necessary when used on open partial thickness wounds with minimal exudate or closed wounds.

IOM: 100-02, 15, 100

⊛ **A6258**	Transparent film, sterile, more than 16 sq. in. but less than or equal to 48 sq. in., each dressing ⓑ Ⓑ Qp ♿	N

IOM: 100-02, 15, 100

⊛ **A6259**	Transparent film, sterile, more than 48 sq. in., each dressing ⓑ Ⓑ Qp Qh ♿	N

IOM: 100-02, 15, 100

⊛ **A6260**	Wound cleansers, any type, any size ⓑ Ⓑ Qp	N

IOM: 100-02, 15, 100

⊛ **A6261**	Wound filler, gel/paste, per fluid ounce, not otherwise specified ⓑ Ⓑ Qp Qh	N

Units of service for wound fillers are 1 gram, 1 fluid ounce, 6 inch length, or 1 yard depending on product.

IOM: 100-02, 15, 100

⊛ **A6262**	Wound filler, dry form, per gram, not otherwise specified ⓑ Ⓑ Qp Qh	N

Dry forms (e.g., powder, granules, beads) are used to eliminate dead space in an open wound.

IOM: 100-02, 15, 100

⊛ **A6266**	Gauze, impregnated, other than water, normal saline, or zinc paste, sterile, any width, per linear yard ⓑ Ⓑ Qp ♿	N

IOM: 100-02, 15, 100

⊛ **A6402**	Gauze, non-impregnated, sterile, pad size 16 sq. in. or less, without adhesive border, each dressing ⓑ Ⓑ Qp ♿	N

IOM: 100-02, 15, 100

⊛ **A6403**	Gauze, non-impregnated, sterile, pad size more than 16 sq. in., less than or equal to 48 sq. in., without adhesive border, each dressing ⓑ Ⓑ Qp ♿	N

IOM: 100-02, 15, 100

⊛ **A6404**	Gauze, non-impregnated, sterile, pad size more than 48 sq. in., without adhesive border, each dressing ⓑ Ⓑ Qp Qh	N

IOM: 100-02, 15, 100

✱ **A6407**	Packing strips, non-impregnated, sterile, up to 2 inches in width, per linear yard ⓑ Ⓑ ♿	N

IOM: 100-02, 15, 100

⊛ **A6410**	Eye pad, sterile, each ⓑ Ⓑ Qp Qh ♿	N

IOM: 100-02, 15, 100

⊛ **A6411**	Eye pad, non-sterile, each ⓑ Ⓑ Qh ♿	N

IOM: 100-02, 15, 100

✱ **A6412**	Eye patch, occlusive, each Ⓑ	N

Bandages

⊘ **A6413**	Adhesive bandage, first-aid type, any size, each ⓑ Ⓑ Qp Qh	E1

First aid type bandage is a wound cover with a pad size of less than 4 sq. in. Does not meet the definition of the surgical dressing benefit and will be denied as non-covered.

Medicare Statute 1861(s)(5)

✱ **A6441**	Padding bandage, non-elastic, non-woven/non-knitted, width greater than or equal to three inches and less than five inches, per yard ⓑ Ⓑ ♿	N
✱ **A6442**	Conforming bandage, non-elastic, knitted/woven, non-sterile, width less than three inches, per yard ⓑ Ⓑ ♿	N

Non-elastic, moderate or high compression that is typically sustained for one week

✱ **A6443**	Conforming bandage, non-elastic, knitted/woven, non-sterile, width greater than or equal to three inches and less than five inches, per yard ⓑ Ⓑ ♿	N
✱ **A6444**	Conforming bandage, non-elastic, knitted/woven, non-sterile, width greater than or equal to five inches, per yard ⓑ Ⓑ ♿	N
✱ **A6445**	Conforming bandage, non-elastic, knitted/woven, sterile, width less than three inches, per yard ⓑ Ⓑ ♿	N
✱ **A6446**	Conforming bandage, non-elastic, knitted/woven, sterile, width greater than or equal to three inches and less than five inches, per yard ⓑ Ⓑ ♿	N
✱ **A6447**	Conforming bandage, non-elastic, knitted/woven, sterile, width greater than or equal to five inches, per yard ⓑ Ⓑ	N
✱ **A6448**	Light compression bandage, elastic, knitted/woven, width less than three inches, per yard ⓑ Ⓑ ♿	N

Used to hold wound cover dressings in place over a wound. Example is an ACE type elastic bandage.

✱ **A6449**	Light compression bandage, elastic, knitted/woven, width greater than or equal to three inches and less than five inches, per yard ⓑ Ⓑ ♿	N

▶ New	↻ Revised	✓ Reinstated	~~deleted~~ Deleted	⊘ Not covered or valid by Medicare
⊛ Special coverage instructions		✱ Carrier discretion	ⓑ Bill Part B MAC	Ⓑ Bill DME MAC

MEDICAL AND SURGICAL SUPPLIES

* **A6450** Light compression bandage, elastic, knitted/woven, width greater than or equal to five inches, per yard N

* **A6451** Moderate compression bandage, elastic, knitted/woven, load resistance of 1.25 to 1.34 foot pounds at 50% maximum stretch, width greater than or equal to three inches and less than five inches, per yard N

  Elastic bandages that produce moderate compression that is typically sustained for one week

  Medicare considers coverage if part of a multi-layer compression bandage system for the treatment of a venous stasis ulcer. Do not assign for strains or sprains.

* **A6452** High compression bandage, elastic, knitted/woven, load resistance greater than or equal to 1.35 foot pounds at 50% maximum stretch, width greater than or equal to three inches and less than five inches, per yard N

  Elastic bandages that produce high compression that is typically sustained for one week

* **A6453** Self-adherent bandage, elastic, non-knitted/non-woven, width less than three inches, per yard N

* **A6454** Self-adherent bandage, elastic, non-knitted/non-woven, width greater than or equal to three inches and less than five inches, per yard N

* **A6455** Self-adherent bandage, elastic, non-knitted/non-woven, width greater than or equal to five inches, per yard N

* **A6456** Zinc paste impregnated bandage, non-elastic, knitted/woven, width greater than or equal to three inches and less than five inches, per yard N

* **A6457** Tubular dressing with or without elastic, any width, per linear yard N

* **A6460** Synthetic resorbable wound dressing, sterile, pad size 16 sq. in. or less, without adhesive border, each dressing N

* **A6461** Synthetic resorbable wound dressing, sterile, pad size more than 16 sq. in. but less than or equal to 48 sq. in., without adhesive border, each dressing N

Compression Garments

* **A6501** Compression burn garment, bodysuit (head to foot), custom fabricated N

  Garments used to reduce hypertrophic scarring and joint contractures following burn injury

  IOM: 100-02, 15, 100

* **A6502** Compression burn garment, chin strap, custom fabricated N

  IOM: 100-02, 15, 100

* **A6503** Compression burn garment, facial hood, custom fabricated N

  IOM: 100-02, 15, 100

* **A6504** Compression burn garment, glove to wrist, custom fabricated N

  IOM: 100-02, 15, 100

* **A6505** Compression burn garment, glove to elbow, custom fabricated N

  IOM: 100-02, 15, 100

* **A6506** Compression burn garment, glove to axilla, custom fabricated N

  IOM: 100-02, 15, 100

* **A6507** Compression burn garment, foot to knee length, custom fabricated N

  IOM: 100-02, 15, 100

* **A6508** Compression burn garment, foot to thigh length, custom fabricated N

  IOM: 100-02, 15, 100

* **A6509** Compression burn garment, upper trunk to waist including arm openings (vest), custom fabricated N

  IOM: 100-02, 15, 100

* **A6510** Compression burn garment, trunk, including arms down to leg openings (leotard), custom fabricated N

  IOM: 100-02, 15, 100

* **A6511** Compression burn garment, lower trunk including leg openings (panty), custom fabricated N

  IOM: 100-02, 15, 100

* **A6512** Compression burn garment, not otherwise classified N

  IOM: 100-02, 15, 100

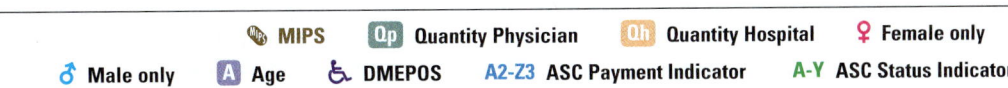

* **A6513** Compression burn mask, face and/or neck, plastic or equal, custom fabricated Ⓑ Qp Qh ♿ B

▶ * **A6515** Gradient compression wrap with adjustable straps, full leg, each, custom Ⓑ Qp Qh ♿ A

▶ * **A6516** Gradient compression wrap with adjustable straps, foot, each, custom Ⓑ Qp Qh ♿ A

▶ * **A6517** Gradient compression wrap with adjustable straps, below knee, each, custom Ⓑ Qp Qh ♿ A

▶ * **A6518** Gradient compression wrap with adjustable straps, arm, each, custom Ⓑ Qp Qh ♿ A

▶ * **A6519** Gradient compression garment, not otherwise specified, for nighttime use, each Ⓑ Qp Qh ♿ A

* **A6520** Gradient compression garment, glove, padded, for nighttime use, each Ⓑ Qp Qh ♿ A

* **A6521** Gradient compression garment, glove, padded, for nighttime use, custom, each Ⓑ Qp Qh ♿ A

* **A6522** Gradient compression garment, arm, padded, for nighttime use, each Ⓑ Qp Qh ♿ A

* **A6523** Gradient compression garment, arm, padded, for nighttime use, custom, each Ⓑ Qp Qh ♿ A

* **A6524** Gradient compression garment, lower leg and foot, padded, for nighttime use, each Ⓑ Qp Qh ♿ A

* **A6525** Gradient compression garment, lower leg and foot, padded, for nighttime use, custom, each Ⓑ Qp Qh ♿ A

* **A6526** Gradient compression garment, full leg and foot, padded, for nighttime use, each Ⓑ Qp Qh ♿ A

* **A6527** Gradient compression garment, full leg and foot, padded, for nighttime use, custom, each Ⓑ Qp Qh ♿ A

* **A6528** Gradient compression garment, bra, for nighttime use, each Ⓑ Qp Qh ♿ A

* **A6529** Gradient compression garment, bra, for nighttime use, custom, each Ⓑ Qp Qh ♿ A

⊘ **A6530** Gradient compression stocking, below knee, 18-30 mmHg, each Ⓑ Qp Qh ♿ A

IOM: 100-03, 4, 280.1

⊛ **A6531** Gradient compression stocking, below knee, 30-40 mmHg, used as a surgical dressing, each Ⓑ Qp Qh ♿ A

Covered when used in treatment of open venous stasis ulcer. Modifiers A1-A9 are not assigned. Must be billed with AW, RT, or LT.

IOM: 100-02, 15, 100

⊛ **A6532** Gradient compression stocking, below knee, 40-50 mmHg, used as a surgical dressing, each Ⓑ Qp Qh ♿ A

Covered when used in treatment of open venous stasis ulcer. Modifiers A1-A9 are not assigned. Must be billed with AW, RT, or LT.

IOM: 100-02, 15, 100

⊘ **A6533** Gradient compression stocking, thigh length, 18-30 mmHg, each Ⓑ Qp Qh ♿ A

IOM: 100-02, 15, 130; 100-03, 4, 280.1

⊘ **A6534** Gradient compression stocking, thigh length, 30-40 mmHg, each Ⓑ Qp Qh ♿ A

IOM: 100-02, 15, 130; 100-03, 4, 280.1

⊘ **A6535** Gradient compression stocking, thigh length, 40-50 mmHg, each Ⓑ Qp Qh ♿ A

IOM: 100-02, 15, 130; 100-03, 4, 280.1

⊘ **A6536** Gradient compression stocking, full length/chap style, 18-30 mmHg, each Ⓑ Qp Qh ♿ A

IOM: 100-02, 15, 130; 100-03, 4, 280.1

⊘ **A6537** Gradient compression stocking, full length/chap style, 30-40 mmHg, each Ⓑ Qp Qh ♿ A

IOM: 100-02, 15, 130; 100-03, 4, 280.1

⊘ **A6538** Gradient compression stocking, full length/chap style, 40-50 mmHg, each Ⓑ Qp Qh ♿ A

IOM: 100-02, 15, 130; 100-03, 4, 280.1

⊘ **A6539** Gradient compression stocking, waist length, 18-30 mmHg, each Ⓑ Qp Qh ♿ A

IOM: 100-02, 15, 130; 100-03, 4, 280.1

⊘ **A6540** Gradient compression stocking, waist length, 30-40 mmHg, each Ⓑ Qp Qh ♿ A

IOM: 100-02, 15, 130; 100-03, 4, 280.1

⊘ **A6541** Gradient compression stocking, waist length, 40-50 mmHg, each Ⓑ Qp Qh ♿ A

IOM: 100-02, 15, 130; 100-03, 4, 280.1

⊘ **A6544** Gradient compression stocking, garter belt Ⓑ Qp Qh E1

IOM: 100-02, 15, 130; 100-03, 4, 280.1

▶ New	⮂ Revised	✓ Reinstated	deleted Deleted	⊘ Not covered or valid by Medicare
⊛ Special coverage instructions		* Carrier discretion	Ⓑ Bill Part B MAC	Ⓑ Bill DME MAC

MEDICAL AND SURGICAL SUPPLIES

◎ **A6545** Gradient compression wrap, non-elastic, below knee, 30-50 mmHg, used as a surgical dressing, each ⒷQpQh♿ A

Modifiers RT and/or LT must be appended. When assigned for bilateral items (left/right) on the same date of service, bill both items on the same claim line using RT/LT modifiers and 2 units of service.

IOM: 10-02, 15, 100

↺⊘ **A6549** Gradient compression garment, not otherwise specified, for daytime use, each ⒷQpQh A

IOM: 100-02, 15, 130; 100-03, 4, 280.1

Wound Care

✳ **A6550** Wound care set, for negative pressure wound therapy electrical pump, includes all supplies and accessories ⒷQh♿ N

✳ **A6552** Gradient compression stocking, below knee, 30-40 mmhg, each ⒷQh♿ A

✳ **A6553** Gradient compression stocking, below knee, 30-40 mmhg, custom, each ⒷQh♿ A

✳ **A6554** Gradient compression stocking, below knee, 40 mmhg or greater, each ⒷQh♿ A

✳ **A6555** Gradient compression stocking, below knee, 40 mmhg or greater, custom, each ⒷQh♿ A

✳ **A6556** Gradient compression stocking, thigh length, 18-30 mmhg, custom, each ⒷQh♿ A

✳ **A6557** Gradient compression stocking, thigh length, 30-40 mmhg, custom, each ⒷQh♿ A

✳ **A6558** Gradient compression stocking, thigh length, 40 mmhg or greater, custom, each ⒷQh♿ A

✳ **A6559** Gradient compression stocking, full length/chap style, 18-30 mmhg, custom, each ⒷQh♿ A

✳ **A6560** Gradient compression stocking, full length/chap style, 30-40 mmhg, custom, each ⒷQh♿ A

✳ **A6561** Gradient compression stocking, full length/chap style, 40 mmhg or greater, custom, each ⒷQh♿ A

✳ **A6562** Gradient compression stocking, waist length, 18-30 mmhg, custom, each ⒷQh♿ A

✳ **A6563** Gradient compression stocking, waist length, 30-40 mmhg, custom, each ⒷQh♿ A

✳ **A6564** Gradient compression stocking, waist length, 40 mmhg or greater, custom, each ⒷQh♿ A

✳ **A6565** Gradient compression gauntlet, custom, each ⒷQh♿ A

✳ **A6566** Gradient compression garment, neck/head, each ⒷQh♿ A

✳ **A6567** Gradient compression garment, neck/head, custom, each ⒷQh♿ A

✳ **A6568** Gradient compression garment, torso and shoulder, each ⒷQh♿ A

✳ **A6569** Gradient compression garment, torso/shoulder, custom, each ⒷQh♿ A

✳ **A6570** Gradient compression garment, genital region, each ⒷQh♿ A

✳ **A6571** Gradient compression garment, genital region, custom, each ⒷQh♿ A

✳ **A6572** Gradient compression garment, toe caps, each ⒷQh♿ A

✳ **A6573** Gradient compression garment, toe caps, custom, each ⒷQh♿ A

✳ **A6574** Gradient compression arm sleeve and glove combination, custom, each ⒷQh♿ A

✳ **A6575** Gradient compression arm sleeve and glove combination, each ⒷQh♿ A

✳ **A6576** Gradient compression arm sleeve, custom, medium weight, each ⒷQh♿ A

✳ **A6577** Gradient compression arm sleeve, custom, heavy weight, each ⒷQh♿ A

✳ **A6578** Gradient compression arm sleeve, each ⒷQh♿ A

✳ **A6579** Gradient compression glove, custom, medium weight, each ⒷQh♿ A

✳ **A6580** Gradient compression glove, custom, heavy weight, each ⒷQh♿ A

✳ **A6581** Gradient compression glove, each ⒷQh♿ A

✳ **A6582** Gradient compression gauntlet, each ⒷQh♿ A

↺✳ **A6583** Gradient compression wrap with adjustable straps, below knee, each ⒷQh♿ A

✳ **A6584** Gradient compression wrap with adjustable straps, not otherwise specified ⒷQh♿ A

↺✳ **A6585** Gradient compression wrap with adjustable straps, above knee, each ⒷQh♿ A

↺✳ **A6586** Gradient compression wrap with adjustable straps, full leg, each ⒷQh♿ A

↺✳ **A6587** Gradient compression wrap with adjustable straps, foot, each ⒷQh♿ A

| MIPS | Qp Quantity Physician | Qh Quantity Hospital | ♀ Female only |
| ♂ Male only | Ⓐ Age | ♿ DMEPOS | A2-Z3 ASC Payment Indicator | A-Y ASC Status Indicator | Coding Clinic |

↻ * A6588 Gradient compression wrap with adjustable straps, arm, each Ⓑ Qh ♿ A

* A6589 Gradient pressure wrap with adjustable straps, bra, each Ⓑ Qh ♿ A

Urinary Catheters

* A6590 External urinary catheters; disposable, with wicking material, for use with suction pump, per month Ⓑ Qh ♿ N

* A6591 External urinary catheter; non-disposable, for use with suction pump, per month Ⓑ Qh ♿ N

* A6593 Accessory for gradient compression garment or wrap with adjustable straps, not-otherwise specified Ⓑ A

* A6594 Gradient compression bandaging supply, bandage liner, lower extremity, any size or length, each Ⓑ Qh ♿ A

* A6595 Gradient compression bandaging supply, bandage liner, upper extremity, any size or length, each Ⓑ Qh ♿ A

* A6596 Gradient compression bandaging supply, conforming gauze, per linear yard, any width, each Ⓑ Qh ♿ A

* A6597 Gradient compression bandage roll, elastic long stretch, linear yard, any width, each Qh ♿ A

* A6598 Gradient compression bandage roll, elastic medium stretch, per linear yard, any width, each Ⓑ Qh ♿ A

* A6599 Gradient compression bandage roll, inelastic short stretch, per linear yard, any width, each Ⓑ Qh ♿ A

* A6600 Gradient compression bandaging supply, high density foam sheet, per 250 square centimeters, each Ⓑ Qh ♿ A

* A6601 Gradient compression bandaging supply, high density foam pad, any size or shape, each Ⓑ Qh ♿ A

* A6602 Gradient compression bandaging supply, high density foam roll for bandage, per linear yard, any width, each Ⓑ Qh ♿ A

* A6603 Gradient compression bandaging supply, low density channel foam sheet, per 250 square centimeters, each Ⓑ Qh ♿ A

* A6604 Gradient compression bandaging supply, low density flat foam sheet, per 250 square centimeters, each Ⓑ Qh ♿ A

* A6605 Gradient compression bandaging supply, padded foam, per linear yard, any width, each Ⓑ Qh ♿ A

* A6606 Gradient compression bandaging supply, padded textile, per linear yard, any width, each Ⓑ Qh ♿ A

* A6607 Gradient compression bandaging supply, tubular protective absorption layer, per linear yard, any width, each Ⓑ Qh ♿ A

* A6608 Gradient compression bandaging supply, tubular protective absorption padded layer, per linear yard, any width, each Ⓑ Qh ♿ A

* A6609 Gradient compression bandaging supply, not otherwise specified Ⓑ Qh ♿ A

* A6610 Gradient compression stocking, below knee, 18-30 mmhg, custom, each Ⓑ Qh ♿ A

▶ * A6611 Gradient compression wrap with adjustable straps, above knee, each, custom Ⓑ Qh ♿ A

Respiratory Supplies

* A7000 Canister, disposable, used with suction pump, each Qp Qh ♿ Y

* A7001 Canister, non-disposable, used with suction pump, each Ⓑ Qh ♿ Y

* A7002 Tubing, used with suction pump, each Ⓑ Qh ♿ Y

* A7003 Administration set, with small volume nonfiltered pneumatic nebulizer, disposable Ⓑ Qp Qh ♿ Y

A7004 Small volume nonfiltered pneumatic nebulizer, disposable Ⓑ Qh ♿ Y

* A7005 Administration set, with small volume nonfiltered pneumatic nebulizer, non-disposable Ⓑ Qp Qh ♿ Y

* A7006 Administration set, with small volume filtered pneumatic nebulizer Qp Qh ♿ Y

* A7007 Large volume nebulizer, disposable, unfilled, used with aerosol compressor Ⓑ Qh ♿ Y

* A7008 Large volume nebulizer, disposable, prefilled, used with aerosol compressor Ⓑ ♿ Y

* A7009 Reservoir bottle, nondisposable, used with large volume ultrasonic nebulizer Ⓑ ♿ Y

* A7010 Corrugated tubing, disposable, used with large volume nebulizer, 100 feet Ⓑ Qh ♿ Y

* A7012 Water collection device, used with large volume nebulizer Ⓑ Qh ♿ Y

* A7013 Filter, disposable, used with aerosol compressor or ultrasonic generator Ⓑ Qp Qh ♿ Y

▶ New   ↻ Revised   ✓ Reinstated   ~~deleted~~ Deleted   ⊘ Not covered or valid by Medicare
✻ Special coverage instructions   * Carrier discretion   Ⓑ Bill Part B MAC   Ⓑ Bill DME MAC

MEDICAL AND SURGICAL SUPPLIES

* A7014	Filter, non-disposable, used with aerosol compressor or ultrasonic generator ⓑ Qp Qh ♿	Y
* A7015	Aerosol mask, used with DME nebulizer ⓑ Qh ♿	Y
* A7016	Dome and mouthpiece, used with small volume ultrasonic nebulizer ⓑ Qp Qh ♿	Y
⊛ A7017	Nebulizer, durable, glass or autoclavable plastic, bottle type, not used with oxygen ⓑ Qp Qh ♿	Y
	IOM: 100-03, 4, 280.1	
* A7018	Water, distilled, used with large volume nebulizer, 1000 ml ⓑ Qh ♿	Y
* A7020	Interface for cough stimulating device, includes all components, replacement only ⓑ Qp Qh ♿	Y
A7021	Supplies and accessories for lung expansion airway clearance, continuous high frequency oscillation, and nebulization device (e.g., handset, nebulizer kit, biofilter) ⓑ Qp Qh ♿	Y
* A7023	Mechanical allergen particle barrier/inhalation filter, cream, nasal, topical	E1
* A7025	High frequency chest wall oscillation system vest, replacement for use with patient owned equipment, each ⓑ Qp Qh ♿	N
* A7026	High frequency chest wall oscillation system hose, replacement for use with patient owned equipment, each ⓑ Qp Qh ♿	Y
* A7027	Combination oral/nasal mask, used with continuous positive airway pressure device, each ⓑ Qp Qh ♿	Y
* A7028	Oral cushion for combination oral/nasal mask, replacement only, each ⓑ Qp Qh ♿	Y
* A7029	Nasal pillows for combination oral/nasal mask, replacement only, pair ⓑ Qp Qh ♿	Y
* A7030	Full face mask used with positive airway pressure device, each ⓑ Qh ♿	Y
* A7031	Face mask interface, replacement for full face mask, each ⓑ Qh ♿	Y
* A7032	Cushion for use on nasal mask interface, replacement only, each ⓑ Qp Qh ♿	Y
* A7033	Pillow for use on nasal cannula type interface, replacement only, pair ⓑ Qh ♿	Y
* A7034	Nasal interface (mask or cannula type) used with positive airway pressure device, with or without head strap ⓑ Qh ♿	Y
* A7035	Headgear used with positive airway pressure device ⓑ Qp Qh ♿	Y
* A7036	Chinstrap used with positive airway pressure device ⓑ Qp Qh ♿	Y
* A7037	Tubing used with positive airway pressure device ⓑ Qp Qh ♿	Y
* A7038	Filter, disposable, used with positive airway pressure device ⓑ Qh ♿	Y
* A7039	Filter, non disposable, used with positive airway pressure device ⓑ Qp Qh ♿	Y
* A7040	One way chest drain valve ⓜ Qp Qh ♿	N
* A7041	Water seal drainage container and tubing for use with implanted chest tube ⓜ Qp Qh ♿	N
* A7044	Oral interface used with positive airway pressure device, each ⓑ Qp Qh ♿	Y
⊛ A7045	Exhalation port with or without swivel used with accessories for positive airway devices, replacement only ⓑ Qh ♿	Y
	IOM: 100-03, 4, 230.17	
⊛ A7046	Water chamber for humidifier, used with positive airway pressure device, replacement, each ⓑ Qh ♿	Y
	IOM: 100-03, 4, 230.17	
* A7047	Oral interface used with respiratory suction pump, each ⓑ Qp Qh ♿	N
* A7048	Vacuum drainage collection unit and tubing kit, including all supplies needed for collection unit change, for use with implanted catheter, each ⓑ Qp Qh ♿	N
* A7049	Expiratory positive airway pressure intranasal resistance valve ⓑ	E1

Tracheostomy Supplies

⊛ A7501	Tracheostoma valve, including diaphragm, each ⓑ Qp Qh ♿	N
	IOM: 100-02, 15, 120	
⊛ A7502	Replacement diaphragm/faceplate for tracheostoma valve, each ⓑ Qh ♿	N
	IOM: 100-02, 15, 120	
⊛ A7503	Filter holder or filter cap, reusable, for use in a tracheostoma heat and moisture exchange system, each ⓑ Qh ♿	N
	IOM: 100-02, 15, 120	
⊛ A7504	Filter for use in a tracheostoma heat and moisture exchange system, each ⓑ Qp Qh ♿	N
	IOM: 100-02, 15, 120	

🍃 MIPS   Qp Quantity Physician   Qh Quantity Hospital   ♀ Female only
♂ Male only   Ⓐ Age   ♿ DMEPOS   A2-Z3 ASC Payment Indicator   A-Y ASC Status Indicator   Coding Clinic

2026 HCPCS LEVEL II NATIONAL CODES

✹ **A7505**   Housing, reusable without adhesive, for use in a heat and moisture exchange system and/or with a tracheostoma valve, each Ⓑ Qh ♿ N
  IOM: 100-02, 15, 120

✹ **A7506**   Adhesive disc for use in a heat and moisture exchange system and/or with tracheostoma valve, any type, each Ⓑ Qh ♿ N
  IOM: 100-02, 15, 120

✹ **A7507**   Filter holder and integrated filter without adhesive, for use in a tracheostoma heat and moisture exchange system, each Ⓑ Qp Qh ♿ N
  IOM: 100-02, 15, 120

✹ **A7508**   Housing and integrated adhesive, for use in a tracheostoma heat and moisture exchange system and/or with a tracheostoma valve, each Ⓑ Qh ♿ N
  IOM: 100-02, 15, 120

✹ **A7509**   Filter holder and integrated filter housing, and adhesive, for use as a tracheostoma heat and moisture exchange system, each Ⓑ Qh ♿ N
  IOM: 100-02, 15, 120

✴ **A7520**   Tracheostomy/laryngectomy tube, non-cuffed, polyvinylchloride (PVC), silicone or equal, each Ⓑ Qp Qh ♿ N

✴ **A7521**   Tracheostomy/laryngectomy tube, cuffed, polyvinylchloride (PVC), silicone or equal, each Ⓑ Qh ♿ N

✴ **A7522**   Tracheostomy/laryngectomy tube, stainless steel or equal (sterilizable and reusable), each Ⓑ Qh ♿ N

✴ **A7523**   Tracheostomy shower protector, each Ⓑ N

✴ **A7524**   Tracheostoma stent/stud/button, each Ⓑ Qp Qh ♿ N

✴ **A7525**   Tracheostomy mask, each Ⓑ Qh ♿ N

✴ **A7526**   Tracheostomy tube collar/holder, each Ⓑ Qh ♿ N

✴ **A7527**   Tracheostomy/laryngectomy tube plug/stop, each Ⓑ Qp Qh ♿ N

Helmets

✴ **A8000**   Helmet, protective, soft, prefabricated, includes all components and accessories Ⓑ ♿ Y

✴ **A8001**   Helmet, protective, hard, prefabricated, includes all components and accessories Ⓑ ♿ Y

✴ **A8002**   Helmet, protective, soft, custom fabricated, includes all components and accessories Ⓑ ♿ Y

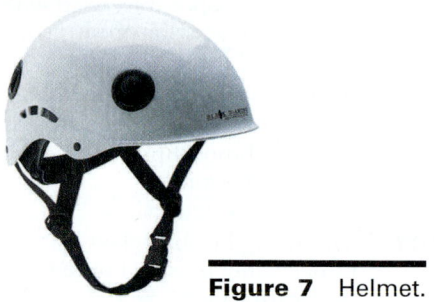

Figure 7 Helmet.

✴ **A8003**   Helmet, protective, hard, custom fabricated, includes all components and accessories Ⓑ ♿ Y

✴ **A8004**   Soft interface for helmet, replacement only Ⓑ ♿ Y

ADMINISTRATIVE, MISCELLANEOUS, AND INVESTIGATIONAL (A9000-A9999)

NOTE: The following codes do not imply that codes in other sections are necessarily covered.

Miscellaneous Supplies

✹ **A9150**   Non-prescription drugs Ⓑ B
  IOM: 100-02, 15, 50

⊘ **A9152**   Single vitamin/mineral/trace element, oral, per dose, not otherwise specified Ⓑ Qp Qh E1

⊘ **A9153**   Multiple vitamins, with or without minerals and trace elements, oral, per dose, not otherwise specified Ⓑ Qp Qh E1

▶ ✴ **A9154**   Artificial saliva, 1 ml Ⓑ Qp Qh B

~~A9155~~   ~~Artificial saliva, 30 ml~~

  A9156   Oral mucoadhesive, any type (liquid, gel, paste, etc.), per 1 ml Ⓑ N1 N

⊘ **A9180**   Pediculosis (lice infestation) treatment, topical, for administration by patient/caretaker Ⓑ Qp Qh E1

⊘ **A9268**   Programmer for transient, orally ingested capsule Ⓑ E1

⊘ **A9269**   Programable, transient, orally ingested capsule, for use with external programmer, per month Ⓑ E1

⊘ **A9270**   Non-covered item or service Ⓑ Qp Qh E1
  IOM: 100-02, 16, 20

⊘ **A9272**   Wound suction, disposable, includes dressing, all accessories and components, any type, each Ⓑ Qp Qh A
  Medicare Statute 1861(n)

▶ New   ⟲ Revised   ✓ Reinstated   ~~deleted~~ Deleted   ⊘ Not covered or valid by Medicare
✹ Special coverage instructions   ✴ Carrier discretion   Ⓑ Bill Part B MAC   Ⓑ Bill DME MAC

ADMINISTRATIVE, MISCELLANEOUS, AND INVESTIGATIONAL

⊘ **A9273** Cold or hot water bottle, ice cap or collar, heat and/or cold wrap, any type ⑧ Qp Qh   E1

⊘ **A9274** External ambulatory insulin delivery system, disposable, each, includes all supplies and accessories ⑧ Qp Qh   E1

Medicare Statute 1861(n)

⊘ **A9275** Home glucose disposable monitor, includes test strips ⑧ Qp Qh   E1

⊘ **A9276** Sensor; invasive (e.g., subcutaneous), disposable, for use with non-durable medical equipment interstitial continuous glucose monitoring system, one unit = 1 day supply ⑧ Qp Qh   E1

Medicare Statute 1861(n)

⊘ **A9277** Transmitter; external, for use with non-durable medical equipment interstitial continuous glucose monitoring system ⑧ Qp Qh   E1

Medicare Statute 1861(n)

⊘ **A9278** Receiver (monitor); external, for use with non-durable medical equipment interstitial continuous glucose monitoring system ⑧ Qp Qh   E1

Medicare Statute 1861(n)

⊘ **A9279** Monitoring feature/device, stand-alone or integrated, any type, includes all accessories, components and electronics, not otherwise classified ⑧ Qp Qh   E1

Medicare Statute 1861(n)

⊘ **A9280** Alert or alarm device, not otherwise classified ⑧ Qp Qh   E1

Medicare Statute 1861

⊘ **A9281** Reaching/grabbing device, any type, any length, each ⑧ Qp Qh   E1

Medicare Statute 1862 SSA

⊘ **A9282** Wig, any type, each ⑧ Qp Qh   E1

Medicare Statute 1862 SSA

⊘ **A9283** Foot pressure off loading/supportive device, any type, each ⑧ Qp Qh   E1

Medicare Statute 1862A(i)13

✺ **A9284** Spirometer, non-electronic, includes all accessories ⑧ Qp Qh   N

* **A9285** Inversion/eversion correction device ⑧ Qp Qh   A

⊘ **A9286** Hygienic item or device, disposable or non-disposable, any type, each ⑧ Qp Qh   E1

Medicare Statute 1834

⊘ **A9291** Prescription digital cognitive and/or behavioral therapy, FDA cleared, per course of treatment   E1

⊘ **A9292** Prescription digital visual therapy, software-only, FDA cleared, per course of treatment

⊘ **A9293** Fertility cycle (contraception & conception) tracking software application, FDA cleared, per month, includes accessories (e.g., thermometer) ⑧   E1

⊘ **A9300** Exercise equipment ⑧ Qp Qh   E1

IOM: 100-02, 15, 110.1; 100-03, 4, 280.1

Supplies for Radiology Procedures (Radiopharmaceuticals)

* **A9500** Technetium Tc-99m sestamibi, diagnostic, per study dose ⑧ Qp Qh   N1 N

Should be filed on same claim as procedure code reporting radiopharmaceutical. Verify with payer definition of a "study."

Coding Clinic: 2006, Q2, P5

* **A9501** Technetium Tc-99m teboroxime, diagnostic, per study dose ⑧ Qp Qh   N1 N

* **A9502** Technetium Tc-99m tetrofosmin, diagnostic, per study dose ⑧ Qp Qh   N1 N

Coding Clinic: 2006, Q2, P5

* **A9503** Technetium Tc-99m medronate, diagnostic, per study dose, up to 30 millicuries ⑧ Qp Qh   N1 N

* **A9504** Technetium Tc-99m apcitide, diagnostic, per study dose, up to 20 millicuries ⑨ Qp Qh   N1 N

* **A9505** Thallium Tl-201 thallous chloride, diagnostic, per millicurie ⑧ Qp Qh   N1 N

A9506 Graphite crucible for preparation of technetium Tc-99m labeled carbon aerosol, one crucible   G

* **A9507** Indium In-111 capromab pendetide, diagnostic, per study dose, up to 10 millicuries ⑧ Qp Qh   N1 N

* **A9508** Iodine I-131 iobenguane sulfate, diagnostic, per 0.5 millicurie ⑧ Qp Qh   N1 N

* **A9509** Iodine I-123 sodium iodide, diagnostic, per millicurie ⑧ Qp Qh   N1 N

* **A9510** Technetium Tc-99m disofenin, diagnostic, per study dose, up to 15 millicuries ⑧ Qp Qh   N1 N

* **A9512** Technetium Tc-99m pertechnetate, diagnostic, per millicurie ⑧ Qp Qh   N1 N

🏷 MIPS	Qp Quantity Physician	Qh Quantity Hospital	♀ Female only
♂ Male only	Ⓐ Age	♿ DMEPOS	A2-Z3 ASC Payment Indicator A-Y ASC Status Indicator Coding Clinic

⊛ A9513	Lutetium lu 177, dotatate, therapeutic, 1 millicurie	K
* A9515	Choline C-11, diagnostic, per study dose up to 20 millicuries Qp Qh	K2 K
* A9516	Iodine I-123 sodium iodide, diagnostic, per 100 microcuries, up to 999 microcuries B Qp Qh	N1 N
* A9517	Iodine I-131 sodium iodide capsule(s), therapeutic, per millicurie B Qp Qh	K
* A9520	Technetium Tc-99m tilmanocept, diagnostic, up to 0.5 millicuries B Qp Qh	N1 N
* A9521	Technetium Tc-99m exametazime, diagnostic, per study dose, up to 25 millicuries B Qp Qh	N1 K
* A9524	Iodine I-131 iodinated serum albumin, diagnostic, per 5 microcuries B Qp Qh	N1 N
* A9526	Nitrogen N-13 ammonia, diagnostic, per study dose, up to 40 millicuries B Qp Qh	N1 N
* A9527	Iodine I-125, sodium iodide solution, therapeutic, per millicurie B Qp Qh	H2 U
* A9528	Iodine I-131 sodium iodide capsule(s), diagnostic, per millicurie B Qp Qh	N1 N
* A9529	Iodine I-131 sodium iodide solution, diagnostic, per millicurie B Qp Qh	N1 N
* A9530	Iodine I-131 sodium iodide solution, therapeutic, per millicurie B Qp Qh	K
* A9531	Iodine I-131 sodium iodide, diagnostic, per microcurie (up to 100 microcuries) B Qp Qh	N1 N
* A9532	Iodine I-125 serum albumin, diagnostic, per 5 microcuries B Qp Qh	N1 N
* A9536	Technetium Tc-99m depreotide, diagnostic, per study dose, up to 35 millicuries B Qp Qh	N1 N
* A9537	Technetium Tc-99m mebrofenin, diagnostic, per study dose, up to 15 millicuries B Qp Qh	N1 N
* A9538	Technetium Tc-99m pyrophosphate, diagnostic, per study dose, up to 25 millicuries B Qp Qh	N1 N
* A9539	Technetium Tc-99m pentetate, diagnostic, per study dose, up to 25 millicuries B Qp Qh	N1 N
* A9540	Technetium Tc-99m macroaggregated albumin, diagnostic, per study dose, up to 10 millicuries B Qp Qh	N1 N
* A9541	Technetium Tc-99m sulfur colloid, diagnostic, per study dose, up to 20 millicuries Qp Qh	N1 N
* A9542	Indium In-111 ibritumomab tiuxetan, diagnostic, per study dose, up to 5 millicuries Qp Qh	N1 K
	Specifically for diagnostic use.	
* A9543	Yttrium Y-90 ibritumomab tiuxetan, therapeutic, per treatment dose, up to 40 millicuries B Qp Qh	K
	Specifically for therapeutic use.	
* A9546	Cobalt Co-57/58, cyanocobalamin, diagnostic, per study dose, up to 1 microcurie B Qp Qh	N1 N
* A9547	Indium In-111 oxyquinoline, diagnostic, per 0.5 microcurie B Qp Qh	N1 K
* A9548	Indium In-111 pentetate, diagnostic, per 0.5 millicurie B Qp Qh	N1 K
* A9550	Technetium Tc-99m sodium gluceptate, diagnostic, per study dose, up to 25 millicuries Qp Qh	N1 N
* A9551	Technetium Tc-99m succimer, diagnostic, per study dose, up to 10 millicuries Qp Qh	N1 N
* A9552	Fluorodeoxyglucose F-18 FDG, diagnostic, per study dose, up to 45 millicuries B Qp Qh	N1 N
	Coding Clinic: 2008, Q3, P7	
* A9553	Chromium Cr-51 sodium chromate, diagnostic, per study dose, up to 250 microcuries B Qp Qh	N1 N
* A9554	Iodine I-125 sodium Iothalamate, diagnostic, per study dose, up to 10 microcuries B Qp Qh	N1 N
* A9555	Rubidium Rb-82, diagnostic, per study dose, up to 60 millicuries B Qp Qh	N1 N
* A9556	Gallium Ga-67 citrate, diagnostic, per millicurie B Qp Qh	N1 N
* A9557	Technetium Tc-99m bicisate, diagnostic, per study dose, up to 25 millicuries Qp Qh	N1 K
* A9558	Xenon Xe-133 gas, diagnostic, per 10 millicuries B Qp Qh	N1 N
* A9559	Cobalt Co-57 cyanocobalamin, oral, diagnostic, per study dose, up to 1 microcurie B Qp Qh	N1 N
* A9560	Technetium Tc-99m labeled red blood cells, diagnostic, per study dose, up to 30 millicuries B Qp Qh	N1 N
	Coding Clinic: 2008, Q3, P7	

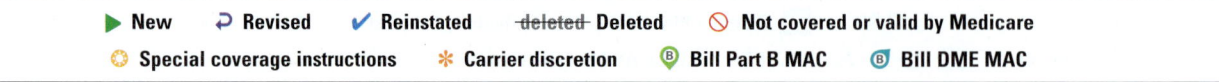

ADMINISTRATIVE, MISCELLANEOUS, AND INVESTIGATIONAL

* **A9561** Technetium Tc-99m oxidronate, diagnostic, per study dose, up to 30 millicuries ⓑ Qp Qh   N1 N

* **A9562** Technetium Tc-99m mertiatide, diagnostic, per study dose, up to 15 millicuries ⓑ Qp Qh   N1 N

* **A9563** Sodium phosphate P-32, therapeutic, per millicurie ⓑ Qp Qh   K

* **A9564** Chromic phosphate P-32 suspension, therapeutic, per millicurie ⓑ Qp Qh   E1

* **A9566** Technetium Tc-99m fanolesomab, diagnostic, per study dose, up to 25 millicuries ⓑ Qp Qh   N1 N

* **A9567** Technetium Tc-99m pentetate, diagnostic, aerosol, per study dose, up to 75 millicuries ⓑ Qp Qh   N1 N

* **A9568** Technetium TC-99m arcitumomab, diagnostic, per study dose, up to 45 millicuries ⓑ Qp Qh   N1 K

* **A9569** Technetium Tc-99m exametazime labeled autologous white blood cells, diagnostic, per study dose ⓑ Qp Qh   N1 K

* **A9570** Indium In-111 labeled autologous white blood cells, diagnostic, per study dose ⓑ Qp Qh   N1 K

* **A9571** Indium In-111 labeled autologous platelets, diagnostic, per study dose ⓑ Qp Qh   N1 K

* **A9572** Indium In-111 pentetreotide, diagnostic, per study dose, up to 6 millicuries ⓑ Qp Qh   N1 K

* **A9573** Injection, gadopiclenol, 1 ml   N1 N

   Other: Clariscan, Elucirem, Vueway

* **A9575** Injection, gadoterate meglumine, 0.1 ml ⓑ Qp Qh   N1 N

   Other: Clariscan, Gadoterate Meglumine, Dotarem

* **A9576** Injection, gadoteridol, (ProHance Multipack), per ml ⓑ Qp Qh   N1 N

* **A9577** Injection, gadobenate dimeglumine (MultiHance), per ml ⓑ Qp Qh   N1 N

* **A9578** Injection, gadobenate dimeglumine (MultiHance Multipack), per ml ⓑ Qp Qh   N1 N

* **A9579** Injection, gadolinium-based magnetic resonance contrast agent, not otherwise specified (NOS), per ml ⓑ Qp Qh   N1 N

   Other: Magnevist, Prohance, Omniscan

* **A9580** Sodium fluoride F-18, diagnostic, per study dose, up to 30 millicuries ⓑ Qp Qh   N1 N

* **A9581** Injection, gadoxetate disodium, 1 ml ⓑ Qp Qh   N1 N

   Local Medicare contractors may require the use of modifier JW to identify unused product from single-dose vials that are appropriately discarded.

   Other: Eovist

* **A9582** Iodine I-123 iobenguane, diagnostic, per study dose, up to 15 millicuries ⓑ Qp Qh   N1 K

   Molecular imaging agent that assists in the identification of rare neuroendocrine tumors.

* **A9583** Injection, gadofosveset trisodium, 1 ml ⓑ Qp Qh   N1 N

* **A9584** Iodine 1-123 ioflupane, diagnostic, per study dose, up to 5 millicuries ⓑ Qp Qh   N1 K

   Coding Clinic: 2012, Q1, P9

* **A9585** Injection, gadobutrol, 0.1 ml ⓑ Qp Qh   N1 N

   Other: Gadavist

   Coding Clinic: 2012, Q1, P8

* **A9586** Florbetapir F18, diagnostic, per study dose, up to 10 millicuries ⓑ Qp Qh   N1 K

* **A9587** Gallium Ga-68, dotatate, diagnostic, 0.1 millicurie Qp Qh   K2 K

   Coding Clinic: 2017, Q1, P9

* **A9588** Fluciclovine F-18, diagnostic, 1 millicurie Qp Qh   K2 K

   Coding Clinic: 2017, Q1, P9

* **A9589** Instillation, hexaminolevulinate hydrochloride, 100 mg   N1 N

* **A9590** Iodine I-131, iobenguane, 1 millicurie   N

* **A9591** Fluoroestradiol F 18, diagnostic, 1 millicurie   K2 K

* **A9592** Copper cu-64, dotatate, diagnostic, 1 millicurie   K2 K

* **A9593** Gallium ga-68 psma-11, diagnostic, (ucsf), 1 millicurie   K2 K

* **A9594** Gallium ga-68 psma-11, diagnostic, (ucla), 1 millicurie   K2 K

* **A9595** Piflufolastat f-18, diagnostic, 1 millicurie   K2 K

   A9596 Gallium GA-68 gozetotide, diagnostic, (illuccix), 1 millicurie   K

* **A9597** Positron emission tomography radiopharmaceutical, diagnostic, for tumor identification, not otherwise classified N1 N

  Coding Clinic: 2017, Q1, P8-9

* **A9598** Positron emission tomography radiopharmaceutical, diagnostic, for non-tumor identification, not otherwise classified N1 N

  Coding Clinic: 2017, Q1, P8-9

* **A9600** Strontium Sr-89 chloride, therapeutic, per millicurie ⓑ Qp Qh K

  A9601 Flortaucipir F 18 injection, diagnostic, 1 millicurie K5 G

  A9602 Fluorodopa F-18, diagnostic, per millicurie K2 G

  A9603 Injection, pafolacianine, 0.1 mg N

* **A9604** Samarium SM-153 lexidronam, therapeutic, per treatment dose, up to 150 millicuries ⓑ Qp Qh K

* **A9606** Radium Ra-223 dichloride, therapeutic, per microcurie Qp Qh K

* **A9607** Lutetium LU 177 vipivotide tetraxetan, therapeutic, 1 millicurie G

* **A9608** Flotufolastat f18, diagnostic, 1 millicurie G

* **A9609** Fludeoxyglucose f18 up to 15 millicuries N

* **A9610** Xenon xe-129 hyperpolarized gas, diagnostic, per study dose N

▶ * **A9611** Flurpiridaz f18, diagnostic, 1 millicurie G

▶ * **A9612** Injection, fluorescein, 1 mg N

▶ * **A9615** Injection, pegulicianine, 1 mg G

▶ * **A9616** Gallium gozetotide, diagnostic, 1 millicurie G

* **A9697** Injection, carboxydextran-coated superparamagnetic iron oxide, per study dose N1 G

◎ **A9698** Non-radioactive contrast imaging material, not otherwise classified, per study ⓑ N1 N

  IOM: 100-04, 12, 70; 100-04, 13, 20

  Coding Clinic: 2017, Q1, P8

* **A9699** Radiopharmaceutical, therapeutic, not otherwise classified ⓑ N

◎ **A9700** Supply of injectable contrast material for use in echocardiography, per study ⓑ Qp Qh N1 N

  IOM: 100-04, 12, 30.4

  Coding Clinic: 2017, Q1, P8

* **A9800** Gallium GA-68 gozetotide, diagnostic, (locametz), 1 millicurie K2 G

Miscellaneous Service Component

* **A9900** Miscellaneous DME supply, accessory, and/or service component of another HCPCS code ⓑ ⓑ Y

  On DMEPOS fee schedule as a payable replacement for miscellaneous implanted or non-implanted items.

* **A9901** DME delivery, set up, and/or dispensing service component of another HCPCS code ⓑ A

* **A9999** Miscellaneous DME supply or accessory, not otherwise specified ⓑ ⓑ Y

  On DMEPOS fee schedule as a payable replacement for miscellaneous implanted or non-implanted items.

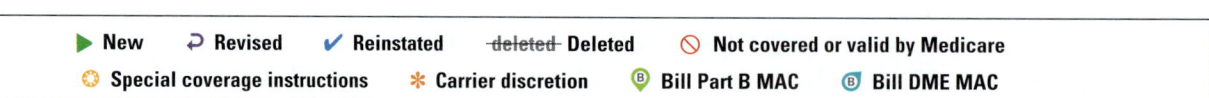

ENTERAL AND PARENTERAL THERAPY
(B4000-B9999)

Enteral Feeding Supplies

B4034 Enteral feeding supply kit; syringe fed, per day, includes but not limited to feeding/flushing syringe, administration set tubing, dressings, tape   Y

Dressings used with gastrostomy tubes for enteral nutrition (covered under the prosthetic device benefit) are included in the payment.

IOM: 100-02, 15, 120; 100-03, 3, 180.2; 100-04, 20, 100.2.2

PEN: On Fee Schedule

B4035 Enteral feeding supply kit; pump fed, per day, includes but not limited to feeding/flushing syringe, administration set tubing, dressings, tape   Y

IOM: 100-02, 15, 120; 100-03, 3, 180.2; 100-04, 20, 100.2.2

PEN: On Fee Schedule

B4036 Enteral feeding supply kit; gravity fed, per day, includes but not limited to feeding/flushing syringe, administration set tubing, dressings, tape   Y

IOM: 100-02, 15, 120; 100-03, 3, 180.2; 100-04, 20, 100.2.2

PEN: On Fee Schedule

B4081 Nasogastric tubing with stylet   Y

More than 3 nasogastric tubes (B4081-B4083), or 1 gastrostomy/jejunostomy tube (B4087-B4088) every three months is rarely medically necessary.

IOM: 100-02, 15, 120; 100-03, 3, 180.2; 100-04, 20, 100.2.2

PEN: On Fee Schedule

B4082 Nasogastric tubing without stylet   Y

IOM: 100-02, 15, 120; 100-03, 3, 180.2; 100-04, 20, 100.2.2

PEN: On Fee Schedule

B4083 Stomach tube - Levine type   Y

IOM: 100-02, 15, 120; 100-03, 3, 180.2; 100-04, 20, 100.2.2

PEN: On Fee Schedule

* **B4087** Gastrostomy/jejunostomy tube, standard, any material, any type, each   Y

PEN: On Fee Schedule

* **B4088** Gastrostomy/jejunostomy tube, low-profile, any material, any type, each   Y

PEN: On Fee Schedule

Enteral Formulas and Additives

B4100 Food thickener, administered orally, per ounce   E1

B4102 Enteral formula, for adults, used to replace fluids and electrolytes (e.g., clear liquids), 500 ml = 1 unit   Y

IOM: 100-03, 3, 180.2

B4103 Enteral formula, for pediatrics, used to replace fluids and electrolytes (e.g., clear liquids), 500 ml = 1 unit   Y

IOM: 100-03, 3, 180.2

B4104 Additive for enteral formula (e.g., fiber)   E1

IOM: 100-03, 3, 180.2

B4105 In-line cartridge containing digestive enzyme(s) for enteral feeding, each   Y

Cross Reference Q9994

B4148 Enteral feeding supply kit; elastomeric control fed, per day, includes but not limited to feeding/flushing syringe, administration set tubing, dressings, tape   Y

B4149 Enteral formula, manufactured blenderized natural foods with intact nutrients, includes proteins, fats, carbohydrates, vitamins and minerals, may include fiber, administered through an enteral feeding tube, 100 calories = 1 unit   Y

Produced to meet unique nutrient needs for specific disease conditions; medical record must document specific condition and need for special nutrient.

IOM: 100-02, 15, 120; 100-03, 3, 180.2; 100-04, 20, 100.2.2

PEN: On Fee Schedule

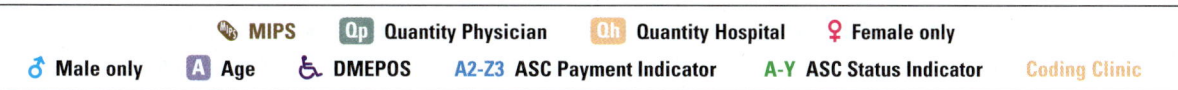

MIPS — Qp Quantity Physician — Qh Quantity Hospital — ♀ Female only
♂ Male only — A Age — & DMEPOS — A2-Z3 ASC Payment Indicator — A-Y ASC Status Indicator — Coding Clinic

B4150 – B4161 ENTERAL AND PARENTERAL THERAPY

⊛ **B4150** Enteral formulae, nutritionally complete with intact nutrients, includes proteins, fats, carbohydrates, vitamins, and minerals, may include fiber, administered through an enteral feeding tube, 100 calories = 1 unit ⓑ Qh   Y

IOM: 100-02, 15, 120; 100-03, 3, 180.2; 100-04, 20, 100.2.2

PEN: On Fee Schedule

⊛ **B4152** Enteral formula, nutritionally complete, calorically dense (equal to or greater than 1.5 kcal/ml) with intact nutrients, includes proteins, fats, carbohydrates, vitamins and minerals, may include fiber, administered through an enteral feeding tube, 100 calories = 1 unit ⓑ Qh   Y

IOM: 100-02, 15, 120; 100-03, 3, 180.2; 100-04, 20, 100.2.2

PEN: On Fee Schedule

⊛ **B4153** Enteral formula, nutritionally complete, hydrolyzed proteins (amino acids and peptide chain), includes fats, carbohydrates, vitamins and minerals, may include fiber, administered through an enteral feeding tube, 100 calories = 1 unit ⓑ Qp Qh   Y

If 2 enteral nutrition products described by same HCPCS code and provided at same time billed on single claim line with units of service reflecting total calories of both nutrients

IOM: 100-02, 15, 120; 100-03, 3, 180.2; 100-04, 20, 100.2.2

PEN: On Fee Schedule

⊛ **B4154** Enteral formula, nutritionally complete, for special metabolic needs, excludes inherited disease of metabolism, includes altered composition of proteins, fats, carbohydrates, vitamins and/or minerals, may include fiber, administered through an enteral feeding tube, 100 calories = 1 unit ⓑ Qh   Y

IOM: 100-02, 15, 120; 100-03, 3, 180.2; 100-04, 20, 100.2.2

PEN: On Fee Schedule

⊛ **B4155** Enteral formula, nutritionally incomplete/modular nutrients, includes specific nutrients, carbohydrates (e.g., glucose polymers), proteins/amino acids (e.g., glutamine, arginine), fat (e.g., medium chain triglycerides) or combination, administered through an enteral feeding tube, 100 calories = 1 unit ⓑ Qh   Y

IOM: 100-02, 15, 120; 100-03, 3, 180.2; 100-04, 20, 100.2.2

PEN: On Fee Schedule

⊛ **B4157** Enteral formula, nutritionally complete, for special metabolic needs for inherited disease of metabolism, includes proteins, fats, carbohydrates, vitamins and minerals, may include fiber, administered through an enteral feeding tube, 100 calories = 1 unit ⓑ Qp Qh   Y

IOM: 100-03, 3, 180.2

⊛ **B4158** Enteral formula, for pediatrics, nutritionally complete with intact nutrients, includes proteins, fats, carbohydrates, vitamins and minerals, may include fiber and/or iron, administered through an enteral feeding tube, 100 calories = 1 unit ⓑ Qh A   Y

IOM: 100-03, 3, 180.2

⊛ **B4159** Enteral formula, for pediatrics, nutritionally complete soy based with intact nutrients, includes proteins, fats, carbohydrates, vitamins and minerals, may include fiber and/or iron, administered through an enteral feeding tube, 100 calories = 1 unit ⓑ Qh A   Y

IOM: 100-03, 3, 180.2

⊛ **B4160** Enteral formula, for pediatrics, nutritionally complete calorically dense (equal to or greater than 0.7 kcal/ml) with intact nutrients, includes proteins, fats, carbohydrates, vitamins and minerals, may include fiber, administered through an enteral feeding tube, 100 calories = 1 unit ⓑ Qp Qh A   Y

IOM: 100-03, 3, 180.2

⊛ **B4161** Enteral formula, for pediatrics, hydrolyzed/amino acids and peptide chain proteins, includes fats, carbohydrates, vitamins and minerals, may include fiber, administered through an enteral feeding tube, 100 calories = 1 unit ⓑ Qh A   Y

IOM: 100-03, 3, 180.2

▶ New ↻ Revised ✓ Reinstated ~~deleted~~ Deleted ⊘ Not covered or valid by Medicare
✦ Special coverage instructions ✱ Carrier discretion ⓑ Bill Part B MAC ⓑ Bill DME MAC

ENTERAL AND PARENTERAL THERAPY

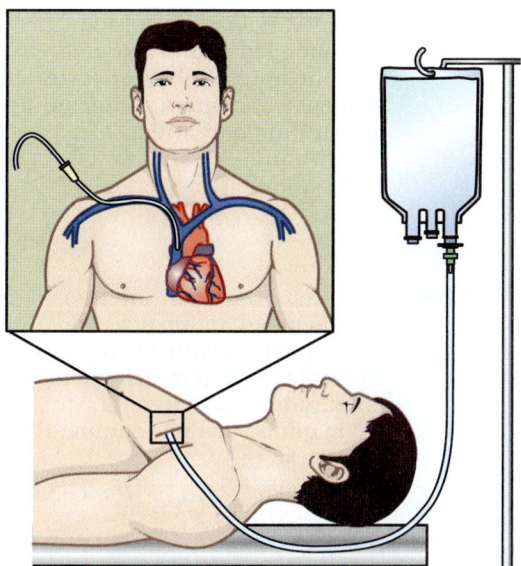

Figure 8 Total Parenteral Nutrition (TPN) involves percutaneous placement of central venous catheter into vena cava or right atrium.

- **B4162** Enteral formula, for pediatrics, special metabolic needs for inherited disease of metabolism, includes proteins, fats, carbohydrates, vitamins and minerals, may include fiber, administered through an enteral feeding tube, 100 calories = 1 unit ⓑ Qh A Y

  IOM: 100-03, 3, 180.2

Parenteral Nutritional Solutions and Supplies

- **B4164** Parenteral nutrition solution: carbohydrates (dextrose), 50% or less (500 ml = 1 unit) - home mix ⓑ Qp Qh Y

  IOM: 100-02, 15, 120; 100-03, 3, 180.2; 100-04, 20, 100.2.2

  PEN: On Fee Schedule

- **B4168** Parenteral nutrition solution; amino acid, 3.5%, (500 ml = 1 unit) - home mix ⓑ Qp Qh Y

  IOM: 100-02, 15, 120; 100-03, 3, 180.2; 100-04, 20, 100.2.2

  PEN: On Fee Schedule

- **B4172** Parenteral nutrition solution; amino acid, 5.5% through 7%, (500 ml = 1 unit) - home mix ⓑ Qp Qh Y

  IOM: 100-02, 15, 120; 100-03, 3, 180.2; 100-04, 20, 100.2.2

- **B4176** Parenteral nutrition solution; amino acid, 7% through 8.5%, (500 ml = 1 unit) - home mix ⓑ Qp Qh Y

  IOM: 100-02, 15, 120; 100-03, 3, 180.2; 100-04, 20, 100.2.2

  PEN: On Fee Schedule

- **B4178** Parenteral nutrition solution: amino acid, greater than 8.5% (500 ml = 1 unit) - home mix ⓑ Qp Qh Y

  IOM: 100-02, 15, 120; 100-03, 3, 180.2; 100-04, 20, 100.2.2

  PEN: On Fee Schedule

- **B4180** Parenteral nutrition solution; carbohydrates (dextrose), greater than 50% (500 ml = 1 unit) - home mix ⓑ Qp Qh Y

  IOM: 100-02, 15, 120; 100-03, 3, 180.2; 100-04, 20, 100.2.2

  PEN: On Fee Schedule

- **B4185** Parenteral nutrition solution, not otherwise specified, 10 grams lipids ⓑ B

  PEN: On Fee Schedule

- **B4187** Omegaven, 10 grams lipids B

- **B4189** Parenteral nutrition solution; compounded amino acid and carbohydrates with electrolytes, trace elements, and vitamins, including preparation, any strength, 10 to 51 grams of protein - premix ⓑ Qp Qh Y

  IOM: 100-02, 15, 120; 100-03, 3, 180.2; 100-04, 20, 100.2.2

  PEN: On Fee Schedule

- **B4193** Parenteral nutrition solution; compounded amino acid and carbohydrates with electrolytes, trace elements, and vitamins, including preparation, any strength, 52 to 73 grams of protein - premix ⓑ Qh Y

  IOM: 100-02, 15, 120; 100-03, 3, 180.2; 100-04, 20, 100.2.2

  PEN: On Fee Schedule

- **B4197** Parenteral nutrition solution; compounded amino acid and carbohydrates with electrolytes, trace elements and vitamins, including preparation, any strength, 74 to 100 grams of protein - premix ⓑ Qh Y

  IOM: 100-02, 15, 120; 100-03, 3, 180.2; 100-04, 20, 100.2.2

  PEN: On Fee Schedule

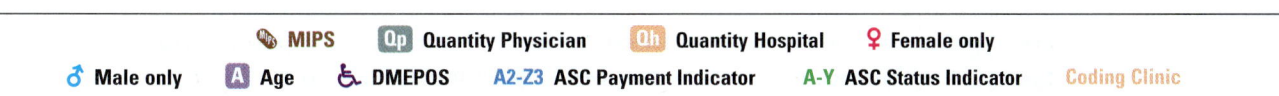

- **B4199** Parenteral nutrition solution; compounded amino acid and carbohydrates with electrolytes, trace elements and vitamins, including preparation, any strength, over 100 grams of protein - premix ⓑ Qp Qh Y

  IOM: 100-02, 15, 120; 100-03, 3, 180.2; 100-04, 20, 100.2.2

  PEN: On Fee Schedule

- **B4216** Parenteral nutrition; additives (vitamins, trace elements, heparin, electrolytes) home mix per day ⓑ Qh Y

  IOM: 100-02, 15, 120; 100-03, 3, 180.2; 100-04, 20, 100.2.2

  PEN: On Fee Schedule

- **B4220** Parenteral nutrition supply kit; premix, per day ⓑ Qh Y

  IOM: 100-02, 15, 120; 100-03, 3, 180.2; 100-04, 20, 100.2.2

  PEN: On Fee Schedule

- **B4222** Parenteral nutrition supply kit; home mix, per day ⓑ Qh Y

  IOM: 100-02, 15, 120; 100-03, 3, 180.2; 100-04, 20, 100.2.2

  PEN: On Fee Schedule

- **B4224** Parenteral nutrition administration kit, per day ⓑ Qh Y

  Dressings used with parenteral nutrition (covered under the prosthetic device benefit) are included in the payment. (www.cms.gov/medicare-coverage-database/)

  IOM: 100-02, 15, 120; 100-03, 3, 180.2; 100-04, 20, 100.2.2

  PEN: On Fee Schedule

- **B5000** Parenteral nutrition solution compounded amino acid and carbohydrates with electrolytes, trace elements, and vitamins, including preparation, any strength, renal - Aminosyn-RF, NephrAmine, RenAmine - premix ⓑ Qp Qh Y

  IOM: 100-02, 15, 120; 100-03, 3, 180.2; 100-04, 20, 100.2.2

  PEN: On Fee Schedule

- **B5100** Parenteral nutrition solution compounded amino acid and carbohydrates with electrolytes, trace elements, and vitamins, including preparation, any strength, hepatic, HepatAmine - premix ⓑ Qp Qh Y

  IOM: 100-02, 15, 120; 100-03, 3, 180.2; 100-04, 20, 100.2.2

  PEN: On Fee Schedule

- **B5200** Parenteral nutrition solution compounded amino acid and carbohydrates with electrolytes, trace elements, and vitamins, including preparation, any strength, stress-branch chain amino acids-FreAmine-HBC - premix ⓑ Qp Qh Y

  IOM: 100-02, 15, 120; 100-03, 3, 180.2; 100-04, 20, 100.2.2

Enteral and Parenteral Pumps

- **B9002** Enteral nutrition infusion pump, any type ⓑ Qh Y

  IOM: 100-02, 15, 120; 100-03, 3, 180.2; 100-04, 20, 100.2.2

  PEN: On Fee Schedule

- **B9004** Parenteral nutrition infusion pump, portable ⓑ Qh Y

  IOM: 100-02, 15, 120; 100-03, 3, 180.2; 100-04, 20, 100.2.2

  PEN: On Fee Schedule

- **B9006** Parenteral nutrition infusion pump, stationary ⓑ Qh Y

  IOM: 100-02, 15, 120; 100-03, 3, 180.2; 100-04, 20, 100.2.2

  PEN: On Fee Schedule

- **B9998** NOC for enteral supplies ⓑ Y

  IOM: 100-02, 15, 120; 100-03, 3, 180.2; 100-04, 20, 100.2.2

- **B9999** NOC for parenteral supplies ⓑ Y

  Determine if an alternative HCPCS Level II or a CPT code better describes the service being reported. This code should be reported only if a more specific code is unavailable.

  IOM: 100-02, 15, 120; 100-03, 3, 180.2; 100-04, 20, 100.2.2

▶ New ↻ Revised ✓ Reinstated ~~deleted~~ Deleted ⊘ Not covered or valid by Medicare
✷ Special coverage instructions ✱ Carrier discretion ⓑ Bill Part B MAC ⓑ Bill DME MAC

CMS HOSPITAL OUTPATIENT PAYMENT SYSTEM (C1000-C9999)

NOTE: C-codes are used on Medicare Ambulatory Surgical Center (ASC) and Hospital Outpatient Prospective Payment System (OPPS) claims, but may also be recognized on claims from other providers or by other payment systems. As of 10/01/2006, the following non-OPPS providers have been able to bill Medicare using the C-codes, or an appropriate CPT code on Types of Bill (TOBs) 12X, 13X, or 85X:

- Critical Access Hospitals (CAHs);
- Indian Health Service Hospitals (IHS);
- Hospitals located in American Samoa, Guam, Saipan or the Virgin Islands; and
- Maryland waiver hospitals.

The billing of C-codes by Method I and Method II Critical Access Hospitals (CAHs) is limited to the billing for facility (technical) services. The C-codes shall not be billed by Method II CAHs for professional services with revenue codes (RCs) 96X, 97X, or 98X.

C codes are updated quarterly by the Centers for Medicare and Medicaid Services (CMS).

Devices and Supplies

- **C1052** Hemostatic agent, gastrointestinal, topical J7 N
- **C1062** Intravertebral body fracture augmentation with implant (e.g., metal, polymer) J7 N
- **C1600** Catheter, transluminal intravascular lesion preparation device, bladed, sheathed (insertable) H
- **C1601** Endoscope, single-use (i.e. disposable), pulmonary, imaging/illumination device (insertable) H
- **C1602** Orthopedic/device/drug matrix/absorbable bone void filler, antimicrobial-eluting (implantable) H
- **C1603** Retrieval device, insertable, laser (used to retrieve intravascular inferior vena cava filter) H
- **C1604** Graft, transmural transvenous arterial bypass (implantable), with all delivery system components H
- C1605 Pacemaker, leadless, dual chamber (right atrial and right ventricular implantable components), rate-responsive, including all necessary components for implantation H

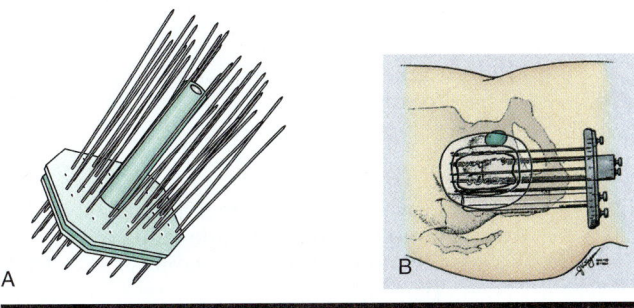

Figure 9 (A) Brachytherapy device, (B) Brachytherapy device inserted.

- **C1606** Adapter, single-use (i.e. disposable), for attaching ultrasound system to upper gastrointestinal endoscope H
- **C1713** Anchor/Screw for opposing bone-to-bone or soft tissue-to-bone (implantable) Qh N1 N
  Medicare Statute 1833(t)
  Coding Clinic: 2022, Q4, P13; 2022, Q3, P9; 2021, Q1, P9-10; 2020, Q4, P7-8; 2018, Q2, P5; Q1, P4; 2016, Q3, P16; 2015, Q3, P2; 2010, Q2, P3
- **C1714** Catheter, transluminal atherectomy, directional Qh N1 N
  Medicare Statute 1833(t)
- **C1715** Brachytherapy needle Qh N1 N
  Medicare Statute 1833(t)

Brachytherapy Sources

- **C1716** Brachytherapy source, non-stranded, gold-198, per source Qp Qh H2 U
  Medicare Statute 1833(t)
- **C1717** Brachytherapy source, non-stranded, high dose rate iridium 192, per source Qp Qh H2 U
  Medicare Statute 1833(t)
- **C1719** Brachytherapy source, non-stranded, non-high dose rate iridium-192, per source Qp Qh H2 U
  Medicare Statute 1833(t)

Cardioverter-Defibrillators

- **C1721** Cardioverter-defibrillator, dual chamber (implantable) Qp Qh N1 N
  Related CPT codes: 33224, 33240, 33249.
  Medicare Statute 1833(t)
- **C1722** Cardioverter-defibrillator, single chamber (implantable) Qp Qh N1 N
  Related CPT codes: 33240, 33249.
  Medicare Statute 1833(t)
  Coding Clinic: 2017, Q2, P5; 2006, Q2, P9

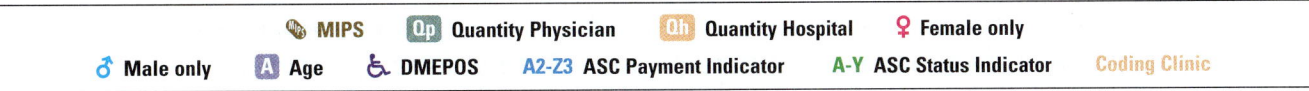

Catheters

C1724 Catheter, transluminal atherectomy, rotational [Qh] N1 N
Medicare Statute 1833(t)
Coding Clinic: 2016, Q3, P9

C1725 Catheter, transluminal angioplasty, non-laser (may include guidance, infusion/perfusion capability) [Qh] N1 N
Medicare Statute 1833(t)
Coding Clinic: 2016, Q3, P16, P19

C1726 Catheter, balloon dilatation, non-vascular [Qh] N1 N
Medicare Statute 1833(t)
Coding Clinic: 2016, Q3, P16, P19

C1727 Catheter, balloon tissue dissector, non-vascular (insertable) [Qh] N1 N
Medicare Statute 1833(t)
Coding Clinic: 2016, Q3, P16

C1728 Catheter, brachytherapy seed administration [Qh] N1 N
Medicare Statute 1833(t)

C1729 Catheter, drainage [Qh] N1 N
Medicare Statute 1833(t)
Coding Clinic: 2016, Q3, P17

C1730 Catheter, electrophysiology, diagnostic, other than 3D mapping (19 or fewer electrodes) [Qp] [Qh] N1 N
Medicare Statute 1833(t)
Coding Clinic: 2016, Q3, P17

C1731 Catheter, electrophysiology, diagnostic, other than 3D mapping (20 or more electrodes) [Qp] [Qh] N1 N
Medicare Statute 1833(t)
Coding Clinic: 2016, Q3, P17

C1732 Catheter, electrophysiology, diagnostic/ablation, 3D or vector mapping [Qp] [Qh] N1 N
Medicare Statute 1833(t)
Coding Clinic: 2016, Q3, P15, P17, P19

C1733 Catheter, electrophysiology, diagnostic/ablation, other than 3D or vector mapping, other than cool-tip [Qp] [Qh] N1 N
Medicare Statute 1833(t)
Coding Clinic: 2016, Q3, P17

C1734 Orthopedic/device/drug matrix for opposing bone-to-bone or soft tissue-to-bone (implantable) N1 N

▶ **C1735** Catheter(s), intravascular for renal denervation, radiofrequency, including all single use system components H

▶ **C1736** Catheter(s), intravascular for renal denervation, ultrasound, including all single use system components H

▶ **C1737** Joint fusion and fixation device(s), sacroiliac and pelvis, including all system components (implantable) H

▶ **C1738** Powered, single-use (i.e. disposable) endoscopic ultrasound-guided biopsy device H

▶ **C1739** Tissue marker, uniquely detectable and identifiable with probe/sensor, any method (implantable), with delivery system H

▶ **C1740** Leadless electrode, transmitter, battery (all implantable), for sequential left ventricular pacing H

▶ **C1741** Anchor/screw for bone fixation, absorbable (implantable) H

▶ **C1742** Pressure monitoring system, compartmental intramuscular (implantable), continuous, including all components (e.g., introducer, sensor), excludes mobile (wireless) software application H

C1747 Endoscope, single-use (i.e. disposable), urinary tract, imaging/illumination device (insertable) J7 H

C1748 Endoscope, single-use (i.e. disposable), upper gi, imaging/illumination device (insertable) J7 N

C1749 Endoscope, retrograde imaging/illumination colonoscope device (implantable) [Qp] [Qh] N1 N
Medicare Statute 1833(t)

C1750 Catheter, hemodialysis/peritoneal, long-term [Qh] N1 N
Medicare Statute 1833(t)
Coding Clinic: 2015, Q4, P6

C1751 Catheter, infusion, inserted peripherally, centrally, or midline (other than hemodialysis) [Qh] N1 N
Medicare Statute 1833(t)

C1752 Catheter, hemodialysis/peritoneal, short-term [Qh] N1 N
Medicare Statute 1833(t)

C1753 Catheter, intravascular ultrasound [Qh] N1 N
Medicare Statute 1833(t)

C1754 Catheter, intradiscal [Qh] N1 N
Medicare Statute 1833(t)

C1755 Catheter, instraspinal [Qh] N1 N
Medicare Statute 1833(t)

C1756 Catheter, pacing, transesophageal [Qh] N1 N
Medicare Statute 1833(t)

▶ New　⟲ Revised　✓ Reinstated　~~deleted~~ Deleted　⊘ Not covered or valid by Medicare
✺ Special coverage instructions　✱ Carrier discretion　Ⓑ Bill Part B MAC　Ⓓ Bill DME MAC

CMS HOSPITAL OUTPATIENT PAYMENT SYSTEM

○ **C1757** Catheter, thrombectomy/embolectomy **Qh** — N1 N
Medicare Statute 1833(t)

○ **C1758** Catheter, ureteral **Qh** — N1 N
Medicare Statute 1833(t)

○ **C1759** Catheter, intracardiac echocardiography **Qh** — N1 N
Medicare Statute 1833(t)

Devices

○ **C1760** Closure device, vascular (implantable/insertable) **Qh** — N1 N
Medicare Statute 1833(t)
Coding Clinic: 2016, Q3, P19

○ **C1761** Catheter, transluminal intravascular lithotripsy, coronary — J7 N
Coding Clinic: 2023, Q2, P19

○ **C1762** Connective tissue, human (includes fascia lata) **Qh** — N1 N
Medicare Statute 1833(t)
Coding Clinic: 2025, Q3, P17; 2016, Q3, P9, P16, P19; 2015, Q3, P2; 2003, Q3, P12

○ **C1763** Connective tissue, non-human (includes synthetic) **Qh** — N1 N
Medicare Statute 1833(t)
Coding Clinic: 2016, Q3, P9, P17, P19; 2010, Q4, P3; Q2, P3; 2003, Q3, P12

○ **C1764** Event recorder, cardiac (implantable) **Qp Qh** — N1 N
Medicare Statute 1833(t)
Coding Clinic: 2015, Q2, P8

○ **C1765** Adhesion barrier **Qh** — N1 N
Medicare Statute 1833(t)
Coding Clinic: 2016, Q3, P16

○ **C1766** Introducer/sheath, guiding, intracardiac electrophysiological, steerable, other than peel-away **Qh** — N1 N
Medicare Statute 1833(t)

○ **C1767** Generator, neurostimulator (implantable), nonrechargeable **Qp Qh** — N1 N
Related CPT codes: 61885, 61886, 63685, 64590.
Medicare Statute 1833(t)
Coding Clinic: 2021, Q1, P8; 2007, Q1, P8

○ **C1768** Graft, vascular **Qh** — N1 N
Medicare Statute 1833(t)

○ **C1769** Guide wire **Qh** — N1 N
Medicare Statute 1833(t)
Coding Clinic: 2019, Q3, P10; 2016, Q3, P3; 2007, Q2, P7-8

○ **C1770** Imaging coil, magnetic reasonance (insertable) **Qh** — N1 N
Medicare Statute 1833(t)

○ **C1771** Repair device, urinary, incontinence, with sling graft **Qp Qh** — N1 N
Medicare Statute 1833(t)
Coding Clinic: 2016, Q3, P19; 2008, Q3, P7

○ **C1772** Infusion pump, programmable (implantable) **Qp Qh** — N1 N
Medicare Statute 1833(t)

○ **C1773** Retrieval device, insertable (used to retrieve fractured medical devices) **Qh** — N1 N
Medicare Statute 1833(t)
Coding Clinic: 2016, Q3, P19

○ **C1776** Joint device (implantable) **Qp Qh** — N1 N
Medicare Statute 1833(t)
Coding Clinic: 2024, Q1, P25; 2020, Q1, P16; 2018, Q3, P6; 2016, Q3, P3, P18; 2010, Q3, P6; 2008, Q4, P10

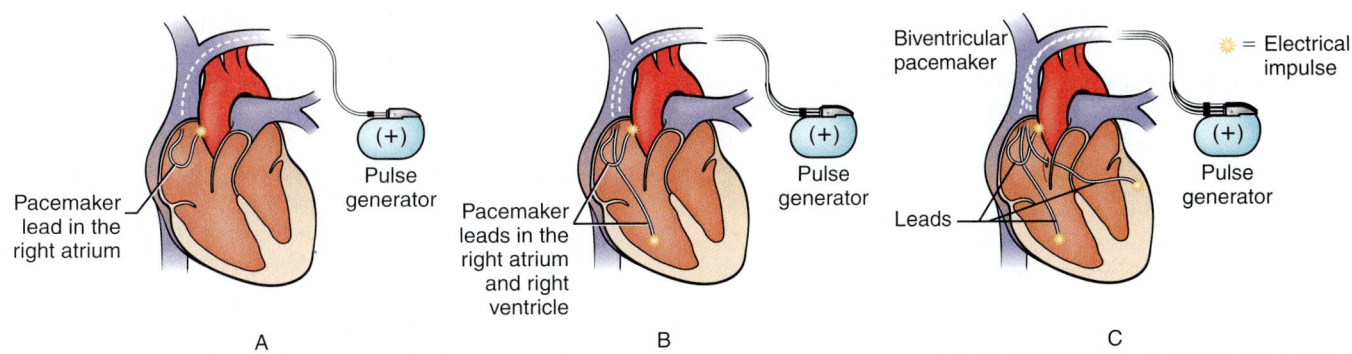

Figure 10 (A) Single pacemaker, (B) Dual pacemaker, (C) Biventricular pacemaker.

| 🪙 MIPS | **Qp** Quantity Physician | **Qh** Quantity Hospital | ♀ Female only |
| ♂ Male only | **A** Age | ♿ DMEPOS | A2-Z3 ASC Payment Indicator | A-Y ASC Status Indicator | Coding Clinic |

149

2026 HCPCS LEVEL II NATIONAL CODES

○ **C1777** Lead, cardioverter-defibrillator, endocardial single coil (implantable) Qh N1 N
Related CPT codes: 33216, 33217, 33249.
Medicare Statute 1833(t)
Coding Clinic: 2017, Q2, P5; 2006, Q2, P9

○ **C1778** Lead, neurostimulator (implantable) Qp Qh N1 N
Related CPT codes: 43647, 63650, 63655, 63663, 63664, 64553, 64555, 64560, 64561, 64565, 64573, 64575, 64577, 64580, 64581.
Medicare Statute 1833(t)
Coding Clinic: 2022, Q4, P16; 2021, Q1, P8; 2019, Q1, P5; 2007, Q1, P8

○ **C1779** Lead, pacemaker, trasvenous VDD single pass Qh N1 N
Related CPT codes: 33206, 33207, 33208, 33210, 33211, 33214, 33216, 33217, 33249.
Medicare Statute 1833(t)
Coding Clinic: 2016, Q3, P19

○ **C1780** Lens, intraocular (new technology) Qh N1 N
Medicare Statute 1833(t)
Coding Clinic: 2016, Q3, P18

○ **C1781** Mesh (implantable) Qh N1 N
Medicare Statute 1833(t)
Coding Clinic: 2022, Q4, P16-17; 2019, Q1, P5; 2016, Q3, P18-19; 2012, Q2, P3; 2010, Q2, P2-3

○ **C1782** Morcellator Qp Qh N1 N
Medicare Statute 1833(t)
Coding Clinic: 2016, Q3, P18

○ **C1783** Ocular implant, aqueous drainage assist device Qh N1 N
Medicare Statute 1833(t)
Coding Clinic: 2017, Q1, P5

○ **C1784** Ocular device, intraoperative, detached retina Qh N1 N
Medicare Statute 1833(t)
Coding Clinic: 2016, Q3, P18

○ **C1785** Pacemaker, dual chamber, rate-responsive (implantable) Qp Qh N1 N
Related CPT codes: 33206, 33207, 33208, 33213, 33214, 33224.
Medicare Statute 1833(t)

○ **C1786** Pacemaker, single chamber, rate-responsive (implantable) Qp Qh N1 N
Related CPT codes: 33206, 33207, 33212.
Medicare Statute 1833(t)

○ **C1787** Patient programmer, neurostimulator Qh N1 N
Medicare Statute 1833(t)
Coding Clinic: 2016, Q3, P19

○ **C1788** Port, indwelling (implantable) Qh N1 N
Medicare Statute 1833(t)

○ **C1789** Prosthesis, breast (implantable) Qh N1 N
Medicare Statute 1833(t)

○ **C1813** Prosthesis, penile, inflatable Qp Qh ♂ N1 N
Medicare Statute 1833(t)

○ **C1814** Retinal tamponade device, silicone oil Qh N1 N
Medicare Statute 1833(t)
Coding Clinic: 2016, Q3, P19; 2006, Q2, P9

○ **C1815** Prosthesis, urinary sphincter (implantable) Qp Qh N1 N
Medicare Statute 1833(t)

○ **C1816** Receiver and/or transmitter, neurostimulator (implantable) Qh N1 N
Medicare Statute 1833(t)
Coding Clinic: 2022, Q4, P16

○ **C1817** Septal defect implant system, intracardiac Qp Qh N1 N
Medicare Statute 1833(t)
Coding Clinic: 2016, Q3, P19

○ **C1818** Integrated keratoprosthesic Qh N1 N
Medicare Statute 1833(t)
Coding Clinic: 2016, Q3, P18

○ **C1819** Surgical tissue localization and excision device (implantable) Qh N1 N
Medicare Statute 1833(t)

○ **C1820** Generator, neurostimulator (implantable), with rechargeable battery and charging system Qp Qh N1 N
Related CPT codes: 61885, 61886, 63685, 64590.
Medicare Statute 1833(t)
Coding Clinic: 2016, Q2, P7

○ **C1821** Interspinous process distraction device (implantable) Qh N1 N
Medicare Statute 1833(t)

○ **C1822** Generator, neurostimulator (implantable), high frequency, with rechargeable battery and charging system Qp Qh N1 N
Medicare Statute 1833(T)
Coding Clinic: 2016, Q2, P7

○ **C1823** Generator, neurostimulator (implantable), non-rechargeable, with transvenous sensing and stimulation leads N
Medicare Statute 1833(t)

▶ New   ↻ Revised   ✓ Reinstated   ~~deleted~~ Deleted   ⊘ Not covered or valid by Medicare
○ Special coverage instructions   ✱ Carrier discretion   Ⓑ Bill Part B MAC   Ⓑ Bill DME MAC

CMS HOSPITAL OUTPATIENT PAYMENT SYSTEM

◎ **C1824** Generator, cardiac contractility modulation (implantable) **N1 N**

◎ **C1825** Generator, neurostimulator (implantable), non-rechargeable with carotid sinus baroreceptor stimulation lead(s) **J7 N**

◎ **C1826** Generator, neurostimulator (implantable), includes closed feedback loop leads and all implantable components, with rechargeable battery and charging system **J7 H**

◎ **C1827** Generator, neurostimulator (implantable), non-rechargeable, with implantable stimulation lead and external paired stimulation controller **J7 H**

◎ **C1830** Powered bone marrow biopsy needle Qp Qh **N1 N**

Medicare Statute 1833(t)

◎ **C1831** Interbody cage, anterior, lateral or posterior, personalized (implantable) **J7 N**

◎ **C1832** Autograft suspension, including cell processing and application, and all system components **J7 N**

◎ **C1833** Monitor, cardiac, including intracardiac lead and all system components (implantable) **J7 N**

◎ **C1839** Iris prosthesis **N1 N**

◎ **C1840** Lens, intraocular (telescopic) Qp Qh **N1 N**

Medicare Statute 1833(t)

Coding Clinic: 2012, Q3, P10

◎ **C1874** Stent, coated/covered, with delivery system Qh **N1 N**

Medicare Statute 1833(t)

Coding Clinic: 2023, Q2, P17,19; 2016, Q3, P16-17, P19

◎ **C1875** Stent, coated/covered, without delivery system Qh **N1 N**

Medicare Statute 1833(t)

Coding Clinic: 2023, Q2, P17; 2020, Q2, P9; 2016, Q3, P16-17

◎ **C1876** Stent, non-coated/non-covered, with delivery system Qh **N1 N**

Medicare Statute 1833(t)

Coding Clinic: 2016, Q3, P19

◎ **C1877** Stent, non-coated/non-covered, without delivery system Qh **N1 N**

Medicare Statute 1833(t)

◎ **C1878** Material for vocal cord medialization, synthetic (implantable) Qh **N1 N**

Medicare Statute 1833(t)

Coding Clinic: 2016, Q3, P18

◎ **C1880** Vena cava filter Qh **N1 N**

Medicare Statute 1833(t)

◎ **C1881** Dialysis access system (implantable) Qh **N1 N**

Medicare Statute 1833(t)

◎ **C1882** Cardioverter-defibrillator, other than single or dual chamber (implantable) Qp Qh **N1 N**

Related CPT codes: 33224, 33240, 33249.

Medicare Statute 1833(t)

Coding Clinic: 2016, Q3, P16; 2012, Q2, P9; 2006, Q2, P9

◎ **C1883** Adapter/Extension, pacing lead or neurostimulator lead (implantable) Qh **N1 N**

Medicare Statute 1833(t)

Coding Clinic: 2016, Q3, P15, P17; 2007, Q1, P8

◎ **C1884** Embolization protective system Qh **N1 N**

Medicare Statute 1833(t)

Coding Clinic: 2016, Q3, P17

◎ **C1885** Catheter, transluminal angioplasty, laser Qh **N1 N**

Medicare Statute 1833(t)

Coding Clinic: 2016, Q3, p16, Q1, P5

◎ **C1886** Catheter, extravascular tissue ablation, any modality (insertable) Qp Qh **N1 N**

Medicare Statute 1833(t)

◎ **C1887** Catheter, guiding (may include infusion/perfusion capability) Qh **N1 N**

Medicare Statute 1833(t)

Coding Clinic: 2016, Q3, P17

◎ **C1888** Catheter, ablation, non-cardiac, endovascular (implantable) Qh **N1 N**

Medicare Statute 1833(t)

Coding Clinic: 2016, Q3, P16

◎ **C1889** Implantable/insertable device, not otherwise classified **N1 N**

Medicare Statute 1833(T)

◎ **C1891** Infusion pump, non-programmable, permanent (implantable) Qp Qh **N1 N**

Medicare Statute 1833(t)

◎ **C1892** Introducer/sheath, guiding, intracardiac electrophysiological, fixed-curve, peel-away Qh **N1 N**

Medicare Statute 1833(t)

Coding Clinic: 2016, Q3, P19

◎ **C1893** Introducer/sheath, guiding, intracardiac electrophysiological, fixed-curve, other than peel-away Qh **N1 N**

Medicare Statute 1833(t)

| ⚬ MIPS | Qp Quantity Physician | Qh Quantity Hospital | ♀ Female only |
| ♂ Male only | A Age | ♿ DMEPOS | A2-Z3 ASC Payment Indicator | A-Y ASC Status Indicator | Coding Clinic |

⊛ **C1894** Introducer/sheath, other than guiding, other than intracardiac electrophysiological, non-laser Qh　　N1 N
Medicare Statute 1833(t)

⊛ **C1895** Lead, cardioverter-defibrillator, endocardial dual coil (implantable) Qh　　N1 N
Related CPT codes: 33216, 33217, 33249.
Medicare Statute 1833(t)
Coding Clinic: 2006, Q2, P9

⊛ **C1896** Lead, cardioverter-defibrillator, other than endocardial single or dual coil (implantable) Qh　　N1 N
Related CPT codes: 33216, 33217, 33249.
Medicare Statute 1833(t)

⊛ **C1897** Lead, neurostimulator test kit (implantable) Qh　　N1 N
Related CPT codes: 43647, 63650, 63655, 63663, 63664, 64553, 64555, 64560, 64561, 64565, 64575, 64577, 64580, 64581.
Medicare Statute 1833(t)
Coding Clinic: 2007, Q1, P8

⊛ **C1898** Lead, pacemaker, other than transvenous VDD single pass Qh　　N1 N
Related CPT codes: 33206, 33207, 33208, 33210, 33211, 33214, 33216, 33217, 33249.
Medicare Statute 1833(t)
Coding Clinic: 2002, Q3, P8

⊛ **C1899** Lead, pacemaker/cardioverter-defibrillator combination (implantable) Qh　　N1 N
Related CPT codes: 33216, 33217, 33249.
Medicare Statute 1833(t)

⊛ **C1900** Lead, left ventricular coronary venous system Qp Qh　　N1 N
Related CPT codes: 33224, 33225.
Medicare Statute 1833(t)
Coding Clinic: 2016, Q3, P18

↻ **C1982** Catheter, pressure-generating, (e.g., one-way valve, intermittently occlusive)　　N1 N

⊛ **C2596** Probe, image-guided, robotic, waterjet ablation　　N1 N

⊛ **C2613** Lung biopsy plug with delivery system Qp Qh　　N1 N
Medicare Statute 1833(t)
Coding Clinic: 2015, Q2, P11

⊛ **C2614** Probe, percutaneous lumbar discectomy Qh　　N1 N
Medicare Statute 1833(t)

⊛ **C2615** Sealant, pulmonary, liquid Qh　　N1 N
Medicare Statute 1833(t)
Coding Clinic: 2016, Q3, P18

Brachytherapy Source

⊛ **C2616** Brachytherapy source, non-stranded, yttrium-90, per source Qp Qh　　H2 U
Medicare Statute 1833(t)

Cardiovascular and Genitourinary Devices

⊛ **C2617** Stent, non-coronary, temporary, without delivery system Qh　　N1 N
Medicare Statute 1833(t)
Coding Clinic: 2018, Q1, P4; 2016, Q3, P3, P19

⊛ **C2618** Probe/needle, cryoablation Qh　　N1 N
Medicare Statute 1833(t)

⊛ **C2619** Pacemaker, dual chamber, non rate-responsive (implantable) Qp Qh　　N1 N
Related CPT codes: 33206, 33207, 33208, 33213, 33214, 33224.
Medicare Statute 1833(t)

⊛ **C2620** Pacemaker, single chamber, non rate-responsive (implantable) Qp Qh　　N1 N
Related CPT codes: 33206, 33207, 33212, 33224.
Medicare Statute 1833(t)

⊛ **C2621** Pacemaker, other than single or dual chamber (implantable) Qp Qh　　N1 N
Related CPT codes: 33206, 33207, 33208, 33212, 33213, 33214, 33224.
Medicare Statute 1833(t)
Coding Clinic: 2016, Q3, P18; 2002, Q3, P8

⊛ **C2622** Prosthesis, penile, non-inflatable Qp Qh ♂　　N1 N
Medicare Statute 1833(t)

⊛ **C2623** Catheter, transluminal angioplasty, drug-coated, non-laser Qp Qh　　N1 N
Medicare Statute 1833(t)

⊛ **C2624** Implantable wireless pulmonary artery pressure sensor with delivery catheter, including all system components Qp Qh　　N1 N
Medicare Statute 1833(t)
Coding Clinic: 2015, Q3, P2

⊛ **C2625** Stent, non-coronary, temporary, with delivery system Qh　　N1 N
Medicare Statute 1833(t)
Coding Clinic: 2016, Q3, P19; 2015, Q2, P9

▶ New　　↻ Revised　　✓ Reinstated　　deleted Deleted　　⊘ Not covered or valid by Medicare
⊛ Special coverage instructions　　✱ Carrier discretion　　Ⓑ Bill Part B MAC　　Ⓑ Bill DME MAC

CMS HOSPITAL OUTPATIENT PAYMENT SYSTEM

- ❂ **C2626** Infusion pump, non-programmable, temporary (implantable) Qp Qh N1 N

  Medicare Statute 1833(t)

  Coding Clinic: 2016, Q3, P18

- ❂ **C2627** Catheter, suprapubic/cystoscopic Qh N1 N

  Medicare Statute 1833(t)

- ❂ **C2628** Catheter, occlusion Qh N1 N

  Medicare Statute 1833(t)

- ❂ **C2629** Introducer/Sheath, other than guiding, other than intracardiac electrophysiological, laser Qh N1 N

  Medicare Statute 1833(t)

- ❂ **C2630** Catheter, electrophysiology, diagnostic/ablation, other than 3D or vector mapping, cool-tip Qp Qh N1 N

  Medicare Statute 1833(t)

  Coding Clinic: 2016, Q3, P17

- ❂ **C2631** Repair device, urinary, incontinence, without sling graft Qp Qh N1 N

  Medicare Statute 1833(t)

Brachytherapy Sources

- ❂ **C2634** Brachytherapy source, non-stranded, high activity, iodine-125, greater than 1.01 mci (NIST), per source Qp Qh H2 U

  Medicare Statute 1833(t)

- ❂ **C2635** Brachytherapy source, non-stranded, high activity, palladium-103, greater than 2.2 mci (NIST), per source Qp Qh H2 U

  Medicare Statute 1833(t)

- ❂ **C2636** Brachytherapy linear source, non-stranded, palladium-103, per 1 mm Qp Qh H2 U

- ❂ **C2637** Brachytherapy source, non-stranded, Ytterbium-169, per source Qp Qh B

  Medicare Statute 1833(t)

- ❂ **C2638** Brachytherapy source, stranded, iodine-125, per source Qp Qh H2 U

  Medicare Statute 1833(t)(2)

- ❂ **C2639** Brachytherapy source, non-stranded, iodine-125, per source Qp Qh H2 U

  Medicare Statute 1833(t)(2)

- ❂ **C2640** Brachytherapy source, stranded, palladium-103, per source Qp Qh H2 U

  Medicare Statute 1833(t)(2)

- ❂ **C2641** Brachytherapy source, non-stranded, palladium-103, per source Qp Qh H2 U

  Medicare Statute 1833(t)(2)

- ❂ **C2642** Brachytherapy source, stranded, cesium-131, per source Qp Qh H2 U

  Medicare Statute 1833(t)(2)

- ❂ **C2643** Brachytherapy source, non-stranded, cesium-131, per source Qp Qh H2 U

  Medicare Statute 1833(t)(2)

- ❂ **C2644** Brachytherapy source, Cesium-131 chloride solution, per millicurie Qp Qh H2 E2

  Medicare Statute 1833(t)

- ❂ **C2645** Brachytherapy planar source, palladium-103, per square millimeter Qp Qh H2 U

  Medicare Statute 1833(T)

- ❂ **C2698** Brachytherapy source, stranded, not otherwise specified, per source H2 U

  Medicare Statute 1833(t)(2)

- ❂ **C2699** Brachytherapy source, non-stranded, not otherwise specified, per source H2 U

  Medicare Statute 1833(t)(2)

Skin Substitute Graft Application

- ❂ **C5271** Application of low cost skin substitute graft to trunk, arms, legs, total wound surface area up to 100 sq cm; first 25 sq cm or less wound surface area Qp Qh G2 T

  Medicare Statute 1833(t)

- ❂ **C5272** Application of low cost skin substitute graft to trunk, arms, legs, total wound surface area up to 100 sq cm; each additional 25 sq cm wound surface area, or part thereof (list separately in addition to code for primary procedure) Qp Qh N1 N

  Medicare Statute 1833(t)

- ❂ **C5273** Application of low cost skin substitute graft to trunk, arms, legs, total wound surface area greater than or equal to 100 sq cm; first 100 sq cm wound surface area, or 1% of body area of infants and children Qp Qh A G2 T

  Medicare Statute 1833(t)

- ❂ **C5274** Application of low cost skin substitute graft to trunk, arms, legs, total wound surface area greater than or equal to 100 sq cm; each additional 100 sq cm wound surface area, or part thereof, or each additional 1% of body area of infants and children, or part thereof (list separately in addition to code for primary procedure) Qp Qh A N1 N

  Medicare Statute 1833(t)

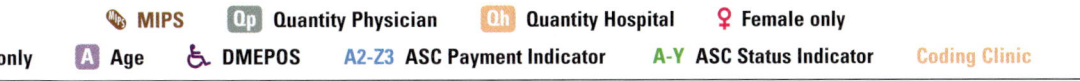

◎ **C5275** Application of low cost skin substitute graft to face, scalp, eyelids, mouth, neck, ears, orbits, genitalia, hands, feet, and/or multiple digits, total wound surface area up to 100 sq cm; first 25 sq cm or less wound surface area Qp Qh G2 T

Medicare Statute 1833(t)

◎ **C5276** Application of low cost skin substitute graft to face, scalp, eyelids, mouth, neck, ears, orbits, genitalia, hands, feet, and/or multiple digits, total wound surface area up to 100 sq cm; each additional 25 sq cm wound surface area, or part thereof (list separately in addition to code for primary procedure) Qp Qh N1 N

Medicare Statute 1833(t)

◎ **C5277** Application of low cost skin substitute graft to face, scalp, eyelids, mouth, neck, ears, orbits, genitalia, hands, feet, and/or multiple digits, total wound surface area greater than or equal to 100 sq cm; first 100 sq cm wound surface area, or 1% of body area of infants and children Qp Qh A G2 T

Medicare Statute 1833(t)

◎ **C5278** Application of low cost skin substitute graft to face, scalp, eyelids, mouth, neck, ears, orbits, genitalia, hands, feet, and/or multiple digits, total wound surface area greater than or equal to 100 sq cm; each additional 100 sq cm wound surface area, or part thereof, or each additional 1% of body area of infants and children, or part thereof (list separately in addition to code for primary procedure) Qp Qh A N1 N

Medicare Statute 1833(t)

C7500 Debridement, bone including epidermis, dermis, subcutaneous tissue, muscle and/or fascia, if performed, first 20 sq cm or less with manual preparation and insertion of deep (eg, subfacial) drug-delivery device(s) Ⓑ G2 E1

C7501 Percutaneous breast biopsies using stereotactic guidance, with placement of breast localization device(s) (eg, clip, metallic pellet), when performed, and imaging of the biopsy specimen, when performed, all lesions unilateral and bilateral (for single lesion biopsy, use appropriate code) Ⓑ G2 E1

C7502 Percutaneous breast biopsies using magnetic resonance guidance, with placement of breast localization device(s) (eg, clip, metallic pellet), when performed, and imaging of the biopsy specimen, when performed, all lesions unilateral or bilateral (for single lesion biopsy, use appropriate code) Ⓑ G2 E1

C7503 Open biopsy or excision of deep cervical node(s) with intraoperative identification (eg, mapping) of sentinel lymph node(s) including injection of non-radioactive dye when performed Ⓑ G2 E1

C7504 Percutaneous vertebroplasties (bone biopsies included when performed), first cervicothoracic and any additional cervicothoracic or lumbosacral vertebral bodies, unilateral or bilateral injection, inclusive of all imaging guidance Ⓑ G2 E1

C7505 Percutaneous vertebroplasties (bone biopsies included when performed), first lumbosacral and any additional cervicothoracic or lumbosacral vertebral bodies, unilateral or bilateral injection, inclusive of all imaging guidance Ⓑ G2 E1

C7506 Arthrodesis, interphalangeal joints, with or without internal fixation Ⓑ G2 E1

C7507 Percutaneous vertebral augmentations, first thoracic and any additional thoracic or lumbar vertebral bodies, including cavity creations (fracture reductions and bone biopsies included when performed) using mechanical device (eg, kyphoplasty), unilateral or bilateral cannulations, inclusive of all imaging guidance Ⓑ G2 E1

C7508 Percutaneous vertebral augmentations, first lumbar and any additional thoracic or lumbar vertebral bodies, including cavity creations (fracture reductions and bone biopsies included when performed) using mechanical device (eg, kyphoplasty), unilateral or bilateral cannulations, inclusive of all imaging guidance Ⓑ E1

C7509 Bronchoscopy, rigid or flexible, diagnostic with cell washing(s) when performed, with computer-assisted image-guided navigation, including fluoroscopic guidance when performed Ⓑ G2 E1

▶ New	↻ Revised	✓ Reinstated	~~deleted~~ Deleted	⊘ Not covered or valid by Medicare
◎ Special coverage instructions		✱ Carrier discretion	Ⓑ Bill Part B MAC	Ⓑ Bill DME MAC

C7510 Bronchoscopy, rigid or flexible, with bronchial alveolar lavage(s), with computer-assisted image-guided navigation, including fluoroscopic guidance when performed ⒷG2 E1

C7511 Bronchoscopy, rigid or flexible, with single or multiple bronchial or endobronchial biopsy(ies), single or multiple sites, with computer-assisted image-guided navigation, including fluoroscopic guidance when performed Ⓑ E1

C7512 Bronchoscopy, rigid or flexible, with single or multiple bronchial or endobronchial biopsy(ies), single or multiple sites, with transendoscopic endobronchial ultrasound (EBUS) during bronchoscopic diagnostic or therapeutic intervention(s) for peripheral lesion(s), including fluoroscopic guidance when performed Ⓑ G2 E1

C7513 Dialysis circuit, introduction of needle(s) and/or catheter(s), with diagnostic angiography of the dialysis circuit, including all direct puncture(s) and catheter placement(s), injection(s) of contrast, all necessary imaging from the arterial anastomosis and adjacent artery through entire venous outflow including the inferior or superior vena cava, fluoroscopic guidance, with transluminal balloon angioplasty of central dialysis segment, performed through dialysis circuit, including all required imaging, radiological supervision and interpretation, image documentation and report Ⓑ G2 E1

Coding Clinic: 2024, Q2, P33-34

C7514 Dialysis circuit, introduction of needle(s) and/or catheter(s), with diagnostic angiography of the dialysis circuit, including all direct puncture(s) and catheter placement(s), injection(s) of contrast, all necessary imaging from the arterial anastomosis and adjacent artery through entire venous outflow including the inferior or superior vena cava, fluoroscopic guidance, with all angioplasty in the central dialysis segment, and transcatheter placement of intravascular stent(s), central dialysis segment, performed through dialysis circuit, including all required imaging, radiological supervision and interpretation, image documentation and report Ⓑ G2 E1

C7515 Dialysis circuit, introduction of needle(s) and/or catheter(s), with diagnostic angiography of the dialysis circuit, including all direct puncture(s) and catheter placement(s), injection(s) of contrast, all necessary imaging from the arterial anastomosis and adjacent artery through entire venous outflow including the inferior or superior vena cava, fluoroscopic guidance, with dialysis circuit permanent endovascular embolization or occlusion of main circuit or any accessory veins, including all required imaging, radiological supervision and interpretation, image documentation and report Ⓑ G2 E1

C7516 Catheter placement in coronary artery(s) for coronary angiography, including intraprocedural injection(s) for coronary angiography, with endoluminal imaging of initial coronary vessel or graft using intravascular ultrasound (IVUS) or optical coherence tomography (OCT) during diagnostic evaluation and/or therapeutic intervention including imaging supervision, interpretation and report Ⓑ G2 E1

C7517 Catheter placement in coronary artery(s) for coronary angiography, including intraprocedural injection(s) for coronary angiography, with iliac and/or femoral artery angiography, non-selective, bilateral or ipsilateral to catheter insertion, performed at the same time as cardiac catheterization and/or coronary angiography, includes positioning or placement of the catheter in the distal aorta or ipsilateral femoral or iliac artery, injection of dye, production of permanent images, and radiologic supervision and interpretation Ⓑ G2 E1

C7518 Catheter placement in coronary artery(ies) for coronary angiography, including intraprocedural injection(s) for coronary angiography, imaging supervision and interpretation, with catheter placement(s) in bypass graft(s) (internal mammary, free arterial, venous grafts) including intraprocedural injection(s) for bypass graft angiography with endoluminal imaging of initial coronary vessel or graft using intravascular ultrasound (IVUS) or optical coherence tomography (OCT) during diagnostic evaluation and/or therapeutic intervention including imaging, supervision, interpretation and report Ⓑ G2 E1

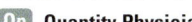 MIPS   Quantity Physician   Quantity Hospital   ♀ Female only
♂ Male only   Ⓐ Age   ♿ DMEPOS   A2-Z3 ASC Payment Indicator   A-Y ASC Status Indicator   *Coding Clinic*

C7519 Catheter placement in coronary artery(ies) for coronary angiography, including intraprocedural injection(s) for coronary angiography, imaging supervision and interpretation, with catheter placement(s) in bypass graft(s) (internal mammary, free arterial, venous grafts) including intraprocedural injection(s) for bypass graft angiography with intravascular doppler velocity and/or pressure derived coronary flow reserve measurement (initial coronary vessel or graft) during coronary angiography including pharmacologically induced stress ⓑ   G2 E1

C7520 Catheter placement in coronary artery(ies) for coronary angiography, including intraprocedural injection(s) for coronary angiography, imaging supervision and interpretation, with catheter placement(s) in bypass graft(s) (internal mammary, free arterial, venous grafts) includes intraprocedural injection(s) for bypass graft angiography with iliac and/or femoral artery angiography, non-selective, bilateral or ipsilateral to catheter insertion, performed at the same time as cardiac catheterization and/or coronary angiography, includes positioning or placement of the catheter in the distal aorta or ipsilateral femoral or iliac artery, injection of dye, production of permanent images, and radiologic supervision and interpretation ⓑ   E1

C7521 Catheter placement in coronary artery(ies) for coronary angiography, including intraprocedural injection(s) for coronary angiography with right heart catheterization with endoluminal imaging of initial coronary vessel or graft using intravascular ultrasound (IVUS) or optical coherence tomography (OCT) during diagnostic evaluation and/or therapeutic intervention including imaging supervision, interpretation and report ⓑ   G2 E1

C7522 Catheter placement in coronary artery(ies) for coronary angiography, including intraprocedural injection(s) for coronary angiography, imaging supervision and interpretation with right heart catheterization, with intravascular doppler velocity and/or pressure derived coronary flow reserve measurement (initial coronary vessel or graft) during coronary angiography including pharmacologically induced stress ⓑ   G2 E1

C7523 Catheter placement in coronary artery(ies) for coronary angiography, including intraprocedural injection(s) for coronary angiography, imaging supervision and interpretation, with left heart catheterization including intraprocedural injection(s) for left ventriculography, when performed, with endoluminal imaging of initial coronary vessel or graft using intravascular ultrasound (IVUS) or optical coherence tomography (OCT) during diagnostic evaluation and/or therapeutic intervention including imaging supervision, interpretation and report ⓑ   G2 E1

C7524 Catheter placement in coronary artery(ies) for coronary angiography, including intraprocedural injection(s) for coronary angiography, imaging supervision and interpretation, with left heart catheterization including intraprocedural injection(s) for left ventriculography, when performed, with intravascular doppler velocity and/or pressure derived coronary flow reserve measurement (initial coronary vessel or graft) during coronary angiography including pharmacologically induced stress ⓑ   G2 E1

C7525 Catheter placement in coronary artery(ies) for coronary angiography, including intraprocedural injection(s) for coronary angiography, imaging supervision and interpretation, with left heart catheterization including intraprocedural injection(s) for left ventriculography, when performed, catheter placement(s) in bypass graft(s) (internal mammary, free arterial, venous grafts) with bypass graft angiography with endoluminal imaging of initial coronary vessel or graft using intravascular ultrasound (IVUS) or optical coherence tomography (OCT) during diagnostic evaluation and/or therapeutic intervention including imaging supervision, interpretation and report ⓑ   G2 E1

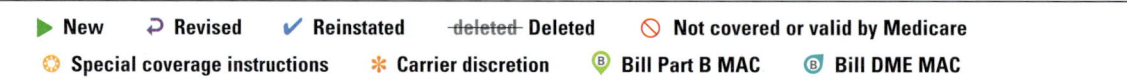

C7526 Catheter placement in coronary artery(ies) for coronary angiography, including intraprocedural injection(s) for coronary angiography, imaging supervision and interpretation, with left heart catheterization including intraprocedural injection(s) for left ventriculography, when performed, catheter placement(s) in bypass graft(s) (internal mammary, free arterial, venous grafts) with bypass graft angiography with intravascular doppler velocity and/or pressure derived coronary flow reserve measurement (initial coronary vessel or graft) during coronary angiography including pharmacologically induced stress ⓑ G2 E1

C7527 Catheter placement in coronary artery(ies) for coronary angiography, including intraprocedural injection(s) for coronary angiography, imaging supervision and interpretation, with right and left heart catheterization including intraprocedural injection(s) for left ventriculography, when performed, with endoluminal imaging of initial coronary vessel or graft using intravascular ultrasound (IVUS) or optical coherence tomography (OCT) during diagnostic evaluation and/or therapeutic intervention including imaging supervision, interpretation and report ⓑ G2 E1

C7528 Catheter placement in coronary artery(ies) for coronary angiography, including intraprocedural injection(s) for coronary angiography, imaging supervision and interpretation, with right and left heart catheterization including intraprocedural injection(s) for left ventriculography, when performed, with intravascular doppler velocity and/or pressure derived coronary flow reserve measurement (initial coronary vessel or graft) during coronary angiography including pharmacologically induced stress ⓑ G2 E1

C7529 Catheter placement in coronary artery(ies) for coronary angiography, including intraprocedural injection(s) for coronary angiography, imaging supervision and interpretation, with right and left heart catheterization including intraprocedural injection(s) for left ventriculography, when performed, catheter placement(s) in bypass graft(s) (internal mammary, free arterial, venous grafts) with bypass graft angiography with intravascular doppler velocity and/or pressure derived coronary flow reserve measurement (initial coronary vessel or graft) during coronary angiography including pharmacologically induced stress ⓑ G2 E1

C7530 Dialysis circuit, introduction of needle(s) and/or catheter(s), with diagnostic angiography of the dialysis circuit, including all direct puncture(s) and catheter placement(s), injection(s) of contrast, all necessary imaging from the arterial anastomosis and adjacent artery through entire venous outflow including the inferior or superior vena cava, fluoroscopic guidance, with transluminal balloon angioplasty, peripheral dialysis segment, including all imaging and radiological supervision and interpretation necessary to perform the angioplasty and all angioplasty in the central dialysis segment, with transcatheter placement of intravascular stent(s), central dialysis segment, performed through dialysis circuit, including all imaging, radiological supervision and interpretation, documentation and report ⓑ E1

C7531 Revascularization, endovascular, open or percutaneous, femoral, popliteal artery(ies), unilateral, with transluminal angioplasty with intravascular ultrasound (initial noncoronary vessel) during diagnostic evaluation and/or therapeutic intervention, including radiological supervision and interpretation ⓑ J8 E1

♂ Male only   Age 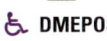 DMEPOS **A2-Z3** ASC Payment Indicator **A-Y** ASC Status Indicator *Coding Clinic*

 MIPS 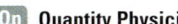 Quantity Physician   Quantity Hospital ♀ Female only

C7532 Transluminal balloon angioplasty (except lower extremity artery(ies) for occlusive disease, intracranial, coronary, pulmonary, or dialysis circuit), initial artery, open or percutaneous, including all imaging and radiological supervision and interpretation necessary to perform the angioplasty within the same artery, with intravascular ultrasound (initial noncoronary vessel) during diagnostic evaluation and/or therapeutic intervention, including radiological supervision and interpretation ⓑ J8 E1

C7533 Percutaneous transluminal coronary angioplasty, single major coronary artery or branch with transcatheter placement of radiation delivery device for subsequent coronary intravascular brachytherapy ⓑ E1

C7534 Revascularization, endovascular, open or percutaneous, femoral, popliteal artery(ies), unilateral, with atherectomy, includes angioplasty within the same vessel, when performed with intravascular ultrasound (initial noncoronary vessel) during diagnostic evaluation and/or therapeutic intervention, including radiological supervision and interpretation ⓑ E1

C7535 Revascularization, endovascular, open or percutaneous, femoral, popliteal artery(ies), unilateral, with transluminal stent placement(s), includes angioplasty within the same vessel, when performed, with intravascular ultrasound (initial noncoronary vessel) during diagnostic evaluation and/or therapeutic intervention, including radiological supervision and interpretation ⓑ E1

C7537 Insertion of new or replacement of permanent pacemaker with atrial transvenous electrode(s), with insertion of pacing electrode, cardiac venous system, for left ventricular pacing, at time of insertion of implantable debribrillator or pacemake pulse generator (eg, for upgrade to dual chamber system) ⓑ E1

C7538 Insertion of new or replacement of permanent pacemaker with ventricular transvenous electrode(s), with insertion of pacing electrode, cardiac venous system, for left ventricular pacing, at time of insertion of implantable defribrillator or pacemaker pulse generator (eg, for upgrade to dual chamber system) ⓑ E1

C7539 Insertion of new or replacement of permanent pacemaker with atrial and ventricular transvenous electrode(s), with insertion of pacing electrode, cardiac venous system, for left ventricular pacing, at time of insertion of implantable defibrillator or pacemaker pulse generator (eg, for upgrade to dual chamber system) ⓑ E1

C7540 Removal of permanent pacemaker pulse generator with replacement of pacemaker pulse generator, dual lead system, with insertion of pacing electrode, cardiac venous system, for left ventricular pacing, at time of insertion of implantable defibrillator or pacemaker pulse generator (eg, for upgrade to dual chamber system) ⓑ E1

C7541 Diagnostic endoscopic retrograde cholangiopancreatography (ERCP), including collection of specimen(s) by brushing or washing, when performed, with endoscopic cannulation of papilla with direct visualization of pancreatic/common bile ducts(s) ⓑ E1

C7542 Endoscopic retrograde cholangiopancreatography (ercp) with biopsy, single or multiple, with endoscopic cannulation of papilla with direct visualization of pancreatic/common bile ducts(s) ⓑ E1

C7543 Endoscopic retrograde cholangiopancreatography (ERCP) with sphincterotomy/papillotomy, with endoscopic cannulation of papilla with direct visualization of pancreatic/common bile ducts(s) ⓑ E1

C7544 Endoscopic retrograde cholangiopancreatography (ERCP) with removal of calculi/debris from biliary/pancreatic duct(s), with endoscopic cannulation of papilla with direct visualization of pancreatic/common bile ducts(s) ⓑ E1

C7545 Percutaneous exchange of biliary drainage catheter (eg, external, internal-external, or conversion of internal-external to external only), with removal of calculi/debris from biliary duct(s) and/or gallbladder, including destruction of calculi by any method (eg, mechanical, electrohydraulic, lithotripsy) when performed, including diagnostic cholangiography(ies) when performed, imaging guidance (eg, fluoroscopy), and all associated radiological supervision and interpretation ⓑ E1

▶ New ↻ Revised ✓ Reinstated ~~deleted~~ Deleted ⊘ Not covered or valid by Medicare ⊛ Special coverage instructions ∗ Carrier discretion ⓑ Bill Part B MAC ⓑ Bill DME MAC

C7546 Removal and replacement of externally accessible nephroureteral catheter (eg, external/internal stent) requiring fluoroscopic guidance, with ureteral stricture balloon dilation, including imaging guidance and all associated radiological supervision and interpretation Ⓑ E1

C7547 Convert nephrostomy catheter to nephroureteral catheter, percutaneous via pre-existing nephrostomy tract, with ureteral stricture balloon dialation, including diagnostic nephrostogram and/or ureterogram when performed, imaging guidance (eg, ultrasound and/or fluoroscopy) and all associated radiological supervision and interpretation Ⓑ E1

C7548 Exchange nephrostomy catheter, percutaneous, with ureteral stricture balloon dilation, including diagnostic nephrostogram and/or ureterogram when performed, imaging guidance (eg, ultrasound and/or fluoroscopy) and all associated radiological supervision and interpretation Ⓑ E1

C7549 Change of ureterostomy tube or externally accessible ureteral stent via ileal conduit with ureteral stricture balloon dilation, including imaging guidance (eg, ultrasound and/or fluoroscopy) and all associated radiological supervision and interpretation Ⓑ E1

C7550 Cystourethroscopy, with biopsy(ies) with adjuctive blue light cystoscopy with fluorescent imaging agent Ⓑ E1

C7551 Excision of major peripheral nerve neuroma, except sciatic, with implantation of nerve end into bone or muscle Ⓑ E1

C7552 Catheter placement in coronary artery(s) for coronary angiography, including intraprocedural injection(s) for coronary angiography, imaging supervision and interpretation; with catheter placement(s) in bypass graft(s) (internal mammary, free arterial, venous grafts) including intraprocedural injection(s) for bypass graft angiography and right heart catheterization with intravascular doppler velocity and/or pressure derived coronary flow reserve measurement (coronary vessel or graft) during coronary angiography including pharmacologically induced stress, initial vessel Ⓑ E1

C7553 Catheter placement in coronary artery(s) for coronary angiography, including intraprocedural injection(s) for coronary angiography, imaging supervision and interpretation; with right and left heart catheterization including intraprocedural injection(s) for left ventriculography, when performed, catheter placement(s) in bypass graft(s) (internal mammary, free arterial, venous grafts) with bypass graft angiography with pharmacologic agent administration (eg, inhaled nitric oxide, intravenous infusion of nitroprusside, dobutamine, milrinone, or other agent) including assessing hemodynamic measurements before, during, after and repeat pharmacologic agent administration, when performed Ⓑ E1

C7554 Cystourethroscopy with adjunctive blue light cystoscopy with fluorescent imaging agent Ⓑ E1

C7555 Thyroidectomy, total or complete with parathyroid autotransplantation Ⓑ E1

C7556 Bronchoscopy, rigid or flexible, with bronchial alveolar lavage and transendoscopic endobronchial ultrasound (EBUS) during bronchoscopic diagnostic or therapeutic intervention(s) for peripheral lesion(s), including fluoroscopic guidance, when performed Ⓑ E1

C7557 Catheter placement in coronary artery(s) for coronary angiography, including intraprocedural injection(s) for coronary angiography, imaging supervision and interpretation with left heart catheterization including intraprocedural injection(s) for left ventriculography, when performed and intraprocedural coronary fractional flow reserve (FFR) with 3d functional mapping of color-coded FFR values for the coronary tree, derived from coronary angiogram data, for real-time review and interpretation of possible atherosclerotic stenosis(es) intervention Ⓑ E1

🏷️ **MIPS**   **Qp** Quantity Physician   **Qh** Quantity Hospital   ♀ Female only
♂ Male only   Ⓐ Age   ♿ DMEPOS   A2-Z3 ASC Payment Indicator   A-Y ASC Status Indicator   Coding Clinic

~~C7558~~ ~~Catheter placement in coronary artery(s) for coronary angiography, including intraprocedural injection(s) for coronary angiography, imaging supervision and interpretation with right and left heart catheterization including intraprocedural injection(s) for left ventriculography, when performed, catheter placement(s) in bypass graft(s) (internal mammary, free arterial, venous grafts) with bypass graft angiography with pharmacologic agent administration (eg, inhaled nitric oxide, intravenous infusion of nitroprusside, dobutamine, milrinone, or other agent) including assessing hemodynamic measurements before, during, after and repeat pharmacologic agent administration, when performed~~

C7560 Endoscopic retrograde cholangiopancreatography (ERCP) with removal of foreign body(s) or stent(s) from biliary/pancreatic duct(s) and endoscopic cannulation of papilla with direct visualization of pancreatic/common bile duct(s) ⓑ E1

▶ C7562 Catheter placement in coronary artery(s) for coronary angiography, including intraprocedural injection(s) for coronary angiography, imaging supervision and interpretation; with right and left heart catheterization including intraprocedural injection(s) for left ventriculography, when performed with intraprocedural coronary fractional flow reserve (FFR) with 3D functional mapping of color-coded FFR values for the coronary tree, derived from coronary angiogram data, for real-time review and interpretation of possible atherosclerotic stenosis(es) intervention ⓑ E1

▶ C7563 Transluminal balloon angioplasty (except lower extremity artery(ies) for occlusive disease, intracranial, coronary, pulmonary, or dialysis circuit), open or percutaneous, including all imaging and radiological supervision and interpretation necessary to perform the angioplasty within the same artery, initial artery and all additional arteries ⓑ E1

▶ C7564 Percutaneous transluminal mechanical thrombectomy, vein(s), including intraprocedural pharmacological thrombolytic injections and fluoroscopic guidance with intravascular ultrasound (noncoronary vessel(s)) during diagnostic evaluation and/or therapeutic intervention, including radiological supervision and interpretation ⓑ E1

▶ C7565 Repair of anterior abdominal hernia(s) (ie, epigastric, incisional, ventral, umbilical, spigelian), any approach (i.e., open, laparoscopic, robotic), recurrent, including implantation of mesh or other prosthesis when performed, total length of defect(s) less than 3 cm, reducible with removal of total or near total non-infected mesh or other prosthesis at the time of initial or recurrent anterior abdominal hernia repair or parastomal hernia repair ⓑ E1

C7900 Service for diagnosis, evaluation, or treatment of a mental health or substance use disorder, 15-29 minutes, provided remotely by hospital staff who are licensed to provide mental health services under applicable state law(s), when the patient is in their home, and there is no associated professional service ⓑ S

C7901 Service for diagnosis, evaluation, or treatment of a mental health or substance use disorder, 30-60 minutes, provided remotely by hospital staff who are licensed to provided mental health services under applicable state law(s), when the patient is in their home, and there is no associated professional service ⓑ S

C7902 Service for diagnosis, evaluation, or treatment of a mental health or substance use disorder, each additional 15 minutes, provided remotely by hospital staff who are licensed to provide mental health services under applicable state law(s), when the patient is in their home, and there is no associated professional service (list separately in addition to code for primary service) ⓑ N

C7903 Group psychotherapy service for diagnosis, evaluation, or treatment of a mental health or substance use disorder provided remotely by hospital staff who are licensed to provide mental health services under applicable state law(s), when the patient is in their home, and there is no associated professional service ⓑ S

C8000 Support device, extravascular, for arteriovenous fistula (implantable) H

▶ ⊛ C8001 3D anatomical segmentation imaging for preoperative planning, data preparation and transmission, obtained from previous diagnostic computed tomographic or magnetic resonance examination of the same anatomy Qp Qh S

▶ New   ⟲ Revised   ✓ Reinstated   ~~deleted~~ Deleted   ⊘ Not covered or valid by Medicare
⊛ Special coverage instructions   ✱ Carrier discretion   ⓑ Bill Part B MAC   ⓑ Bill DME MAC

CMS HOSPITAL OUTPATIENT PAYMENT SYSTEM

▶ ⊛ **C8002** Preparation of skin cell suspension autograft, automated, including all enzymatic processing and device components (do not report with manual suspension preparation) Qp Qh **S**

▶ ⊛ **C8003** Implantation of medial knee extraarticular implantable shock absorber spanning the knee joint from distal femur to proximal tibia, open, includes measurements, positioning and adjustments, with imaging guidance (e.g., fluoroscopy) Qp Qh **S**

▶ ⊛ **C8004** Simulation angiogram with use of a pressure-generating catheter (e.g., one-way valve, intermittently occluding), inclusive of all radiological supervision and interpretation, intraprocedural roadmapping, and imaging guidance necessary to complete the angiogram, for subsequent therapeutic radioembolization of tumors Qp Qh **J1**

▶ ⊛ **C8005** Bronchoscopy, rigid or flexible, non-thermal transbronchial ablation of lesion(s) by pulsed electric field (PEF) energy, including fluoroscopic and/or ultrasound guidance, when performed, with computed tomography acquisition(s) and 3D rendering, computer-assisted, image-guided navigation, and endobronchial ultrasound (EBUS) guided transtracheal and/or transbronchial sampling (e.g., aspiration[s]/biopsy[ies]) of all mediastinal and/or hilar lymph node stations or structures, and therapeutic intervention(s) Qp Qh **S**

▶ ⊛ **C8006** Insertion of pleural-peritoneal shunt with intercostal pump chamber, including imaging, injection(s) of contrast with radiological supervision and interpretation, when performed Qp Qh **J1**

Magnetic Resonance Angiography: Trunk and Lower Extremities

⊛ **C8900** Magnetic resonance angiography with contrast, abdomen Qp Qh **Z2 Q3**
Medicare Statute 1833(t)(2)

⊛ **C8901** Magnetic resonance angiography without contrast, abdomen Qp Qh **Z2 Q3**
Medicare Statute 1833(t)(2)

⊛ **C8902** Magnetic resonance angiography without contrast followed by with contrast, abdomen Qp Qh **Z2 Q3**
Medicare Statute 1833(t)(2)

⊛ **C8903** Magnetic resonance imaging with contrast, breast; unilateral Qp Qh **Z2 Q3**
Medicare Statute 1833(t)(2)

⊛ **C8905** Magnetic resonance imaging without contrast followed by with contrast, breast; unilateral Qp Qh **Z2 Q3**
Medicare Statute 1833(t)(2)

⊛ **C8906** Magnetic resonance imaging with contrast, breast; bilateral Qp Qh **Z2 Q3**
Medicare Statute 1833(t)(2)

⊛ **C8908** Magnetic resonance imaging without contrast followed by with contrast, breast; bilateral Qp Qh **Z2 Q3**
Medicare Statute 1833(t)(2)

⊛ **C8909** Magnetic resonance angiography with contrast, chest (excluding myocardium) Qp Qh **Z2 Q3**
Medicare Statute 1833(t)(2)

⊛ **C8910** Magnetic resonance angiography without contrast, chest (excluding myocardium) Qp Qh **Z2 Q3**
Medicare Statute 1833(t)(2)

⊛ **C8911** Magnetic resonance angiography without contrast followed by with contrast, chest (excluding myocardium) Qp Qh **Z2 Q3**
Medicare Statute 1833(t)(2)

⊛ **C8912** Magnetic resonance angiography with contrast, lower extremity Qp Qh **Z2 Q3**
Medicare Statute 1833(t)(2)

⊛ **C8913** Magnetic resonance angiography without contrast, lower extremity Qp Qh **Z2 Q3**
Medicare Statute 1833(t)(2)

⊛ **C8914** Magnetic resonance angiography without contrast followed by with contrast, lower extremity Qp Qh **Z2 Q3**
Medicare Statute 1833(t)(2)

⊛ **C8918** Magnetic resonance angiography with contrast, pelvis Qp Qh **Z2 Q3**
Medicare Statute 1833(t)(2)

⊛ **C8919** Magnetic resonance angiography without contrast, pelvis Qp Qh **Z2 Q3**
Medicare Statute 1833(t)(2)

⊛ **C8920** Magnetic resonance angiography without contrast followed by with contrast, pelvis Qp Qh **Z2 Q3**
Medicare Statute 1833(t)(2)

MIPS	Qp Quantity Physician	Qh Quantity Hospital	♀ Female only
♂ Male only	A Age	DMEPOS	A2-Z3 ASC Payment Indicator	A-Y ASC Status Indicator	Coding Clinic

Transthoracic and Transesophageal Echocardiography

◎ **C8921** Transthoracic echocardiography with contrast, or without contrast followed by with contrast, for congenital cardiac anomalies; complete Qp Qh S

Medicare Statute 1833(t)(2)

Coding Clinic: 2012, Q3, P8

◎ **C8922** Transthoracic echocardiography with contrast, or without contrast followed by with contrast, for congenital cardiac anomalies; follow-up or limited study Qp Qh S

Medicare Statute 1833(t)(2)

Coding Clinic: 2012, Q3, P8

◎ **C8923** Transthoracic echocardiography with contrast, or without contrast followed by with contrast, real-time with image documentation (2D), includes M-mode recording, when performed, complete, without spectral or color Doppler echocardiography Qp Qh S

Medicare Statute 1833(t)(2)

Coding Clinic: 2012, Q3, P8

◎ **C8924** Transthoracic echocardiography with contrast, or without contrast followed by with contrast, real-time with image documentation (2D), includes M-mode recording, when performed, follow-up or limited study Qp Qh S

Medicare Statute 1833(t)(2)

Coding Clinic: 2012, Q3, P8

◎ **C8925** Transesophageal echocardiography (TEE) with contrast, or without contrast followed by with contrast, real time with image documentation (2D) (with or without M-mode recording); including probe placement, image acquisition, interpretation and report Qp Qh S

Medicare Statute 1833(t)(2)

Coding Clinic: 2012, Q3, P8

◎ **C8926** Transesophageal echocardiography (TEE) with contrast, or without contrast followed by with contrast, for congenital cardiac anomalies; including probe placement, image acquisition, interpretation and report Qp Qh S

Medicare Statute 1833(t)(2)

Coding Clinic: 2012, Q3, P8

◎ **C8927** Transesophageal echocardiography (TEE) with contrast, or without contrast followed by with contrast, for monitoring purposes, including probe placement, real time 2-dimensional image acquisition and interpretation leading to ongoing (continuous) assessment of (dynamically changing) cardiac pumping function and to therapeutic measures on an immediate time basis Qp Qh S

Medicare Statute 1833(t)(2)

Coding Clinic: 2012, Q3, P8

◎ **C8928** Transthoracic echocardiography with contrast, or without contrast followed by with contrast, real-time with image documentation (2D), includes M-mode recording, when performed, during rest and cardiovascular stress test using treadmill, bicycle exercise and/or pharmacologically induced stress, with interpretation and report Qp Qh S

Medicare Statute 1833(t)(2)

Coding Clinic: 2012, Q3, P8

◎ **C8929** Transthoracic echocardiography with contrast, or without contrast followed by with contrast, real-time with image documentation (2D), includes M-mode recording, when performed, complete, with spectral Doppler echocardiography, and with color flow Doppler echocardiography Qp Qh S

Medicare Statute 1833(t)(2)

Coding Clinic: 2012, Q3, P8

◎ **C8930** Transthoracic echocardiography, with contrast, or without contrast followed by with contrast, real-time with image documentation (2D), includes M-mode recording, when performed, during rest and cardiovascular stress test using treadmill, bicycle exercise and/or pharmacologically induced stress, with interpretation and report; including performance of continuous electrocardiographic monitoring, with physician supervision Qp Qh S

Medicare Statute 1833(t)(2)

Coding Clinic: 2012, Q3, P8

Magnetic Resonance Angiography: Spine and Upper Extremities

◎ **C8931** Magnetic resonance angiography with contrast, spinal canal and contents Qp Qh Z2 Q3

Medicare Statute 1833(t)

▶ New ↻ Revised ✓ Reinstated ~~deleted~~ Deleted ⊘ Not covered or valid by Medicare
◎ Special coverage instructions ✱ Carrier discretion Ⓑ Bill Part B MAC Ⓑ Bill DME MAC

◉ **C8932** Magnetic resonance angiography without contrast, spinal canal and contents Qp Qh Z2 Q3

Medicare Statute 1833(t)

◉ **C8933** Magnetic resonance angiography without contrast followed by with contrast, spinal canal and contents Qp Qh Z2 Q3

Medicare Statute 1833(t)

◉ **C8934** Magnetic resonance angiography with contrast, upper extremity Qh Z2 Q3

Medicare Statute 1833(t)

◉ **C8935** Magnetic resonance angiography without contrast, upper extremity Qh Z2 Q3

Medicare Statute 1833(t)

◉ **C8936** Magnetic resonance angiography without contrast followed by with contrast, upper extremity Qh Z2 Q3

Medicare Statute 1833(t)

◉ **C8937** Computer-aided detection, including computer algorithm analysis of breast MRI image data for lesion detection/characterization, pharmacokinetic analysis, with further physician review for interpretation (list separately in addition to code for primary procedure) N

Medicare Statute 1833(t)

Drugs and Biologicals

◉ **C8957** Intravenous infusion for therapy/diagnosis; initiation of prolonged infusion (more than 8 hours), requiring use of portable or implantable pump Qp Qh S

Medicare Statute 1833(t)

Coding Clinic: 2008, Q3, P8

◉ **C9034** Injection, dexamethasone 9%, intraocular, 1 mcg G

Medicare Statute 1833(t)

◉ **C9046** Cocaine hydrochloride nasal solution for topical administration, 1 mg K2 N

◉ **C9047** Injection, caplacizumab-yhdp, 1 mg K2 N

◉ **C9061** Injection, teprotumumab-trbw, 10 mg

◉ **C9063** Injection, eptinezumab-jjmr, 1 mg

◉ **C9067** Gallium ga-68, dotatoc, diagnostic, 0.01 mci K2 K

◉ **C9084** injection, loncastuximab tesirine-lpyl, 0.1 mg K2 D

◉ **C9085** Injection, avalglucosidase alfa-ngpt, 4 mg K2 G

◉ **C9086** Injection, anifrolumab-fnia, 1 mg K2 G

◉ **C9087** Injection, cyclophosphamide, (auromedics), 10 mg K2 G

~~C9088 Instillation, bupivacaine and meloxicam, 1 mg/0.03 mg~~

◉ **C9089** Bupivacaine, collagen-matrix implant, 1 mg K2 K1

✱ **C9101** Injection, oliceridine, 0.1 mg K2 G

✱ **C9143** Cocaine hydrochloride nasal solution (numbrino), 1 mg N

✱ **C9144** Injection, bupivacaine (posimir), 1 mg K2 G

C9166 Injection, secukinumab, intravenous, 1 mg

C9167 Injection, adamts13, recombinant-krhn, 10 iu

C9168 Injection, mirikizumab-mrkz, 1 mg

~~C9169 Injection, nogapendekin alfa-inbakicept-pmln, for intravesical use, 1 mcg~~

~~C9170 Injection, tarlatamab-dlle, 1 mg~~

~~C9171 Injection, pegulicianine, 1 mg~~

~~C9172 Injection, fidanacogene elaparvovec-dzkt, per therapeutic dose~~

~~C9248 Injection, clevidipine butyrate, 1 mg~~ K

◉ **C9250** Human plasma fibrin sealant, vapor-heated, solvent-detergent (ARTISS), 2 ml Qp Qh K2 K

Example of diagnosis codes to be reported with C9250: T20.00-T25.799.

Medicare Statute 621MMA

◉ **C9254** Injection, lacosamide, 1 mg Qp Qh N1 N

Medicare Statute 621MMA

◉ **C9257** injection, bevacizumab, 0.25 mg Qp Qh K2 K

Medicare Statute 1833(t)

◉ **C9285** Lidocaine 70 mg/tetracaine 70 mg, per patch Qp Qh N1 N

Medicare Statute 1833(t)

Coding Clinic: 2011, Q3, P9

~~C9290 Injection, bupivacine liposome, 1 mg~~

◉ **C9293** Injection, glucarpidase, 10 units Qp Qh K2 E2

Medicare Statute 1833(t)

▶ ◉ **C9305** Injection, nipocalimab-aahu, 3 mg Qp Qh G

▶ ◉ **C9306** Injection, telisotuzumab vedotin-tllv, 1 mg Qp Qh G

◈ MIPS   Qp Quantity Physician   Qh Quantity Hospital   ♀ Female only   ♂ Male only   A Age   ♿ DMEPOS   A2-Z3 ASC Payment Indicator   A-Y ASC Status Indicator   Coding Clinic

◎ **C9352** Microporous collagen implantable tube (NeuraGen Nerve Guide), per centimeter length Qp Qh N1 N
Medicare Statute 621MMA

◎ **C9353** Microporous collagen implantable slit tube (NeuraWrap Nerve Protector), per centimeter length Qp Qh N1 N
Medicare Statute 621MMA

◎ **C9354** Acellular pericardial tissue matrix of non-human origin (Veritas), per square centimeter Qp Qh N1 N
Medicare Statute 621MMA

◎ **C9355** Collagen nerve cuff (NeuroMatrix), per 0.5 centimeter length Qp Qh N1 N
Medicare Statute 621MMA

◎ **C9356** Tendon, porous matrix of cross-linked collagen and glycosaminoglycan matrix (TenoGlide Tendon Protector Sheet), per square centimeter Qp Qh N1 N
Medicare Statute 621MMA

◎ **C9358** Dermal substitute, native, non-denatured collagen, fetal bovine origin (SurgiMend Collagen Matrix), per 0.5 square centimeters Qp Qh N1 N
Medicare Statute 621MMA
Coding Clinic: 2024, Q1, P23; 2013, Q3, P9; 2012, Q2, P7

◎ **C9359** Porous purified collagen matrix bone void filler (Integra Mozaik Osteoconductive Scaffold Putty, Integra OS Osteoconductive Scaffold Putty), per 0.5 cc Qp Qh N1 N
Medicare Statute 1833(t)
Coding Clinic: 2015, Q3, P2

◎ **C9360** Dermal substitute, native, non-denatured collagen, neonatal bovine origin (SurgiMend Collagen Matrix), per 0.5 square centimeters Qp Qh N1 N
Medicare Statute 621MMA
Coding Clinic: 2024, Q1, P23; 2012, Q2, P7

◎ **C9361** Collagen matrix nerve wrap (NeuroMend Collagen Nerve Wrap), per 0.5 centimeter length Qp Qh N1 N
Medicare Statute 621MMA

◎ **C9362** Porous purified collagen matrix bone void filler (Integra Mozaik Osteoconductive Scaffold Strip), per 0.5 cc Qp Qh N1 N
Medicare Statute 621MMA
Coding Clinic: 2010, Q2, P8

◎ **C9363** Skin substitute, Integra Meshed Bilayer Wound Matrix, per square centimeter Qp Qh N1 N
Medicare Statute 621MMA
Coding Clinic: 2012, Q2, P7; 2010, Q2, P8

◎ **C9364** Porcine implant, Permacol, per square centimeter Qp Qh N1 N
Medicare Statute 621MMA

◎ **C9399** Unclassified drugs or biologicals K7 A
Medicare Statute 621MMA
Coding Clinic: 2017, Q1, P1-3, P8; 2016, Q4, P10; 2014, Q2, P8; 2013, Q2, P3; 2010, Q3, P8

◎ **C9460** Injection, cangrelor, 1 mg Qp Qh K2 K
Medicare Statute 1833(t)

◎ **C9462** Injection, delafloxacin, 1 mg K2 E2
Medicare Statute 1833(t)

◎ **C9482** Injection, sotalol hydrochloride, 1 mg Qp Qh K2 K
Medicare Statute 1833(t)
Coding Clinic: 2016, Q4, P9

◎ **C9488** Injection, conivaptan hydrochloride, 1 mg K2 N
Medicare Statute 1833(t)

C9507 Plasma, high titer covid-19 convalescent, each unit R

Percutaneous Transcatheter and Transluminal Coronary Procedures

◎ **C9600** Percutaneous transcatheter placement of drug-eluting intracoronary stent(s), with coronary angioplasty when performed; a single major coronary artery or branch Qp Qh J1
Medicare Statute 1833(t)
Coding Clinic: 2023, Q2, P18-19

◎ **C9601** Percutaneous transcatheter placement of drug-eluting intracoronary stent(s), with coronary angioplasty when performed; each additional branch of a major coronary artery (list separately in addition to code for primary procedure) Qp Qh N
Medicare Statute 1833(t)
Coding Clinic: 2023, Q2, P18-19

◎ **C9602** Percutaneous transluminal coronary atherectomy, with drug-eluting intracoronary stent, with coronary angioplasty when performed; a single major coronary artery or branch Qp Qh J1
Medicare Statute 1833(t)
Coding Clinic: 2023, Q2, P18-19

▶ New ⟳ Revised ✓ Reinstated ~~deleted~~ Deleted ⊘ Not covered or valid by Medicare
◎ Special coverage instructions ✱ Carrier discretion Ⓑ Bill Part B MAC Ⓑ Bill DME MAC

CMS HOSPITAL OUTPATIENT PAYMENT SYSTEM

○ **C9603** Percutaneous transluminal coronary atherectomy, with drug-eluting intracoronary stent, with coronary angioplasty when performed; each additional branch of a major coronary artery (list separately in addition to code for primary procedure) Qp Qh   N

Medicare Statute 1833(t)

Coding Clinic: 2023, Q2, P18-19

○ **C9604** Percutaneous transluminal revascularization of or through coronary artery bypass graft (internal mammary, free arterial, venous), any combination of drug-eluting intracoronary stent, atherectomy and angioplasty, including distal protection when performed; a single vessel Qp Qh   J1

Coding Clinic: 2023, Q2, P18-19

○ **C9605** Percutaneous transluminal revascularization of or through coronary artery bypass graft (internal mammary, free arterial, venous), any combination of drug-eluting intracoronary stent, atherectomy and angioplasty, including distal protection when performed; each additional branch subtended by the bypass graft (list separately in addition to code for primary procedure) Qp Qh   N

Medicare Statute 1833(t)

Coding Clinic: 2023, Q2, P18-19

○ **C9606** Percutaneous transluminal revascularization of acute total/subtotal occlusion during acute myocardial infarction, coronary artery or coronary artery bypass graft, any combination of drug-eluting intracoronary stent, atherectomy and angioplasty, including aspiration thrombectomy when performed, single vessel Qp Qh   C

Medicare Statute 1833(t)

Coding Clinic: 2023, Q2, P18-19

○ **C9607** Percutaneous transluminal revascularization of chronic total occlusion, coronary artery, coronary artery branch, or coronary artery bypass graft, any combination of drug-eluting intracoronary stent, atherectomy and angioplasty; single vessel Qp Qh   J1

Medicare Statute 1833(t)

Coding Clinic: 2023, Q2, P18-19

○ **C9608** Percutaneous transluminal revascularization of chronic total occlusion, coronary artery, coronary artery branch, or coronary artery bypass graft, any combination of drug-eluting intracoronary stent, atherectomy and angioplasty; each additional coronary artery, coronary artery branch, or bypass graft (list separately in addition to code for primary procedure) Qp Qh   N

Medicare Statute 1833(t)

Coding Clinic: 2023, Q2, P18-19

▶ ○ **C9610** Catheter, transluminal drug delivery with or without angioplasty, coronary, non-laser (insertable) Qp Qh   N

Medicare Statute 1833(t)

Therapeutic Services and Supplies

○ **C9725** Placement of endorectal intracavitary applicator for high intensity brachytherapy Qp Qh   T

Medicare Statute 1833(t)

○ **C9726** Placement and removal (if performed) of applicator into breast for intraoperative radiation therapy, add-on to primary breast procedure Qh   N

Medicare Statute 1833(t)

○ **C9727** Insertion of implants into the soft palate; minimum of three implants Qp Qh   J1

Medicare Statute 1833(t)

○ **C9728** Placement of interstitial device(s) for radiation therapy/surgery guidance (e.g., fiducial markers, dosimeter), for other than the following sites (any approach): abdomen, pelvis, prostate, retroperitoneum, thorax, single or multiple Qp Qh   S

Medicare Statute 1833(t)

Coding Clinic: 2018, Q2, P4

○ **C9733** Non-ophthalmic fluorescent vascular angiography Qp Qh   Q2

Medicare Statute 1833(t)

Coding Clinic: 2023, Q1, P22; 2012, Q1, P7

○ **C9734** Focused ultrasound ablation/therapeutic intervention, other than uterine leiomyomata, with magnetic resonance (MR) guidance Qp Qh   H

Medicare Statute 1833(t)

○ **C9738** Adjunctive blue light cystoscopy with fluorescent imaging agent (list separately in addition to code for primary procedure)   N1 N

Medicare Statute 1833(t)

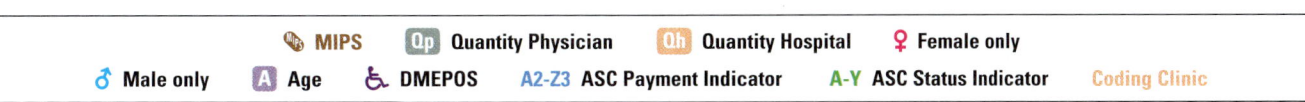

◉ **C9739** Cystourethroscopy, with insertion of transprostatic implant; 1 to 3 implants Qp Qh **J1**
Medicare Statute 1833(t)
Coding Clinic: 2014, Q2, P6

◉ **C9740** Cystourethroscopy, with insertion of transprostatic implant; 4 or more implants Qp Qh **J1**
Medicare Statute 1833(t)
Coding Clinic: 2014, Q2, P6

◉ **C9751** Bronchoscopy, rigid or flexible, transbronchial ablation of lesion(s) by microwave energy, including fluoroscopic guidance, when performed, with computed tomography acquisition(s) and 3-D rendering, computer-assisted, image-guided navigation, and endobronchial ultrasound (EBUS) guided transtracheal and/or transbronchial sampling (e.g., aspiration[s]/biopsy[ies]) and all mediastinal and/or hilar lymph node stations or structures and therapeutic intervention(s) **T**
Medicare Statute 1833(t)

◉ **C9756** Intraoperative near-infrared fluorescence lymphatic mapping of lymph node(s) (sentinel or tumor draining) with administration of indocyanine green (ICG) (list separately in addition to code for primary procedure) **N**
Coding Clinic: 2021, Q1, P9

◉ **C9757** Laminotomy (hemilaminectomy), with decompression of nerve root(s), including partial facetectomy, foraminotomy and excision of herniated intervertebral disc, and repair of annular defect with implantation of bone anchored annular closure device, including annular defect measurement, alignment and sizing assessment, and image guidance; 1 interspace, lumbar **J1**

◉ **C9758** Blinded procedure for NYHA class III/IV heart failure; transcatheter implantation of interatrial shunt or placebo control, including right heart catheterization, trans-esophageal echocardiography (TEE)/intracardiac echocardiography (ICE), and all imaging with or without guidance (e.g., ultrasound, fluoroscopy), performed in an approved investigational device exemption (IDE) study **T**

◉ **C9759** Transcatheter intraoperative blood vessel microinfusion(s) (e.g., intraluminal, vascular wall and/or perivascular) therapy, any vessel, including radiological supervision and interpretation, when performed **N**

◉ **C9760** Non-randomized, non-blinded procedure for NYHA class ii, iii, iv heart failure; transcatheter implantation of interatrial shunt, including right and left heart catheterization, transeptal puncture, trans-esophageal echocardiography (tee)/intracardiac echocardiography (ice), and all imaging with or without guidance (e.g., ultrasound, fluoroscopy), performed in an approved investigational device exemption (ide) study **T**

◉ **C9761** Cystourethroscopy, with ureteroscopy and/or pyeloscopy, with lithotripsy, and ureteral catheterization for steerable vacuum aspiration of the kidney, collecting system, ureter, bladder, and urethra if applicable (must use a steerable ureteral catheter) **J1**

◉ **C9762** Cardiac magnetic resonance imaging for morphology and function, quantification of segmental dysfunction; with strain imaging **Z2 Q3**

◉ **C9763** Cardiac magnetic resonance imaging for morphology and function, quantification of segmental dysfunction; with stress imaging **Z2 Q3**

◉ **C9764** Revascularization, endovascular, open or percutaneous, any vessel(s); with intravascular lithotripsy, includes angioplasty within the same vessel(s), when performed **J1**

◉ **C9765** Revascularization, endovascular, open or percutaneous, any vessel(s); with intravascular lithotripsy, and transluminal stent placement(s), includes angioplasty within the same vessel(s), when performed **J1**

◉ **C9766** Revascularization, endovascular, open or percutaneous, any vessel(s); with intravascular lithotripsy and atherectomy, includes angioplasty within the same vessel(s), when performed **J1**

◉ **C9767** Revascularization, endovascular, open or percutaneous, any vessel(s); with intravascular lithotripsy and transluminal stent placement(s), and atherectomy, includes angioplasty within the same vessel(s), when performed **J1**

▶ New ⇌ Revised ✔ Reinstated ~~deleted~~ Deleted ⊘ Not covered or valid by Medicare
◉ Special coverage instructions ✱ Carrier discretion Ⓑ Bill Part B MAC Ⓑ Bill DME MAC

CMS HOSPITAL OUTPATIENT PAYMENT SYSTEM

- ⊛ **C9768** Endoscopic ultrasound-guided direct measurement of hepatic portosystemic pressure gradient by any method (list separately in addition to code for primary procedure) **N**

- ~~C9769~~ ~~Cystourethroscopy, with insertion of temporary prostatic implant/stent with fixation/anchor and incisional struts~~

- ⊛ **C9772** Revascularization, endovascular, open or percutaneous, tibial/peroneal artery(ies), with intravascular lithotripsy, includes angioplasty within the same vessel(s), when performed **J1**

- ⊛ **C9973** Revascularization, endovascular, open or percutaneous, tibial/peroneal artery(ies); with intravascular lithotripsy, and transluminal stent placement(s), includes angioplasty within the same vessel(s), when performed **J1**

- ⊛ **C9774** Revascularization, endovascular, open or percutaneous, tibial/peroneal artery(ies); with intravascular lithotripsy and atherectomy, includes angioplasty within the same vessel(s), when performed **J1**

- ⊛ **C9775** Revascularization, endovascular, open or percutaneous, tibial/peroneal artery(ies); with intravascular lithotripsy and transluminal stent placement(s), and atherectomy, includes angioplasty within the same vessel(s), when performed **J1**

- ⊛ **C9776** Intraoperative near-infrared fluorescence imaging of major extra-hepatic bile duct(s) (e.g., cystic duct, common bile duct and common hepatic duct) with intravenous administration of indocyanine green (icg) (list separately in addition to code for primary procedure) **N**

   Coding Clinic: 2023, Q2, P19

- ⊛ **C9777** Esophageal mucosal integrity testing by electrical impedance, transoral, includes esophagoscopy or esophagogastroduodenoscopy **J1**

- ⊛ **C9778** Colpopexy, vaginal; minimally invasive extra-peritoneal approach (sacrospinous) **J1**

- ⊛ **C9779** Endoscopic submucosal dissection (esd), including endoscopy or colonoscopy, mucosal closure, when performed **J1**

   Coding Clinic: 2025, Q3, P15; 2023, Q3, P9-10; 2023, Q3, P9-10

- ⊛ **C9780** Insertion of central venous catheter through central venous occlusion via inferior and superior approaches (e.g., inside-out technique), including imaging guidance **S**

- **C9781** Arthroscopy, shoulder, surgical; with implantation of subacromial spacer (e.g., balloon), includes debridement (e.g., limited or extensive), subacromial decompression, acromioplasty, and biceps tenodesis when performed **J1**

- **C9782** Blinded procedure for New York heart association (NYHA) class ii or iii heart failure, or Canadian cardiovascular society (ccs) class iii or iv chronic refractory angina; transcatheter intramyocardial transplantation of autologous bone marrow cells (e.g., mononuclear) or placebo control, autologous bone marrow harvesting and preparation for transplantation, left heart catheterization including ventriculography, all laboratory services, and all imaging with or without guidance (e.g., transthoracic echocardiography, ultrasound, fluoroscopy), performed in an approved investigational device exemption (IDE) study **T**

- **C9783** Blinded procedure for transcatheter implantation of coronary sinus reduction device or placebo control, including vascular access and closure, right heart catherization, venous and coronary sinus angiography, imaging guidance and supervision and interpretation when performed in an approved investigational device exemption (IDE) study **J1**

- ⊛ **C9784** Gastric restrictive procedure, endoscopic sleeve gastroplasty, with esophagogastroduodenoscopy and intraluminal tube insertion, if performed, including all system and tissue anchoring components **J1**

- ⊛ **C9785** Endoscopic outlet reduction, gastric pouch application, with endoscopy and intraluminal tube insertion, if performed, including all system and tissue anchoring components **J1**

- ~~C9786~~ ~~Echocardiography image post processing for computer aided detection of heart failure with preserved ejection fraction, including interpretation and report~~

- ⊛ **C9789** Instillation of anti-neoplastic pharmacologic/biologic agent into renal pelvis, any method, including all imaging guidance, including volumetric measurement if performed **T**

♂ Male only | **A** Age | ♿ DMEPOS | **A2-Z3** ASC Payment Indicator | **A-Y** ASC Status Indicator | *Coding Clinic*

 MIPS | **Qp** Quantity Physician | **Qh** Quantity Hospital | ♀ Female only

C9791 Magnetic resonance imaging with inhaled hyperpolarized xenon-129 contrast agent, chest, including preparation and administration of agent T

C9792 Blinded or nonblinded procedure for symptomatic new york heart association (nyha) class ii, iii, iva heart failure; transcatheter implantation of left atrial to coronary sinus shunt using jugular vein access, including all imaging necessary to intra procedurally map the coronary sinus for optimal shunt placement (e.g., tee or ice ultrasound, fluoroscopy), performed under general anesthesia in an approved investigational device exemption (ide) study S

C9793 3D predictive model generation for pre-planning of a cardiac procedure, using data from cardiac computed tomographic angiography and/or magnetic resonance imaging with report S

~~C9794 Therapeutic radiology simulation aided field setting; complex, including acquisition of pet and ct imaging data required for radiopharmaceutical directed radiation therapy treatment planning (i.e., modeling)~~

~~C9795 Stereotactic body radiation therapy, treatment delivery, per fraction to 1 or more lesions, including image guidance and real-time positron emissions-based delivery adjustments to 1 or more lesions, entire course not to exceed 5 fractions~~

C9796 Repair of enterocutaneous fistula small intestine or colon (excluding anorectal fistula) with plug (e.g., porcine small intestine submucosa [sis]) J1

C9797 Vascular embolization or occlusion procedure with use of a pressure-generating catheter (e.g., one-way valve, intermittently occluding), inclusive of all radiological supervision and interpretation, intraprocedural roadmapping, and imaging guidance necessary to complete the intervention; for tumors, organ ischemia, or infarction J1

▶ **C9804** Elastomeric infusion pump (e.g., on-q* pump with bolus), including catheter and all disposable system components, non-opioid medical device (must be a qualifying Medicare non-opioid medical device for post-surgical pain relief in accordance with section 4135 of the CAA, 2023) H1

▶ **C9806** Rotary peristaltic infusion pump (e.g., ambit pump), including catheter and all disposable system components, non-opioid medical device (must be a qualifying Medicare non-opioid medical device for post-surgical pain relief in accordance with section 4135 of the CAA, 2023) H1

▶ **C9807** Nerve stimulator, percutaneous, peripheral (e.g., sprint peripheral nerve stimulation system), including electrode and all disposable system components, non-opioid medical device (must be a qualifying Medicare non-opioid medical device for post-surgical pain relief in accordance with section 4135 of the CAA, 2023) H1

▶ **C9808** Nerve cryoablation probe (e.g., cryoice, cryosphere, cryosphere max, cryoice cryosphere, cryoice cryo2), including probe and all disposable system components, non-opioid medical device (must be a qualifying Medicare non-opioid medical device for post-surgical pain relief in accordance with section 4135 of the CAA, 2023) H1

▶ **C9809** Cryoablation needle (e.g., iovera system), including needle/tip and all disposable system components, non-opioid medical device (must be a qualifying Medicare non-opioid medical device for post-surgical pain relief in accordance with section 4135 of the CAA, 2023) H1

C9898 Radiolabeled product provided during a hospital inpatient stay Qh N

C9899 Implanted prosthetic device, payable only for inpatients who do not have inpatient coverage A

Medicare Statute 1833(t)

C9901 Endoscopic defect closure within the entire gastrointestinal tract, including upper endoscopy (including diagnostic, if performed) or colonoscopy (including diagnostic, if performed), with all system and tissue anchoring components J1

▶ New   ↻ Revised   ✓ Reinstated   ~~deleted~~ Deleted   ⊘ Not covered or valid by Medicare
✺ Special coverage instructions   ✱ Carrier discretion   Ⓑ Bill Part B MAC   Ⓑ Bill DME MAC

DURABLE MEDICAL EQUIPMENT (E0100-E8002)

Canes

- **E0100** Cane, includes canes of all materials, adjustable or fixed, with tip Y

  IOM: 100-02, 15, 110.1; 100-03, 4, 280.1; 100-03, 4, 280.2

- **E0105** Cane, quad or three prong, includes canes of all materials, adjustable or fixed, with tips Y

  IOM: 100-02, 15, 110.1; 100-03, 4, 280.1; 100-03, 4, 280.2

  Coding Clinic: 2016, Q3, P3

Crutches

- **E0110** Crutches, forearm, includes crutches of various materials, adjustable or fixed, pair, complete with tips and handgrips Y

  Crutches are covered when prescribed for a patient who is normally ambulatory but suffers from a condition that impairs ambulation. Provides minimal to moderate weight support while ambulating.

  IOM: 100-02, 15, 110.1; 100-03, 4, 280.1

- **E0111** Crutch forearm, includes crutches of various materials, adjustable or fixed, each, with tips and handgrips Y

  IOM: 100-02, 15, 110.1; 100-03, 4, 280.1

- **E0112** Crutches, underarm, wood, adjustable or fixed, pair, with pads, tips, and handgrips Y

  IOM: 100-02, 15, 110.1; 100-03, 4, 280.1

- **E0113** Crutch underarm, wood, adjustable or fixed, each, with pad, tip, and handgrip Y

  IOM: 100-02, 15, 110.1; 100-03, 4, 280.1

- **E0114** Crutches, underarm, other than wood, adjustable or fixed, pair, with pads, tips and handgrips Y

  IOM: 100-02, 15, 110.1; 100-03, 4, 280.1

- **E0116** Crutch, underarm, other than wood, adjustable or fixed, with pad, tip, handgrip, with or without shock absorber, each Y

  IOM: 100-02, 15, 110.1; 100-03, 4, 280.1

- **E0117** Crutch, underarm, articulating, spring assisted, each Y

  IOM: 100-02, 15, 110.1

- **E0118** Crutch substitute, lower leg platform, with or without wheels, each E1

Walkers

- **E0130** Walker, rigid (pickup), adjustable or fixed height Y

  Standard walker criteria for payment: Individual has a mobility limitation that significantly impairs ability to participate in mobility-related activities of daily living that cannot be adequately or safely addressed by a cane. The patient is able to use the walker safely; the functional mobility deficit can be resolved with use of a standard walker.

  IOM: 100-02, 15, 110.1; 100-03, 4, 280.1

- **E0135** Walker, folding (pickup), adjustable or fixed height Y

  IOM: 100-02, 15, 110.1; 100-03, 4, 280.1

- **E0140** Walker, with trunk support, adjustable or fixed height, any type Y

  IOM: 100-02, 15, 110.1; 100-03, 4, 280.1

- **E0141** Walker, rigid, wheeled, adjustable or fixed height Y

  IOM: 100-02, 15, 110.1; 100-03, 4, 280.1

- **E0143** Walker, folding, wheeled, adjustable or fixed height Y

  IOM: 100-02, 15, 110.1; 100-03, 4, 280.1

- **E0144** Walker, enclosed, four sided framed, rigid or folding, wheeled, with posterior seat Y

  IOM: 100-02, 15, 110.1; 100-03, 4, 280.1

- **E0147** Walker, heavy duty, multiple braking system, variable wheel resistance Y

  Heavy-duty walker is labeled as capable of supporting more than 300 pounds

  IOM: 100-02, 15, 110.1; 100-03, 4, 280.1

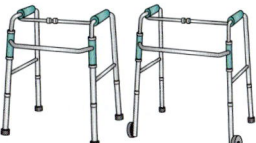

Figure 11 Walkers.

* **E0148** Walker, heavy duty, without wheels, rigid or folding, any type, each Ⓑ Qp Qh ♿ Y

    Heavy-duty walker is labeled as capable of supporting more than 300 pounds

* **E0149** Walker, heavy duty, wheeled, rigid or folding, any type Ⓑ Qp Qh ♿ Y

    Heavy-duty walker is labeled as capable of supporting more than 300 pounds

▶ * **E0150** Combination wheeled walker with seat and transport chair, folding, adjustable or fixed height Ⓑ Qp Qh ♿ E1

* **E0152** Walker, battery powered, wheeled, folding, adjustable or fixed height Ⓑ Qp Qh ♿ E1

* **E0153** Platform attachment, forearm crutch, each Ⓑ Qp Qh ♿ Y

* **E0154** Platform attachment, walker, each Ⓑ Qp Qh ♿ Y

* **E0155** Wheel attachment, rigid pick-up walker, per pair Ⓑ Qp Qh ♿ Y

Attachments

* **E0156** Seat attachment, walker Ⓑ Qp Qh ♿ Y

* **E0157** Crutch attachment, walker, each Ⓑ Qp Qh ♿ Y

* **E0158** Leg extensions for walker, per set of four (4) Ⓑ Qp Qh ♿ Y

    Leg extensions are considered medically necessary DME for patients 6 feet tall or more.

* **E0159** Brake attachment for wheeled walker, replacement, each Ⓑ Qp Qh ♿ Y

Sitz Bath/Equipment

✹ **E0160** Sitz type bath or equipment, portable, used with or without commode Ⓑ Qp Qh ♿ Y

    IOM: 100-03, 4, 280.1

✹ **E0161** Sitz type bath or equipment, portable, used with or without commode, with faucet attachment/s Ⓑ Qp Qh ♿ Y

    IOM: 100-03, 4, 280.1

✹ **E0162** Sitz bath chair Ⓑ Qp Qh ♿ Y

    IOM: 100-03, 4, 280.1

Commodes

✹ **E0163** Commode chair, mobile or stationary, with fixed arms Ⓑ Qp Qh ♿ Y

    IOM: 100-02, 15, 110.1; 100-03, 4, 280.1

✹ **E0165** Commode chair, mobile or stationary, with detachable arms Ⓑ Qp Qh ♿ Y

    IOM: 100-02, 15, 110.1; 100-03, 4, 280.1

✹ **E0167** Pail or pan for use with commode chair, replacement only Ⓑ Qp Qh ♿ Y

    IOM: 100-03, 4, 280.1

* **E0168** Commode chair, extra wide and/or heavy duty, stationary or mobile, with or without arms, any type, each Ⓑ Qp Qh ♿ Y

    Extra-wide or heavy duty commode chair is labeled as capable of supporting more than 300 pounds

* **E0170** Commode chair with integrated seat lift mechanism, electric, any type Ⓑ Qp Qh ♿ Y

* **E0171** Commode chair with integrated seat lift mechanism, non-electric, any type Ⓑ Qp Qh ♿ Y

⊘ **E0172** Seat lift mechanism placed over or on top of toilet, any type Ⓑ Qp Qh E1

    Medicare Statute 1861 SSA

* **E0175** Foot rest, for use with commode chair, each Ⓑ Qp Qh ♿ Y

Decubitus Care Equipment

✹ **E0181** Powered pressure reducing mattress overlay/pad, alternating, with pump, includes heavy duty Ⓑ Qp Qh ♿ Y

    Requires the provider to determine medical necessity compliance. To demonstrate the requirements in the medical policy were met, attach KX.

    IOM: 100-03, 4, 280.1; 100-08, 5, 5.2.3

✹ **E0182** Pump for alternating pressure pad, for replacement only Ⓑ Qp Qh ♿ Y

    IOM: 100-03, 4, 280.1; 100-08, 5, 5.2.3

* **E0183** Powered pressure reducing underlay/pad, alternating, with pump, includes heavy duty Ⓑ Qp Qh ♿ Y

✹ **E0184** Dry pressure mattress Ⓑ Qp Qh ♿ Y

    IOM: 100-03, 4, 280.1; 100-08, 5, 5.2.3

✹ **E0185** Gel or gel-like pressure pad for mattress, standard mattress length and width Ⓑ Qp Qh ♿ Y

    IOM: 100-03, 4, 280.1; 100-08, 5, 5.2.3

✹ **E0186** Air pressure mattress Ⓑ Qp Qh ♿ Y

    IOM: 100-03, 4, 280.1

✹ **E0187** Water pressure mattress Ⓑ Qp Qh ♿ Y

    IOM: 100-03, 4, 280.1

▶ New ⤾ Revised ✓ Reinstated ~~deleted~~ Deleted ⊘ Not covered or valid by Medicare
✹ Special coverage instructions * Carrier discretion Ⓑ Bill Part B MAC Ⓑ Bill DME MAC

DURABLE MEDICAL EQUIPMENT

⊛ **E0188** Synthetic sheepskin pad Ⓑ Qp Qh ♿ Y
IOM: 100-03, 4, 280.1; 100-08, 5, 5.2.3

⊛ **E0189** Lambswool sheepskin pad, any size Ⓑ Qp Qh ♿ Y
IOM: 100-03, 4, 280.1; 100-08, 5, 5.2.3

⊛ **E0190** Positioning cushion/pillow/wedge, any shape or size, includes all components and accessories Ⓑ Qp Qh E1
IOM: 100-02, 15, 110.1

✱ **E0191** Heel or elbow protector, each Ⓑ Qp Qh ♿ Y

✱ **E0193** Powered air flotation bed (low air loss therapy) Ⓑ Qp Qh ♿ Y

⊛ **E0194** Air fluidized bed Ⓑ Qp Qh ♿ Y
IOM: 100-03, 4, 280.1

⊛ **E0196** Gel pressure mattress Ⓑ Qp Qh ♿ Y
IOM: 100-03, 4, 280.1

⊛ **E0197** Air pressure pad for mattress, standard mattress length and width Ⓑ Qp Qh ♿ Y
IOM: 100-03, 4, 280.1

⊛ **E0198** Water pressure pad for mattress, standard mattress length and width Ⓑ Qp Qh ♿ Y
IOM: 100-03, 4, 280.1

⊛ **E0199** Dry pressure pad for mattress, standard mattress length and width Ⓑ Qp Qh ♿ Y
IOM: 100-03, 4, 280.1

Heat/Cold Application

⊛ **E0200** Heat lamp, without stand (table model), includes bulb, or infrared element Ⓑ Qp Qh ♿ Y

Covered when medical review determines patient's medical condition is one for which application of heat by heat lamp is therapeutically effective

IOM: 100-02, 15, 110.1; 100-03, 4, 280.1

▶ **E0201** Penile contracture device, manual, greater than 3 lbs traction force Y

✱ **E0202** Phototherapy (bilirubin) light with photometer Ⓑ Qp Qh ♿ Y

⊘ **E0203** Therapeutic lightbox, minimum 10,000 lux, table top model Ⓑ Qp Qh E1
IOM: 100-03, 4, 280.1

⊛ **E0205** Heat lamp, with stand, includes bulb, or infrared element Ⓑ Qp Qh ♿ Y
IOM: 100-02, 15, 110.1; 100-03, 4, 280.1

⊛ **E0210** Electric heat pad, standard Ⓑ Qp Qh ♿ Y

Flexible device containing electric resistive elements producing heat; has fabric cover to prevent burns; with or without timing devices for automatic shut-off

IOM: 100-03, 4, 280.1

⊛ **E0215** Electric heat pad, moist Ⓑ Qp Qh ♿ Y

Flexible device containing electric resistive elements producing heat. Must have component that will absorb and retain liquid (water).

IOM: 100-03, 4, 280.1

⊛ **E0217** Water circulating heat pad with pump Ⓑ Qp Qh ♿ Y

Consists of flexible pad containing series of channels through which water is circulated by means of electrical pumping mechanism and heated in external reservoir

IOM: 100-03, 4, 280.1

⊛ **E0218** Fluid circulating cold pad with pump, any type Ⓑ Qp Qh Y
IOM: 100-03, 4, 280.1

✱ **E0221** Infrared heating pad system Ⓑ Qp Qh Y

⊛ **E0225** Hydrocollator unit, includes pads Ⓑ Qp Qh ♿ Y
IOM: 100-02, 15, 230; 100-03, 4, 280.1

⊘ **E0231** Non-contact wound warming device (temperature control unit, AC adapter and power cord) for use with warming card and wound cover Ⓑ Qp Qh E1
IOM: 100-02, 16, 20

⊘ **E0232** Warming card for use with the non-contact wound warming device and non-contact wound warming wound cover Ⓑ Qp Qh E1
IOM: 100-02, 16, 20

⊛ **E0235** Paraffin bath unit, portable, (see medical supply code A4265 for paraffin) Ⓑ Qp Qh Y

Ordered by physician and patient's condition expected to be relieved by long-term use of modality

IOM: 100-02, 15, 230; 100-03, 4, 280.1

⊛ **E0236** Pump for water circulating pad Ⓑ Qp Qh ♿ Y
IOM: 100-03, 4, 280.1

⊛ **E0239** Hydrocollator unit, portable Ⓑ Qp Qh ♿ Y
IOM: 100-02, 15, 230; 100-03, 4, 280.1

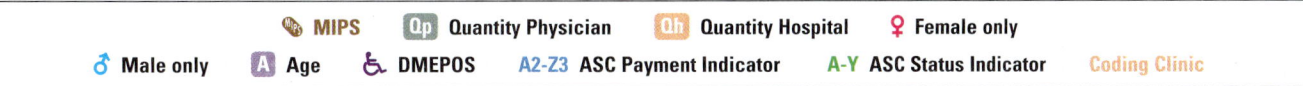

 MIPS   Qp Quantity Physician   Qh Quantity Hospital   ♀ Female only
♂ Male only   Ⓐ Age   ♿ DMEPOS   A2-Z3 ASC Payment Indicator   A-Y ASC Status Indicator   Coding Clinic

Bath and Toilet Aids

⊘ **E0240** Bath/shower chair, with or without wheels, any size ⒷQp Qh E1
IOM: 100-03, 4, 280.1

⊘ **E0241** Bath tub wall rail, each ⒷQp Qh E1
IOM: 100-02, 15, 110.1; 100-03, 4, 280.1

⊘ **E0242** Bath tub rail, floor base ⒷQp Qh E1
IOM: 100-02, 15, 110.1; 100-03, 4, 280.1

⊘ **E0243** Toilet rail, each ⒷQp Qh E1
IOM: 100-02, 15, 110.1; 100-03, 4, 280.1

⊘ **E0244** Raised toilet seat ⒷQp Qh E1
IOM: 100-03, 4, 280.1

⊘ **E0245** Tub stool or bench ⒷQp Qh E1
IOM: 100-03, 4, 280.1

✱ **E0246** Transfer tub rail attachment ⒷQp Qh E1

✽ **E0247** Transfer bench for tub or toilet with or without commode opening ⒷQp Qh E1
IOM: 100-03, 4, 280.1

✽ **E0248** Transfer bench, heavy duty, for tub or toilet with or without commode opening ⒷQp Qh E1

Heavy duty transfer bench is labeled as capable of supporting more than 300 pounds

IOM: 100-03, 4, 280.1

Pad for Heating Unit

✽ **E0249** Pad for water circulating heat unit, for replacement only ⒷQp Qh ♿ Y

Describes durable replacement pad used with water circulating heat pump system

IOM: 100-03, 4, 280.1

Hospital Beds and Accessories

✽ **E0250** Hospital bed, fixed height, with any type side rails, with mattress ⒷQp Qh ♿ Y
IOM: 100-02, 15, 110.1; 100-03, 4, 280.7

✽ **E0251** Hospital bed, fixed height, with any type side rails, without mattress ⒷQp Qh ♿ Y
IOM: 100-02, 15, 110.1; 100-03, 4, 280.7

✽ **E0255** Hospital bed, variable height, hi-lo, with any type side rails, with mattress ⒷQp Qh ♿ Y
IOM: 100-02, 15, 110.1; 100-03, 4, 280.7

✽ **E0256** Hospital bed, variable height, hi-lo, with any type side rails, without mattress ⒷQp Qh ♿ Y
IOM: 100-02, 15, 110.1; 100-03, 4, 280.7

✽ **E0260** Hospital bed, semi-electric (head and foot adjustment), with any type side rails, with mattress ⒷQp Qh ♿ Y
IOM: 100-02, 15, 110.1; 100-03, 4, 280.7

✽ **E0261** Hospital bed, semi-electric (head and foot adjustment), with any type side rails, without mattress ⒷQp Qh ♿ Y
IOM: 100-02, 15, 110.1; 100-03, 4, 280.7

✽ **E0265** Hospital bed, total electric (head, foot and height adjustments), with any type side rails, with mattress ⒷQp Qh ♿ Y
IOM: 100-02, 15, 110.1; 100-03, 4, 280.7

✽ **E0266** Hospital bed, total electric (head, foot and height adjustments), with any type side rails, without mattress ⒷQp Qh ♿ Y
IOM: 100-02, 15, 110.1; 100-03, 4, 280.7

⊘ **E0270** Hospital bed, institutional type includes: oscillating, circulating and Stryker frame, with mattress ⒷQp Qh E1
IOM: 100-03, 4, 280.1

✽ **E0271** Mattress, innerspring ⒷQp Qh ♿ Y
IOM: 100-03, 4, 280.1; 100-03, 4, 280.7

✽ **E0272** Mattress, foam rubber ⒷQp Qh ♿ Y
IOM: 100-03, 4, 280.1; 100-03, 4, 280.7

⊘ **E0273** Bed board ⒷQp Qh E1
IOM: 100-03, 4, 280.1

⊘ **E0274** Over-bed table ⒷQp Qh E1
IOM: 100-03, 4, 280.1

✽ **E0275** Bed pan, standard, metal or plastic ⒷQp Qh ♿ Y
IOM: 100-03, 4, 280.1

✽ **E0276** Bed pan, fracture, metal or plastic ⒷQp Qh ♿ Y
IOM: 100-03, 4, 280.1

✽ **E0277** Powered pressure-reducing air mattress ⒷQp Qh ♿ Y
IOM: 100-03, 4, 280.1

✱ **E0280** Bed cradle, any type ⒷQp Qh ♿ Y

✽ **E0290** Hospital bed, fixed height, without side rails, with mattress ⒷQp Qh ♿ Y
IOM: 100-02, 15, 110.1; 100-03, 4, 280.7

✽ **E0291** Hospital bed, fixed height, without side rails, without mattress ⒷQp Qh ♿ Y
IOM: 100-02, 15, 110.1; 100-03, 4, 280.7

▶ New   ↻ Revised   ✓ Reinstated   ~~deleted~~ Deleted   ⊘ Not covered or valid by Medicare
✽ Special coverage instructions   ✱ Carrier discretion   Ⓑ Bill Part B MAC   Ⓑ Bill DME MAC

DURABLE MEDICAL EQUIPMENT

○ **E0292** Hospital bed, variable height, hi-lo, without side rails, with mattress ⓑ Qp Qh ♿ Y

IOM: 100-02, 15, 110.1; 100-03, 4, 280.7

○ **E0293** Hospital bed, variable height, hi-lo, without side rails, without mattress ⓑ Qp Qh ♿ Y

IOM: 100-02, 15, 110.1; 100-03, 4, 280.7

○ **E0294** Hospital bed, semi-electric (head and foot adjustment), without side rails, with mattress ⓑ Qp Qh ♿ Y

IOM: 100-02, 15, 110.1; 100-03, 4, 280.7

○ **E0295** Hospital bed, semi-electric (head and foot adjustment), without side rails, without mattress ⓑ Qp Qh ♿ Y

IOM: 100-02, 15, 110.1; 100-03, 4, 280.7

○ **E0296** Hospital bed, total electric (head, foot and height adjustments), without side rails, with mattress ⓑ Qp Qh ♿ Y

IOM: 100-02, 15, 110.1; 100-03, 4, 280.7

○ **E0297** Hospital bed, total electric (head, foot and height adjustments), without side rails, without mattress ⓑ Qp Qh ♿ Y

IOM: 100-02, 15, 110.1; 100-03, 4, 280.7

✱ **E0300** Pediatric crib, hospital grade, fully enclosed, with or without top enclosure ⓑ Qp Qh A ♿ Y

○ **E0301** Hospital bed, heavy duty, extra wide, with weight capacity greater than 350 pounds, but less than or equal to 600 pounds, with any type side rails, without mattress ⓑ Qp Qh ♿ Y

IOM: 100-03, 4, 280.7

○ **E0302** Hospital bed, extra heavy duty, extra wide, with weight capacity greater than 600 pounds, with any type side rails, without mattress ⓑ Qp Qh ♿ Y

IOM: 100-03, 4, 280.7

○ **E0303** Hospital bed, heavy duty, extra wide, with weight capacity greater than 350 pounds, but less than or equal to 600 pounds, with any type side rails, with mattress ⓑ Qp Qh ♿ Y

IOM: 100-03, 4, 280.7

○ **E0304** Hospital bed, extra heavy duty, extra wide, with weight capacity greater than 600 pounds, with any type side rails, with mattress ⓑ Qp Qh ♿ Y

IOM: 100-03, 4, 280.7

○ **E0305** Bed side rails, half length ⓑ Qp Qh ♿ Y

IOM: 100-03, 4, 280.7

○ **E0310** Bed side rails, full length ⓑ Qp Qh ♿ Y

IOM: 100-03, 4, 280.7

⊘ **E0315** Bed accessory: board, table, or support device, any type ⓑ Qp Qh E1

IOM: 100-03, 4, 280.1

✱ **E0316** Safety enclosure frame/canopy for use with hospital bed, any type ⓑ Qp Qh ♿ Y

○ **E0325** Urinal; male, jug-type, any material ⓑ Qp Qh ♂ ♿ Y

IOM: 100-03, 4, 280.1

○ **E0326** Urinal; female, jug-type, any material ⓑ Qp Qh ♀ ♿ Y

IOM: 100-03, 4, 280.1

✱ **E0328** Hospital bed, pediatric, manual, 360 degree side enclosures, top of headboard, footboard and side rails up to 24 inches above the spring, includes mattress ⓑ Qp Qh A Y

✱ **E0329** Hospital bed, pediatric, electric or semi-electric, 360 degree side enclosures, top of headboard, footboard and side rails up to 24 inches above the spring, includes mattress ⓑ Qp Qh A Y

✱ **E0350** Control unit for electronic bowel irrigation/evacuation system ⓑ Qp Qh E1

Pulsed Irrigation Enhanced Evacuation (PIEE) is pulsed irrigation of severely impacted fecal material and may be necessary for patients who have not responded to traditional bowel program.

✱ **E0352** Disposable pack (water reservoir bag, speculum, valving mechanism and collection bag/box) for use with the electronic bowel irrigation/evacuation system ⓑ Qp Qh E1

Therapy kit includes 1 B-Valve circuit, 2 containment bags, 1 lubricating jelly, 1 bed pad, 1 tray liner-waste disposable bag, and 2 hose clamps

✱ **E0370** Air pressure elevator for heel ⓑ Qp Qh E1

✱ **E0371** Non powered advanced pressure reducing overlay for mattress, standard mattress length and width ⓑ Qp Qh ♿ Y

Patient has at least one large Stage III or Stage IV pressure sore (greater than 2 × 2 cm.) on trunk, with only two turning surfaces on which to lie

* **E0372** Powered air overlay for mattress, standard mattress length and width ⓑ Qp Qh ♿ Y
* **E0373** Non powered advanced pressure reducing mattress ⓑ Qp Qh ♿ Y

Oxygen and Related Respiratory Equipment

○ **E0424** Stationary compressed gaseous oxygen system, rental; includes container, contents, regulator, flowmeter, humidifier, nebulizer, cannula or mask, and tubing ⓑ Qp Qh ♿ Y

IOM: 100-03, 4, 280.1; 100-04, 20, 30.6

○ **E0425** Stationary compressed gas system, purchase; includes regulator, flowmeter, humidifier, nebulizer, cannula or mask, and tubing ⓑ Qp Qh E1

IOM: 100-03, 4, 280.1; 100-04, 20, 30.6

○ **E0430** Portable gaseous oxygen system, purchase; includes regulator, flowmeter, humidifier, cannula or mask, and tubing ⓑ Qp Qh E1

IOM: 100-03, 4, 280.1; 100-04, 20, 30.6

○ **E0431** Portable gaseous oxygen system, rental; includes portable container, regulator, flowmeter, humidifier, cannula or mask, and tubing ⓑ Qp Qh ♿ Y

IOM: 100-03, 4, 280.1; 100-04, 20, 30.6

* **E0433** Portable liquid oxygen system, rental; home liquefier used to fill portable liquid oxygen containers, includes portable containers, regulator, flowmeter, humidifier, cannula or mask and tubing, with or without supply reservoir and contents gauge ⓑ Qh ♿ Y

○ **E0434** Portable liquid oxygen system, rental; includes portable container, supply reservoir, humidifier, flowmeter, refill adaptor, contents gauge, cannula or mask, and tubing ⓑ Qp Qh ♿ Y

Fee schedule payments for stationary oxygen system rentals are all-inclusive and represent monthly allowance for beneficiary. Non-Medicare payers may rent device to beneficiaries, or arrange for purchase of device.

IOM: 100-03, 4, 280.1; 100-04, 20, 30.6

○ **E0435** Portable liquid oxygen system, purchase; includes portable container, supply reservoir, flowmeter, humidifier, contents gauge, cannula or mask, tubing and refill adaptor ⓑ Qp Qh E1

IOM: 100-03, 4, 280.1; 100-04, 20, 30.6

○ **E0439** Stationary liquid oxygen system, rental; includes container, contents, regulator, flowmeter, humidifier, nebulizer, cannula or mask, and tubing ⓑ Qp Qh ♿ Y

This allowance includes payment for equipment, contents, and accessories furnished during rental month

IOM: 100-03, 4, 280.1; 100-04, 20, 30.6

○ **E0440** Stationary liquid oxygen system, purchase; includes use of reservoir, contents indicator, regulator, flowmeter, humidifier, nebulizer, cannula or mask, and tubing ⓑ Qp Qh E1

IOM: 100-03, 4, 280.1; 100-04, 20, 30.6

○ **E0441** Stationary oxygen contents, gaseous, 1 month's supply = 1 unit ⓑ Qp Qh ♿ Y

IOM: 100-03, 4, 280.1; 100-04, 20, 30.6

○ **E0442** Stationary oxygen contents, liquid, 1 month's supply = 1 unit ⓑ Qp Qh ♿ Y

IOM: 100-03, 4, 280.1; 100-04, 20, 30.6

○ **E0443** Portable oxygen contents, gaseous, 1 month's supply = 1 unit ⓑ Qp Qh ♿ Y

IOM: 100-03, 4, 280.1; 100-04, 20, 30.6

○ **E0444** Portable oxygen contents, liquid, 1 month's supply = 1 unit ⓑ Qp Qh ♿ Y

IOM: 100-03, 4, 280.1; 100-04, 20, 30.6

* **E0445** Oximeter device for measuring blood oxygen levels non-invasively ⓑ Qp Qh N

* **E0446** Topical oxygen delivery system, not otherwise specified, includes all supplies and accessories ⓑ Qp Qh A

○ **E0447** Portable oxygen contents, liquid, 1 month's supply = 1 unit, prescribed amount at rest or nighttime exceeds 4 liters per minute (lpm) ⓑ ♿ Y

○ **E0455** Oxygen tent, excluding croup or pediatric tents ⓑ Qp Qh Y

IOM: 100-03, 4, 280.1; 100-04, 20, 30.6

⊘ **E0457** Chest shell (cuirass) ⓑ Qp Qh E1
⊘ **E0459** Chest wrap ⓑ Qp Qh E1

* **E0462** Rocking bed with or without side rails ⓑ Qp Qh ♿ Y

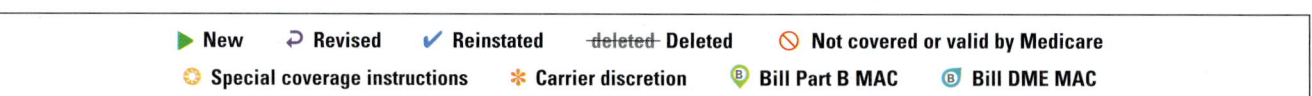

Figure 12 Oximeter device.

▶ New ⟲ Revised ✓ Reinstated ~~deleted~~ Deleted ⊘ Not covered or valid by Medicare
○ Special coverage instructions * Carrier discretion ⓑ Bill Part B MAC ⓑ Bill DME MAC

DURABLE MEDICAL EQUIPMENT

E0465 Home ventilator, any type, used with invasive interface (e.g., tracheostomy tube) ⑧ Qp Qh ⚕ Y
IOM: 100-03, 4, 280.1

E0466 Home ventilator, any type, used with non-invasive interface (e.g., mask, chest shell) ⑧ Qp Qh ⚕ Y
IOM: 100-03, 4, 280.1

E0467 Home ventilator, multi-function respiratory device, also performs any or all of the additional functions of oxygen concentration, drug nebulization, aspiration, and cough stimulation, includes all accessories, components and supplies for all functions ⑧ ⚕ Y

E0468 Home ventilator, dual-function respiratory device, also performs additional function of cough stimulation, includes all accessories, components and supplies for all functions ⑧ Qp Qh ⚕ Y

E0469 Lung expansion airway clearance, continuous high frequency oscillation, and nebulization device ⑧ Qp Qh ⚕ Y

E0470 Respiratory assist device, bi-level pressure capability, without backup rate feature, used with noninvasive interface, e.g., nasal or facial mask (intermittent assist device with continuous positive airway pressure device) ⑧ Qp Qh ⚕ Y
IOM: 100-03, 4, 240.2

E0471 Respiratory assist device, bi-level pressure capability, with back-up rate feature, used with noninvasive interface, e.g., nasal or facial mask (intermittent assist device with continuous positive airway pressure device) ⑧ Qp Qh ⚕ Y
IOM: 100-03, 4, 240.2

E0472 Respiratory assist device, bi-level pressure capability, with backup rate feature, used with invasive interface, e.g., tracheostomy tube (intermittent assist device with continuous positive airway pressure device) ⑧ Qp Qh ⚕ Y
IOM: 100-03, 4, 240.2

E0480 Percussor, electric or pneumatic, home model ⑧ Qp Qh ⚕ Y
IOM: 100-03, 4, 240.2

E0481 Intrapulmonary percussive ventilation system and related accessories ⑧ Qp Qh E1
IOM: 100-03, 4, 240.2

E0482 Cough stimulating device, alternating positive and negative airway pressure ⑧ Qp Qh ⚕ Y

E0483 High frequency chest wall oscillation system, with full anterior and/or posterior thoracic region receiving simultaneous external oscillation, includes all accessories and supplies, each ⑧ Qp Qh ⚕ Y

E0484 Oscillatory positive expiratory pressure device, non-electric, any type, each ⑧ Qp Qh ⚕ Y

E0485 Oral device/appliance used to reduce upper airway collapsibility, adjustable or non-adjustable, prefabricated, includes fitting and adjustment ⑧ Qp Qh ⚕ Y

E0486 Oral device/appliance used to reduce upper airway collapsibility, adjustable or non-adjustable, custom fabricated, includes fitting and adjustment ⑧ Qp Qh ⚕ Y

E0487 Spirometer, electronic, includes all accessories ⑧ Qp Qh N

E0490 Power source and control electronics unit for oral device/appliance for neuromuscular electrical stimulation of the tongue muscle, controlled by hardware remote ⑧ Qp Qh E1

E0491 Oral device/appliance for neuromuscular electrical stimulation of the tongue muscle, used in conjunction with the power source and control electronics unit, controlled by hardware remote, 90-day supply ⑧ Qp Qh E1

E0492 Power source and control electronics unit for oral device/appliance for neuromuscular electrical stimulation of the tongue muscle, controlled by phone application ⑧ Qp Qh E1

E0493 Oral device/appliance for neuromuscular electrical stimulation of the tongue muscle, used in conjunction with the power source and control electronics unit, controlled by phone application, 90-day supply ⑧ Qp Qh E1

IPPB Machines

E0500 IPPB machine, all types, with built-in nebulization; manual or automatic valves; internal or external power source ⑧ Qp Qh ⚕ Y
IOM: 100-03, 4, 240.2

E0530 Electronic positional obstructive sleep apnea treatment, with sensor, includes all components and accessories, any type ⑧ Qp Qh ⚕ Y

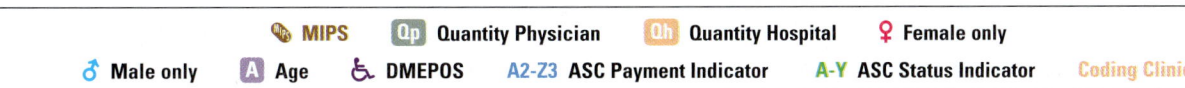

Humidifiers/Nebulizers/Compressors for Use with Oxygen IPPB Equipment

○ **E0550** Humidifier, durable for extensive supplemental humidification during IPPB treatments or oxygen delivery ⓑ Qp Qh ♿ Y
IOM: 100-03, 4, 240.2

○ **E0555** Humidifier, durable, glass or autoclavable plastic bottle type, for use with regulator or flowmeter ⓑ Qp Qh Y
IOM: 100-03, 4, 280.1; 100-04, 20, 30.6

○ **E0560** Humidifier, durable for supplemental humidification during IPPB treatment or oxygen delivery ⓑ Qp Qh ♿ Y
IOM: 100-03, 4, 280.1

* **E0561** Humidifier, non-heated, used with positive airway pressure device ⓑ Qp Qh ♿ Y

* **E0562** Humidifier, heated, used with positive airway pressure device ⓑ Qp Qh ♿ Y

* **E0565** Compressor, air power source for equipment which is not self-contained or cylinder driven ⓑ Qp Qh ♿ Y

E0570 Nebulizer, with compressor ⓑ Qp Qh ♿ Y
IOM: 100-03, 4, 240.2; 100-03, 4, 280.1

* **E0572** Aerosol compressor, adjustable pressure, light duty for intermittent use ⓑ Qp Qh ♿ Y

* **E0574** Ultrasonic/electronic aerosol generator with small volume nebulizer ⓑ Qp Qh ♿ Y

○ **E0575** Nebulizer, ultrasonic, large volume ⓑ Qp Qh ♿ Y
IOM: 100-03, 4, 240.2

○ **E0580** Nebulizer, durable, glass or autoclavable plastic, bottle type, for use with regulator or flowmeter ⓑ Qp Qh ♿ Y
IOM: 100-03, 4, 240.2; 100-03, 4, 280.1

○ **E0585** Nebulizer, with compressor and heater ⓑ Qp Qh ♿ Y
IOM: 100-03, 4, 240.2; 100-03, 4, 280.1

Suction Pump/CPAP

○ **E0600** Respiratory suction pump, home model, portable or stationary, electric ⓑ Qp Qh ♿ Y
IOM: 100-03, 4, 240.2

○ **E0601** Continuous positive airway pressure (CPAP) device ⓑ Qp Qh ♿ Y
IOM: 100-03, 4, 240.4

Breast Pump

* **E0602** Breast pump, manual, any type ⓑ Qp Qh ♀ ♿ Y
Bill either manual breast pump or breast pump kit

* **E0603** Breast pump, electric (AC and/or DC), any type ⓑ Qp Qh ♀ N

* **E0604** Breast pump, hospital grade, electric (AC and/or DC), any type ⓑ Qp Qh ♀ A

Other Breathing Aids

○ **E0605** Vaporizer, room type ⓑ Qp Qh ♿ Y
IOM: 100-03, 4, 240.2

○ **E0606** Postural drainage board ⓑ Qp Qh ♿ Y
IOM: 100-03, 4, 240.2

Monitoring Equipment

○ **E0607** Home blood glucose monitor ⓑ Qp Qh ♿ Y

Document recipient or caregiver is competent to monitor equipment and that device is designed for home rather than clinical use

IOM: 100-03, 4, 280.1; 100-03, 1, 40.2

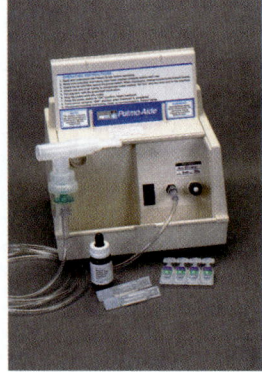

Figure 13 Nebulizer

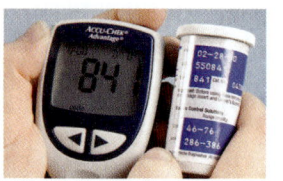

Figure 14 Glucose monitor.

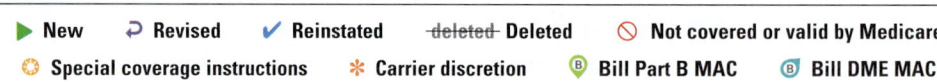

▶ New ⤺ Revised ✓ Reinstated ~~deleted~~ Deleted ⊘ Not covered or valid by Medicare
○ Special coverage instructions * Carrier discretion ⓑ Bill Part B MAC ⓑ Bill DME MAC

DURABLE MEDICAL EQUIPMENT

✺ **E0610** Pacemaker monitor, self-contained, (checks battery depletion, includes audible and visible check systems) ⓑ Qp Qh ♿ Y
IOM: 100-03, 1, 20.8

E0615 Pacemaker monitor, self-contained, checks battery depletion and other pacemaker components, includes digital/visible check systems ⓑ Qp Qh ♿ Y
IOM: 100-03, 1, 20.8

✱ **E0616** Implantable cardiac event recorder with memory, activator and programmer ⓑ Qp Qh N
Assign when two 30-day pre-symptom external loop recordings fail to establish a definitive diagnosis

✱ **E0617** External defibrillator with integrated electrocardiogram analysis ⓑ Qp Qh ♿ Y

✱ **E0618** Apnea monitor, without recording feature ⓑ Qp Qh ♿ Y

✱ **E0619** Apnea monitor, with recording feature ⓑ Qp Qh ♿ Y

✱ **E0620** Skin piercing device for collection of capillary blood, laser, each ⓑ Qp Qh ♿ Y

Patient Lifts

✺ **E0621** Sling or seat, patient lift, canvas or nylon ⓑ Qp Qh ♿ Y
IOM: 100-03, 4, 240.2, 280.4

⊘ **E0625** Patient lift, bathroom or toilet, not otherwise classified ⓑ Qp Qh E1
IOM: 100-03, 4, 240.2

✺ **E0627** Seat lift mechanism, electric, any type ⓑ Qp Qh ♿ Y
IOM: 100-03, 4, 280.4; 100-04, 4, 20

✺ **E0629** Seat lift mechanism, non-electric, any type ⓑ Qp Qh ♿ Y
IOM: 100-04, 4, 20

✺ **E0630** Patient lift, hydraulic or mechanical, includes any seat, sling, strap(s) or pad(s) ⓑ Qp Qh ♿ Y
IOM: 100-03, 4, 240.2

✺ **E0635** Patient lift, electric, with seat or sling ⓑ Qp Qh ♿ Y
IOM: 100-03, 4, 240.2

✱ **E0636** Multipositional patient support system, with integrated lift, patient accessible controls ⓑ Qp Qh ♿ Y

⊘ **E0637** Combination sit to stand frame/table system, any size including pediatric, with seat lift feature, with or without wheels ⓑ Qp Qh E1
IOM: 100-03, 4, 240.2

⊘ **E0638** Standing frame/table system, one position (e.g., upright, supine or prone stander), any size including pediatric, with or without wheels ⓑ Qp Qh E1
IOM: 100-03, 4, 240.2

✱ **E0639** Patient lift, moveable from room to room with disassembly and reassembly, includes all components/accessories ⓑ Qp Qh ♿ E1

✱ **E0640** Patient lift, fixed system, includes all components/accessories ⓑ Qp Qh ♿ E1

⊘ **E0641** Standing frame/table system, multi-position (e.g., three-way stander), any size including pediatric, with or without wheels ⓑ Qp Qh E1
IOM: 100-03, 4, 240.2

⊘ **E0642** Standing frame/table system, mobile (dynamic stander), any size including pediatric ⓑ Qp Qh E1
IOM: 100-03, 4, 240.2

Pneumatic Compressor and Appliances

✺ **E0650** Pneumatic compressor, non-segmental home model ⓑ Qp Qh ♿ Y
Lymphedema pumps are classified as segmented or nonsegmented, depending on whether distinct segments of devices can be inflated sequentially.
IOM: 100-03, 4, 280.6

✺ **E0651** Pneumatic compressor, segmental home model without calibrated gradient pressure ⓑ Qp Qh ♿ Y
IOM: 100-03, 4, 280.6

✺ **E0652** Pneumatic compressor, segmental home model with calibrated gradient pressure ⓑ Qp Qh ♿ Y
IOM: 100-03, 4, 280.6

✺ **E0655** Non-segmental pneumatic appliance for use with pneumatic compressor, half arm ⓑ Qp Qh ♿ Y
IOM: 100-03, 4, 280.6

✺ **E0656** Segmental pneumatic appliance for use with pneumatic compressor, trunk ⓑ Qp Qh ♿ Y

✺ **E0657** Segmental pneumatic appliance for use with pneumatic compressor, chest ⓑ Qp Qh ♿ Y

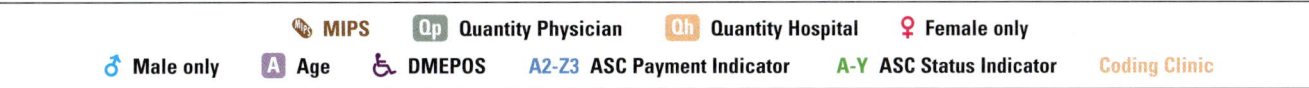

| 🎗 MIPS | Qp Quantity Physician | Qh Quantity Hospital | ♀ Female only |
| ♂ Male only | Ⓐ Age | ♿ DMEPOS | A2-Z3 ASC Payment Indicator | A-Y ASC Status Indicator | Coding Clinic |

- ▶ ⊛ **E0658** Segmental pneumatic appliance for use with pneumatic compressor, integrated, 2 full arms and chest Ⓑ Qp Qh ♿ Y
- ▶ ⊛ **E0659** Segmental pneumatic appliance for use with pneumatic compressor, integrated, head, neck and chest Ⓑ Qp Qh ♿ Y
- ⊛ **E0660** Non-segmental pneumatic appliance for use with pneumatic compressor, full leg Ⓑ Qp Qh ♿ Y
  IOM: 100-03, 4, 280.6
- ⊛ **E0665** Non-segmental pneumatic appliance for use with pneumatic compressor, full arm Ⓑ Qp Qh ♿ Y
  IOM: 100-03, 4, 280.6
- ⊛ **E0666** Non-segmental pneumatic appliance for use with pneumatic compressor, half leg Ⓑ Qp Qh ♿ Y
  IOM: 100-03, 4, 280.6
- ⊛ **E0667** Segmental pneumatic appliance for use with pneumatic compressor, full leg Ⓑ Qp Qh ♿ Y
  IOM: 100-03, 4, 280.6
- ⊛ **E0668** Segmental pneumatic appliance for use with pneumatic compressor, full arm Ⓑ Qp Qh ♿ Y
  IOM: 100-03, 4, 280.6
- ⊛ **E0669** Segmental pneumatic appliance for use with pneumatic compressor, half leg Ⓑ Qp Qh ♿ Y
  IOM: 100-03, 4, 280.6
- ⊛ **E0670** Segmental pneumatic appliance for use with pneumatic compressor, integrated, 2 full legs and trunk Ⓑ Qp Qh ♿ Y
  IOM: 100-03, 4, 280.6
- ⊛ **E0671** Segmental gradient pressure pneumatic appliance, full leg Ⓑ Qp Qh ♿ Y
  IOM: 100-03, 4, 280.6
- ⊛ **E0672** Segmental gradient pressure pneumatic appliance, full arm Ⓑ Qp Qh ♿ Y
  IOM: 100-03, 4, 280.6
- ⊛ **E0673** Segmental gradient pressure pneumatic appliance, half leg Ⓑ Qp Qh ♿ Y
  IOM: 100-03, 4, 280.6
- ✱ **E0675** Pneumatic compression device, high pressure, rapid inflation/deflation cycle, for arterial insufficiency (unilateral or bilateral system) Ⓑ Qp Qh ♿ Y
- ✱ **E0676** Intermittent limb compression device (includes all accessories), not otherwise specified Ⓑ Qp Qh Y
- **E0677** Non-pneumatic sequential compression garment, trunk Ⓑ Qp Qh Y
- **E0678** Non-pneumatic sequential compression garment, full leg Ⓑ Qp Qh Y
- **E0679** Non-pneumatic sequential compression garment, half leg Ⓑ Qp Qh Y
- **E0680** Non-pneumatic compression controller with sequential calibrated gradient pressure Ⓑ Qp Qh Y
- **E0681** Non-pneumatic compression controller without calibrated gradient pressure Ⓑ Qp Qh Y
- **E0682** Non-pneumatic sequential compression garment, full arm Ⓑ Qp Qh Y
- **E0683** Non-pneumatic, non-sequential, peristaltic wave compression pump Ⓑ Qp Qh Y

Ultraviolet Light Therapy Systems

- ✱ **E0691** Ultraviolet light therapy system, includes bulbs/lamps, timer and eye protection; treatment area 2 square feet or less Ⓑ Qp Qh ♿ Y
- ✱ **E0692** Ultraviolet light therapy system panel, includes bulbs/lamps, timer and eye protection, 4 foot panel Ⓑ Qp Qh ♿ Y
- ✱ **E0693** Ultraviolet light therapy system panel, includes bulbs/lamps, timer and eye protection, 6 foot panel Ⓑ Qp Qh ♿ Y
- ✱ **E0694** Ultraviolet multidirectional light therapy system in 6 foot cabinet, includes bulbs/lamps, timer and eye protection Ⓑ Qp Qh ♿ Y

Safety Equipment

- ✱ **E0700** Safety equipment, device or accessory, any type Ⓑ Qp Qh E1
- ⊛ **E0705** Transfer device, any type, each Ⓑ Qp Qh ♿ B

Restraints/Enclosures; Pelvic Device

- ✱ **E0710** Restraints, any type (body, chest, wrist or ankle) Ⓑ Qp Qh E1
- **E0711** Upper extremity medical tubing/lines enclosure or covering device, restricts elbow range of motion Ⓑ Qp Qh E1
- **E0715** Intravaginal device intended to strengthen pelvic floor muscles during kegel exercises Ⓑ Qp Qh E1

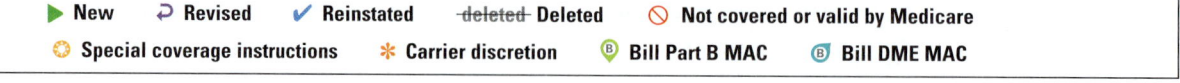

▶ New   ⟳ Revised   ✓ Reinstated   ~~deleted~~ Deleted   ⊘ Not covered or valid by Medicare
⊛ Special coverage instructions   ✱ Carrier discretion   Ⓑ Bill Part B MAC   Ⓑ Bill DME MAC

E0716	Supplies and accessories for intravaginal device intended to strengthen pelvic floor muscles during kegel exercises ⓑ Qp Qh		E1

Transcutaneous and/or Neuromuscular Electrical Nerve Stimulators (TENS)

E0720 Transcutaneous electrical nerve stimulation (TENS) device, two lead, localized stimulation ⓑ Qp Qh ♿ Y

A Certificate of Medical Necessity (CMN) is not needed for a TENS rental, but is needed for purchase.

IOM: 100-03, 2, 160.2; 100-03, 4, 280.1

E0721 Transcutaneous electrical nerve stimulator for nerves in the auricular region ⓑ Qp Qh ♿ Y

E0730 Transcutaneous electrical nerve stimulation (TENS) device, four or more leads, for multiple nerve stimulation ⓑ Qp Qh ♿ Y

IOM: 100-03, 2, 160.2; 100-03, 4, 280.1

E0731 Form-fitting conductive garment for delivery of TENS or NMES (with conductive fibers separated from the patient's skin by layers of fabric) ⓑ Qp Qh ♿ Y

IOM: 100-03, 2, 160.13

E0732 Cranial electrotherapy stimulation (ces) system, any type ⓑ Qp Qh ♿ Y

E0733 Transcutaneous electrical nerve stimulator for electrical stimulation of the trigeminal nerve ⓑ Qp Qh ♿ Y

E0734 External upper limb tremor stimulator of the peripheral nerves of the wrist ⓑ Qp Qh ♿ Y

E0735 Non-invasive vagus nerve stimulator ⓑ Qp Qh ♿ Y

E0736 Transcutaneous tibial nerve stimulator ⓑ Qp Qh ♿ A

E0737 Transcutaneous tibial nerve stimulator, controlled by phone application ⓑ Qp Qh ♿ E1

E0738 Upper extremity rehabilitation system providing active assistance to facilitate muscle re-education, include microprocessor, all components and accessories ⓑ Qp Qh ♿ A

E0739 Rehabilitation system with interactive interface providing active assistance in rehabilitation therapy, includes all components and accessories, motors, microprocessors, sensors ⓑ Qp Qh ♿ A

E0740 Non-implanted pelvic floor electrical stimulator, complete system ⓑ Qp Qh ♿ Y

IOM: 100-03, 4, 230.8

✻ E0743 External lower extremity nerve stimulator for restless legs syndrome, each ⓑ Qp Qh Y

✻ E0744 Neuromuscular stimulator for scoliosis ⓑ Qp Qh ♿ Y

E0745 Neuromuscular stimulator, electronic shock unit ⓑ Qp Qh ♿ Y

IOM: 100-03, 2, 160.12

E0746 Electromyography (EMG), biofeedback device ⓑ Qp Qh N

IOM: 100-03, 1, 30.1

E0747 Osteogenesis stimulator, electrical, non-invasive, other than spinal applications ⓑ Qp Qh ♿ Y

Devices are composed of two basic parts: Coils that wrap around cast and pulse generator that produces electric current

E0748 Osteogenesis stimulator, electrical, non-invasive, spinal applications ⓑ Qp Qh ♿ Y

Device should be applied within 30 days as adjunct to spinal fusion surgery

E0749 Osteogenesis stimulator, electrical, surgically implanted ⓑ Qp Qh ♿ N

✻ E0755 Electronic salivary reflex stimulator (intra-oral/non-invasive) ⓑ Qp Qh E1

✻ E0760 Osteogenesis stimulator, low intensity ultrasound, non-invasive ⓑ Qp Qh ♿ Y

Ultrasonic osteogenesis stimulator may not be used concurrently with other noninvasive stimulators

E0761 Non-thermal pulsed high frequency radiowaves, high peak power electromagnetic energy treatment device ⓑ Qp Qh E1

✻ E0762 Transcutaneous electrical joint stimulation device system, includes all accessories ⓑ Qp Qh ♿ B

E0764 Functional neuromuscular stimulator, transcutaneous stimulation of sequential muscle groups of ambulation with computer control, used for walking by spinal cord injured, entire system, after completion of training program ⓑ Qp Qh ♿ Y

IOM: 100-03, 2, 160.12

↺ ✻ E0765 FDA approved nerve stimulator, for treatment of nausea and vomiting ⓑ Qp Qh ♿ Y

 MIPS　Qp Quantity Physician　Qh Quantity Hospital　♀ Female only
♂ Male only　A Age　♿ DMEPOS　A2-Z3 ASC Payment Indicator　A-Y ASC Status Indicator　Coding Clinic

Code	Description	Status
* E0766	Electrical stimulation device used for cancer treatment, includes all accessories, any type	Y
* E0767	Intrabuccal, systemic delivery of amplitude-modulated, radiofrequency electromagnetic field device, for cancer treatment, includes all accessories	Y
E0769	Electrical stimulation or electromagnetic wound treatment device, not otherwise classified	B

IOM: 100-04, 32, 11.1

Code	Description	Status
E0770	Functional electrical stimulator, transcutaneous stimulation of nerve and/or muscle groups, any type, complete system, not otherwise specified	Y

Infusion Supplies

Code	Description	Status
* E0776	IV pole	Y

PEN: On Fee Schedule

Code	Description	Status
* E0779	Ambulatory infusion pump, mechanical, reusable, for infusion 8 hours or greater	Y

Requires prior authorization and copy of invoice

This is a capped rental infusion pump modifier. The correct monthly modifier (KH, KI, KJ) is used to indicate which month the rental is for (i.e., KH, month 1; KI, months 2 and 3; KJ, months 4 through 13).

Code	Description	Status
* E0780	Ambulatory infusion pump, mechanical, reusable, for infusion less than 8 hours	Y

Requires prior authorization and copy of invoice

Code	Description	Status
E0781	Ambulatory infusion pump, single or multiple channels, electric or battery operated with administrative equipment, worn by patient	Y

IOM: 100-03, 1, 50.3

Code	Description	Status
E0782	Infusion pump, implantable, non-programmable (includes all components, e.g., pump, cathether, connectors, etc.)	N

IOM: 100-03, 1, 50.3

Code	Description	Status
E0783	Infusion pump system, implantable, programmable (includes all components, e.g., pump, catheter, connectors, etc.)	N

IOM: 100-03, 1, 50.3

Code	Description	Status
E0784	External ambulatory infusion pump, insulin	Y

IOM: 100-03, 4, 280.14

Code	Description	Status
E0785	Implantable intraspinal (epidural/intrathecal) catheter used with implantable infusion pump, replacement	N

IOM: 100-03, 1, 50.3

Code	Description	Status
E0786	Implantable programmable infusion pump, replacement (excludes implantable intraspinal catheter)	N

IOM: 100-03, 1, 50.3

Code	Description	Status
* E0787	External ambulatory infusion pump, insulin, dosage rate adjustment using therapeutic continuous glucose sensing	E1
E0791	Parenteral infusion pump, stationary, single or multi-channel	Y

IOM: 100-02, 15, 120; 100-03, 3, 180.2; 100-04, 20, 100.2.2

Traction Equipment and Orthopedic Devices

Code	Description	Status
E0830	Ambulatory traction device, all types, each	N

IOM: 100-03, 4, 280.1

Code	Description	Status
E0840	Traction frame, attached to headboard, cervical traction	Y

IOM: 100-03, 4, 280.1

Code	Description	Status
* E0849	Traction equipment, cervical, free-standing stand/frame, pneumatic, applying traction force to other than mandible	Y
E0850	Traction stand, free standing, cervical traction	Y

IOM: 100-03, 4, 280.1

Code	Description	Status
* E0855	Cervical traction equipment not requiring additional stand or frame	Y
* E0856	Cervical traction device, with inflatable air bladder(s)	Y
E0860	Traction equipment, overdoor, cervical	Y

IOM: 100-03, 4, 280.1

Code	Description	Status
E0870	Traction frame, attached to footboard, extremity traction, (e.g., Buck's)	Y

IOM: 100-03, 4, 280.1

Code	Description	Status
E0880	Traction stand, free standing, extremity traction	Y

IOM: 100-03, 4, 280.1

▶ New ⤶ Revised ✓ Reinstated ~~deleted~~ Deleted 🚫 Not covered or valid by Medicare ◉ Special coverage instructions * Carrier discretion ⓑ Bill Part B MAC ⓑ Bill DME MAC

DURABLE MEDICAL EQUIPMENT

- **E0890** Traction frame, attached to footboard, pelvic traction Ⓑ Qp Qh ♿ Y
  IOM: 100-03, 4, 280.1
- **E0900** Traction stand, free standing, pelvic traction (e.g., Buck's) Ⓑ Qp Qh ♿ Y
  IOM: 100-03, 4, 280.1
- **E0910** Trapeze bars, A/K/A patient helper, attached to bed, with grab bar Ⓑ Qp Qh ♿ Y
  IOM: 100-03, 4, 280.1
- **E0911** Trapeze bar, heavy duty, for patient weight capacity greater than 250 pounds, attached to bed, with grab bar Ⓑ Qp Qh ♿ Y
  IOM: 100-03, 4, 280.1
- **E0912** Trapeze bar, heavy duty, for patient weight capacity greater than 250 pounds, free standing, complete with grab bar Ⓑ Qp Qh ♿ Y
- **E0920** Fracture frame, attached to bed, includes weights Ⓑ Qp Qh ♿ Y
  IOM: 100-03, 4, 280.1
- **E0930** Fracture frame, free standing, includes weights Ⓑ Qp Qh ♿ Y
  IOM: 100-03, 4, 280.1
- **E0935** Continuous passive motion exercise device for use on knee only Ⓑ Qp Qh ♿ Y
  To qualify for coverage, use of device must commence within two days following surgery
  IOM: 100-03, 4, 280.1
- ⊘ **E0936** Continuous passive motion exercise device for use other than knee Ⓑ Qp Qh E1
- **E0940** Trapeze bar, free standing, complete with grab bar Ⓑ Qp Qh ♿ Y
  IOM: 100-03, 4, 280.1
- **E0941** Gravity assisted traction device, any type Ⓑ Qp Qh ♿ Y
  IOM: 100-03, 4, 280.1
- ∗ **E0942** Cervical head harness/halter Ⓑ Qp Qh ♿ Y
- ∗ **E0944** Pelvic belt/harness/boot Ⓑ Qp Qh ♿ Y
- ∗ **E0945** Extremity belt/harness Ⓑ Qp Qh ♿ Y
- **E0946** Fracture, frame, dual with cross bars, attached to bed (e.g., Balken, 4 poster) Ⓑ Qp Qh ♿ Y
  IOM: 100-03, 4, 280.1
- **E0947** Fracture frame, attachments for complex pelvic traction Ⓑ Qp Qh ♿ Y
  IOM: 100-03, 4, 280.1
- **E0948** Fracture frame, attachments for complex cervical traction Ⓑ Qp Qh ♿ Y
  IOM: 100-03, 4, 280.1

Wheelchair Accessories

- **E0950** Wheelchair accessory, tray, each Ⓑ Qp Qh ♿ Y
  IOM: 100-03, 4, 280.1
- ∗ **E0951** Heel loop/holder, any type, with or without ankle strap, each Ⓑ Qp Qh ♿ Y
- **E0952** Toe loop/holder, any type, each Ⓑ Qp Qh ♿ Y
  IOM: 100-03, 4, 280.1
- ∗ **E0953** Wheelchair accessory, lateral thigh or knee support, any type, including fixed mounting hardware, each ♿ Y
- ∗ **E0954** Wheelchair accessory, foot box, any type, includes attachment and mounting hardware, each foot ♿ Y
- ∗ **E0955** Wheelchair accessory, headrest, cushioned, any type, including fixed mounting hardware, each Ⓑ Qp Qh ♿ Y
- ∗ **E0956** Wheelchair accessory, lateral trunk or hip support, any type, including fixed mounting hardware, each Ⓑ Qp Qh ♿ Y
- ∗ **E0957** Wheelchair accessory, medial thigh support, any type, including fixed mounting hardware, each Ⓑ Qp Qh ♿ Y
- **E0958** Manual wheelchair accessory, one-arm drive attachment, each Ⓑ Qp Qh ♿ Y
  IOM: 100-03, 4, 280.1
- ∗ **E0959** Manual wheelchair accessory, adapter for amputee, each Ⓑ Qp Qh ♿ B
  IOM: 100-03, 4, 280.1
- ∗ **E0960** Wheelchair accessory, shoulder harness/straps or chest strap, including any type mounting hardware Ⓑ Qp Qh ♿ Y
- ∗ **E0961** Manual wheelchair accessory, wheel lock brake extension (handle), each Ⓑ Qp Qh ♿ B
  IOM: 100-03, 4, 280.1

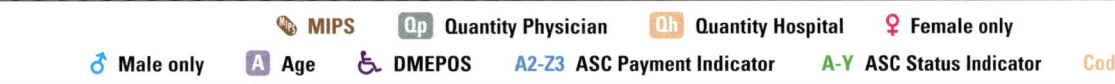

MIPS Qp Quantity Physician Qh Quantity Hospital ♀ Female only
♂ Male only A Age ♿ DMEPOS A2-Z3 ASC Payment Indicator A-Y ASC Status Indicator Coding Clinic

* E0966	Manual wheelchair accessory, headrest extension, each	B
	IOM: 100-03, 4, 280.1	
⊛ E0967	Manual wheelchair accessory, hand rim with projections, any type, replacement only, each	Y
	IOM: 100-03, 4, 280.1	
⊛ E0968	Commode seat, wheelchair	Y
	IOM: 100-03, 4, 280.1	
⊛ E0969	Narrowing device, wheelchair	Y
⊘ E0970	No. 2 footplates, except for elevating leg rest	E1
	IOM: 100-03, 4, 280.1	
	Cross Reference K0037, K0042	
* E0971	Manual wheelchair accessory, anti-tipping device, each	B
	IOM: 100-03, 4, 280.1	
	Cross Reference K0021	
⊛ E0973	Wheelchair accessory, adjustable height, detachable armrest, complete assembly, each	B
	IOM: 100-03, 4, 280.1	
⊛ E0974	Manual wheelchair accessory, anti-rollback device, each	B
	IOM: 100-03, 4, 280.1	
* E0978	Wheelchair accessory, positioning belt/safety belt/pelvic strap, each	B
* E0980	Safety vest, wheelchair	Y
* E0981	Wheelchair accessory, seat upholstery, replacement only, each	Y
* E0982	Wheelchair accessory, back upholstery, replacement only, each	Y
* E0983	Manual wheelchair accessory, power add-on to convert manual wheelchair to motorized wheelchair, joystick control	Y
* E0984	Manual wheelchair accessory, power add-on to convert manual wheelchair to motorized wheelchair, tiller control	Y
* E0985	Wheelchair accessory, seat lift mechanism	Y
⇄ E0986	Manual wheelchair accessory, power assist system	Y
* E0988	Manual wheelchair accessory, lever-activated, wheel drive, pair	Y
* E0990	Wheelchair accessory, elevating leg rest, complete assembly, each	B
	IOM: 100-03, 4, 280.1	
* E0992	Manual wheelchair accessory, solid seat insert	B
⊛ E0994	Arm rest, each	Y
	IOM: 100-03, 4, 280.1	
* E0995	Wheelchair accessory, calf rest/pad, replacement only, each	B
	IOM: 100-03, 4, 280.1	
* E1002	Wheelchair accessory, power seating system, tilt only	Y
* E1003	Wheelchair accessory, power seating system, recline only, without shear reduction	Y
* E1004	Wheelchair accessory, power seating system, recline only, with mechanical shear reduction	Y
* E1005	Wheelchair accessory, power seating system, recline only, with power shear reduction	Y
* E1006	Wheelchair accessory, power seating system, combination tilt and recline, without shear reduction	Y
* E1007	Wheelchair accessory, power seating system, combination tilt and recline, with mechanical shear reduction	Y
* E1008	Wheelchair accessory, power seating system, combination tilt and recline, with power shear reduction	Y
* E1009	Wheelchair accessory, addition to power seating system, mechanically linked leg elevation system, including pushrod and leg rest, each	Y
* E1010	Wheelchair accessory, addition to power seating system, power leg elevation system, including leg rest, pair	Y
⊛ E1011	Modification to pediatric size wheelchair, width adjustment package (not to be dispensed with initial chair)	Y
	IOM: 100-03, 4, 280.1	
* E1012	Wheelchair accessory, addition to power seating system, center mount power elevating leg rest/platform, complete system, any type, each	Y

▶ New ⤺ Revised ✔ Reinstated ~~deleted~~ Deleted ⊘ Not covered or valid by Medicare
⊛ Special coverage instructions * Carrier discretion Ⓑ Bill Part B MAC Ⓑ Bill DME MAC

DURABLE MEDICAL EQUIPMENT

E1014 Reclining back, addition to pediatric size wheelchair ⓑ Qp Qh A & Y
IOM: 100-03, 4, 280.1

E1015 Shock absorber for manual wheelchair, each ⓑ Qp Qh & Y
IOM: 100-03, 4, 280.1

E1016 Shock absorber for power wheelchair, each ⓑ Qp Qh & Y
IOM: 100-03, 4, 280.1

E1017 Heavy duty shock absorber for heavy duty or extra heavy duty manual wheelchair, each ⓑ Qp Qh & Y
IOM: 100-03, 4, 280.1

E1018 Heavy duty shock absorber for heavy duty or extra heavy duty power wheelchair, each ⓑ Qp Qh & Y
IOM: 100-03, 4, 280.1

E1020 Residual limb support system for wheelchair, any type ⓑ Qp Qh & Y
IOM: 100-03, 3, 280.3

▶ **E1022** Wheelchair transportation securement system, any type includes all components and accessories ⓑ Qp Qh & Y

▶ **E1023** Wheelchair transit securement system, includes all components and accessories ⓑ Qp Qh & Y

↩ * **E1028** Wheelchair accessory, manual swing-away, retractable or removable mounting, other ⓑ Qp Qh & Y

* **E1029** Wheelchair accessory, ventilator tray, fixed ⓑ Qp Qh & Y

* **E1030** Wheelchair accessory, ventilator tray, gimbaled ⓑ Qp Qh & Y

Rollabout Chair, Transfer System, Transport Chair

E1031 Rollabout chair, any and all types with casters 5" or greater ⓑ Qp Qh & Y
IOM: 100-03, 4, 280.1

▶ **E1032** Wheelchair accessory, manual swingaway, retractable or removable mounting hardware used with joystick or other drive control interface ⓑ Qp Qh & Y

▶ **E1033** Wheelchair accessory, manual swingaway, retractable or removable mounting hardware for headrest, cushioned, any type ⓑ Qp Qh & Y

▶ **E1034** Wheelchair accessory, manual swingaway, retractable or removable mounting hardware for lateral trunk or hip support, any type ⓑ Qp Qh & Y

E1035 Multi-positional patient transfer system, with integrated seat, operated by care giver, patient weight capacity up to and including 300 lbs ⓑ Qp Qh & Y
IOM: 100-02, 15, 110

* **E1036** Multi-positional patient transfer system, extra-wide, with integrated seat, operated by caregiver, patient weight capacity greater than 300 lbs ⓑ Qh & Y

E1037 Transport chair, pediatric size ⓑ Qp Qh A & Y
IOM: 100-03, 4, 280.1

E1038 Transport chair, adult size, patient weight capacity up to and including 300 pounds ⓑ Qp Qh A & Y
IOM: 100-03, 4, 280.1

* **E1039** Transport chair, adult size, heavy duty, patient weight capacity greater than 300 pounds ⓑ Qp Qh A & Y

Wheelchair: Fully Reclining

E1050 Fully-reclining wheelchair, fixed full length arms, swing away detachable elevating leg rests ⓑ Qp Qh & Y
IOM: 100-03, 4, 280.1

E1060 Fully-reclining wheelchair, detachable arms, desk or full length, swing away detachable elevating legrests ⓑ Qp Qh & Y
IOM: 100-03, 4, 280.1

E1070 Fully-reclining wheelchair, detachable arms (desk or full length), swing away detachable footrests ⓑ Qp Qh & Y
IOM: 100-03, 4, 280.1

Wheelchair: Hemi

E1083 Hemi-wheelchair, fixed full length arms, swing away detachable elevating leg rest ⓑ Qp Qh & Y
IOM: 100-03, 4, 280.1

E1084 Hemi-wheelchair, detachable arms desk or full length arms, swing away detachable elevating leg rests ⓑ Qp Qh & Y
IOM: 100-03, 4, 280.1

⊘ **E1085** Hemi-wheelchair, fixed full length arms, swing away detachable foot rests ⓑ Qp Qh E1
IOM: 100-03, 4, 280.1
Cross Reference K0002

| 🌀 MIPS | Qp Quantity Physician | Qh Quantity Hospital | ♀ Female only |
| ♂ Male only | A Age | & DMEPOS | A2-Z3 ASC Payment Indicator | A-Y ASC Status Indicator | Coding Clinic |

183

⊘ **E1086** Hemi-wheelchair, detachable arms desk or full length, swing away detachable footrests Ⓑ Qp Qh E1
  IOM: 100-03, 4, 280.1
  Cross Reference K0002

Wheelchair: High-strength Lightweight

✺ **E1087** High strength lightweight wheelchair, fixed full length arms, swing away detachable elevating leg rests Ⓑ Qp Qh ♿ Y
  IOM: 100-03, 4, 280.1

✺ **E1088** High strength lightweight wheelchair, detachable arms desk or full length, swing away detachable elevating leg rests Ⓑ Qp Qh ♿ Y
  IOM: 100-03, 4, 280.1

⊘ **E1089** High strength lightweight wheelchair, fixed length arms, swing away detachable footrest Ⓑ Qp Qh E1
  IOM: 100-03, 4, 280.1
  Cross Reference K0004

⊘ **E1090** High strength lightweight wheelchair, detachable arms desk or full length, swing away detachable foot rests Ⓑ Qp Qh E1
  IOM: 100-03, 4, 280.1
  Cross Reference K0004

Wheelchair: Wide Heavy Duty

✺ **E1092** Wide heavy duty wheelchair, detachable arms (desk or full length), swing away detachable elevating leg rests Ⓑ Qp Qh ♿ Y
  IOM: 100-03, 4, 280.1

✺ **E1093** Wide heavy duty wheelchair, detachable arms (desk or full length arms), swing away detachable foot rests Ⓑ Qp Qh ♿ Y
  IOM: 100-03, 4, 280.1

Wheelchair: Semi-reclining

✺ **E1100** Semi-reclining wheelchair, fixed full length arms, swing away detachable elevating leg rests Ⓑ Qp Qh ♿ Y
  IOM: 100-03, 4, 280.1

✺ **E1110** Semi-reclining wheelchair, detachable arms (desk or full length), elevating leg rest Ⓑ Qp Qh ♿ Y
  IOM: 100-03, 4, 280.1

Wheelchair: Standard

⊘ **E1130** Standard wheelchair, fixed full length arms, fixed or swing away detachable footrests Ⓑ Qp Qh E1
  IOM: 100-03, 4, 280.1
  Cross Reference K0001

⊘ **E1140** Wheelchair, detachable arms, desk or full length, swing away detachable footrests Ⓑ Qp Qh E1
  IOM: 100-03, 4, 280.1
  Cross Reference K0001

✺ **E1150** Wheelchair, detachable arms, desk or full length, swing away detachable elevating legrests Ⓑ Qp Qh ♿ Y
  IOM: 100-03, 4, 280.1

✺ **E1160** Wheelchair, fixed full length arms, swing away detachable elevating legrests Ⓑ Qp Qh ♿ Y
  IOM: 100-03, 4, 280.1

∗ **E1161** Manual adult size wheelchair, includes tilt in space Ⓑ Qp Qh Ⓐ ♿ Y

Wheelchair: Amputee

✺ **E1170** Amputee wheelchair, fixed full length arms, swing away detachable elevating legrests Ⓑ Qp Qh ♿ Y
  IOM: 100-03, 4, 280.1

✺ **E1171** Amputee wheelchair, fixed full length arms, without footrests or legrest Ⓑ Qp Qh ♿ Y
  IOM: 100-03, 4, 280.1

✺ **E1172** Amputee wheelchair, detachable arms (desk or full length) without footrests or legrest Ⓑ Qp Qh ♿ Y
  IOM: 100-03, 4, 280.1

✺ **E1180** Amputee wheelchair, detachable arms (desk or full length) swing away detachable footrests Ⓑ Qp Qh ♿ Y
  IOM: 100-03, 4, 280.1

✺ **E1190** Amputee wheelchair, detachable arms (desk or full length), swing away detachable elevating legrests Ⓑ Qp Qh ♿ Y
  IOM: 100-03, 4, 280.1

✺ **E1195** Heavy duty wheelchair, fixed full length arms, swing away detachable elevating legrests Ⓑ Qp Qh ♿ Y
  IOM: 100-03, 4, 280.1

✺ **E1200** Amputee wheelchair, fixed full length arms, swing away detachable footrest Ⓑ Qp Qh ♿ Y
  IOM: 100-03, 4, 280.1

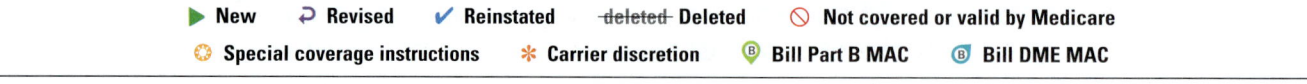

▶ New ⤴ Revised ✓ Reinstated ~~deleted~~ Deleted ⊘ Not covered or valid by Medicare
✺ Special coverage instructions ∗ Carrier discretion Ⓑ Bill Part B MAC Ⓑ Bill DME MAC

DURABLE MEDICAL EQUIPMENT

Wheelchair: Other and Accessories

- ⊛ **E1220** Wheelchair; specially sized or constructed (indicate brand name, model number, if any) and justification ⓑ Qp Qh Y
  IOM: 100-03, 4, 280.3

- ⊛ **E1221** Wheelchair with fixed arm, footrests ⓑ Qp Qh ♿ Y
  IOM: 100-03, 4, 280.3

- ⊛ **E1222** Wheelchair with fixed arm, elevating legrests ⓑ Qp Qh ♿ Y
  IOM: 100-03, 4, 280.3

- ⊛ **E1223** Wheelchair with detachable arms, footrests ⓑ Qp Qh ♿ Y
  IOM: 100-03, 4, 280.3

- ⊛ **E1224** Wheelchair with detachable arms, elevating legrests ⓑ Qp Qh ♿ Y
  IOM: 100-03, 4, 280.3

- ⊛ **E1225** Wheelchair accessory, manual semi-reclining back, (recline greater than 15 degrees, but less than 80 degrees), each ⓑ Qp Qh ♿ Y
  IOM: 100-03, 4, 280.3

- ⊛ **E1226** Wheelchair accessory, manual fully reclining back, (recline greater than 80 degrees), each ⓑ Qp Qh ♿ B
  IOM: 100-03, 4, 280.1

- ⊛ **E1227** Special height arms for wheelchair ⓑ ♿ Y
  IOM: 100-03, 4, 280.3

- ⊛ **E1228** Special back height for wheelchair ⓑ Qp Qh ♿ Y
  IOM: 100-03, 4, 280.3

Wheelchair: Pediatric

- ✱ **E1229** Wheelchair, pediatric size, not otherwise specified ⓑ Qp Qh A Y

- ⊛ **E1230** Power operated vehicle (three or four wheel non-highway), specify brand name and model number ⓑ Qp Qh ♿ Y

  Patient is unable to operate manual wheelchair; patient capable of safely operating controls for scooter; patient can transfer safely in and out of scooter
  IOM: 100-08, 5, 5.2.3

- ⊛ **E1231** Wheelchair, pediatric size, tilt-in-space, rigid, adjustable, with seating system ⓑ Qp Qh A ♿ Y
  IOM: 100-03, 4, 280.1

- ⊛ **E1232** Wheelchair, pediatric size, tilt-in-space, folding, adjustable, with seating system ⓑ Qp Qh A ♿ Y
  IOM: 100-03, 4, 280.1

- ⊛ **E1233** Wheelchair, pediatric size, tilt-in-space, rigid, adjustable, without seating system ⓑ Qp Qh A ♿ Y
  IOM: 100-03, 4, 280.1

- ⊛ **E1234** Wheelchair, pediatric size, tilt-in-space, folding, adjustable, without seating system ⓑ Qp Qh A ♿ Y
  IOM: 100-03, 4, 280.1

- ⊛ **E1235** Wheelchair, pediatric size, rigid, adjustable, with seating system ⓑ Qp Qh A ♿ Y
  IOM: 100-03, 4, 280.1

- ⊛ **E1236** Wheelchair, pediatric size, folding, adjustable, with seating system ⓑ Qp Qh A ♿ Y
  IOM: 100-03, 4, 280.1

- ⊛ **E1237** Wheelchair, pediatric size, rigid, adjustable, without seating system ⓑ Qp Qh A ♿ Y
  IOM: 100-03, 4, 280.1

- ⊛ **E1238** Wheelchair, pediatric size, folding, adjustable, without seating system ⓑ Qp Qh A ♿ Y
  IOM: 100-03, 4, 280.1

- ✱ **E1239** Power wheelchair, pediatric size, not otherwise specified ⓑ Qh A Y

Wheelchair: Lightweight

- ⊛ **E1240** Lightweight wheelchair, detachable arms (desk or full length), swing-away detachable elevating leg rests ⓑ Qp Qh ♿ Y
  IOM: 100-03, 4, 280.1

- ⊘ **E1250** Lightweight wheelchair, fixed full length arms, swing away detachable footrest ⓑ Qp Qh E1
  IOM: 100-03, 4, 280.1
  Cross Reference K0003

- ⊘ **E1260** Lightweight wheelchair, detachable arms (desk or full length), swing-away detachable footrest ⓑ Qp Qh E1
  IOM: 100-03, 4, 280.1
  Cross Reference K0003

- ⊛ **E1270** Lightweight wheelchair, fixed full length arms, swing away detachable elevating legrests ⓑ Qp Qh ♿ Y
  IOM: 100-03, 4, 280.1

MIPS Qp Quantity Physician Qh Quantity Hospital ♀ Female only ♂ Male only A Age ♿ DMEPOS A2-Z3 ASC Payment Indicator A-Y ASC Status Indicator Coding Clinic

185

Wheelchair: Heavy Duty

- **E1280** Heavy duty wheelchair, detachable arms (desk or full length), elevating legrests ⓑ Qp Qh ♿ Y
  IOM: 100-03, 4, 280.1

- ⊘ **E1285** Heavy duty wheelchair, fixed full length arms, swing away detachable footrest ⓑ Qp Qh E1
  IOM: 100-03, 4, 280.1
  Cross Reference K0006

- ⊘ **E1290** Heavy duty wheelchair, detachable arms (desk or full length), swing-away detachable footrest ⓑ Qp Qh E1
  IOM: 100-03, 4, 280.1
  Cross Reference K0006

- **E1295** Heavy duty wheelchair, fixed full length arms, elevating legrest ⓑ Qp Qh ♿ Y
  IOM: 100-03, 4, 280.1

- **E1296** Special wheelchair seat height from floor ⓑ ♿ Y
  IOM: 100-03, 4, 280.3

- **E1297** Special wheelchair seat depth, by upholstery ⓑ ♿ Y
  IOM: 100-03, 4, 280.3

- **E1298** Special wheelchair seat depth and/or width, by construction ⓑ ♿ Y
  IOM: 100-03, 4, 280.3

Whirlpool Equipment

- ⊘ **E1300** Whirlpool, portable (overtub type) ⓑ Qp Qh E1
  IOM: 100-03, 4, 280.1

- **E1301** Whirlpool tub, walk-in, portable ⓑ Qp Qh E1

- **E1310** Whirlpool, non-portable (built-in type) ⓑ Qp Qh ♿ Y
  IOM: 100-03, 4, 280.1

Additional Oxygen Related Equipment

- ✱ **E1352** Oxygen accessory, flow regulator capable of positive inspiratory pressure ⓑ Qp Qh Y

- **E1353** Regulator ⓑ Qp Qh ♿ Y
  IOM: 100-03, 4, 240.2

- ✱ **E1354** Oxygen accessory, wheeled cart for portable cylinder or portable concentrator, any type, replacement only, each ⓑ Qp Qh Y

- **E1355** Stand/rack ⓑ Qp Qh ♿ Y
  IOM: 100-03, 4, 240.2

- ✱ **E1356** Oxygen accessory, battery pack/cartridge for portable concentrator, any type, replacement only, each ⓑ Qp Qh Y

- ✱ **E1357** Oxygen accessory, battery charger for portable concentrator, any type, replacement only, each ⓑ Qp Qh Y

- **E1358** Oxygen accessory, DC power adapter for portable concentrator, any type, replacement only, each ⓑ Qp Qh Y

- **E1372** Immersion external heater for nebulizer ⓑ Qp Qh ♿ Y
  IOM: 100-03, 4, 240.2

- **E1390** Oxygen concentrator, single delivery port, capable of delivering 85 percent or greater oxygen concentration at the prescribed flow rate ⓑ Qp Qh ♿ Y
  IOM: 100-03, 4, 240.2

- **E1391** Oxygen concentrator, dual delivery port, capable of delivering 85 percent or greater oxygen concentration at the prescribed flow rate, each ⓑ Qp Qh ♿ Y
  IOM: 100-03, 4, 240.2

- **E1392** Portable oxygen concentrator, rental ⓑ Qp Qh ♿ Y
  IOM: 100-03, 4, 240.2

- ✱ **E1399** Durable medical equipment, miscellaneous ⓑ ⓑ Y

  Example: Therapeutic exercise putty; rubber exercise tubing; anti-vibration gloves

  On DMEPOS fee schedule as a payable replacement for miscellaneous implanted or non-implanted items

- **E1405** Oxygen and water vapor enriching system with heated delivery ⓑ Qp Qh ♿ Y
  IOM: 100-03, 4, 240.2

- **E1406** Oxygen and water vapor enriching system without heated delivery ⓑ Qp Qh ♿ Y
  IOM: 100-03, 4, 240.2

Artificial Kidney Machines and Accessories

- **E1500** Centrifuge, for dialysis ⓑ Qp Qh A

- **E1510** Kidney, dialysate delivery system, kidney machine, pump recirculating, air removal system, flowrate meter, power off, heater and temperature control with alarm, I.V. poles, pressure gauge, concentrate container ⓑ Qp Qh A

▶ New ↻ Revised ✓ Reinstated ~~deleted~~ Deleted ⊘ Not covered or valid by Medicare
⊛ Special coverage instructions ✱ Carrier discretion ⓑ Bill Part B MAC ⓑ Bill DME MAC

DURABLE MEDICAL EQUIPMENT

Code	Description	Indicator
✪ E1520	Heparin infusion pump for hemodialysis ⑧ Qp Qh	A
✪ E1530	Air bubble detector for hemodialysis, each, replacement ⑧ Qp Qh	A
✪ E1540	Pressure alarm for hemodialysis, each, replacement ⑧ Qp Qh	A
✪ E1550	Bath conductivity meter for hemodialysis, each ⑧ Qp Qh	A
✪ E1560	Blood leak detector for hemodialysis, each, replacement ⑧ Qp Qh	A
✪ E1570	Adjustable chair, for ESRD patients ⑧ Qp Qh	A
✪ E1575	Transducer protectors/fluid barriers for hemodialysis, any size, per 10 ⑧ Qp Qh	A
✪ E1580	Unipuncture control system for hemodialysis ⑧ Qp Qh	A
✪ E1590	Hemodialysis machine ⑧ Qp Qh	A
✪ E1592	Automatic intermittent peritoneal dialysis system ⑧ Qp Qh	A
✪ E1594	Cycler dialysis machine for peritoneal dialysis ⑧ Qp Qh	A
✪ E1600	Delivery and/or installation charges for hemodialysis equipment ⑧ Qp Qh	A
✪ E1610	Reverse osmosis water purification system, for hemodialysis ⑧ Qp Qh	A
	IOM: 100-03, 4, 230.7	
✪ E1615	Deionizer water purification system, for hemodialysis ⑧ Qp Qh	A
	IOM: 100-03, 4, 230.7	
✪ E1620	Blood pump for hemodialysis replacement ⑧ Qp Qh	A
✪ E1625	Water softening system, for hemodialysis ⑧ Qp Qh	A
	IOM: 100-03, 4, 230.7	
✪ E1629	Tablo hemodialysis system for the billable dialysis service	A
✴ E1630	Reciprocating peritoneal dialysis system ⑧ Qp Qh	A
✪ E1632	Wearable artificial kidney, each ⑧ Qp Qh	A
✪ E1634	Peritoneal dialysis clamps, each ⑧ Qp Qh	B
	IOM: 100-04, 8, 60.4.2; 100-04, 8, 90.1; 100-04, 18, 80; 100-04, 18, 90	
✪ E1635	Compact (portable) travel hemodialyzer system ⑧ Qp Qh	A
✪ E1636	Sorbent cartridges, for hemodialysis, per 10 ⑧ Qp Qh	A
✪ E1637	Hemostats, each ⑧ Qp Qh	A
✪ E1639	Scale, each ⑧ Qp Qh	A
✪ E1699	Dialysis equipment, not otherwise specified ⑧	A

Jaw Motion Rehabilitation System

Code	Description	Indicator
✴ E1700	Jaw motion rehabilitation system ⑧ Qp Qh ♿	Y
	Must be prescribed by physician	
✴ E1701	Replacement cushions for jaw motion rehabilitation system, pkg. of 6 ⑧ Qp Qh ♿	Y
✴ E1702	Replacement measuring scales for jaw motion rehabilitation system, pkg. of 200 ⑧ Qp Qh ♿	Y

Other Orthopedic Devices

Code	Description	Indicator
⟲ ✴ E1800	Dynamic adjustable elbow extension and flexion device, includes soft interface material ⑧ Qp Qh ♿	Y
⟲ ✴ E1801	Static progressive stretch/patient actualized serial stretch elbow device, extension and/or flexion, with or without range of motion adjustment, includes all components and accessories ⑧ Qp Qh ♿	Y
✴ E1802	Dynamic adjustable forearm pronation/supination device, includes soft interface material ⑧ Qp Qh ♿	Y
▶ ✴ E1803	Dynamic adjustable elbow extension only device, includes soft interface material ⑧ Qp Qh ♿	Y
▶ ✴ E1804	Dynamic adjustable elbow flexion only device, includes soft interface material ⑧ Qp Qh ♿	Y
⟲ ✴ E1805	Dynamic adjustable wrist extension and flexion device, includes soft interface material ⑧ Qp Qh ♿	Y
✴ E1806	Static progressive stretch wrist device, flexion and/or extension, with or without range of motion adjustment, includes all components and accessories ⑧ Qp Qh ♿	Y
▶ ✴ E1807	Dynamic adjustable wrist extension only device, includes soft interface material ⑧ Qp Qh ♿	Y
▶ ✴ E1808	Dynamic adjustable wrist flexion only device, includes soft interface material ⑧ Qp Qh ♿	Y
✴ E1810	Dynamic adjustable knee extension and flexion device, includes soft interface material ⑧ Qp Qh ♿	Y
⟲ ✴ E1811	Static progressive stretch/patient actualized serial stretch knee device, extension and/or flexion, with or without range of motion adjustment, includes all components and accessories ⑧ Qp Qh ♿	Y
✴ E1812	Dynamic knee, extension/flexion device with active resistance control ⑧ Qp Qh ♿	Y

🪙 MIPS   Qp Quantity Physician   Qh Quantity Hospital   ♀ Female only
♂ Male only   Ⓐ Age   ♿ DMEPOS   A2-Z3 ASC Payment Indicator   A-Y ASC Status Indicator   Coding Clinic

▶ * E1813	Dynamic adjustable knee extension only device, includes soft interface material Ⓑ Qp Qh ♿	Y
▶ * E1814	Dynamic adjustable knee flexion only device, includes soft interface material Ⓑ Qp Qh ♿	Y
↻ * E1815	Dynamic adjustable ankle extension and flexion device, includes soft interface material Ⓑ Qp Qh ♿	Y
↻ * E1816	Static progressive stretch/patient actualized serial stretch ankle device, flexion and/or extension, with or without range of motion adjustment, includes all components and accessories Ⓑ Qp Qh ♿	Y
↻ * E1818	Static progressive stretch/patient actualized serial stretch forearm pronation/supination device with or without range of motion adjustment, includes all components and accessories Ⓑ Qp Qh ♿	Y
* E1820	Replacement soft interface material, dynamic adjustable extension/flexion device Ⓑ Qp Qh ♿	Y
* E1821	Replacement soft interface material/cuffs for bi-directional static progressive stretch device Ⓑ Qp Qh ♿	Y
▶ * E1822	Dynamic adjustable ankle extension only device, includes soft interface material Ⓑ Qp Qh ♿	Y
▶ * E1823	Dynamic adjustable ankle flexion only device, includes soft interface material Ⓑ Qp Qh ♿	Y
↻ * E1825	Dynamic adjustable finger extension and flexion device, includes soft interface material Ⓑ Qp Qh ♿	Y
▶ * E1826	Dynamic adjustable finger extension only device, includes soft interface material Ⓑ Qp Qh ♿	Y
▶ * E1827	Dynamic adjustable finger flexion only device, includes soft interface material Ⓑ Qp Qh ♿	Y
▶ * E1828	Dynamic adjustable toe extension only device, includes soft interface material Ⓑ Qp Qh ♿	Y
▶ * E1829	Dynamic adjustable toe flexion only device, includes soft interface material Ⓑ Qp Qh ♿	Y
↻ * E1830	Dynamic adjustable toe extension and flexion device, includes soft interface material Ⓑ Qp Qh ♿	Y
* E1831	Static progressive stretch toe device, extension and/or flexion, with or without range of motion adjustment, includes all components and accessories Ⓑ Qp Qh ♿	Y
▶ * E1832	Static progressive stretch finger device, extension and/or flexion, with or without range of motion adjustment, includes all components and accessories Ⓑ Qp Qh ♿	Y
* E1840	Dynamic adjustable shoulder flexion/abduction/rotation device, includes soft interface material Ⓑ Qp Qh ♿	Y
↻ * E1841	Static progressive stretch /patient actualized serial stretch shoulder device, with or without range of motion adjustment, includes all components and accessories Ⓑ Qp Qh ♿	Y

Miscellaneous

* E1902	Communication board, non-electronic augmentative or alternative communication device Ⓑ Qp Qh	Y
E1905	Virtual reality cognitive behavioral therapy device (cbt), including pre-programmed therapy software Ⓑ Qp Qh	A
* E2000	Gastric suction pump, home model, portable or stationary, electric Ⓑ Qp Qh ♿	Y
E2001	Suction pump, home model, portable or stationary, electric, any type, for use with external urine and/or fecal management system Ⓑ Qp Qh	Y
⊙ E2100	Blood glucose monitor with integrated voice synthesizer Ⓑ Qp Qh ♿	Y
	IOM: 100-03, 4, 230.16	
⊙ E2101	Blood glucose monitor with integrated lancing/blood sample Ⓑ Qp Qh ♿	Y
	IOM: 100-03, 4, 230.16	
* E2102	Adjunctive, non-implanted continuous glucose monitor or receiver Ⓑ ♿	Y
* E2103	Non-adjunctive, non-implanted continuous glucose monitor or receiver Ⓑ ♿	Y
E2104	Home blood glucose monitor for use with integrated lancing/blood sample testing cartridge Ⓑ	A
* E2120	Pulse generator system for tympanic treatment of inner ear endolymphatic fluid Ⓑ Qp Qh ♿	Y

Wheelchair Assessories: Manual and Power

* E2201	Manual wheelchair accessory, nonstandard seat frame, width greater than or equal to 20 inches and less than 24 inches Ⓑ Qp Qh ♿	Y
* E2202	Manual wheelchair accessory, nonstandard seat frame width, 24-27 inches Ⓑ Qp Qh ♿	Y

▶ New ↻ Revised ✓ Reinstated ~~deleted~~ Deleted ⊘ Not covered or valid by Medicare
⊙ Special coverage instructions * Carrier discretion Ⓑ Bill Part B MAC Ⓑ Bill DME MAC

DURABLE MEDICAL EQUIPMENT

* **E2203** Manual wheelchair accessory, nonstandard seat frame depth, 20 to less than 22 inches ⓑ Qp Qh ♿ Y
* **E2204** Manual wheelchair accessory, nonstandard seat frame depth, 22 to 25 inches ⓑ Qp Qh ♿ Y
* **E2205** Manual wheelchair accessory, handrim without projections (includes ergonomic or contoured), any type, replacement only, each ⓑ Qp Qh ♿ Y
* **E2206** Manual wheelchair accessory, wheel lock assembly, complete, replacement only, each ⓑ Qp Qh ♿ Y
* **E2207** Wheelchair accessory, crutch and cane holder, each ⓑ Qp Qh ♿ Y
* **E2208** Wheelchair accessory, cylinder tank carrier, each ⓑ Qp Qh ♿ Y
* **E2209** Accessory arm trough, with or without hand support, each ⓑ Qp Qh ♿ Y
* **E2210** Wheelchair accessory, bearings, any type, replacement only, each ⓑ Qp Qh ♿ Y
* **E2211** Manual wheelchair accessory, pneumatic propulsion tire, any size, each ⓑ Qp Qh ♿ Y
* **E2212** Manual wheelchair accessory, tube for pneumatic propulsion tire, any size, each ⓑ Qp Qh ♿ Y
* **E2213** Manual wheelchair accessory, insert for pneumatic propulsion tire (removable), any type, any size, each ⓑ Qp Qh ♿ Y
* **E2214** Manual wheelchair accessory, pneumatic caster tire, any size, each ⓑ Qp Qh ♿ Y
* **E2215** Manual wheelchair accessory, tube for pneumatic caster tire, any size, each ⓑ Qp Qh ♿ Y
* **E2216** Manual wheelchair accessory, foam filled propulsion tire, any size, each ⓑ Qp Qh ♿ Y
* **E2217** Manual wheelchair accessory, foam filled caster tire, any size, each ⓑ Qp Qh ♿ Y
* **E2218** Manual wheelchair accessory, foam propulsion tire, any size, each ⓑ Qp Qh ♿ Y
* **E2219** Manual wheelchair accessory, foam caster tire, any size, each ⓑ Qp Qh ♿ Y
* **E2220** Manual wheelchair accessory, solid (rubber/plastic) propulsion tire, any size, replacement only, each ⓑ Qp Qh ♿ Y
* **E2221** Manual wheelchair accessory, solid (rubber/plastic) caster tire (removable), any size, replacement only, each ⓑ Qp Qh ♿ Y
* **E2222** Manual wheelchair accessory, solid (rubber/plastic) caster tire with integrated wheel, any size, replacement only, each ⓑ Qp Qh ♿ Y
* **E2224** Manual wheelchair accessory, propulsion wheel excludes tire, any size, replacement only, each ⓑ Qp Qh ♿ Y
* **E2225** Manual wheelchair accessory, caster wheel excludes tire, any size, replacement only, each ⓑ Qp Qh ♿ Y
* **E2226** Manual wheelchair accessory, caster fork, any size, replacement only, each ⓑ Qp Qh ♿ Y
* **E2227** Manual wheelchair accessory, gear reduction drive wheel, each ⓑ Qp Qh ♿ Y
* **E2228** Manual wheelchair accessory, wheel braking system and lock, complete, each ⓑ Qp Qh ♿ Y
* **E2230** Manual wheelchair accessory, manual standing system ⓑ Qp Qh
* **E2231** Manual wheelchair accessory, solid seat support base (replaces sling seat), includes any type mounting hardware ⓑ Qp Qh ♿ Y
* **E2291** Back, planar, for pediatric size wheelchair including fixed attaching hardware ⓑ Qp Qh Ⓐ Y
* **E2292** Seat, planar, for pediatric size wheelchair including fixed attaching hardware ⓑ Qp Qh Ⓐ Y
* **E2293** Back, contoured, for pediatric size wheelchair including fixed attaching hardware ⓑ Qp Qh Ⓐ Y
* **E2294** Seat, contoured, for pediatric size wheelchair including fixed attaching hardware ⓑ Qp Qh Ⓐ Y
* **E2295** Manual wheelchair accessory, for pediatric size wheelchair, dynamic seating frame, allows coordinated movement of multiple positioning features ⓑ Qp Qh Ⓐ Y
* **E2298** Complex rehabilitative power wheelchair accessory, power seat elevation system, any type ⓑ Y
* **E2301** Wheelchair accessory, power standing system, any type ⓑ Qp Qh Y
* **E2310** Power wheelchair accessory, electronic connection between wheelchair controller and one power seating system motor, including all related electronics, indicator feature, mechanical function selection switch, and fixed mounting hardware ⓑ Qp Qh ♿ Y

🔗 MIPS	Qp Quantity Physician	Qh Quantity Hospital	♀ Female only	
♂ Male only	Ⓐ Age	♿ DMEPOS	A2-Z3 ASC Payment Indicator	A-Y ASC Status Indicator	Coding Clinic

* **E2311** Power wheelchair accessory, electronic connection between wheelchair controller and two or more power seating system motors, including all related electronics, indicator feature, mechanical function selection switch, and fixed mounting hardware Ⓑ Qp Qh ♿ Y

* **E2312** Power wheelchair accessory, hand or chin control interface, mini-proportional remote joystick, proportional, including fixed mounting hardware Ⓑ Qp Qh ♿ Y

* **E2313** Power wheelchair accessory, harness for upgrade to expandable controller, including all fasteners, connectors and mounting hardware, each Ⓑ Qp Qh ♿ Y

* **E2321** Power wheelchair accessory, hand control interface, remote joystick, nonproportional, including all related electronics, mechanical stop switch, and fixed mounting hardware Ⓑ Qp Qh ♿ Y

* **E2322** Power wheelchair accessory, hand control interface, multiple mechanical switches, nonproportional, including all related electronics, mechanical stop switch, and fixed mounting hardware Ⓑ Qp Qh ♿ Y

* **E2323** Power wheelchair accessory, specialty joystick handle for hand control interface, prefabricated Ⓑ Qp Qh ♿ Y

* **E2324** Power wheelchair accessory, chin cup for chin control interface Ⓑ Qp Qh ♿ Y

* **E2325** Power wheelchair accessory, sip and puff interface, nonproportional, including all related electronics, mechanical stop switch, and manual swingaway mounting hardware Ⓑ Qp Qh ♿ Y

* **E2326** Power wheelchair accessory, breath tube kit for sip and puff interface Ⓑ Qp Qh ♿ Y

* **E2327** Power wheelchair accessory, head control interface, mechanical, proportional, including all related electronics, mechanical direction change switch, and fixed mounting hardware Ⓑ Qp Qh ♿ Y

* **E2328** Power wheelchair accessory, head control or extremity control interface, electronic, proportional, including all related electronics and fixed mounting hardware Ⓑ Qp Qh ♿ Y

* **E2329** Power wheelchair accessory, head control interface, contact switch mechanism, nonproportional, including all related electronics, mechanical stop switch, mechanical direction change switch, head array, and fixed mounting hardware Ⓑ Qp Qh ♿ Y

* **E2330** Power wheelchair accessory, head control interface, proximity switch mechanism, nonproportional, including all related electronics, mechanical stop switch, mechanical direction change switch, head array, and fixed mounting hardware Ⓑ Qp Qh ♿ Y

* **E2331** Power wheelchair accessory, attendant control, proportional, including all related electronics and fixed mounting hardware Ⓑ Qp Qh Y

* **E2340** Power wheelchair accessory, nonstandard seat frame width, 20-23 inches Qp Qh ♿ Y

* **E2341** Power wheelchair accessory, nonstandard seat frame width, 24-27 inches Ⓑ Qp Qh ♿ Y

* **E2342** Power wheelchair accessory, nonstandard seat frame depth, 20 or 21 inches Ⓑ Qp Qh ♿ Y

* **E2343** Power wheelchair accessory, nonstandard seat frame depth, 22-25 inches Ⓑ Qp Qh ♿ Y

* **E2351** Power wheelchair accessory, electronic interface to operate speech generating device using power wheelchair control interface Ⓑ Qp Qh ♿ Y

* **E2358** Power wheelchair accessory, Group 34 non-sealed lead acid battery, each Ⓑ Qp Qh Y

* **E2359** Power wheelchair accessory, Group 34 sealed lead acid battery, each (e.g., gel cell, absorbed glassmat) Ⓑ Qp Qh ♿ Y

* **E2360** Power wheelchair accessory, 22 NF non-sealed lead acid battery, each Ⓑ ♿ Y

* **E2361** Power wheelchair accessory, 22NF sealed lead acid battery, each (e.g., gel cell, absorbed glassmat) Ⓑ Qp Qh Y

* **E2362** Power wheelchair accessory, group 24 non-sealed lead acid battery, each Ⓑ ♿ Y

* **E2363** Power wheelchair accessory, group 24 sealed lead acid battery, each (e.g., gel cell, absorbed glassmat) Ⓑ Qp Qh Y

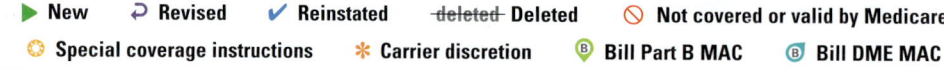

▶ New ⤺ Revised ✓ Reinstated ~~deleted~~ Deleted ⊘ Not covered or valid by Medicare
✹ Special coverage instructions ✶ Carrier discretion Ⓑ Bill Part B MAC Ⓑ Bill DME MAC

DURABLE MEDICAL EQUIPMENT

* **E2364** Power wheelchair accessory, U-1 non-sealed lead acid battery, each ♿ Y
* **E2365** Power wheelchair accessory, U-1 sealed lead acid battery, each (e.g., gel cell, absorbed glassmat) ⓑ Qp Qh ♿ Y
* **E2366** Power wheelchair accessory, battery charger, single mode, for use with only one battery type, sealed or non-sealed, each ⓑ Qp Qh ♿ Y
* **E2367** Power wheelchair accessory, battery charger, dual mode, for use with either battery type, sealed or non-sealed, each ⓑ Qp Qh ♿ Y
* **E2368** Power wheelchair component, drive wheel motor, replacement only ⓑ Qp Qh ♿ Y
* **E2369** Power wheelchair component, drive wheel gear box, replacement only ⓑ Qp Qh ♿ Y
* **E2370** Power wheelchair component, integrated drive wheel motor and gear box combination, replacement only ⓑ Qp Qh ♿ Y
* **E2371** Power wheelchair accessory, group 27 sealed lead acid battery, (e.g., gel cell, absorbed glass mat), each ⓑ Qp Qh ♿ Y
* **E2372** Power wheelchair accessory, group 27 non-sealed lead acid battery, each ⓑ ♿ Y
* **E2373** Power wheelchair accessory, hand or chin control interface, compact remote joystick, proportional, including fixed mounting hardware ⓑ Qp Qh ♿ Y
* **E2374** Power wheelchair accessory, hand or chin control interface, standard remote joystick (not including controller), proportional, including all related electronics and fixed mounting hardware, replacement only ⓑ Qp Qh ♿ Y
* **E2375** Power wheelchair accessory, non-expandable controller, including all related electronics and mounting hardware, replacement only ⓑ Qp Qh ♿ Y
* **E2376** Power wheelchair accessory, expandable controller, including all related electronics and mounting hardware, replacement only ⓑ Qp Qh ♿ Y
* **E2377** Power wheelchair accessory, expandable controller, including all related electronics and mounting hardware, upgrade provided at initial issue ⓑ Qp Qh ♿ Y
* **E2378** Power wheelchair component, actuator, replacement only ⓑ Qp Qh ♿ Y
* **E2381** Power wheelchair accessory, pneumatic drive wheel tire, any size, replacement only, each ⓑ Qp Qh ♿ Y
* **E2382** Power wheelchair accessory, tube for pneumatic drive wheel tire, any size, replacement only, each ⓑ Qp Qh ♿ Y
* **E2383** Power wheelchair accessory, insert for pneumatic drive wheel tire (removable), any type, any size, replacement only, each ⓑ Qp Qh ♿ Y
* **E2384** Power wheelchair accessory, pneumatic caster tire, any size, replacement only, each ⓑ Qp Qh ♿ Y
* **E2385** Power wheelchair accessory, tube for pneumatic caster tire, any size, replacement only, each ⓑ Qp Qh ♿ Y
* **E2386** Power wheelchair accessory, foam filled drive wheel tire, any size, replacement only, each ⓑ Qp Qh ♿ Y
* **E2387** Power wheelchair accessory, foam filled caster tire, any size, replacement only, each ⓑ Qp Qh ♿ Y
* **E2388** Power wheelchair accessory, foam drive wheel tire, any size, replacement only, each ⓑ Qp Qh ♿ Y
* **E2389** Power wheelchair accessory, foam caster tire, any size, replacement only, each ⓑ Qp Qh ♿ Y
* **E2390** Power wheelchair accessory, solid (rubber/plastic) drive wheel tire, any size, replacement only, each ⓑ Qp Qh ♿ Y
* **E2391** Power wheelchair accessory, solid (rubber/plastic) caster tire (removable), any size, replacement only, each ⓑ Qp Qh ♿ Y
* **E2392** Power wheelchair accessory, solid (rubber/plastic) caster tire with integrated wheel, any size, replacement only, each ⓑ Qp Qh ♿ Y
* **E2394** Power wheelchair accessory, drive wheel excludes tire, any size, replacement only, each ⓑ Qp Qh ♿ Y
* **E2395** Power wheelchair accessory, caster wheel excludes tire, any size, replacement only, each ⓑ Qp Qh ♿ Y
* **E2396** Power wheelchair accessory, caster fork, any size, replacement only, each ⓑ Qp Qh ♿ Y
* **E2397** Power wheelchair accessory, lithium-based battery, each ⓑ Qp Qh ♿ Y
* **E2398** Wheelchair accessory, dynamic positioning hardware for back ⓑ Qp Qh ♿ Y

🏅 MIPS   Qp Quantity Physician   Qh Quantity Hospital   ♀ Female only
♂ Male only   A Age   ♿ DMEPOS   A2-Z3 ASC Payment Indicator   A-Y ASC Status Indicator   Coding Clinic

Negative Pressure

* **E2402** Negative pressure wound therapy electrical pump, stationary or portable Y

  Document at least every 30 calendar days the quantitative wound characteristics, including wound surface area (length, width and depth).

  Medicare coverage up to a maximum of 15 dressing kits (A6550) per wound per month unless documentation states that the wound size requires more than one dressing kit for each dressing change.

Speech Device

* **E2500** Speech generating device, digitized speech, using pre-recorded messages, less than or equal to 8 minutes recording time Y

  IOM: 100-03, 1, 50.1

* **E2502** Speech generating device, digitized speech, using pre-recorded messages, greater than 8 minutes but less than or equal to 20 minutes recording time Y

  IOM: 100-03, 1, 50.1

* **E2504** Speech generating device, digitized speech, using pre-recorded messages, greater than 20 minutes but less than or equal to 40 minutes recording time Y

  IOM: 100-03, 1, 50.1

* **E2506** Speech generating device, digitized speech, using pre-recorded messages, greater than 40 minutes recording time Y

  IOM: 100-03, 1, 50.1

* **E2508** Speech generating device, synthesized speech, requiring message formulation by spelling and access by physical contact with the device Y

  IOM: 100-03, 1, 50.1

* **E2510** Speech generating device, synthesized speech, permitting multiple methods of message formulation and multiple methods of device access Y

  IOM: 100-03, 1, 50.1

* **E2511** Speech generating software program, for personal computer or personal digital assistant Y

  IOM: 100-03, 1, 50.1

* **E2512** Accessory for speech generating device, mounting system Y

  IOM: 100-03, 1, 50.1

  E2513 Accessory for speech generating device, electromyographic sensor Y

* **E2599** Accessory for speech generating device, not otherwise classified Y

  IOM: 100-03, 1, 50.1

Wheelchair: Cushion

* **E2601** General use wheelchair seat cushion, width less than 22 inches, any depth Y

* **E2602** General use wheelchair seat cushion, width 22 inches or greater, any depth Y

* **E2603** Skin protection wheelchair seat cushion, width less than 22 inches, any depth Y

* **E2604** Skin protection wheelchair seat cushion, width 22 inches or greater, any depth Y

* **E2605** Positioning wheelchair seat cushion, width less than 22 inches, any depth Y

* **E2606** Positioning wheelchair seat cushion, width 22 inches or greater, any depth Y

* **E2607** Skin protection and positioning wheelchair seat cushion, width less than 22 inches, any depth Y

* **E2608** Skin protection and positioning wheelchair seat cushion, width 22 inches or greater, any depth Y

* **E2609** Custom fabricated wheelchair seat cushion, any size Y

* **E2610** Wheelchair seat cushion, powered B

* **E2611** General use wheelchair back cushion, width less than 22 inches, any height, including any type mounting hardware Y

* **E2612** General use wheelchair back cushion, width 22 inches or greater, any height, including any type mounting hardware Y

* **E2613** Positioning wheelchair back cushion, posterior, width less than 22 inches, any height, including any type mounting hardware Y

▶ New   ↻ Revised   ✓ Reinstated   ~~deleted~~ Deleted   ⊘ Not covered or valid by Medicare

✺ Special coverage instructions   ✱ Carrier discretion   Ⓑ Bill Part B MAC   Ⓑ Bill DME MAC

DURABLE MEDICAL EQUIPMENT

* **E2614** Positioning wheelchair back cushion, posterior, width 22 inches or greater, any height, including any type mounting hardware ⑧ Qp Qh   Y

* **E2615** Positioning wheelchair back cushion, posterior-lateral, width less than 22 inches, any height, including any type mounting hardware ⑧ Qp Qh   Y

* **E2616** Positioning wheelchair back cushion, posterior-lateral, width 22 inches or greater, any height, including any type mounting hardware ⑧ Qp Qh   Y

* **E2617** Custom fabricated wheelchair back cushion, any size, including any type mounting hardware ⑧ Qp Qh   Y

* **E2619** Replacement cover for wheelchair seat cushion or back cushion, each ⑧ Qp Qh   Y

* **E2620** Positioning wheelchair back cushion, planar back with lateral supports, width less than 22 inches, any height, including any type mounting hardware ⑧ Qp Qh   Y

* **E2621** Positioning wheelchair back cushion, planar back with lateral supports, width 22 inches or greater, any height, including any type mounting hardware ⑧ Qp Qh   Y

Wheelchair: Skin Protection

* **E2622** Skin protection wheelchair seat cushion, adjustable, width less than 22 inches, any depth ⑧ Qp Qh   Y

* **E2623** Skin protection wheelchair seat cushion, adjustable, width 22 inches or greater, any depth ⑧ Qp Qh   Y

* **E2624** Skin protection and positioning wheelchair seat cushion, adjustable, width less than 22 inches, any depth ⑧ Qp Qh   Y

* **E2625** Skin protection and positioning wheelchair seat cushion, adjustable, width 22 inches or greater, any depth ⑧ Qp Qh   Y

Wheelchair: Arm Support

* **E2626** Wheelchair accessory, shoulder elbow, mobile arm support attached to wheelchair, balanced, adjustable ⑧ Qp Qh   Y

* **E2627** Wheelchair accessory, shoulder elbow, mobile arm support attached to wheelchair, balanced, adjustable rancho type ⑧ Qp Qh   Y

* **E2628** Wheelchair accessory, shoulder elbow, mobile arm support attached to wheelchair, balanced, reclining ⑧ Qp Qh   Y

* **E2629** Wheelchair accessory, shoulder elbow, mobile arm support attached to wheelchair, balanced, friction arm support (friction dampening to proximal and distal joints) ⑧ Qp Qh   Y

* **E2630** Wheelchair accessory, shoulder elbow, mobile arm support, monosuspension arm and hand support, overhead elbow forearm hand sling support, yoke type suspension support ⑧ Qp Qh   Y

* **E2631** Wheelchair accessory, addition to mobile arm support, elevating proximal arm ⑧ Qp Qh   Y

* **E2632** Wheelchair accessory, addition to mobile arm support, offset or lateral rocker arm with elastic balance control ⑧ Qp Qh   Y

* **E2633** Wheelchair accessory, addition to mobile arm support, supinator ⑧ Qp Qh   Y

Speech Volume System

E3000 Speech volume modulation system, any type, including all components and accessories ⑧ Qp Qh   Y

E3200 Gait modulation system, rhythmic auditory stimulation, including restricted therapy software, all components and accessories, prescription only ⑧ Qp Qh   Y

Pediatric Gait Trainer

⊘ **E8000** Gait trainer, pediatric size, posterior support, includes all accessories and components ⑧ A   E1

⊘ **E8001** Gait trainer, pediatric size, upright support, includes all accessories and components ⑧ A   E1

⊘ **E8002** Gait trainer, pediatric size, anterior support, includes all accessories and components ⑧ A   E1

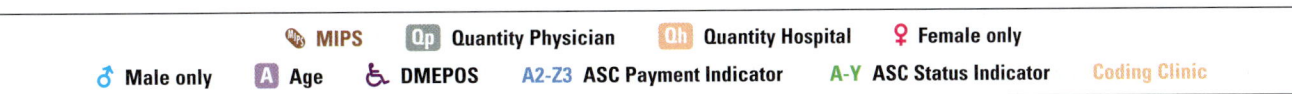

 MIPS   Qp Quantity Physician   Qh Quantity Hospital   ♀ Female only   ♂ Male only   A Age   & DMEPOS   A2-Z3 ASC Payment Indicator   A-Y ASC Status Indicator   Coding Clinic

2026 HCPCS LEVEL II NATIONAL CODES

TEMPORARY PROCEDURES/ PROFESSIONAL SERVICES (G0000-G9999)

NOTE: Series "G", "K", and "Q" in the Level II coding are reserved for CMS assignment. "G", "K", and "Q" codes are temporary national codes for items or services requiring uniform national coding between one year's update and the next. Sometimes "temporary" codes remain for more than one update. If "G", "K", and "Q" codes are not converted to permanent codes in Level I or Level II series in the following update, they will remain active until converted in following years or until CMS notifies contractors to delete them. All active "G", "K", and "Q" codes at the time of update will be included on the update file for contractors. In addition, deleted codes are retained on the file for informational purposes, with a deleted indicator, for four years.

Vaccine Administration

* **G0008** Administration of influenza virus vaccine Ⓑ Qp Qh S

   Coinsurance and deductible do not apply. If provided, report significant, separately identifiable E/M for medically necessary services (Z23).

   Coding Clinic: 2016, Q4, P3

* **G0009** Administration of pneumococcal vaccine Ⓑ Qp Qh S

   Reported once in a lifetime based on risk; Medicare covers cost of vaccine and administration (Z23)

   Copayment, coinsurance, and deductible waived. (https://www.cms.gov/MLNProducts/downloads/MPS_QuickReferenceChart_1.pdf)

   Coding Clinic: 2016, Q4, P3

* **G0010** Administration of hepatitis B vaccine Ⓑ Qp Qh S

   Report for other than OPPs. Coinsurance and deductible apply; Medicare covers both cost of vaccine and administration (Z23)

   Copayment/coinsurance and deductible are waived. (https://www.cms.gov/MLNProducts/downloads/MPS_QuickReferenceChart_1.pdf)

   Coding Clinic: 2016, Q4, P3

* **G0011** Individual counseling for pre-exposure prophylaxis (prep) by physician or qualified health care professional (QHP) to prevent human immunodeficiency virus (HIV), includes HIV risk assessment (initial or continued assessment of risk), HIV risk reduction and medication adherence, 15-30 minutes M

* **G0012** Injection of pre-exposure prophylaxis (prep) drug for HIV prevention, under skin or into muscle S

* **G0013** Individual counseling for pre-exposure prophylaxis (prep) by clinical staff to prevent human immunodeficiency virus (HIV), includes: HIV risk assessment (initial or continued assessment of risk), HIV risk reduction and medication adherence S

Crisis Psychotherapy

* **G0017** Psychotherapy for crisis furnished in an applicable site of service (any place of service at which the non-facility rate for psychotherapy for crisis services applies, other than the office setting); first 60 minutes M

* **G0018** Psychotherapy for crisis furnished in an applicable site of service (any place of service at which the non-facility rate for psychotherapy for crisis services applies, other than the office setting); each additional 30 minutes (list separately in addition to code for primary service) M

Integration and Navigation Services

* **G0019** Community health integration services performed by certified or trained auxiliary personnel, including a community health worker, under the direction of a physician or other practitioner; 60 minutes per calendar month, in the following activities to address social determinants of health (SDOH) need(s) that are significantly limiting the ability to diagnose or treat problem(s) addressed in an initiating visit: person-centered assessment, performed to better understand the individualized context of the intersection between the SDOH need(s) and the problem(s) addressed in the initiating visit. ++conducting a person-centered assessment to understand patient's life story, strengths, needs,

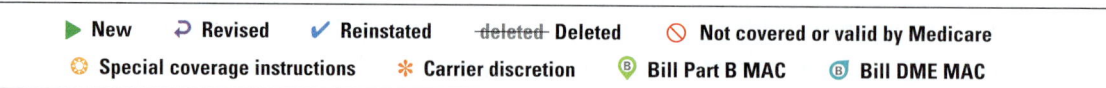

▶ New   ⟳ Revised   ✓ Reinstated   ~~deleted~~ Deleted   ⊘ Not covered or valid by Medicare
⊛ Special coverage instructions   * Carrier discretion   Ⓑ Bill Part B MAC   Ⓑ Bill DME MAC

TEMPORARY PROCEDURES/PROFESSIONAL SERVICES

goals, preferences and desired outcomes, including understanding cultural and linguistic factors and including unmet SDOH needs (that are not separately billed). ++ facilitating patient-driven goal-setting and establishing an action plan.
++providing tailored support to the patient as needed to accomplish the practitioner's treatment plan. practitioner, home-, and community-based care coordination.
++coordinating receipt of needed services from healthcare practitioners, providers, and facilities; and from home- and community-based service providers, social service providers, and caregiver (if applicable).
++communication with practitioners, home- and community-based service providers, hospitals, and skilled nursing facilities (or other health care facilities) regarding the patient's psychosocial strengths and needs, functional deficits, goals, preferences, and desired outcomes, including cultural and linguistic factors. ++coordination of care transitions between and among health care practitioners and settings, including transitions involving referral to other clinicians; follow-up after an emergency department visit; or follow-up after discharges from hospitals, skilled nursing facilities or other health care facilities.
++facilitating access to community-based social services (e.g., housing, utilities, transportation, food assistance) to address the SDOH need(s). health education- helping the patient contextualize health education provided by the patient's treatment team with the patient's individual needs, goals, and preferences, in the context of the SDOH need(s), and educating the patient on how to best participate in medical decision-making. building patient self-advocacy skills, so that the patient can interact with members of the health care team and related community-based services addressing the SDOH need(s), in ways that are more likely to promote personalized and effective diagnosis or treatment. health care access / health system navigation. ++helping the patient access healthcare, including identifying appropriate practitioners or providers for clinical care and helping secure appointments with them. facilitating behavioral change as necessary for meeting diagnosis and treatment goals, including promoting patient motivation to participate in care and reach person-centered diagnosis or treatment goals. facilitating and providing social and emotional support to help the patient cope with the problem(s) addressed in the initiating visit, the SDOH need(s), and adjust daily routines to better meet diagnosis and treatment goals. leveraging lived experience when applicable to provide support, mentorship, or inspiration to meet treatment goals **S**

* **G0022** Community health integration services, each additional 30 minutes per calendar month (list separately in addition to G0019) **N**

* **G0023** Principal illness navigation services by certified or trained auxiliary personnel under the direction of a physician or other practitioner, including a patient navigator; 60 minutes per calendar month, in the following activities: person-centered assessment, performed to better understand the individual context of the serious, high-risk condition. ++ conducting a person-centered assessment to understand the patient's life story, strengths, needs, goals, preferences, and desired outcomes, including understanding cultural and linguistic factors and including unmet SDOH needs (that are not separately billed). ++ facilitating patient-driven goal setting and establishing an action plan. ++ providing tailored support as needed to accomplish the practitioner's treatment plan. identifying or referring patient (and caregiver or family, if applicable) to appropriate supportive services. practitioner, home, and community-based care coordination. ++ coordinating receipt of needed services from healthcare practitioners, providers, and facilities; home- and community-based service providers; and caregiver (if applicable). ++ communication with practitioners, home-, and community-based service providers, hospitals, and skilled nursing facilities (or other health care facilities) regarding the patient's psychosocial strengths and needs, functional deficits, goals, preferences, and desired outcomes, including cultural and linguistic factors. ++ coordination of care transitions between and among health care practitioners and settings, including transitions involving referral

---

MIPS	**Qp** Quantity Physician	**Qh** Quantity Hospital	♀ Female only
♂ Male only	**A** Age	DMEPOS	**A2-Z3** ASC Payment Indicator	**A-Y** ASC Status Indicator	Coding Clinic

to other clinicians; follow-up after an emergency department visit; or follow-up after discharges from hospitals, skilled nursing facilities or other health care facilities. ++ facilitating access to community-based social services (e.g., housing, utilities, transportation, food assistance) as needed to address SDOH need(s). health education- helping the patient contextualize health education provided by the patient's treatment team with the patient's individual needs, goals, preferences, and SDOH need(s), and educating the patient (and caregiver if applicable) on how to best participate in medical decision-making. building patient self-advocacy skills, so that the patient can interact with members of the health care team and related community-based services (as needed), in ways that are more likely to promote personalized and effective treatment of their condition. health care access / health system navigation. ++ helping the patient access healthcare, including identifying appropriate practitioners or providers for clinical care, and helping secure appointments with them. ++ providing the patient with information/ resources to consider participation in clinical trials or clinical research as applicable. facilitating behavioral change as necessary for meeting diagnosis and treatment goals, including promoting patient motivation to participate in care and reach person-centered diagnosis or treatment goals. facilitating and providing social and emotional support to help the patient cope with the condition, SDOH need(s), and adjust daily routines to better meet diagnosis and treatment goals. leverage knowledge of the serious, high-risk condition and/or lived experience when applicable to provide support, mentorship, or inspiration to meet treatment goals   S

* G0024   Principal illness navigation services, additional 30 minutes per calendar month (list separately in addition to G0023)   N

Semen Analysis

* G0027   Semen analysis; presence and/or motility of sperm excluding Huhner Ⓑ Qp Qh ♂   Q4
           Laboratory Certification: Hematology

* G0029   Tobacco screening not performed or tobacco cessation intervention not provided during the measurement period or in the six months prior to the measurement period   M

* G0030   Patient screened for tobacco use and received tobacco cessation intervention during the measurement period or in the six months prior to the measurement period (counseling, pharmacotherapy, or both), if identified as a tobacco user   M

* G0031   Palliative care services given to patient any time during the measurement period   M

* G0032   Two or more antipsychotic prescriptions ordered for patients who had a diagnosis of schizophrenia, schizoaffective disorder, or bipolar disorder on or between January 1 of the year prior to the measurement period and the index prescription start date (ipsd) for antipsychotics   M

* G0033   Two or more benzodiazepine prescriptions ordered for patients who had a diagnosis of seizure disorders, rapid eye movement sleep behavior disorder, benzodiazepine withdrawal, ethanol withdrawal, or severe generalized anxiety disorder on or between January 1 of the year prior to the measurement period and the ipsd for benzodiazepines   M

* G0034   Patients receiving palliative care during the measurement period   M

* G0035   Patient has any emergency department encounter during the performance period with place of service indicator 23   M

* G0036   Patient or care partner decline assessment   M

* G0037   On date of encounter, patient is not able to participate in assessment or screening, including non-verbal patients, delirious, severely aphasic, severely developmentally delayed, severe visual or hearing impairment and for those patients, no knowledgeable informant available   M

* G0038   Clinician determines patient does not require referral   M

* G0039   Patient not referred, reason not otherwise specified   M

* G0040   Patient already receiving physical/ occupational/speech/recreational therapy during the measurement period   M

* G0041   Patient and/or care partner decline referral   M

* G0042   Referral to physical, occupational, speech, or recreational therapy   M

* G0043   Patients with mechanical prosthetic heart valve   M

TEMPORARY PROCEDURES/PROFESSIONAL SERVICES

* G0044 Patients with moderate or severe mitral stenosis M
* G0045 Clinical follow-up and mrs score assessed at 90 days following endovascular stroke intervention M
* G0046 Clinical follow-up and mrs score not assessed at 90 days following endovascular stroke intervention M
* G0047 Pediatric patient with minor blunt head trauma and pecarn prediction criteria are not assessed M
* G0048 Patients who receive palliative care services any time during the intake period through the end of the measurement year M
* G0049 With maintenance hemodialysis (in-center and home hd) for the complete reporting month M
* G0050 Patients with a catheter that have limited life expectancy M
* G0051 Patients under hospice care in the current reporting month M
* G0052 Patients on peritoneal dialysis for any portion of the reporting month M
* G0053 Advancing rheumatology patient care mips value pathways M
* G0054 Coordinating stroke care to promote prevention and cultivate positive outcomes mips value pathways M
* G0055 Advancing care for heart disease mips value pathways M
* G0057 Proposed adopting best practices and promoting patient safety within emergency medicine mips value pathways M
* G0058 Improving care for lower extremity joint repair mips value pathways M
* G0059 Patient safety and support of positive experiences with anesthesia mips value pathways M
* G0060 Allergy/immunology mips specialty set M
* G0061 Anesthesiology mips specialty set M
* G0062 Audiology mips specialty set M
* G0063 Cardiology mips specialty set M
* G0064 Certified nurse midwife mips specialty set M
* G0065 Chiropractic medicine mips specialty set M
* G0066 Clinical social work mips specialty set M
* G0067 Dentistry mips specialty set M

Administration, Payment and Care Management Services

* G0068 Professional services for the administration of anti-infective, pain management, chelation, pulmonary hypertension, or other intravenous infusion drug or biological (excluding chemotherapy or other highly complex drug or biological) inotropic for each infusion drug administration calendar day in the individual's home, each 15 minutes A
* G0069 Professional services for the administration of subcutaneous immunotherapy or other subcutaneous infusion drug or biological for each infusion drug administration calendar day in the individual's home, each 15 minutes A
* G0070 Professional services for the administration of intravenous chemotherapy or other intravenous highly complex drug or biological infusion for each infusion drug administration calendar day in the individual's home, each 15 minutes A
* G0071 Payment for communication technology-based services for 5 minutes or more of a virtual (non-face-to-face) communication between an rural health clinic (RHC) or federally qualified health center (FQHC) practitioner and RHC or FQHC patient, or 5 minutes or more of remote evaluation of recorded video and/or images by an RHC or FQHC practitioner, occurring in lieu of an office visit; RHC or FQHC only A
* G0076 Brief (20 minutes) care management home visit for a new patient. For use only in a Medicare-approved CMMI model. (Services must be furnished within a beneficiary's home, domiciliary, rest home, assisted living and/or nursing facility.) B
* G0077 Limited (30 minutes) care management home visit for a new patient. For use only in a Medicare-approved CMMI model. (Services must be furnished within a beneficiary's home, domiciliary, rest home, assisted living and/or nursing facility.) B
* G0078 Moderate (45 minutes) care management home visit for a new patient. For use only in a Medicare-approved CMMI model. (Services must be furnished within a beneficiary's home, domiciliary, rest home, assisted living and/or nursing facility.) B

* **G0079** Comprehensive (60 minutes) care management home visit for a new patient. For use only in a Medicare-approved CMMI model. (Services must be furnished within a beneficiary's home, domiciliary, rest home, assisted living and/or nursing facility.) Ⓑ B

* **G0080** Extensive (75 minutes) care management home visit for a new patient. For use only in a Medicare-approved CMMI model. (Services must be furnished within a beneficiary's home, domiciliary, rest home, assisted living and/or nursing facility.) Ⓑ B

* **G0081** Brief (20 minutes) care management home visit for an existing patient. For use only in a Medicare-approved CMMI model. (Services must be furnished within a beneficiary's home, domiciliary, rest home, assisted living and/or nursing facility.) Ⓑ B

* **G0082** Limited (30 minutes) care management home visit for an existing patient. For use only in a Medicare-approved CMMI model. (Services must be furnished within a beneficiary's home, domiciliary, rest home, assisted living and/or nursing facility.) Ⓑ B

* **G0083** Moderate (45 minutes) care management home visit for an existing patient. For use only in a Medicare-approved CMMI model. (Services must be furnished within a beneficiary's home, domiciliary, rest home, assisted living and/or nursing facility.) Ⓑ B

* **G0084** Comprehensive (60 minutes) care management home visit for an existing patient. For use only in a Medicare-approved CMMI model. (Services must be furnished within a beneficiary's home, domiciliary, rest home, assisted living and/or nursing facility.) Ⓑ B

* **G0085** Extensive (75 minutes) care management home visit for an existing patient. For use only in a Medicare-approved CMMI model. (Services must be furnished within a beneficiary's home, domiciliary, rest home, assisted living and/or nursing facility.) Ⓑ B

* **G0086** Limited (30 minutes) care management home care plan oversight. For use only in a Medicare-approved CMMI model. (Services must be furnished within a beneficiary's home, domiciliary, rest home, assisted living and/or nursing facility.) Ⓑ B

* **G0087** Comprehensive (60 minutes) care management home care plan oversight. For use only in a Medicare-approved CMMI model. (Services must be furnished within a beneficiary's home, domiciliary, rest home, assisted living and/or nursing facility.) Ⓑ B

* **G0088** Professional services, initial visit, for the administration of anti-infective, pain management, chelation, pulmonary hypertension, inotropic, or other intravenous infusion drug or biological (excluding chemotherapy or other highly complex drug or biological) for each infusion drug administration calendar day in the individual's home, each 15 minutes A

* **G0089** Professional services, initial visit, for the administration of subcutaneous immunotherapy or other subcutaneous infusion drug or biological for each infusion drug administration calendar day in the individual's home, each 15 minutes A

* **G0090** Professional services, initial visit, for the administration of intravenous chemotherapy or other highly complex infusion drug or biological for each infusion drug administration calendar day in the individual's home, each 15 minutes A

Screening Services

G0101 Cervical or vaginal cancer screening; pelvic and clinical breast examination Ⓑ Qp Qh S

Covered once every two years and annually if high risk for cervical/vaginal cancer, or if childbearing age patient has had an abnormal Pap smear in preceding three years. High risk diagnosis, Z77.9

Coding Clinic: 2024, Q2, P35-36; 2002, Q4, P8

G0102 Prostate cancer screening; digital rectal examination Ⓑ Qp Qh N

Covered annually by Medicare (Z12.5). Not separately payable with an E/M code (99201-99499).

IOM: 100-02, 6, 10; 100-04, 4, 240; 100-04, 18, 50.1

G0103 Prostate cancer screening; prostate specific antigen test (PSA) Ⓑ Qp Qh A

Covered annually by Medicare (Z12.5)

IOM: 100-02, 6, 10; 100-04, 4, 240; 100-04, 18, 50

Laboratory Certification: Routine chemistry

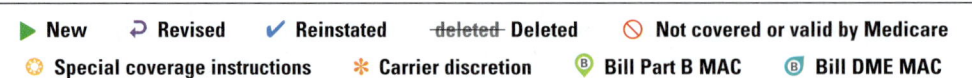

TEMPORARY PROCEDURES/PROFESSIONAL SERVICES

G0104 Colorectal cancer screening; flexible sigmoidoscopy ⓑ Qp Qh T

Covered once every 48 months for beneficiaries age 50+

Co-insurance waived under Section 4104.

Coding Clinic: 2011, Q2, P4

G0105 Colorectal cancer screening; colonoscopy on individual at high risk ⓑ Qp Qh T

Screening colonoscopy covered once every 24 months for high risk for developing colorectal cancer. May use modifier 53 if appropriate (physician fee schedule).

Co-insurance waived under Section 4104.

Coding Clinic: 2023, Q3, P12; 2018, Q2, P4; 2011, Q2, P4

~~G0106 Colorectal cancer screening; alternative to G0104, screening sigmoidoscopy, barium enema~~

Diabetes Management Training Services

G0108 Diabetes outpatient self-management training services, individual, per 30 minutes ⓑ Qp Qh A

Report for beneficiaries diagnosed with diabetes.

Effective January 2011, DSMT will be included in the list of reimbursable Medicare telehealth services.

G0109 Diabetes outpatient self-management training services, group session (2 or more) per 30 minutes Qp Qh A

Report for beneficiaries diagnosed with diabetes.

Effective January 2011, DSMT will be included in the list of reimbursable Medicare telehealth services.

Screening Services

G0117 Glaucoma screening for high risk patients furnished by an optometrist or ophthalmologist ⓑ Qp Qh S

Covered once per year (full 11 months between screenings). Bundled with all other ophthalmic services provided on same day. Diagnosis code Z13.5.

G0118 Glaucoma screening for high risk patient furnished under the direct supervision of an optometrist or ophthalmologist Qp Qh S

Covered once per year (full 11 months between screenings). Diagnosis code Z13.5.

~~G0120 Colorectal cancer screening; alternative to G0105, screening colonoscopy, barium enema.~~

G0121 Colorectal cancer screening; colonoscopy on individual not meeting criteria for high risk ⓑ Qp Qh T

Screening colonoscopy for patients that are not high risk. Covered once every 10 years, but not within 48 months of a G0104. For non-Medicare patients report 45378.

Co-insurance waived under Section 4104.

Coding Clinic: 2023, Q3, P12; 2018, Q2, P4

~~G0122 Colorectal cancer screening; barium enema~~

G0123 Screening cytopathology, cervical or vaginal (any reporting system), collected in preservative fluid, automated thin layer preparation, screening by cytotechnologist under physician supervision ⓑ Qp Qh ♀ A

Use G0123 or G0143 or G0144 or G0145 or G0147 or G0148 or P3000 for Pap smears NOT requiring physician interpretation (technical component).

IOM: 100-03, 3, 190.2; 100-04, 18, 30

Laboratory Certification: Cytology

G0124 Screening cytopathology, cervical or vaginal (any reporting system), collected in preservative fluid, automated thin layer preparation, requiring interpretation by physician ⓑ Qp Qh ♀ B

Report professional component for Pap smears requiring physician interpretation.

IOM: 100-03, 3, 190.2; 100-04, 18, 30

Laboratory Certification: Cytology

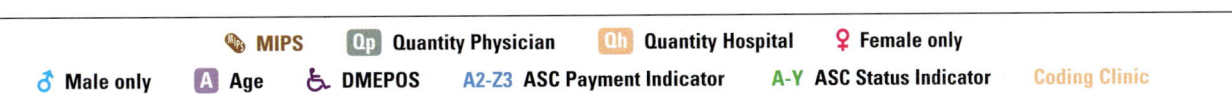

Miscellaneous Services, Diagnostic and Therapeutic

G0127 Trimming of dystrophic nails, any number ⓑ Qp Qh   Q1

Must be used with a modifier (Q7, Q8, or Q9) to show that the foot care service is needed because the beneficiary has a systemic disease. Limit 1 unit of service.

IOM: 100-02, 15, 290

G0128 Direct (face-to-face with patient) skilled nursing services of a registered nurse provided in a comprehensive outpatient rehabilitation facility, each 10 minutes beyond the first 5 minutes ⓑ Qp Qh   B

A separate nursing service that is clearly identifiable in the Plan of Treatment and not part of other services. Documentation must support this service. Examples include: Insertion of a urinary catheter, intramuscular injections, bowel disimpaction, nursing assessment, and education. Restricted coverage by Medicare.

Medicare Statute 1833(a)

G0129 Occupational therapy services requiring the skills of a qualified occupational therapist, furnished as a component of a partial hospitalization or intensive outpatient treatment program, per session (45 minutes or more) ⓑ Qh   P

G0130 Single energy x-ray absorptiometry (SEXA) bone density study, one or more sites; appendicular skeleton (peripheral) (e.g., radius, wrist, heel) ⓑ Qp Qh   Z3 S

Covered every 24 months (more frequently if medically necessary). Use modifier 26 for professional component only.

Preventive service; no deductible

IOM: 100-03, 2, 150.3; 100-04, 13, 140.1

G0136 Administration of a standardized, evidence-based social determinants of health risk assessment tool, 5-15 minutes   S

G0137 Intensive outpatient services; weekly bundle, minimum of 9 services over a 7 contiguous day period, which can include individual and group therapy with physicians or psychologists (or other mental health professionals to the extent authorized under state law); occupational therapy requiring the skills of a qualified occupational therapist; services of social workers, trained psychiatric nurses, and other staff trained to work with psychiatric patients; individualized activity therapies that are not primarily recreational or diversionary; family counseling (the primary purpose of which is treatment of the individual's condition); patient training and education (to the extent that training and educational activities are closely and clearly related to individual's care and treatment); diagnostic services; and such other items and services (excluding meals and transportation) that are reasonable and necessary for the diagnosis or active treatment of the individual's condition, reasonably expected to improve or maintain the individual's condition and functional level and to prevent relapse or hospitalization, and furnished pursuant to such guidelines relating to frequency and duration of services in accordance with a physician certification and plan of treatment (provision of the services by a Medicare-enrolled opioid treatment program); list separately in addition to code for primary procedure   A

G0138 Intravenous infusion of cipaglucosidase alfa-atga, including provider/supplier acquisition and clinical supervision of oral administration of miglustat in preparation of receipt of cipaglucosidase alfa-atga   S

G0140 Principal illness navigation - peer support by certified or trained auxiliary personnel under the direction of a physician or other practitioner, including a certified peer specialist; 60 minutes per calendar month, in the following activities: person-centered interview, performed to better understand the individual context of the serious, high-risk condition. ++ conducting a person-centered interview to understand the patient's life story, strengths, needs, goals, preferences, and desired outcomes, including understanding cultural and linguistic factors, and including unmet SDOH needs (that are not billed separately). ++ facilitating patient-driven goal setting and establishing an action plan. ++ providing tailored support as needed to accomplish the person-centered goals in the practitioner's treatment plan. identifying or referring patient (and caregiver or family, if applicable) to appropriate supportive services. practitioner, home, and community-based care communication. ++ assist the patient in communicating with their practitioners, home-, and community-based service providers, hospitals, and skilled nursing facilities (or other health

---

▶ New   ⟲ Revised   ✓ Reinstated   ~~deleted~~ Deleted   ⊘ Not covered or valid by Medicare
✪ Special coverage instructions   ✻ Carrier discretion   ⓑ Bill Part B MAC   ⓑ Bill DME MAC

TEMPORARY PROCEDURES/PROFESSIONAL SERVICES

care facilities) regarding the patient's psychosocial strengths and needs, goals, preferences, and desired outcomes, including cultural and linguistic factors. ++ facilitating access to community-based social services (e.g., housing, utilities, transportation, food assistance) as needed to address SDOH need(s). health education. helping the patient contextualize health education provided by the patient's treatment team with the patient's individual needs, goals, preferences, and SDOH need(s), and educating the patient (and caregiver if applicable) on how to best participate in medical decision-making. building patient self-advocacy skills, so that the patient can interact with members of the health care team and related community-based services (as needed), in ways that are more likely to promote personalized and effective treatment of their condition. developing and proposing strategies to help meet person-centered treatment goals and supporting the patient in using chosen strategies to reach person-centered treatment goals. facilitating and providing social and emotional support to help the patient cope with the condition, SDOH need(s), and adjust daily routines to better meet person-centered diagnosis and treatment goals. leverage knowledge of the serious, high-risk condition and/or lived experience when applicable to provide support, mentorship, or inspiration to meet treatment goals **S**

* **G0141** Screening cytopathology smears, cervical or vaginal, performed by automated system, with manual rescreening, requiring interpretation by physician ⓑ Qp Qh ♀ **B**

Co-insurance, copay, and deductible waived

Report professional component for Pap smears requiring physician interpretation. Refer to diagnosis of Z92.89, Z12.4, Z12.72, or Z12.89 to report appropriate risk level.

Laboratory Certification: Cytology

* **G0143** Screening cytopathology, cervical or vaginal (any reporting system), collected in preservative fluid, automated thin layer preparation, with manual screening and rescreening by cytotechnologist under physician supervision ⓑ Qp Qh ♀ **A**

Co-insurance, copay, and deductible waived

Laboratory Certification: Cytology

* **G0144** Screening cytopathology, cervical or vaginal (any reporting system), collected in preservative fluid, automated thin layer preparation, with screening by automated system, under physician supervision ⓑ Qp Qh ♀ **A**

Co-insurance, copay, and deductible waived

Laboratory Certification: Cytology

* **G0145** Screening cytopathology, cervical or vaginal (any reporting system), collected in preservative fluid, automated thin layer preparation, with screening by automated system and manual rescreening under physician supervision ⓑ Qp Qh ♀ **A**

Co-insurance, copay, and deductible waived

Laboratory Certification: Cytology

G0146 Principal illness navigation - peer support, additional 30 minutes per calendar month (list separately in addition to G0140) **N**

* **G0147** Screening cytopathology smears, cervical or vaginal; performed by automated system under physician supervision ⓑ Qp Qh ♀ **A**

Co-insurance, copay, and deductible waived

Laboratory Certification: Cytology

* **G0148** Screening cytopathology smears, cervical or vaginal; performed by automated system with manual rescreening ⓑ Qp Qh ♀ **A**

Co-insurance, copay, and deductible waived

Laboratory Certification: Cytology

* **G0151** Services performed by a qualified physical therapist in the home health or hospice setting, each 15 minutes ⓑ **B**

* **G0152** Services performed by a qualified occupational therapist in the home health or hospice setting, each 15 minutes ⓑ **B**

* **G0153** Services performed by a qualified speech-language pathologist in the home health or hospice setting, each 15 minutes ⓑ **B**

 * **G0155** Services of clinical social worker in home health or hospice settings, each 15 minutes ⓑ **B**

* **G0156** Services of home health/health aide in home health or hospice settings, each 15 minutes ⓑ **B**

* **G0157** Services performed by a qualified physical therapist assistant in the home health or hospice setting, each 15 minutes ⓑ **B**

| 🪙 MIPS | Qp Quantity Physician | Qh Quantity Hospital | ♀ Female only |
| ♂ Male only | Ⓐ Age | ♿ DMEPOS | A2-Z3 ASC Payment Indicator | A-Y ASC Status Indicator | Coding Clinic |

* G0158	Services performed by a qualified occupational therapist assistant in the home health or hospice setting, each 15 minutes ⓑ B
* G0159	Services performed by a qualified physical therapist, in the home health setting, in the establishment or delivery of a safe and effective physical therapy maintenance program, each 15 minutes ⓑ B
* G0160	Services performed by a qualified occupational therapist, in the home health setting, in the establishment or delivery of a safe and effective occupational therapy maintenance program, each 15 minutes ⓑ B
* G0161	Services performed by a qualified speech-language pathologist, in the home health setting, in the establishment or delivery of a safe and effective speech-language pathology maintenance program, each 15 minutes ⓑ B
* G0162	Skilled services by a registered nurse (RN) for management and evaluation of the plan of care; each 15 minutes (the patient's underlying condition or complication requires an RN to ensure that essential non-skilled care achieves its purpose in the home health or hospice setting) ⓑ B

Transmittal No. 824 (CR7182)

⊙ G0166	External counterpulsation, per treatment session ⓑ Qp Qh Q1

IOM: 100-03, 1, 20.20

⊙ * G0168	Wound closure utilizing tissue adhesive(s) only ⓑ Qp Qh B

Report for wound closure with only tissue adhesive. If a practitioner utilizes tissue adhesive in addition to staples or sutures to close a wound, HCPCS code G0168 is not separately reportable, but is included in the tissue repair.

The only closure material used for a simple repair, coverage based on payer.

Coding Clinic: 2005, Q1, P5; 2001, Q4, P12; Q3, P13

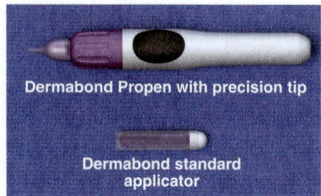

Figure 15 Tissue adhesive.

* G0175	Scheduled interdisciplinary team conference (minimum of three exclusive of patient care nursing staff) with patient present ⓑ Qp Qh V
⊙ G0176	Activity therapy, such as music, dance, art or play therapies not for recreation, related to the care and treatment of patient's disabling mental health problems, per session (45 minutes or more) ⓑ Qh P

Paid in partial hospitalization

⊙ G0177	Training and educational services related to the care and treatment of patient's disabling mental health problems per session (45 minutes or more) ⓑ Qp Qh N

Paid in partial hospitalization

* G0179	Physician recertification for Medicare-covered home health services under a home health plan of care (patient not present), including contacts with home health agency and review of reports of patient status required by physicians to affirm the initial implementation of the plan of care that meets patient's needs, per recertification period ⓑ Qp Qh M

The recertification code is used after a patient has received services for at least 60 days (or one certification period) when the physician signs the certification after the initial certification period.

* G0180	Physician certification for Medicare-covered home health services under a home health plan of care (patient not present), including contacts with home health agency and review of reports of patient status required by physicians to affirm the initial implementation of the plan of care that meets patient's needs, per certification period ⓑ Qp Qh M

This code can be billed only when the patient has not received Medicare covered home health services for at least 60 days.

* G0181	Physician supervision of a patient receiving Medicare-covered services provided by a participating home health agency (patient not present) requiring complex and multidisciplinary care modalities involving regular physician development and/or revision of care plans, review of subsequent reports of patient status, review of laboratory and other studies, communication (including telephone calls) with other health care professionals involved in the patient's care, integration of new information into the medical treatment plan and/or adjustment of medical therapy, within a calendar month, 30 minutes or more ⓑ Qp Qh M

Coding Clinic: 2015, Q2, P10

▶ New ↻ Revised ✓ Reinstated ~~deleted~~ Deleted ⊘ Not covered or valid by Medicare
⊙ Special coverage instructions * Carrier discretion ⓑ Bill Part B MAC Ⓑ Bill DME MAC

TEMPORARY PROCEDURES/PROFESSIONAL SERVICES

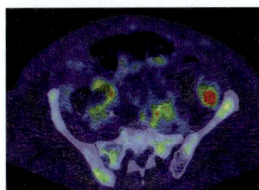

Figure 16 PET scan.

* **G0182** Physician supervision of a patient under a Medicare-approved hospice (patient not present) requiring complex and multidisciplinary care modalities involving regular physician development and/or revision of care plans, review of subsequent reports of patient status, review of laboratory and other studies, communication (including telephone calls) with other health care professionals involved in the patient's care, integration of new information into the medical treatment plan and/or adjustment of medical therapy, within a calendar month, 30 minutes or more ⓑ Qp Qh M

  Coding Clinic: 2015, Q2, P10

▶ * **G0183** Quantitative software measurements of cardiac volume, cardiac chambers volumes and left ventricular wall mass derived from ct scan(s) data of the chest/heart (with or without contrast) ⓑ Qp Qh S

* **G0186** Destruction of localized lesion of choroid (for example, choroidal neovascularization); photocoagulation, feeder vessel technique (one or more sessions) ⓑ Qp Qh T

⊘ **G0219** PET imaging whole body; melanoma for non-covered indications ⓑ E1

  Example: Assessing regional lymph nodes in melanoma.

  IOM: 100-03, 4, 220.6

  Coding Clinic: 2007, Q1, P6

⊘ **G0235** PET imaging, any site, not otherwise specified ⓑ Qp Qh S

  Example: Prostate cancer diagnosis and initial staging.

  IOM: 100-03, 4, 220.6

  Coding Clinic: 2007, Q1, P6

* **G0237** Therapeutic procedures to increase strength or endurance of respiratory muscles, face to face, one on one, each 15 minutes (includes monitoring) ⓑ Qp Qh S

* **G0238** Therapeutic procedures to improve respiratory function, other than described by G0237, one on one, face to face, per 15 minutes (includes monitoring) ⓑ Qp Qh S

* **G0239** Therapeutic procedures to improve respiratory function or increase strength or endurance of respiratory muscles, two or more individuals (includes monitoring) ⓑ Qp Qh S

● ○ **G0245** Initial physician evaluation and management of a diabetic patient with diabetic sensory neuropathy resulting in a loss of protective sensation (LOPS) which must include (1) the diagnosis of LOPS, (2) a patient history, (3) a physical examination that consist of at least the following elements: (A) visual inspection of the forefoot, hindfoot and toe web spaces, (B) evaluation of a protective sensation, (C) evaluation of foot structure and biomechanics, (D) evaluation of vascular status and skin integrity, and (E) evaluation and recommendation of footwear, and (4) patient education ⓑ Qp Qh V

  IOM: 100-03, 1, 70.2.1

● ○ **G0246** Follow-up physician evaluation and management of a diabetic patient with diabetic sensory neuropathy resulting in a loss of protective sensation (LOPS) to include at least the following: (1) a patient history, (2) a physical examination that includes: (A) visual inspection of the forefoot, hindfoot and toe web spaces, (B) evaluation of protective sensation, (C) evaluation of foot structure and biomechanics, (D) evaluation of vascular status and skin integrity, and (E) evaluation and recommendation of footwear, and (3) patient education ⓑ Qp Qh V

  IOM: 100-03, 1, 70.2.1; 100-02, 15, 290

● ○ **G0247** Routine foot care by a physician of a diabetic patient with diabetic sensory neuropathy resulting in a loss of protective sensation (LOPS) to include, the local care of superficial wounds (i.e., superficial to muscle and fascia) and at least the following if present: (1) local care of superficial wounds, (2) debridement of corns and calluses, and (3) trimming and debridement of nails ⓑ Qp Qh Q1

  IOM: 100-03, 1, 70.2.1

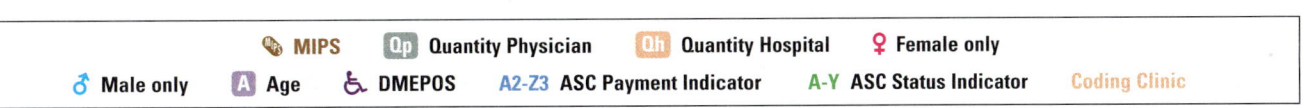

✪ **G0248**	Demonstration, prior to initiation, of home INR monitoring for patient with either mechanical heart valve(s), chronic atrial fibrillation, or venous thromboembolism who meets Medicare coverage criteria, under the direction of a physician; includes: face-to-face demonstration of use and care of the INR monitor, obtaining at least one blood sample, provision of instructions for reporting home INR test results, and documentation of patient's ability to perform testing and report results ⓑ Qp Qh **V**	✪ **G0260**	Injection procedure for sacroiliac joint; provision of anesthetic, steroid and/or other therapeutic agent, with or without arthrography ⓑ Qp Qh **T**

ASCs report when a therapeutic sacroiliac joint injection is administered in ASC |
| | | ✱ **G0268** | Removal of impacted cerumen (one or both ears) by physician on same date of service as audiologic function testing ⓑ Qp Qh **N**

Report only when a physician, not an audiologist, performs the procedure.

Use with DX H61.2- when performed by physician.

Coding Clinic: 2016, Q2, P2-3; 2003, Q1, P12 |
| ✪ **G0249** | Provision of test materials and equipment for home INR monitoring of patient with either mechanical heart valve(s), chronic atrial fibrillation, or venous thromboembolism who meets Medicare coverage criteria; includes provision of materials for use in the home and reporting of test results to physician; testing not occurring more frequently than once a week; testing materials, billing units of service include 4 tests ⓑ Qp Qh **V** | ✪ **G0269** | Placement of occlusive device into either a venous or arterial access site, post surgical or interventional procedure (e.g., angioseal plug, vascular plug) ⓑ Qh **N**

Report for replacement of vasoseal. Hospitals may report the closure device as a supply with C1760. Bundled status on Physician Fee Schedule.

Coding Clinic: 2011, Q3, P4; 2010, Q4, P6 |
| ✪ **G0250** | Physician review, interpretation, and patient management of home INR testing for patient with either mechanical heart valve(s), chronic atrial fibrillation, or venous thromboembolism who meets Medicare coverage criteria; testing not occurring more frequently than once a week; billing units of service include 4 tests ⓑ Qp Qh **M** | ✱ **G0270** | Medical nutrition therapy; reassessment and subsequent intervention(s) following second referral in same year for change in diagnosis, medical condition or treatment regimen (including additional hours needed for renal disease), individual, face to face with the patient, each 15 minutes ⓑ Qp Qh **A**

Requires physician referral for beneficiaries with diabetes or renal disease. Services must be provided by dietitian/nutritionist. Co-insurance and deductible waived. |
| 🚫 **G0252** | PET imaging, full and partial-ring PET scanners only, for initial diagnosis of breast cancer and/or surgical planning for breast cancer (e.g., initial staging of axillary lymph nodes) ⓑ **E1**

IOM: 100-03, 4, 220.6

Coding Clinic: 2007, Q1, P6 | | |
| 🚫 **G0255** | Current perception threshold/sensory nerve conduction test (SNCT), per limb, any nerve ⓑ **E1**

IOM: 100-03, 2, 160.23 | ✱ **G0271** | Medical nutrition therapy, reassessment and subsequent intervention(s) following second referral in same year for change in diagnosis, medical condition, or treatment regimen (including additional hours needed for renal disease), group (2 or more individuals), each 30 minutes ⓑ Qp Qh **A**

Requires physician referral for beneficiaries with diabetes or renal disease. Services must be provided by dietitian/nutritionist. Co-insurance and deductible waived. |
| ✪ **G0257** | Unscheduled or emergency dialysis treatment for an ESRD patient in a hospital outpatient department that is not certified as an ESRD facility ⓑ Qp Qh **S**

Coding Clinic: 2003, Q1, P9 | | |
| ✪ **G0259** | Injection procedure for sacroiliac joint; arthrography ⓑ Qp Qh **N**

Replaces 27096 for reporting injections for Medicare beneficiaries

Used by Part A only (facility), not priced by Part B Medicare. | ✪ **G0276** | Blinded procedure for lumbar stenosis, percutaneous image-guided lumbar decompression (PILD) or placebo-control, performed in an approved coverage with evidence development (CED) clinical trial ⓑ Qp Qh **J1** |

▶ New   ⤻ Revised   ✓ Reinstated   ~~deleted~~ Deleted   🚫 Not covered or valid by Medicare
✪ Special coverage instructions   ✱ Carrier discretion   ⓑ Bill Part B MAC   Ⓑ Bill DME MAC

TEMPORARY PROCEDURES/PROFESSIONAL SERVICES

⊙ **G0277** Hyperbaric oxygen under pressure, full body chamber, per 30 minute interval ⓑ Qp Qh S

IOM: 100-03, 1, 20.29

Coding Clinic: 2015, Q3, P7

◆* **G0278** Iliac and/or femoral artery angiography, non-selective, bilateral or ipsilateral to catheter insertion, performed at the same time as cardiac catheterization and/or coronary angiography, includes positioning or placement of the catheter in the distal aorta or ipsilateral femoral or iliac artery, injection of dye, production of permanent images, and radiologic supervision and interpretation (list separately in addition to primary procedure) ⓑ Qp Qh N

Medicare specific code not reported for iliac injection used as a guiding shot for a closure device

Coding Clinic: 2011, Q3, P4; 2006, Q4, P7

* **G0279** Diagnostic digital breast tomosynthesis, unilateral or bilateral (list separately in addition to 77065 or 77066) ⓑ A

* **G0281** Electrical stimulation, (unattended), to one or more areas, for chronic stage III and stage IV pressure ulcers, arterial ulcers, diabetic ulcers, and venous stasis ulcers not demonstrating measurable signs of healing after 30 days of conventional care, as part of a therapy plan of care ⓑ Qp Qh A

Reported by encounter/areas and not by site. Therapists report G0281 and G0283 rather than 97014.

⊘ **G0282** Electrical stimulation, (unattended), to one or more areas, for wound care other than described in G0281 ⓑ E1

IOM: 100-03, 4, 270.1

* **G0283** Electrical stimulation (unattended), to one or more areas for indication(s) other than wound care, as part of a therapy plan of care ⓑ Qp Qh A

Reported by encounter/areas and not by site. Therapists report G0281 and G0283 rather than 97014.

* **G0288** Reconstruction, computed tomographic angiography of aorta for surgical planning for vascular surgery ⓑ Qp Qh N

* **G0289** Arthroscopy, knee, surgical, for removal of loose body, foreign body, debridement/shaving of articular cartilage (chondroplasty) at the time of other surgical knee arthroscopy in a different compartment of the same knee ⓑ Qp Qh N

Add-on code reported with knee arthroscopy code for major procedure performed-reported once per extra compartment

"The code may be reported twice (or with a unit of two) if the physician performs these procedures in two compartments, in addition to the compartment where the main procedure was performed." (http://www.ama-assn.org/resources/doc/cpt/orthopaedics.pdf)

⊙ **G0293** Noncovered surgical procedure(s) using conscious sedation, regional, general or spinal anesthesia in a Medicare qualifying clinical trial, per day ⓑ Qp Qh Q1

⊙ **G0294** Noncovered procedure(s) using either no anesthesia or local anesthesia only, in a Medicare qualifying clinical trial, per day ⓑ Qp Qh Q1

⊘ **G0295** Electromagnetic therapy, to one or more areas, for wound care other than described in G0329 or for other uses ⓑ E1

IOM: 100-03, 4, 270.1

* **G0296** Counseling visit to discuss need for lung cancer screening (LDCT) using low dose CT scan (service is for eligibility determination and shared decision making) ⓑ Qp Qh S

* **G0299** Direct skilled nursing services of a registered nurse (RN) in the home health or hospice setting, each 15 minutes ⓑ B

* **G0300** Direct skilled nursing services of a licensed practical nurse (LPN) in the home health or hospice setting, each 15 minutes ⓑ B

* **G0302** Pre-operative pulmonary surgery services for preparation for LVRS, complete course of services, to include a minimum of 16 days of services ⓑ Qp Qh S

* **G0303** Pre-operative pulmonary surgery services for preparation for LVRS, 10 to 15 days of services ⓑ Qp Qh S

* **G0304** Pre-operative pulmonary surgery services for preparation for LVRS, 1 to 9 days of services ⓑ Qp Qh S

* **G0305** Post-discharge pulmonary surgery services after LVRS, minimum of 6 days of services ⓑ Qp Qh S

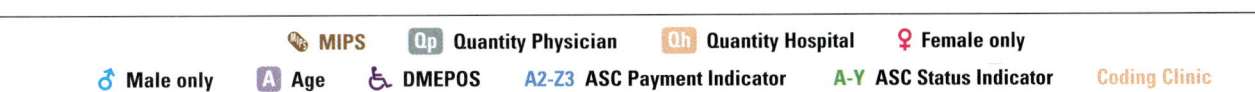

| ♦ MIPS | Qp Quantity Physician | Qh Quantity Hospital | ♀ Female only |
| ♂ Male only | Ⓐ Age | ♿ DMEPOS | A2-Z3 ASC Payment Indicator | A-Y ASC Status Indicator | Coding Clinic |

205

* **G0306** Complete CBC, automated (HgB, HCT, RBC, WBC, without platelet count) and automated WBC differential count ⓑ Qp Qh Q4
Laboratory Certification: Hematology

* **G0307** Complete CBC, automated (HgB, HCT, RBC, WBC; without platelet count) ⓑ Qp Qh Q4
Laboratory Certification: Hematology

G0310 Immunization counseling by a physician or other qualified health care professional when the vaccine(s) is not administered on the same date of service, 5 to 15 mins time (this code is used for Medicaid billing purposes) E1

G0311 Immunization counseling by a physician or other qualified health care professional when the vaccine(s) is not administered on the same date of service, 16-30 mins time (this code is used for Medicaid billing purposes) E1

G0312 Immunization counseling by a physician or other qualify ED health care professional when the vaccine(s) is not administered on the same date of service for ages under 21, 5 to 15 mins time (this code is used for Mcdicaid billing purposes) E1

G0313 Immunization counseling by a physician or other qualified health care professional when the vaccine(s) is not administered on the same date of service for ages under 21, 16-30 mins time (this code is used for Medicaid billing purposes) E1

G0314 Immunization counseling by a physician or other qualified health care professional for covid-19, ages under 21, 16-30 mins time (this code is used for the medicaid early and periodic screening, diagnostic, and treatment benefit [EPSDT]) E1

G0315 Immunization counseling by a physician or other qualified health care professional for covid-19, ages under 21, 5-15 mins time (this code is used for the medicaid early and periodic screening, diagnostic, and treatment benefit [EPSDT]) E1

G0316 Prolonged hospital inpatient or observation care evaluation and management service(s) beyond the total time for the primary service (when the primary service has been selected using time on the date of the primary service); each additional 15 minutes by the physician or qualified healthcare professional, with or without direct patient contact (list separately in addition to CPT codes 99223, 99233, and 99236 for hospital inpatient or observation care evaluation and management services). (do not report G0316 on the same date of service as other prolonged services for evaluation and management 99358, 99359, 99418, 99415, 99416). (do not report G0316 for any time unit less than 15 minutes) N

G0317 Prolonged nursing facility evaluation and management service(s) beyond the total time for the primary service (when the primary service has been selected using time on the date of the primary service); each additional 15 minutes by the physician or qualified healthcare professional, with or without direct patient contact (list separately in addition to CPT codes 99306, 99310 for nursing facility evaluation and management services). (do not report G0317 on the same date of service as other prolonged services for evaluation and management 99358, 99359, 99418). (do not report G0317 for any time unit less than 15 minutes) B

G0318 Prolonged home or residence evaluation and management service(s) beyond the total time for the primary service (when the primary service has been selected using time on the date of the primary service); each additional 15 minutes by the physician or qualified healthcare professional, with or without direct patient contact (list separately in addition to CPT codes 99345, 99350 for home or residence evaluation and management services). (do not report G0318 on the same date of service as other prolonged services for evaluation and management 99358, 99359, 99417). (do not report G0318 for any time unit less than 15 minutes) B

G0320 Home health services furnished using synchronous telemedicine rendered via a real-time two-way audio and video telecommunications system A

▶ New   ⤺ Revised   ✔ Reinstated   ~~deleted~~ Deleted   ⊘ Not covered or valid by Medicare
Ⓢ Special coverage instructions   * Carrier discretion   ⓑ Bill Part B MAC   Ⓑ Bill DME MAC

TEMPORARY PROCEDURES/PROFESSIONAL SERVICES

G0321 Home health services furnished using synchronous telemedicine rendered via telephone or other real-time interactive audio-only telecommunications system A

G0322 The collection of physiologic data digitally stored and/or transmitted by the patient to the home health agency (i.e., remote patient monitoring) A

G0323 Care management services for behavioral health conditions, at least 20 minutes of clinical psychologist, clinical social worker time, mental health counselor, or marriage and family therapist time, per calendar month. (these services include the following required elements: initial assessment or follow-up monitoring, including the use of applicable validated rating scales; behavioral health care planning in relation to behavioral/psychiatric health problems, including revision for patients who are not progressing or whose status changes; facilitating and coordinating treatment such as psychotherapy, coordination with and/or referral to physicians and practitioners who are authorized by Medicare to prescribe medications and furnish E/M services, counseling and/or psychiatric consultation; and continuity of care with a designated member of the care team) S

* G0327 Colorectal cancer screening; blood-based biomarker A

⊛ G0328 Colorectal cancer screening; fecal occult blood test, immunoassay, 1-3 simultaneous ⑧ Qp Qh A

Co-insurance and deductible waived

Reported for Medicare patients 501; one FOBT per year, with either G0107 (guaiac-based) or G0328 (immunoassay-based)

Laboratory Certification: Routine chemistry, Hematology

Coding Clinic: 2023, Q3, P12; 2012, Q2, P9

* G0329 Electromagnetic therapy, to one or more areas for chronic stage III and stage IV pressure ulcers, arterial ulcers, and diabetic ulcers and venous stasis ulcers not demonstrating measurable signs of healing after 30 days of conventional care as part of a therapy plan of care ⑧ Qp Qh A

G0330 Facility services for dental rehabilitation procedure(s) performed on a patient who requires monitored anesthesia (e.g., general, intravenous sedation (monitored anesthesia care) and use of an operating room J1

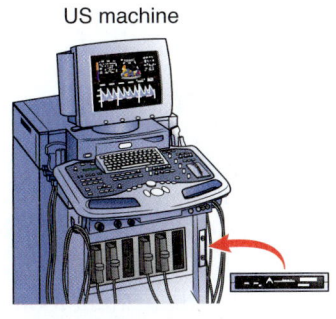

Figure 17 Electromagnetic device.

⊛ G0333 Pharmacy dispensing fee for inhalation drug(s); initial 30-day supply as a beneficiary ⑧ Qp Qh M

Medicare will reimburse an initial dispensing fee to a pharmacy for initial 30-day period of inhalation drugs furnished through DME.

* G0337 Hospice evaluation and counseling services, pre-election ⑧ Qp Qh B

* G0339 Image-guided robotic linear accelerator-based stereotactic radiosurgery, complete course of therapy in one session or first session of fractionated treatment ⑧ Qp Qh B

* G0340 Image-guided robotic linear accelerator-based stereotactic radiosurgery, delivery including collimator changes and custom plugging, fractionated treatment, all lesions, per session, second through fifth sessions, maximum five sessions per course of treatment ⑧ Qp Qh B

⊛ G0341 Percutaneous islet cell transplant, includes portal vein catheterization and infusion ⑧ Qp Qh C

IOM: 100-03, 4, 260.3; 100-04, 32, 70

⊛ G0342 Laparoscopy for islet cell transplant, includes portal vein catheterization and infusion ⑧ Qp Qh C

IOM: 100-03, 4, 260.3

⊛ G0343 Laparotomy for islet cell transplant, includes portal vein catheterization and infusion ⑧ Qp Qh C

IOM: 100-03, 4, 260.3

⊛ G0372 Physician service required to establish and document the need for a power mobility device ⑧ Qp Qh M

Providers should bill the E/M code and G0372 on the same claim.

🟢 MIPS Qp Quantity Physician Qh Quantity Hospital ♀ Female only
♂ Male only A Age ♿ DMEPOS A2-Z3 ASC Payment Indicator A-Y ASC Status Indicator Coding Clinic

Hospital Services: Observation and Emergency Department

○ **G0378** Hospital observation service, per hour Ⓑ Qh N

Report all related services in addition to G0378. Report units of hours spent in observation (rounded to the nearest hour). Hospitals report the ED or clinic visit with a CPT code or, if applicable, G0379 (direct admit to observation) and G0378 (hospital observation services, per hour).

Coding Clinic: 2007, Q1, P10; 2006, Q3, P7-8

○ **G0379** Direct admission of patient for hospital observation care Ⓑ Qp Qh J2

Report all related services in addition to G0379. Report units of hours spent in observation (rounded to the nearest hour). Hospitals report the ED or clinic visit with a CPT code or, if applicable, G0379 (direct admit to observation) and G0378 (hospital observation services, per hour).

Coding Clinic: 2007, Q1, P7

✱ **G0380** Level 1 hospital emergency department visit provided in a type B emergency department; (the ED must meet at least one of the following requirements: (1) it is licensed by the state in which it is located under applicable state law as an emergency room or emergency department; (2) it is held out to the public (by name, posted signs, advertising, or other means) as a place that provides care for emergency medical conditions on an urgent basis without requiring a previously scheduled appointment; or (3) during the calendar year immediately preceding the calendar year in which a determination under 42 CFR 489.24 is being made, based on a representative sample of patient visits that occurred during that calendar year, it provides at least one-third of all of its outpatient visits for the treatment of emergency medical conditions on an urgent basis without requiring a previously scheduled appointment) Ⓑ Qh J2

Coding Clinic: 2009, Q1, P4; 2007, Q2, P1

✱ **G0381** Level 2 hospital emergency department visit provided in a type B emergency department; (the ED must meet at least one of the following requirements: (1) it is licensed by the state in which it is located under applicable state law as an emergency room or emergency department; (2) it is held out to the public (by name, posted signs, advertising, or other means) as a place that provides care for emergency medical conditions on an urgent basis without requiring a previously scheduled appointment; or (3) during the calendar year immediately preceding the calendar year in which a determination under 42 CFR 489.24 is being made, based on a representative sample of patient visits that occurred during that calendar year, it provides at least one-third of all of its outpatient visits for the treatment of emergency medical conditions on an urgent basis without requiring a previously scheduled appointment) Ⓑ Qh J2

Coding Clinic: 2009, Q1, P4; 2007, Q2, P1

✱ **G0382** Level 3 hospital emergency department visit provided in a type B emergency department; (the ED must meet at least one of the following requirements: (1) it is licensed by the state in which it is located under applicable state law as an emergency room or emergency department; (2) it is held out to the public (by name, posted signs, advertising, or other means) as a place that provides care for emergency medical conditions on an urgent basis without requiring a previously scheduled appointment; or (3) during the calendar year immediately preceding the calendar year in which a determination under 42 CFR 489.24 is being made, based on a representative sample of patient visits that occurred during that calendar year, it provides at least one-third of all of its outpatient visits for the treatment of emergency medical conditions on an urgent basis without requiring a previously scheduled appointment) Ⓑ Qh J2

Coding Clinic: 2009, Q1, P4; 2007, Q2, P1

▶ New   ↻ Revised   ✓ Reinstated   ~~deleted~~ Deleted   ⊘ Not covered or valid by Medicare
○ Special coverage instructions   ✱ Carrier discretion   Ⓑ Bill Part B MAC   Ⓑ Bill DME MAC

TEMPORARY PROCEDURES/PROFESSIONAL SERVICES

* **G0383** Level 4 hospital emergency department visit provided in a type B emergency department; (the ED must meet at least one of the following requirements: (1) it is licensed by the state in which it is located under applicable state law as an emergency room or emergency department; (2) it is held out to the public (by name, posted signs, advertising, or other means) as a place that provides care for emergency medical conditions on an urgent basis without requiring a previously scheduled appointment; or (3) during the calendar year immediately preceding the calendar year in which a determination under 42 CFR 489.24 is being made, based on a representative sample of patient visits that occurred during that calendar year, it provides at least one-third of all of its outpatient visits for the treatment of emergency medical conditions on an urgent basis without requiring a previously scheduled appointment) B Qh   J2

  Coding Clinic: 2009, Q1, P4; 2007, Q2, P1

* **G0384** Level 5 hospital emergency department visit provided in a type B emergency department; (the ED must meet at least one of the following requirements: (1) it is licensed by the state in which it is located under applicable state law as an emergency room or emergency department; (2) it is held out to the public (by name, posted signs, advertising, or other means) as a place that provides care for emergency medical conditions on an urgent basis without requiring a previously scheduled appointment; or (3) during the calendar year immediately preceding the calendar year in which a determination under 42 CFR 489.24 is being made, based on a representative sample of patient visits that occurred during that calendar year, it provides at least one-third of all of its outpatient visits for the treatment of emergency medical conditions on an urgent basis without requiring a previously scheduled appointment) B Qh   J2

  Coding Clinic: 2009, Q1, P4; 2007, Q2, P1

Trauma Response Team

* **G0390** Trauma response team associated with hospital critical care service B Qh   S

  Coding Clinic: 2007, Q2, P5

Alcohol Substance Abuse Assessment and Intervention

* **G0396** Alcohol and/or substance (other than tobacco) misuse structured assessment (e.g., audit) and brief intervention 15 to 30 minutes B Qp Qh   S

  Bill instead of 99408 and 99409

* **G0397** Alcohol and/or substance (other than tobacco) misuse structured assessment (e.g., audit) and intervention, greater than 30 minutes B Qp Qh   S

  Bill instead of 99408 and 99409

Home Sleep Study Test

* **G0398** Home sleep study test (HST) with type II portable monitor, unattended; minimum of 7 channels: EEG, EOG, EMG, ECG/heart rate, airflow, respiratory effort and oxygen saturation B Qp Qh   S

* **G0399** Home sleep test (HST) with type III portable monitor, unattended; minimum of 4 channels: 2 respiratory movement/airflow, 1 ECG/heart rate and 1 oxygen saturation B Qp Qh   S

* **G0400** Home sleep test (HST) with type IV portable monitor, unattended; minimum of 3 channels B Qp Qh   S

Initial Examination for Medicare Enrollment

* **G0402** Initial preventive physical examination; face-to-face visit, services limited to new beneficiary during the first 12 months of Medicare enrollment B Qp Qh   V

  Depending on circumstances, 99201-99215 may be assigned with modifier 25 to report an E/M service as a significant, separately identifiable service in addition to the Initial Preventive Physical Examination (IPPE), G0402.

  Copayment and coinsurance waived, deductible waived.

  Coding Clinic: 2009, Q4, P8

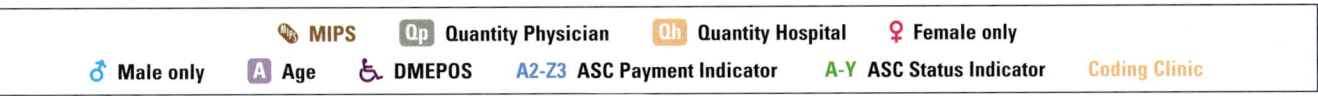

| MIPS | Qp Quantity Physician | Qh Quantity Hospital | ♀ Female only |
| ♂ Male only | A Age | DMEPOS | A2-Z3 ASC Payment Indicator | A-Y ASC Status Indicator | Coding Clinic |

Electrocardiogram

* **G0403** Electrocardiogram, routine ECG with 12 leads; performed as a screening for the initial preventive physical examination with interpretation and report Ⓑ Qp Qh M

   Optional service may be ordered or performed at discretion of physician. Once in a lifetime screening, stemming from a referral from Initial Preventive Physical Examination (IPPE). Both deductible and co-payment apply.

* **G0404** Electrocardiogram, routine ECG with 12 leads; tracing only, without interpretation and report, performed as a screening for the initial preventive physical examination Ⓑ Qp Qh S

* **G0405** Electrocardiogram, routine ECG with 12 leads; interpretation and report only, performed as a screening for the initial preventive physical examination Ⓑ Qp Qh B

Follow-up Telehealth Consultation

* **G0406** Follow-up inpatient consultation, limited, physicians typically spend 15 minutes communicating with the patient via telehealth Ⓑ Qp Qh B

   These telehealth modifiers are required when billing for telehealth services with codes G0406-G0408 and G0425-G0427:
   - GT, via interactive audio and video telecommunications system
   - GQ, via asynchronous telecommunications system

* **G0407** Follow-up inpatient consultation, intermediate, physicians typically spend 25 minutes communicating with the patient via telehealth Ⓑ Qp Qh B

* **G0408** Follow-up inpatient consultation, complex, physicians typically spend 35 minutes communicating with the patient via telehealth Ⓑ Qp Qh B

Psychological Services

* **G0409** Social work and psychological services, directly relating to and/or furthering the patient's rehabilitation goals, each 15 minutes, face-to-face; individual (services provided by a CORF-qualified social worker or psychologist in a CORF) Ⓑ B

* **G0410** Group psychotherapy other than of a multiple-family group, in a partial hospitalization or intensive outpatient setting, approximately 45 to 50 minutes Ⓑ Qp Qh P

   Coding Clinic: 2009, Q4, P9, 10

* **G0411** Interactive group psychotherapy, or intensive outpatient in a partial hospitalization setting, approximately 45 to 50 minutes Ⓑ Qp Qh P

   Coding Clinic: 2009, Q4, P9, 10

Fracture Treatment

* **G0412** Open treatment of iliac spine(s), tuberosity avulsion, or iliac wing fracture(s), unilateral or bilateral for pelvic bone fracture patterns which do not disrupt the pelvic ring, includes internal fixation, when performed Ⓑ Qp Qh C

* **G0413** Percutaneous skeletal fixation of posterior pelvic bone fracture and/or dislocation, for fracture patterns which disrupt the pelvic ring, unilateral or bilateral, (includes ilium, sacroiliac joint and/or sacrum) Ⓑ Qp Qh J1

* **G0414** Open treatment of anterior pelvic bone fracture and/or dislocation for fracture patterns which disrupt the pelvic ring, unilateral or bilateral, includes internal fixation when performed (includes pubic symphysis and/or superior/inferior rami) Ⓑ Qp Qh C

* **G0415** Open treatment of posterior pelvic bone fracture and/or dislocation, for fracture patterns which disrupt the pelvic ring, unilateral or bilateral, includes internal fixation, when performed (includes ilium, sacroiliac joint and/or sacrum) Ⓑ Qp Qh C

▶ New   ↻ Revised   ✓ Reinstated   ~~deleted~~ Deleted   ⊘ Not covered or valid by Medicare
Ⓒ Special coverage instructions   * Carrier discretion   Ⓑ Bill Part B MAC   Ⓑ Bill DME MAC

TEMPORARY PROCEDURES/PROFESSIONAL SERVICES

Surgical Pathology: Prostate Biopsy

* **G0416** Surgical pathology, gross and microscopic examinations for prostate needle biopsy, any method ♂ Q2

  This testing requires a facility to have either a CLIA certificate of registration (certificate type code 9), a CLIA certificate of compliance (certificate type code 1), or a CLIA certificate of accreditation (certificate type code 3). A facility without a valid, current, CLIA certificate, with a current CLIA certificate of waiver (certificate type code 2) or with a current CLIA certificate for provider-performed microscopy procedures (certificate type code 4), must not be permitted to be paid for these tests. This code has a TC, 26 (physician), or global component.

  Laboratory Certification: Histopathology

  Coding Clinic: 2013, Q2, P6

Educational Services

* **G0420** Face-to-face educational services related to the care of chronic kidney disease; individual, per session, per one hour A

  CKD is kidney damage of 3 months or longer, regardless of the cause of kidney damage. Sessions billed in increments of one hour (if session is less than one hour, it must last at least 31 minutes to be billable. Sessions less than one hour and longer than 31 minutes are billable as one session. No more than 6 sessions of KDE services in a beneficiary's lifetime.

* **G0421** Face-to-face educational services related to the care of chronic kidney disease; group, per session, per one hour A

  Group setting: 2 to 20, report codes G0420 and G0421 with diagnosis code N18.4.

Cardiac and Pulmonary Rehabilitation

* **G0422** Intensive cardiac rehabilitation; with or without continuous ECG monitoring with exercise, per session S

  Includes the same service as 93798 but at a greater frequency; may be reported with as many as six hourly sessions on a single date of service. Includes medical nutrition services to reduce cardiac disease risk factors.

* **G0423** Intensive cardiac rehabilitation; with or without continuous ECG monitoring; without exercise, per session S

  Includes the same service as 93797 but at a greater frequency; may be reported with as many as six hourly sessions on a single date of service. Includes medical nutrition services to reduce cardiac disease risk factors.

Initial Telehealth Consultation

* **G0425** Telehealth consultation, emergency department or initial inpatient, typically 30 minutes communicating with the patient via telehealth B

  Problem Focused: Problem focused history and examination, with straightforward medical decision-making complexity. Typically 30 minutes communicating with patient via telehealth.

* **G0426** Initial inpatient telehealth consultation, emergency department or initial inpatient, typically 50 minutes communicating with the patient via telehealth B

  Detailed: Detailed history and examination, with moderate medical decision-making complexity. Typically 50 minutes communicating with patient via telehealth.

* **G0427** Initial inpatient telehealth consultation, emergency department or initial inpatient, typically 70 minutes or more communicating with the patient via telehealth B

  Comprehensive: Comprehensive history and examination, with high medical decision-making complexity. Typically 70 minutes or more communicating with patient via telehealth.

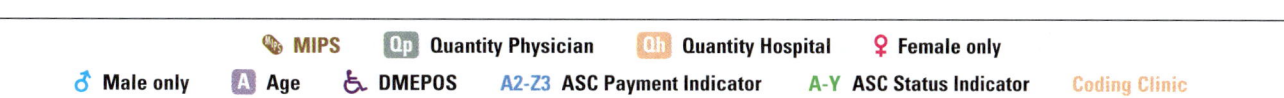

| MIPS | Qp Quantity Physician | Qh Quantity Hospital | ♀ Female only |
| ♂ Male only | A Age | DMEPOS | A2-Z3 ASC Payment Indicator | A-Y ASC Status Indicator | Coding Clinic |

2026 HCPCS LEVEL II NATIONAL CODES

Fillers

⊘ **G0428** Collagen meniscus implant procedure for filling meniscal defects (e.g., cmi, collagen scaffold, menaflex) Ⓑ E1

* **G0429** Dermal filler injection(s) for the treatment of facial lipodystrophy syndrome (LDS) (e.g., as a result of highly active antiretroviral therapy) Ⓑ Qp Qh T

Designated for dermal fillers Sculptra and Radiesse (Medicare). (https://www.cms.gov/ContractorLearningResources/downloads/JA6953.pdf)

Coding Clinic: 2010, Q3, P8

Laboratory Screening

* **G0432** Infectious agent antibody detection by enzyme immunoassay (EIA) technique, HIV-1 and/or HIV-2, screening Ⓑ Qp Qh A

Laboratory Certification: Virology, General immunology

Coding Clinic: 2010, Q2, P10

* **G0433** Infectious agent antibody detection by enzyme-linked immunosorbent assay (ELISA) technique, HIV-1 and/or HIV-2, screening Ⓑ Qp Qh A

Laboratory Certification: Virology, General immunology

Coding Clinic: 2010, Q2, P10

* **G0435** Infectious agent antibody detection by rapid antibody test, HIV-1 and/or HIV-2, screening Ⓑ Qp Qh A

Coding Clinic: 2010, Q2, P10

Counselling, Wellness, and Screening Services

* **G0438** Annual wellness visit; includes a personalized prevention plan of service (pps), initial visit Ⓑ Qp Qh A

* **G0439** Annual wellness visit, includes a personalized prevention plan of service (pps), subsequent visit Ⓑ Qp Qh A

* **G0442** Annual alcohol misuse screening, 5 to 15 minutes Ⓑ Qp Qh S

Coding Clinic: 2012, Q1, P7

* **G0443** Brief face-to-face behavioral counseling for alcohol misuse, 15 minutes Ⓑ Qp Qh S

Coding Clinic: 2012, Q1, P7

* **G0444** Annual depression screening, 5 to 15 minutes Ⓑ Qp Qh S

* **G0445** High intensity behavioral counseling to prevent sexually transmitted infection; face-to-face, individual, includes: education, skills training and guidance on how to change sexual behavior; performed semi-annually, 30 minutes Ⓑ Qp Qh S

* **G0446** Annual, face-to-face intensive behavioral therapy for cardiovascular disease, individual, 15 minutes Ⓑ Qp Qh S

Coding Clinic: 2012, Q2, P8

* **G0447** Face-to-face behavioral counseling for obesity, 15 minutes Ⓑ Qp Qh S

Coding Clinic: 2012, Q1, P8

* **G0448** Insertion or replacement of a permanent pacing cardioverter-defibrillator system with transvenous lead(s), single or dual chamber with insertion of pacing electrode, cardiac venous system, for left ventricular pacing Ⓑ Qp Qh B

* **G0451** Development testing, with interpretation and report, per standardized instrument form Ⓑ Qp Qh Q3

Miscellaneous Services

* **G0452** Molecular pathology procedure; physician interpretation and report Ⓑ Qp Qh B

* **G0453** Continuous intraoperative neurophysiology monitoring, from outside the operating room (remote or nearby), per patient (attention directed exclusively to one patient), each 15 minutes (list in addition to primary procedure) Ⓑ Qp Qh N

* **G0454** Physician documentation of face-to-face visit for durable medical equipment determination performed by nurse practitioner, physician assistant or clinical nurse specialist Ⓑ Qp Qh B

* **G0455** Preparation with instillation of fecal microbiota by any method, including assessment of donor specimen Ⓑ Qp Qh T

Coding Clinic: 2013, Q3, P8

* **G0458** Low dose rate (LDR) prostate brachytherapy services, composite rate Ⓑ Qp Qh B

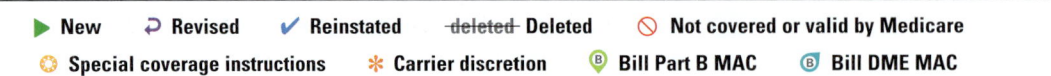

▶ New ⟲ Revised ✓ Reinstated ~~deleted~~ Deleted ⊘ Not covered or valid by Medicare
◉ Special coverage instructions * Carrier discretion Ⓑ Bill Part B MAC Ⓑ Bill DME MAC

TEMPORARY PROCEDURES/PROFESSIONAL SERVICES

* **G0459** Inpatient telehealth pharmacologic management, including prescription, use, and review of medication with no more than minimal medical psychotherapy ⒷQp Qh — B

* **G0460** Autologous platelet rich plasma or other blood-derived product for non-diabetic chronic wounds/ulcers, including phlebotomy, centrifugation or mixing, and all other preparatory procedures, administration and dressings, per treatment ⒷQp Qh — T

* **G0463** Hospital outpatient clinic visit for assessment and management of a patient ⒷQp Qh — J2

* **G0464** Colorectal cancer screening; stool-based DNA and fecal occult hemoglobin (e.g., KRAS, NDRG4 and BMP3) Ⓑ

  Cross Reference 81528

  Laboratory Certification: General immunology, Routine chemistry, Clinical cytogenetics

* **G0465** Autologous platelet rich plasma (prp) or other blood-derived product for diabetic chronic wounds/ulcers, using an FDA-cleared device for this indication, (includes administration, dressings, phlebotomy, centrifugation or mixing, and all other preparatory procedures, per treatment) — T

Federally Qualified Health Center Visits

* **G0466** Federally qualified health center (FQHC) visit, new patient; a medically-necessary, face-to-face encounter (one-on-one) between a new patient and a FQHC practitioner during which time one or more FQHC services are rendered and includes a typical bundle of Medicare-covered services that would be furnished per diem to a patient receiving a FQHC visit ⒷQp Qh — A

* **G0467** Federally qualified health center (FQHC) visit, established patient; a medically-necessary, face-to-face encounter (one-on-one) between an established patient and a FQHC practitioner during which time one or more FQHC services are rendered and includes a typical bundle of Medicare-covered services that would be furnished per diem to a patient receiving a FQHC visit ⒷQp Qh — A

* **G0468** Federally qualified health center (FQHC) visit, IPPE or AWV; a FQHC visit that includes an initial preventive physical examination (IPPE) or annual wellness visit (AWV) and includes a typical bundle of Medicare-covered services that would be furnished per diem to a patient receiving an IPPE or AWV ⒷQp Qh — A

* **G0469** Federally qualified health center (FQHC) visit, mental health, new patient; a medically-necessary, face-to-face mental health encounter (one-on-one) between a new patient and a FQHC practitioner during which time one or more FQHC services are rendered and includes a typical bundle of Medicare-covered services that would be furnished per diem to a patient receiving a mental health visit ⒷQp Qh — A

* **G0470** Federally qualified health center (FQHC) visit, mental health, established patient; a medically-necessary, face-to-face mental health encounter (one-on-one) between an established patient and a FQHC practitioner during which time one or more FQHC services are rendered and includes a typical bundle of Medicare-covered services that would be furnished per diem to a patient receiving a mental health visit ⒷQp Qh — A

Other Miscellaneous Services

* **G0471** Collection of venous blood by venipuncture or urine sample by catheterization from an individual in a skilled nursing facility (SNF) or by a laboratory on behalf of a home health agency (HHA) ⒷQp Qh — A

* **G0472** Hepatitis C antibody screening, for individual at high risk and other covered indication(s) ⒷQp Qh — A

  Medicare Statute 1861SSA

  Laboratory Certification: General immunology

* **G0473** Face-to-face behavioral counseling for obesity, group (2-10), 30 minutes ⒷQp Qh — S

* **G0475** HIV antigen/antibody, combination assay, screening ⒷQp Qh — A

  Laboratory Certification: Virology, General immunology

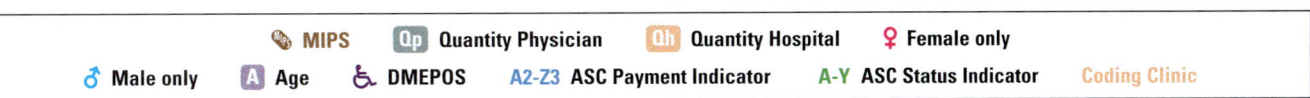

| MIPS | Qp Quantity Physician | Qh Quantity Hospital | ♀ Female only |
| ♂ Male only | A Age | DMEPOS | A2-Z3 ASC Payment Indicator | A-Y ASC Status Indicator | Coding Clinic |

* **G0476** Infectious agent detection by nucleic acid (DNA or RNA); human papillomavirus (HPV), high-risk types (e.g., 16, 18, 31, 33, 35, 39, 45, 51, 52, 56, 58, 59, 68) for cervical cancer screening, must be performed in addition to pap test ⓑ Qp Qh A

    Laboratory Certification: Virology

Drug Tests

* **G0480** Drug test(s), definitive, utilizing drug identification methods able to identify individual drugs and distinguish between structural isomers (but not necessarily stereoisomers), including, but not limited to GC/MS (any type, single or tandem) and LC/MS (any type, single or tandem and excluding immunoassays (e.g., IA, EIA, ELISA, EMIT, FPIA) and enzymatic methods (e.g., alcohol dehydrogenase)); qualitative or quantitative, all sources(s), includes specimen validity testing, per day, 1-7 drug class(es), including metabolite(s) if performed ⓑ Qp Qh Q4

    Coding Clinic: 2018, Q1, P5

* **G0481** Drug test(s), definitive, utilizing drug identification methods able to identify individual drugs and distinguish between structural isomers (but not necessarily stereoisomers), including, but not limited to GC/MS (any type, single or tandem) and LC/MS (any type, single or tandem and excluding immunoassays (e.g., IA, EIA, ELISA, EMIT, FPIA) and enzymatic methods (e.g., alcohol dehydrogenase)); qualitative or quantitative, all sources(s), includes specimen validity testing, per day, 8-14 drug class(es), including metabolite(s) if performed ⓑ Qp Qh Q4

    Coding Clinic: 2018, Q1, P5

* **G0482** Drug test(s), definitive, utilizing drug identification methods able to identify individual drugs and distinguish between structural isomers (but not necessarily stereoisomers), including, but not limited to GC/MS (any type, single or tandem) and LC/MS (any type, single or tandem and excluding immunoassays (e.g., IA, EIA, ELISA, EMIT, FPIA) and enzymatic methods (e.g., alcohol dehydrogenase); qualitative or quantitative, all sources(s), includes specimen validity testing, per day, 15-21 drug class(es), including metabolite(s) if performed ⓑ Qp Qh Q4

    Coding Clinic: 2018, Q1, P5

* **G0483** Drug test(s), definitive, utilizing drug identification methods able to identify individual drugs and distinguish between structural isomers (but not necessarily stereoisomers), including, but not limited to GC/MS (any type, single or tandem) and LC/MS (any type, single or tandem and excluding immunoassays (e.g., IA, EIA, ELISA, EMIT, FPIA) and enzymatic methods (e.g., alcohol dehydrogenase); qualitative or quantitative, all sources(s), includes specimen validity testing, per day, 22 or more drug class(es), including metabolite(s) if performed ⓑ Qp Qh Q4

    Coding Clinic: 2018, Q1, P5

Home Health Nursing Visit: Area of Shortage

* **G0490** Face-to-face home health nursing visit by a rural health clinic (RHC) or federally qualified health center (FQHC) in an area with a shortage of home health agencies (services limited to RN or LPN only) ⓑ A

Dialysis Procedure

* **G0491** Dialysis procedure at a Medicare certified ESRD facility for acute kidney injury without ESRD ⓑ Qp Qh B

* **G0492** Dialysis procedure with single evaluation by a physician or other qualified health care professional for acute kidney injury without ESRD ⓑ Qp Qh B

TEMPORARY PROCEDURES/PROFESSIONAL SERVICES

Home Health or Hospice: Skilled Services

* **G0493** Skilled services of a registered nurse (RN) for the observation and assessment of the patient's condition, each 15 minutes (the change in the patient's condition requires skilled nursing personnel to identify and evaluate the patient's need for possible modification of treatment in the home health or hospice setting) ⓑ B

* **G0494** Skilled services of a licensed practical nurse (LPN) for the observation and assessment of the patient's condition, each 15 minutes (the change in the patient's condition requires skilled nursing personnel to identify and evaluate the patient's need for possible modification of treatment in the home health or hospice setting) ⓑ B

* **G0495** Skilled services of a registered nurse (RN), in the training and/or education of a patient or family member, in the home health or hospice setting, each 15 minutes ⓑ B

* **G0496** Skilled services of a licensed practical nurse (LPN), in the training and/or education of a patient or family member, in the home health or hospice setting, each 15 minutes ⓑ B

Chemotherapy Administration

* **G0498** Chemotherapy administration, intravenous infusion technique; initiation of infusion in the office/clinic setting using office/clinic pump/supplies, with continuation of the infusion in the community setting (e.g., home, domiciliary, rest home or assisted living) using a portable pump provided by the office/clinic, includes follow up office/clinic visit at the conclusion of the infusion ⓑ Qp Qh S

Hepatitis B Screening

* **G0499** Hepatitis B screening in non-pregnant, high risk individual includes hepatitis B surface antigen (HBsAG), antibodies to HBsAG (anti-HBs) and antibodies to hepatitis B core antigen (anti-hbc), and is followed by a neutralizing confirmatory test, when performed, only for an initially reactive HBsAG result ⓑ Qp Qh A

   Laboratory Certification: Virology

Moderate Sedation Services

* **G0500** Moderate sedation services provided by the same physician or other qualified health care professional performing a gastrointestinal endoscopic service that sedation supports, requiring the presence of an independent trained observer to assist in the monitoring of the patient's level of consciousness and physiological status; initial 15 minutes of intra-service time; patient age 5 years or older (additional time may be reported with 99153, as appropriate) ⓑ Qp Qh N

Resource-Intensive Service

* **G0501** Resource-intensive services for patients for whom the use of specialized mobility-assistive technology (such as adjustable height chairs or tables, patient lift, and adjustable padded leg supports) is medically necessary and used during the provision of an office/outpatient, evaluation and management visit (list separately in addition to primary service) ⓑ N

Psychiatric Care Management

* **G0506** Comprehensive assessment of and care planning for patients requiring chronic care management services (list separately in addition to primary monthly care management service) ⓑ Qp Qh N

Critical Care Telehealth Consultation

* **G0508** Telehealth consultation, critical care, initial, physicians typically spend 60 minutes communicating with the patient and providers via telehealth ⓑ Qp Qh B

* **G0509** Telehealth consultation, critical care, subsequent, physicians typically spend 50 minutes communicating with the patient and providers via telehealth ⓑ Qp Qh B

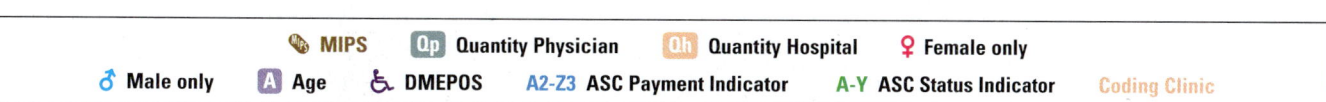

Rural Health Clinic: Management and Care

✺ **G0511** Rural health clinic or federally qualified health center (RHC or FQHC) only, general care management, 20 minutes or more of clinical staff time for chronic care management services or behavioral health integration services directed by an RHC or FQHC practitioner (physician, NP, PA, or CNM), per calendar month   A

✺ **G0512** Rural health clinic or federally qualified health center (RHC/FQHC) only, psychiatric collaborative care model (psychiatric CoCM), 60 minutes or more of clinical staff time for psychiatric CoCM services directed by an RHC or FQHC practitioner (physician, NP, PA, or CNM) and including services furnished by a behavioral health care manager and consultation with a psychiatric consultant, per calendar month   A

Prolonged Preventive Services

∗ **G0513** Prolonged preventive service(s) (beyond the typical service time of the primary procedure), in the office or other outpatient setting requiring direct patient contact beyond the usual service; first 30 minutes (list separately in addition to code for preventive service)   N

∗ **G0514** Prolonged preventive service(s) (beyond the typical service time of the primary procedure), in the office or other outpatient setting requiring direct patient contact beyond the usual service; each additional 30 minutes (list separately in addition to code G0513 for additional 30 minutes of preventive service)   N

Non-biodegradable Drug Delivery Implants: Removal and Insertion

∗ **G0516** Insertion of non-biodegradable drug delivery implants, 4 or more (services for subdermal rod implant)   Q1

∗ **G0517** Removal of non-biodegradable drug delivery implants, 4 or more (services for subdermal implants)   Q1

∗ **G0518** Removal with reinsertion, non-biodegradable drug delivery implants, 4 or more (services for subdermal implants)   Q1

∗ **G0519** Management of new patient-caregiver dyad with dementia, low complexity, for use in CMMI model   Q1

∗ **G0520** Management of new patient-caregiver dyad with dementia, moderate complexity, for use in CMMI model   Q1

∗ **G0521** Management of new patient-caregiver dyad with dementia, high complexity, for use in CMMI model   Q1

∗ **G0522** Management of a new patient with dementia, low complexity, for use in CMMI model   Q1

∗ **G0523** Management of a new patient with dementia, moderate to high complexity, for use in CMMI model   Q1

∗ **G0524** Management of established patient-caregiver dyad with dementia, low complexity, for use in CMMI model   Q1

∗ **G0525** Management of established patient-caregiver dyad with dementia, moderate complexity, for use in CMMI model   Q1

∗ **G0526** Management of established patient-caregiver dyad with dementia, high complexity, for use in CMMI model   Q1

∗ **G0527** Management of established patient with dementia, low complexity, for use in CMMI model   Q1

∗ **G0528** Management of established patient with dementia, moderate to high complexity, for use in CMMI model   Q1

∗ **G0529** In-home respite care, 4-hour unit, for use in CMMI model   Q1

∗ **G0530** Adult day center, 8-hour unit, for use in CMMI model   Q1

∗ **G0531** Facility-based respite, 24-hour unit, for use in CMMI model   Q1

▶ ✺ **G0532** Take-home supply of nasal Nalmefene hydrochloride; one carton of two, 2.7 mg per 0.1 ml nasal sprays (provision of the services by a Medicare-enrolled opioid treatment program); (list separately in addition to each primary code)   A

▶ ✺ **G0533** Medication assisted treatment, buprenorphine (injectable) administered on a weekly basis; weekly bundle including dispensing and/or administration, substance use counseling, individual and group therapy, and toxicology testing if performed (provision of the services by a Medicare-enrolled opioid treatment program)   A

▶ New   ⤳ Revised   ✔ Reinstated   ~~deleted~~ Deleted   ⊘ Not covered or valid by Medicare
✺ Special coverage instructions   ∗ Carrier discretion   Ⓑ Bill Part B MAC   Ⓑ Bill DME MAC

TEMPORARY PROCEDURES/PROFESSIONAL SERVICES

▶ ⊛ **G0534** Coordinated care and/or referral services, such as to adequate and accessible community resources to address unmet health-related social needs, including harm reduction interventions and recovery support services a patient needs and wishes to pursue, which significantly limit the ability to diagnose or treat an opioid use disorder; each additional 30 minutes of services (provision of the services by a Medicare-enrolled opioid treatment program); (list separately in addition to each primary code) **A**

▶ ⊛ **G0535** Patient navigational services, provided directly or by referral; including helping the patient to navigate health systems and identify care providers and supportive services, to build patient self-advocacy and communication skills with care providers, and to promote patient-driven action plans and goals; each additional 30 minutes of services (provision of the services by a Medicare-enrolled opioid treatment program); (list separately in addition to each primary code) **A**

▶ ⊛ **G0536** Peer recovery support services, provided directly or by referral; including leveraging knowledge of the condition or lived experience to provide support, mentorship, or inspiration to meet oud treatment and recovery goals; conducting a person-centered interview to understand the patient's life story, strengths, needs, goals, preferences, and desired outcomes; developing and proposing strategies to help meet person-centered treatment goals; assisting the patient in locating or navigating recovery support services; each additional 30 minutes of services (provision of the services by a Medicare-enrolled opioid treatment program) (list separately in addition to each primary code) **A**

▶ ⊛ **G0537** Administration of a standardized, evidence-based atherosclerotic cardiovascular disease (ASCVD) risk assessment, 5-15 minutes, not more often than every 12 months **S**

▶ ⊛ **G0538** Atherosclerotic cardiovascular disease (ASCVD) risk management services; clinical staff time; per calendar month **S**

▶ ⊛ **G0539** Caregiver training in behavior management/modification for caregiver(s) of patients with a mental or physical health diagnosis, administered by physician or other qualified health care professional (without the patient present), face-to-face; initial 30 minutes **A**

▶ ⊛ **G0540** Caregiver training in behavior management/modification for parent(s)/guardian(s)/caregiver(s) of patients with a mental or physical health diagnosis, administered by physician or other qualified health care professional (without the patient present), face-to-face; each additional 15 minutes **A**

▶ ⊛ **G0541** Caregiver training in direct care strategies and techniques to support care for patients with an ongoing condition or illness and to reduce complications (including, but not limited to, techniques to prevent decubitus ulcer formation, wound care, and infection control) (without the patient present), face-to-face; initial 30 minutes **A**

▶ ⊛ **G0542** Caregiver training in direct care strategies and techniques to support care for patients with an ongoing condition or illness and to reduce complications (including, but not limited to, techniques to prevent decubitus ulcer formation, wound care, and infection control) (without the patient present), face-to-face; each additional 15 minutes (list separately in addition to code for primary service) (use G0542 in conjunction with G0541) **A**

▶ ⊛ **G0543** Group caregiver training in direct care strategies and techniques to support care for patients with an ongoing condition or illness and to reduce complications (including, but not limited to, techniques to prevent decubitus ulcer formation, wound care, and infection control) (without the patient present), face-to-face with multiple sets of caregivers **A**

▶ ⊛ **G0544** Post discharge telephonic follow-up contacts performed in conjunction with a discharge from the emergency department for behavioral health or other crisis encounter, 4 calls per calendar month **S**

| 🍃 MIPS | **Qp** Quantity Physician | **Qh** Quantity Hospital | ♀ Female only |
| ♂ Male only | **A** Age | ♿ DMEPOS | A2-Z3 ASC Payment Indicator | A-Y ASC Status Indicator | Coding Clinic |

▶ ⊛ **G0545** Visit complexity inherent to hospital inpatient or observation care associated with a confirmed or suspected infectious disease by an infectious diseases specialist, including disease transmission risk assessment and mitigation, public health investigation, analysis, and testing, and complex antimicrobial therapy counseling and treatment (add-on code, list separately in addition to hospital inpatient or observation evaluation and management visit, initial, same day discharge, subsequent or discharge) **B**

▶ ⊛ **G0546** Interprofessional telephone/internet/electronic health record assessment and management service provided by a practitioner in a specialty whose covered services are limited by statute to services for the diagnosis and treatment of mental illness, including a verbal and written report to the patient's treating/requesting practitioner; 5-10 minutes of medical consultative discussion and review **M**

▶ ⊛ **G0547** Interprofessional telephone/internet/electronic health record assessment and management service provided by a practitioner in a specialty whose covered services are limited by statute to services for the diagnosis and treatment of mental illness, including a verbal and written report to the patient's treating/requesting practitioner; 11-20 minutes of medical consultative discussion and review **M**

▶ ⊛ **G0548** Interprofessional telephone/internet/electronic health record assessment and management service provided by a practitioner in a specialty whose covered services are limited by statute to services for the diagnosis and treatment of mental illness, including a verbal and written report to the patient's treating/requesting practitioner; 21-30 minutes of medical consultative discussion and review **M**

▶ ⊛ **G0549** Interprofessional telephone/internet/electronic health record assessment and management service provided by a practitioner in a specialty whose covered services are limited by statute to services for the diagnosis and treatment of mental illness, including a verbal and written report to the patient's treating/requesting practitioner; 31 or more minutes of medical consultative discussion and review **M**

▶ ⊛ **G0550** Interprofessional telephone/internet/electronic health record assessment and management service provided by a practitioner in a specialty whose covered services are limited by statute to services for the diagnosis and treatment of mental illness, including a written report to the patient's treating/requesting practitioner, 5 minutes or more of medical consultative time **M**

▶ ⊛ **G0551** Interprofessional telephone/internet/electronic health record referral service(s) provided by a treating/requesting practitioner in a specialty whose covered services are limited by statute to services for the diagnosis and treatment of mental illness, 30 minutes **M**

▶ ⊛ **G0552** Supply of digital mental health treatment device and initial education and onboarding, per course of treatment that augments a behavioral therapy plan **V**

▶ ⊛ **G0553** First 20 minutes of monthly treatment management services directly related to the patient's therapeutic use of the digital mental health treatment (DMHT) device that augments a behavioral therapy plan, physician/other qualified health care professional time reviewing information related to the use of the DMHT device, including patient observations and patient specific inputs in a calendar month and requiring at least one interactive communication with the patient/caregiver during the calendar month **V**

▶ ⊛ **G0554** Each additional 20 minutes of monthly treatment management services directly related to the patient's therapeutic use of the digital mental health treatment (DMHT) device that augments a behavioral therapy plan, physician/other qualified health care professional time reviewing data generated from the DMHT device from patient observations and patient specific inputs in a calendar month and requiring at least one interactive communication with the patient/caregiver during the calendar month **N**

▶ ⊛ **G0555** Provision of replacement patient electronics system (e.g., system pillow, handheld reader) for home pulmonary artery pressure monitoring **S**

▶ New ↻ Revised ✓ Reinstated ~~deleted~~ Deleted ⊘ Not covered or valid by Medicare ⊛ Special coverage instructions * Carrier discretion Ⓑ Bill Part B MAC Ⓑ Bill DME MAC

TEMPORARY PROCEDURES/PROFESSIONAL SERVICES

▶ ⊛ **G0556** Advanced primary care management services for a patient with one chronic condition [expected to last at least 12 months, or until the death of the patient, which place the patient at significant risk of death, acute exacerbation/decompensation, or functional decline], or fewer, provided by clinical staff and directed by a physician or other qualified health care professional who is responsible for all primary care and serves as the continuing focal point for all needed health care services, per calendar month, with the following elements, as appropriate: Consent; ++ inform the patient of the availability of the service; that only one practitioner can furnish and be paid for the service during a calendar month; of the right to stop the services at any time (effective at the end of the calendar month); and that cost sharing may apply. ++ document in patient's medical record that consent was obtained. Initiation during a qualifying visit for new patients or patients not seen within 3 years; provide 24/7 access for urgent needs to care team/practitioner, including providing patients/caregivers with a way to contact health care professionals in the practice to discuss urgent needs regardless of the time of day or day of week; continuity of care with a designated member of the care team with whom the patient is able to schedule successive routine appointments; deliver care in alternative ways to traditional office visits to best meet the patient's needs, such as home visits and/or expanded hours; overall comprehensive care management; ++ systematic needs assessment (medical and psychosocial). ++ system-based approaches to ensure receipt of preventive services. ++ medication reconciliation, management and oversight of self-management. Development, implementation, revision, and maintenance of an electronic patient-centered comprehensive care plan with typical care plan elements when clinically relevant; ++ care plan is available timely within and outside the billing practice as appropriate to individuals involved in the beneficiary's care, can be routinely accessed and updated by care team/practitioner, and copy of care plan to patient/caregiver; coordination of care transitions between and among health care providers and settings, including referrals to other clinicians and follow-up after an emergency department visit and discharges from hospitals, skilled nursing facilities or other health care facilities as applicable; ++ ensure timely exchange of electronic health information with other practitioners and providers to support continuity of care. ++ ensure timely follow-up communication (direct contact, telephone, electronic) with the patient and/or caregiver after an emergency department visit and discharges from hospitals, skilled nursing facilities, or other health care facilities, within 7 calendar days of discharge, as clinically indicated. Ongoing communication and coordinating receipt of needed services from practitioners, home- and community-based service providers, community-based social service providers, hospitals, and skilled nursing facilities (or other health care facilities), and document communication regarding the patient's psychosocial strengths and needs, functional deficits, goals, preferences, and desired outcomes, including cultural and linguistic factors, in the patient's medical record; enhanced opportunities for the beneficiary and any caregiver to communicate with the care team/practitioner regarding the beneficiary's care through the use of asynchronous non-face-to-face consultation methods other than telephone, such as secure messaging, email, internet, or patient portal, and other communication-technology based services, including remote evaluation of pre-recorded patient information and interprofessional telephone/internet/EHR referral service(s), to maintain ongoing communication with patients, as appropriate; ++ ensure access to patient-initiated digital communications that require a clinical decision, such as virtual check-ins and digital online assessment and management and e/m visits (or e-visits). Analyze patient population data to identify gaps in care and offer additional interventions, as appropriate; risk stratify the practice population based on defined diagnoses, claims, or other electronic data to identify and target services to patients; be assessed through performance measurement of primary care quality, total cost of care, and meaningful use of certified EHR technology S

▶ ✴ **G0557** Advanced primary care management services for a patient with multiple (two or more) chronic conditions expected to last at least 12 months, or until the death of the patient, which place the patient at significant risk of death, acute exacerbation/decompensation, or functional decline, provided by clinical staff and directed by a physician or other qualified health care professional who is responsible for all primary care and serves as the continuing focal point for all needed health care services, per calendar month, with the following elements, as appropriate: consent; ++ inform the patient of the availability of the service; that only one practitioner can furnish and be paid for the service during a calendar month; of the right to stop the services at any time (effective at the end of the calendar month); and that cost sharing may apply. ++ document in patient's medical record that consent was obtained. Initiation during a qualifying visit for new patients or patients not seen within 3 years; provide 24/7 access for urgent needs to care team/practitioner, including providing patients/caregivers with a way to contact health care professionals in the practice to discuss urgent needs regardless of the time of day or day of week; continuity of care with a designated member of the care team with whom the patient is able to schedule successive routine appointments; deliver care in alternative ways to traditional office visits to best meet the patient's needs, such as home visits and/or expanded hours; overall comprehensive care management; ++ systematic needs assessment (medical and psychosocial). ++ system-based approaches to ensure receipt of preventive services. ++ medication reconciliation, management and oversight of self-management. Development, implementation, revision, and maintenance of an electronic patient-centered comprehensive care plan; ++ care plan is available timely within and outside the billing practice as appropriate to individuals involved in the beneficiary's care, can be routinely accessed and updated by care team/practitioner, and copy of care plan to patient/caregiver; coordination of care transitions between and among health care providers and settings, including referrals to other clinicians and follow-up after an emergency department visit and discharges from hospitals, skilled nursing facilities or other health care facilities as applicable; ++ ensure timely exchange of electronic health information with other practitioners and providers to support continuity of care. ++ Ensure timely follow-up communication (direct contact, telephone, electronic) with the patient and/or caregiver after an emergency department visit and discharges from hospitals, skilled nursing facilities, or other health care facilities, within 7 calendar days of discharge, as clinically indicated. Ongoing communication and coordinating receipt of needed services from practitioners, home- and community-based service providers, community-based social service providers, hospitals, and skilled nursing facilities (or other health care facilities), and document communication regarding the patient's psychosocial strengths and needs, functional deficits, goals, preferences, and desired outcomes, including cultural and linguistic factors, in the patient's medical record; enhanced opportunities for the beneficiary and any caregiver to communicate with the care team/practitioner regarding the beneficiary's care through the use of asynchronous non-face-to-face consultation methods other than telephone, such as secure messaging, email, internet, or patient portal, and other communication-technology based services, including remote evaluation of pre-recorded patient information and interprofessional telephone/internet/EHR referral service(s), to maintain ongoing communication with patients, as appropriate; ++ ensure access to patient-initiated digital communications that require a clinical decision, such as virtual check-ins and digital online assessment and management and e/m visits (or e-visits). analyze patient population data to identify gaps in care and offer additional interventions, as appropriate; risk stratify the practice population based on defined diagnoses, claims, or other electronic data to identify and target services to patients; be assessed through performance measurement of primary care quality, total cost of care, and meaningful use of certified EHR technology **S**

▶ ⊛ **G0558** Advanced primary care management services for a patient that is a qualified Medicare beneficiary with multiple (two or more) chronic conditions expected to last at least 12 months, or until the death of the patient, which place the patient at significant risk of death, acute exacerbation/decompensation, or functional decline, provided by clinical staff and directed by a physician or other qualified health care professional who is responsible for all primary care and serves as the continuing focal point for all needed health care services, per calendar month, with the following elements, as appropriate: consent; ++ inform the patient of the availability of the service; that only one practitioner can furnish and be paid for the service during a calendar month; of the right to stop the services at any time (effective at the end of the calendar month); and that cost sharing may apply. ++ Document in patient's medical record that consent was obtained. Initiation during a qualifying visit for new patients or patients not seen within 3 years; provide 24/7 access for urgent needs to care team/practitioner, including providing patients/caregivers with a way to contact health care professionals in the practice to discuss urgent needs regardless of the time of day or day of week; continuity of care with a designated member of the care team with whom the patient is able to schedule successive routine appointments; deliver care in alternative ways to traditional office visits to best meet the patient's needs, such as home visits and/or expanded hours; overall comprehensive care management; ++ systematic needs assessment (medical and psychosocial). ++ System-based approaches to ensure receipt of preventive services. ++ Medication reconciliation, management and oversight of self-management. Development, implementation, revision, and maintenance of an electronic patient-centered comprehensive care plan; ++ care plan is available timely within and outside the billing practice as appropriate to individuals involved in the beneficiary's care, can be routinely accessed and updated by care team/practitioner, and copy of care plan to patient/caregiver; coordination of care transitions between and among health care providers and settings, including referrals to other clinicians and follow-up after an emergency department visit and discharges from hospitals, skilled nursing facilities or other health care facilities as applicable; ++ ensure timely exchange of electronic health information with other practitioners and providers to support continuity of care. ++ ensure timely follow-up communication (direct contact, telephone, electronic) with the patient and/or caregiver after an emergency department visit and discharges from hospitals, skilled nursing facilities, or other health care facilities, within 7 calendar days of discharge, as clinically indicated. Ongoing communication and coordinating receipt of needed services from practitioners, home- and community-based service providers, community-based social service providers, hospitals, and skilled nursing facilities (or other health care facilities), and document communication regarding the patient's psychosocial strengths and needs, functional deficits, goals, preferences, and desired outcomes, including cultural and linguistic factors, in the patient's medical record; enhanced opportunities for the beneficiary and any caregiver to communicate with the care team/practitioner regarding the beneficiary's care through the use of asynchronous non-face-to-face consultation methods other than telephone, such as secure messaging, email, internet, or patient portal, and other communication-technology based services, including remote evaluation of pre-recorded patient information and interprofessional telephone/internet/EHR referral service(s), to maintain ongoing communication with patients, as appropriate; ++ ensure access to patient-initiated digital communications that require a clinical decision, such as virtual check-ins and digital online assessment and management and e/m visits (or e-visits). Analyze patient population data to identify gaps in care and offer additional interventions, as appropriate; risk stratify the practice population based on defined diagnoses, claims, or other electronic data to identify and target services to patients; be assessed through performance measurement of primary care quality, total cost of care, and meaningful use of certified HER technology   S

▶ ✪ **G0559** Post-operative follow-up visit complexity inherent to evaluation and management services addressing surgical procedure(s), provided by a physician or qualified health care professional who is not the practitioner who performed the procedure (or in the same group practice) and is of the same or of a different specialty than the practitioner who performed the procedure, within the 90-day global period of the procedure(s), once per 90-day global period, when there has not been a formal transfer of care and requires the following required elements, when possible and applicable: reading available surgical note to understand the relative success of the procedure, the anatomy that was affected, and potential complications that could have arisen due to the unique circumstances of the patient's operation. Research the procedure to determine expected post-operative course and potential complications (in the case of doing a post-op for a procedure outside the specialty). Evaluate and physically examine the patient to determine whether the post-operative course is progressing appropriately. communicate with the practitioner who performed the procedure if any questions or concerns arise. (List separately in addition to office/outpatient evaluation and management visit, new or established) **B**

▶ ✪ **G0560** Safety planning interventions, each 20 minutes personally performed by the billing practitioner, including assisting the patient in the identification of the following personalized elements of a safety plan: recognizing warning signs of an impending suicidal or substance use-related crisis; employing internal coping strategies; utilizing social contacts and social settings as a means of distraction from suicidal thoughts or risky substance use; utilizing family members, significant others, caregivers, and/or friends to help resolve the crisis; contacting mental health or substance use disorder professionals or agencies; and making the environment safe **A**

▶ ✪ **G0561** Tympanostomy with local or topical anesthesia and insertion of a ventilating tube when performed with tympanostomy tube delivery device, unilateral (list separately in addition to 69433) (do not use in conjunction with 0583T) **N**

▶ ✪ **G0562** Therapeutic radiology simulation-aided field setting; complex, including acquisition of pet and CT imaging data required for radiopharmaceutical-directed radiation therapy treatment planning (i.e., modeling) **S**

▶ ✪ **G0563** Stereotactic body radiation therapy, treatment delivery, per fraction to 1 or more lesions, including image guidance and real-time positron emissions-based delivery adjustments to 1 or more lesions, entire course not to exceed 5 fractions **S**

▶ ✪ **G0564** Creation of subcutaneous pocket with insertion of 365-day implantable interstitial glucose sensor, including system activation and patient training

▶ ✪ **G0565** Removal of implantable interstitial glucose sensor with creation of subcutaneous pocket at different anatomic site and insertion of new 365-day implantable sensor, including system activation

▶ ✪ **G0566** 3D radiodensity-value bone imaging, algorithm derived, from previous magnetic resonance examination of the same anatomy **S**

▶ ✪ **G0567** Infectious agent detection by nucleic acid (DNA or RNA); Hepatitis C, screening, amplified probe technique **A**

Drug Test

✱ **G0659** Drug test(s), definitive, utilizing drug identification methods able to identify individual drugs and distinguish between structural isomers (but not necessarily stereoisomers), including but not limited to GC/MS (any type, single or tandem) and LC/MS (any type, single or tandem), excluding immunoassays (e.g., IA, EIA, ELISA, EMIT, FPIA) and enzymatic methods (e.g., alcohol dehydrogenase), performed without method or drug-specific calibration, without matrix-matched quality control material, or without use of stable isotope or other universally recognized internal standard(s) for each drug, drug metabolite or drug class per specimen; qualitative or quantitative, all sources, includes specimen validity testing, per day, any number of drug classes **Q4**

▶ New ↻ Revised ✓ Reinstated ~~deleted~~ Deleted ⊘ Not covered or valid by Medicare
✪ Special coverage instructions ✱ Carrier discretion Ⓑ Bill Part B MAC Ⓑ Bill DME MAC

TEMPORARY PROCEDURES/PROFESSIONAL SERVICES

Quality Care Measures: Cataract Surgery

* **G0913** Improvement in visual function achieved within 90 days following cataract surgery M
* **G0914** Patient care survey was not completed by patient M
* **G0915** Improvement in visual function not achieved within 90 days following cataract surgery M
* **G0916** Satisfaction with care achieved within 90 days following cataract surgery M
* **G0917** Patient care survey was not completed by patient M
* **G0918** Satisfaction with care not achieved within 90 days following cataract surgery M

Clinical Decision Support Mechanism

~~G1001 Clinical decision support mechanism eviCore, as defined by the Medicare Appropriate Use Criteria Program~~

~~G1002 Clinical decision support mechanism MedCurrent, as defined by the Medicare Appropriate Use Criteria Program~~

~~G1003 Clinical decision support mechanism Medicalis, as defined by the Appropriate Use Criteria Program~~

~~G1004 Clinical decision support mechanism National Decision Support Company, as defined by the Medicare Appropriate Use Criteria Program~~

~~G1007 Clinical decision support mechanism AIM Specialty Health, as defined by the Medicare Appropriate Use Criteria Program~~

~~G1008 Clinical decision support mechanism Cranberry Peak, as defined by the Medicare Appropriate Use Criteria Program~~

* **G1009** Clinical decision support mechanism Sage Health Management Solutions, as defined by the Medicare Appropriate Use Criteria Program E1

~~G1010 Clinical decision support mechanism Stanson, as defined by the Medicare Appropriate Use Criteria Program~~

~~G1011 Clinical decision support mechanism, qualified tool not otherwise specified, as defined by the Medicare Appropriate Use Criteria Program~~

~~G1012 Clinical decision support mechanism AgileMD, as defined by the Medicare appropriate use criteria program~~

~~G1013 Clinical decision support mechanism EvidenceCare ImagingCare, as defined by the Medicare appropriate use criteria program~~

~~G1014 Clinical decision support mechanism InveniQA semantic answers in medicine, as defined by the Medicare appropriate use criteria program~~

~~G1015 Clinical decision support mechanism Reliant Medical Group, as defined by the Medicare appropriate use criteria program~~

~~G1016 Clinical decision support mechanism Speed of Care, as defined by the Medicare appropriate use criteria program~~

~~G1017 Clinical decision support mechanism HealthHelp, as defined by the Medicare appropriate use criteria program~~

~~G1018 Clinical decision support mechanism Infinx, as defined by the Medicare appropriate use criteria program~~

~~G1019 Clinical decision support mechanism LogicNets, as defined by the Medicare appropriate use criteria program~~

~~G1020 Clinical decision support mechanism Curbside Clinical Augmented Workflow, as defined by the Medicare appropriate use criteria program~~

~~G1021 Clinical decision support mechanism E*HealthLine clinical decision support mechanism, as defined by the Medicare appropriate use criteria program~~

~~G1022 Clinical decision support mechanism Intermountain clinical decision support mechanism, as defined by the Medicare appropriate use criteria program~~

~~G1023 Clinical decision support mechanism Persivia clinical decision support, as defined by the Medicare appropriate use criteria program~~

~~G1024 Clinical decision support mechanism radrite, as defined by the medicare appropriate use criteria program~~

* **G1025** Patient-months where there are more than one medicare capitated payment (mcp) provider listed for the month M

* **G1026** The number of adult patient-months in the denominator who were on maintenance hemodialysis using a catheter continuously for three months or longer under the care of the same practitioner or group partner as of the last hemodialysis session of the reporting month **M**

* **G1027** The number of adult patient-months in the denominator who were on maintenance hemodialysis under the care of the same practitioner or group partner as of the last hemodialysis session of the reporting month using a catheter continuously for less than three months **M**

* **G1028** Take-home supply of nasal naloxone; 2-pack of 8mg per 0.1 ml nasal spray (provision of the services by a medicare-enrolled opioid treatment program); list separately in addition to code for primary procedure **A**

Therapy, Evaluation and Assessment

* **G2000** Blinded administration of convulsive therapy procedure, either electroconvulsive therapy (ECT, current covered gold standard) or magnetic seizure therapy (MST, non-covered experimental therapy), performed in an approved IDE-based clinical trial, per treatment session **S**

* **G2001** Brief (20 minutes) in-home visit for a new patient post-discharge. for use only in a medicare-approved CMMI model. (services must be furnished within a beneficiary's home, domiciliary, rest home, assisted living and/or nursing facility within 90 days following discharge from an inpatient facility and no more than 9 times.) **B**

* **G2002** Limited (30 minutes) in-home visit for a new patient post-discharge. for use only in a medicare-approved CMMI model. (services must be furnished within a beneficiary's home, domiciliary, rest home, assisted living and/or nursing facility within 90 days following discharge from an inpatient facility and no more than 9 times.) **B**

* **G2003** Moderate (45 minutes) in-home visit for a new patient post-discharge. for use only in a medicare-approved CMMI model. (services must be furnished within a beneficiary's home, domiciliary, rest home, assisted living and/or nursing facility within 90 days following discharge from an inpatient facility and no more than 9 times.) **B**

* **G2004** Comprehensive (60 minutes) in-home visit for a new patient post-discharge. for use only in a medicare-approved CMMI model. (services must be furnished within a beneficiary's home, domiciliary, rest home, assisted living and/or nursing facility within 90 days following discharge from an inpatient facility and no more than 9 times.) **B**

* **G2005** Extensive (75 minutes) in-home visit for a new patient post-discharge. for use only in a medicare-approved CMMI model. (services must be furnished within a beneficiary's home, domiciliary, rest home, assisted living and/or nursing facility within 90 days following discharge from an inpatient facility and no more than 9 times.) **B**

* **G2006** Brief (20 minutes) in-home visit for an existing patient post-discharge. for use only in a medicare-approved CMMI model. (services must be furnished within a beneficiary's home, domiciliary, rest home, assisted living and/or nursing facility within 90 days following discharge from an inpatient facility and no more than 9 times.) **B**

* **G2007** Limited (30 minutes) in-home visit for an existing patient post-discharge. for use only in a medicare-approved CMMI model. (services must be furnished within a beneficiary's home, domiciliary, rest home, assisted living and/or nursing facility within 90 days following discharge from an inpatient facility and no more than 9 times.) **B**

* **G2008** Moderate (45 minutes) in-home visit for an existing patient post-discharge. for use only in a medicare-approved CMMI model. (services must be furnished within a beneficiary's home, domiciliary, rest home, assisted living and/or nursing facility within 90 days following discharge from an inpatient facility and no more than 9 times.) **B**

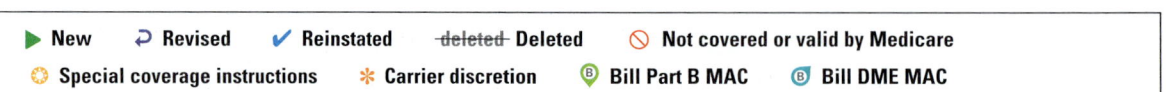

▶ New　↺ Revised　✔ Reinstated　~~deleted~~ Deleted　⊘ Not covered or valid by Medicare
✱ Special coverage instructions　* Carrier discretion　Ⓑ Bill Part B MAC　Ⓑ Bill DME MAC

TEMPORARY PROCEDURES/PROFESSIONAL SERVICES

* **G2009** Comprehensive (60 minutes) in-home visit for an existing patient post-discharge. for use only in a medicare-approved CMMI model. (services must be furnished within a beneficiary's home, domiciliary, rest home, assisted living and/or nursing facility within 90 days following discharge from an inpatient facility and no more than 9 times.) **B**

* **G2010** Remote evaluation of recorded video and/or images submitted by an established patient (e.g., store and forward), including interpretation with follow-up with the patient within 24 business hours, not originating from a related E/M service provided within the previous 7 days nor leading to an E/M service or procedure within the next 24 hours or soonest available appointment **B**

* **G2011** Alcohol and/or substance (other than tobacco) misuse structured assessment (e.g., audit, dast), and brief intervention, 5-14 minutes **S**

~~G2012~~ ~~Brief communication technology-based service, e.g., virtual check-in, by a physician or other qualified health care professional who can report evaluation and management services, provided to an established patient, not originating from a related E/M service provided within the previous 7 days nor leading to an E/M service or procedure within the next 24 hours or soonest available appointment; 5-10 minutes of medical discussion~~

* **G2013** Extensive (75 minutes) in-home visit for an existing patient post-discharge. for use only in a medicare-approved CMMI model. (services must be furnished within a beneficiary's home, domiciliary, rest home, assisted living and/or nursing facility within 90 days following discharge from an inpatient facility and no more than 9 times.) **B**

* **G2014** Limited (30 minutes) care plan oversight. for use only in a medicare-approved CMMI model. (services must be furnished within a beneficiary's home, domiciliary, rest home, assisted living and/or nursing facility within 90 days following discharge from an inpatient facility and no more than 9 times.) **B**

* **G2015** Comprehensive (60 mins) home care plan oversight. for use only in a medicare-approved CMMI model. (services must be furnished within a beneficiary's home, domiciliary, rest home, assisted living and/or nursing facility within 90 days following discharge from an inpatient facility.) **B**

* **G2020** Services for high intensity clinical services associated with the initial engagement and outreach of beneficiaries assigned to the sip component of the pcf model (do not bill with chronic care management codes) **A**

* **G2021** Health care practitioners rendering treatment in place (TIP) **E1**

* **G2022** A model participant (ambulance supplier/provider), the beneficiary refuses services covered under the model (transport to an alternate destination/treatment in place) **E1**

* **G2025** Payment for a telehealth distant site service furnished by a rural health clinic (RHC) or federally qualified health center (FQHC) only **A**

* **G2061** Qualified nonphysician healthcare professional online assessment and management service, for an established patient, for up to seven days, cumulative time during the 7 days; 5-10 minutes **M**

* **G2062** Qualified nonphysician healthcare professional online assessment and management service, for an established patient, for up to seven days, cumulative time during the 7 days; 11-20 minutes **M**

* **G2063** Qualified nonphysician qualified healthcare professional assessment and management service, for an established patient, for up to seven days, cumulative time during the 7 days; 21 or more minutes **M**

* **G2067** Medication assisted treatment, methadone; weekly bundle including dispensing and/or administration, substance use counseling, individual and group therapy, and toxicology testing, if performed (provision of the services by a Medicare-enrolled opioid treatment program) **A**

* **G2068** Medication assisted treatment, buprenorphine (oral); weekly bundle including dispensing and/or administration, substance use counseling, individual and group therapy, and toxicology testing if performed (provision of the services by a Medicare-enrolled opioid treatment program) **A**

MIPS   Quantity Physician   Quantity Hospital   ♀ Female only
♂ Male only   Age   DMEPOS   A2-Z3 ASC Payment Indicator   A-Y ASC Status Indicator   Coding Clinic

↻ * **G2069** Medication assisted treatment, buprenorphine (injectable) administered on a monthly basis; bundle including dispensing and/or administration, substance use counseling, individual and group therapy, and toxicology testing if performed (provision of the services by a Medicare-enrolled opioid treatment program) D

~~G2070~~ ~~Medication assisted treatment, buprenorphine (implant insertion); weekly bundle including dispensing and/or administration, substance use counseling, individual and group therapy, and toxicology testing if performed (provision of the services by a Medicare-enrolled opioid treatment program)~~

~~G2071~~ ~~Medication assisted treatment, buprenorphine (implant removal); weekly bundle including dispensing and/or administration, substance use counseling, individual and group therapy, and toxicology testing if performed (provision of the services by a Medicare-enrolled opioid treatment program)~~

~~G2072~~ ~~Medication assisted treatment, buprenorphine (implant insertion and removal); weekly bundle including dispensing and/or administration, substance use counseling, individual and group therapy, and toxicology testing if performed (provision of the services by a Medicare-enrolled opioid treatment program)~~

* **G2073** Medication assisted treatment, naltrexone; weekly bundle including dispensing and/or administration, substance use counseling, individual and group therapy, and toxicology testing if performed (provision of the services by a Medicare-enrolled opioid treatment program) A

* **G2074** Medication assisted treatment, weekly bundle not including the drug, including substance use counseling, individual and group therapy, and toxicology testing if performed (provision of the services by a Medicare-enrolled opioid treatment program) A

* **G2075** Medication assisted treatment, medication not otherwise specified; weekly bundle including dispensing and/or administration, substance use counseling, individual and group therapy, and toxicology testing, if performed (provision of the services by a Medicare-enrolled opioid treatment program) A

↻ * **G2076** Intake activities, including initial medical examination that is a conducted by an appropriately licensed practitioner and preparation of a care plan, which may be informed by administration of a standardized, evidence-based social determinants of health risk assessment to identify unmet health-related social needs, and that includes the patient's goals and mutually agreed-upon actions for the patient to meet those goals, including harm reduction interventions; the patient's needs and goals in the areas of education, vocational training, and employment; and the medical and psychiatric, psychosocial, economic, legal, housing, and other recovery support services that a patient needs and wishes to pursue, conducted by an appropriately licensed/credentialed personnel personnel (provision of the services by a Medicare-enrolled opioid treatment program); list separately in addition to each primary code A

↻ * **G2077** Periodic assessment; assessing periodically by an otp practitioner and includes a review of moud dosing, treatment response, other substance use disorder treatment needs, responses and patient-identified goals, and other relevant physical and psychiatric treatment needs and goals; assessment may be informed by administration of a standardized, evidence-based social determinants of health risk assessment to identify unmet health-related social needs, or the need and interest for harm reduction interventions and recovery support services (provision of the services by a Medicare-enrolled opioid treatment program); list separately in addition to each primary code A

* **G2078** Take-home supply of methadone; up to 7 additional day supply (provision of the services by a Medicare-enrolled opioid treatment program); list separately in addition to code for primary procedure A

TEMPORARY PROCEDURES/PROFESSIONAL SERVICES

* **G2079** Take-home supply of buprenorphine (oral); up to 7 additional day supply (provision of the services by a Medicare-enrolled opioid treatment program); list separately in addition to code for primary procedure A

* **G2080** Each additional 30 minutes of counseling in a week of medication assisted treatment, (provision of the services by a Medicare-enrolled opioid treatment program); list separately in addition to code for primary procedure A

* **G2081** Patients age 66 and older in institutional special needs plans (SNP) or residing in long-term care with a POS code 32, 33, 34, 54 or 56 for more than 90 consecutive days during the measurement period M

* **G2082** Office or other outpatient visit for the evaluation and management of an established patient that requires the supervision of a physician or other qualified health care professional and provision of up to 56 mg of esketamine nasal self-administration, includes 2 hours post-administration observation S

* **G2083** Office or other outpatient visit for the evaluation and management of an established patient that requires the supervision of a physician or other qualified health care professional and provision of greater than 56 mg esketamine nasal self-administration, includes 2 hours post-administration observation S

* **G2086** Office-based treatment for opioid use disorder, including development of the treatment plan, care coordination, individual therapy and group therapy and counseling; at least 70 minutes in the first calendar month S

* **G2087** Office-based treatment for opioid use disorder, including care coordination, individual therapy and group therapy and counseling; at least 60 minutes in a subsequent calendar month S

* **G2088** Office-based treatment for opioid use disorder, including care coordination, individual therapy and group therapy and counseling; each additional 30 minutes beyond the first 120 minutes (list separately in addition to code for primary procedure) N

* **G2090** Patients 66 years of age and older with at least one claim/encounter for frailty during the measurement period and a dispensed medication for dementia during the measurement period or the year prior to the measurement period N1 M

↩ * **G2091** Patients 66 years of age and older with at least one claim/encounter for frailty during the measurement period and an advanced illness diagnosis during the measurement period or the year prior to the measurement period N1 M

* **G2092** Angiotensin converting enzyme (ACE) inhibitor or angiotensin receptor blocker (ARB) or angiotensin receptor-neprilysin inhibitor (AMI) therapy prescribed or currently being taken N1 M

* **G2093** Documentation of medical reason(s) for not prescribing ACE inhibitor or ARB or AMI therapy (e.g., hypotensive patients who are at immediate risk of cardiogenic shock, hospitalized patients who have experienced marked azotemia, allergy, intolerance, other medical reasons) N1 M

* **G2094** Documentation of patient reason(s) for not prescribing ACE inhibitor or ARB or AMI therapy (e.g., patient declined, other patient reasons) N1 M

* **G2096** Angiotensin converting enzyme (ACE) inhibitor or angiotensin receptor blocker (ARB) or angiotensin receptor-neprilysin inhibitor (AMI) therapy was not prescribed, reason not given N1 M

* **G2097** Episodes where the patient had a competing diagnosis on or within three days after the episode date (e.g., intestinal infection, pertussis, bacterial infection, Lyme disease, otitis media, acute sinusitis, acute pharyngitis, acute tonsillitis, chronic sinusitis, infection of the pharynx/larynx/tonsils/adenoids, prostatitis, cellulitis, mastoiditis, or bone infections, acute lymphadenitis, impetigo, skin staph infections, pneumonia/gonococcal infections, venereal disease (syphilis, chlamydia, inflammatory diseases [female reproductive organs]), infections of the kidney, cystitis or UTI N1 M

MIPS Qp Quantity Physician Qh Quantity Hospital ♀ Female only
♂ Male only A Age ♿ DMEPOS A2-Z3 ASC Payment Indicator A-Y ASC Status Indicator Coding Clinic

* **G2098** Patients 66 years of age and older with at least one claim/encounter for frailty during the measurement period and a dispensed medication for dementia during the measurement period or the year prior to the measurement period N1 M

↪ * **G2099** Patients 66 years of age and older with at least one claim/encounter for frailty during the measurement period and an advanced illness diagnosis during the measurement period or the year prior to the measurement period N1 M

* **G2100** Patients 66 years of age and older with at least one claim/encounter for frailty during the measurement period and a dispensed medication for dementia during the measurement period or the year prior to the measurement period N1 M

↪ * **G2101** Patients 66 years of age and older with at least one claim/encounter for frailty during the measurement period and an advanced illness diagnosis during the measurement period or the year prior to the measurement period N1 M

* **G2105** Patients age 66 or older in institutional special needs plans (SNP) or residing in long-term care with POS code 32, 33, 34, 54 or 56 for more than 90 days consecutive during the measurement period N1 M

* **G2106** Patients 66 years of age and older with at least one claim/encounter for frailty during the measurement period and a dispensed medication for dementia during the measurement period or the year prior to the measurement period N1 M

↪ * **G2107** Patients 66 years of age and older with at least one claim/encounter for frailty during the measurement period and an advanced illness diagnosis during the measurement period or the year prior to the measurement period N1 M

* **G2112** Patient receiving <=5 mg daily prednisone (or equivalent), or RA activity is worsening, or glucocorticoid use is for less than 6 months N1 M

* **G2113** Patient receiving >5 mg daily prednisone (or equivalent) for longer than 6 months, and improvement or no change in disease activity N1 M

* **G2115** Patients 66-80 years of age with at least one claim/encounter for frailty during the measurement period and a dispensed medication for dementia during the measurement period or the year prior to the measurement period N1 M

↪ * **G2116** Patients 66-80 years of age with at least one claim/encounter for frailty during the measurement period and an advanced illness diagnosis during the measurement period or the year prior to the measurement period N1 M

* **G2118** Patients 81 years of age and older with at least one claim/encounter for frailty during the measurement period N1 M

* **G2121** Depression, anxiety, apathy, and psychosis assessed N1 M

* **G2122** Depression, anxiety, apathy, and psychosis not assessed N1 M

* **G2125** Patients 81 years of age and older with at least one claim/encounter for frailty during the six months prior to the measurement period through December 31 of the measurement period N1 M

↪ * **G2126** Patients 66-80 years of age with at least one claim/encounter for frailty during the measurement period and an advanced illness diagnosis during the measurement period or the year prior to the measurement period N1 M

* **G2127** Patients 66-80 years of age with at least one claim/encounter for frailty during the measurement period and a dispensed dementia medication N1 M

* **G2128** Documentation of medical reason(s) for not on a daily aspirin or other antiplatelet (e.g. history of gastrointestinal bleed, intra-cranial bleed, blood disorders, idiopathic thrombocytopenic purpura [ITP], gastric bypass or documentation of active anticoagulant use during the measurement period) N1 M

* **G2129** Procedure-related BP's not taken during an outpatient visit. Examples include same day surgery, ambulatory service center, G.I. lab, dialysis, infusion center, chemotherapy N1 M

▶ New   ↪ Revised   ✔ Reinstated   ~~deleted~~ Deleted   ⊘ Not covered or valid by Medicare
✱ Special coverage instructions   * Carrier discretion   Ⓑ Bill Part B MAC   Ⓑ Bill DME MAC

TEMPORARY PROCEDURES/PROFESSIONAL SERVICES

* **G2136** Back pain measured by the Visual Analog Scale (VAS) or numeric pain scale at three months (6 - 20 weeks) postoperatively was less than or equal to 3.0 or back pain measured by the Visual Analog Scale (VAS) or numeric pain scale within three months preoperatively and at three months (6 - 20 weeks) postoperatively demonstrated an improvement of 5.0 points or greater N1 M

* **G2137** Back pain measured by the Visual Analog Scale (VAS) or numeric pain scale at three months (6 - 20 weeks) postoperatively was greater than 3.0 and back pain measured by the Visual Analog Scale (VAS) or numeric pain scale within three months preoperatively and at three months (6 - 20 weeks) postoperatively demonstrated improvement of less than 5.0 points N1 M

* **G2138** Back pain as measured by the Visual Analog Scale (VAS) or numeric pain scale at one year (9 to 15 months) postoperatively was less than or equal to 3.0 or back pain measured by the Visual Analog Scale (VAS) or numeric pain scale within three months preoperatively and at one year (9 to 15 months) postoperatively demonstrated a change of 5.0 points or greater N1 M

* **G2139** Back pain measured by the Visual Analog Scale (VAS) or numeric pain scale pain at one year (9 to 15 months) postoperatively was greater than 3.0 and back pain measured by the Visual Analog Scale (VAS) or numeric pain scale within three months preoperatively and at one year (9 to 15 months) postoperatively demonstrated improvement of less than 5.0 points N1 M

* **G2140** Leg pain measured by the Visual Analog Scale (VAS) or numeric pain scale at three months (6 - 20 weeks) postoperatively was less than or equal to 3.0 or leg pain measured by the Visual Analog Scale (VAS) or numeric pain scale within three months preoperatively and at three months (6 - 20 weeks) postoperatively demonstrated an improvement of 5.0 points or greater N1 M

* **G2141** Leg pain measured by the Visual Analog Scale (VAS) or numeric pain scale at three months (6 - 20 weeks) postoperatively was greater than 3.0 and leg pain measured by the Visual Analog Scale (VAS) or numeric pain scale within three months preoperatively and at three months (6 - 20 weeks) postoperatively demonstrated improvement of less than 5.0 points N1 M

* **G2142** Functional status measured by the Oswestry Disability Index (ODI version 2.1a) at one year (9 to 15 months) postoperatively was less than or equal to 22 or functional status measured by the ODI version 2.1a within three months preoperatively and at one year (9 to 15 months) postoperatively demonstrated an improvement of 30 points or greater N1 M

* **G2143** Functional status measured by the Oswestry Disability Index (ODI version 2.1a) at one year (9 to 15 months) postoperatively was greater than 22 and functional status measured by the ODI version 2.1a within three months preoperatively and at one year (9 to 15 months) postoperatively demonstrated an improvement of less than 30 points N1 M

* **G2144** Functional status measured by the Oswestry Disability Index (ODI version 2.1a) at three months (6 - 20 weeks) postoperatively was less than or equal to 22 or functional status measured by the ODI version 2.1a within three months preoperatively and at three months (6 - 20 weeks) postoperatively demonstrated an improvement of 30 points or greater N1 M

* **G2145** Functional status measured by the Oswestry Disability Index (ODI version 2.1a) at three months (6 - 20 weeks) postoperatively was greater than 22 and functional status measured by the ODI version 2.1a within three months preoperatively and at three months (6 - 20 weeks) postoperatively demonstrated an improvement of less than 30 points N1 M

* G2146	Leg pain as measured by the Visual Analog Scale (VAS) or numeric pain scale at one year (9 to 15 months) postoperatively was less than or equal to 3.0 or leg pain measured by the Visual Analog Scale (VAS) or numeric pain scale within three months preoperatively and at one year (9 to 15 months) postoperatively demonstrated an improvement of 5.0 points or greater	N1 M
* G2147	Leg pain measured by the Visual Analog Scale (VAS) or numeric pain scale at one year (9 to 15 months) postoperatively was greater than 3.0 and leg pain measured by the Visual Analog Scale (VAS) or numeric pain scale within three months preoperatively and at one year (9 to 15 months) postoperatively demonstrated improvement of less than 5.0 points	N1 M
* G2148	Multimodal pain management was used	N1 M
* G2149	Documentation of medical reason(s) for not using multimodal pain management (e.g., allergy to multiple classes of analgesics, intubated patient, hepatic failure, patient reports no pain during PACU stay, other medical reason(s))	N1 M
* G2150	Multimodal pain management was not used	N1 M
* G2151	Documentation stating patient has a diagnosis of a degenerative neurological condition such as ALS, MS, Parkinson's diagnosed at any time before or during the episode of care	N1 M
* G2152	Residual score for the neck impairment successfully calculated and the score was equal to zero (0) or greater than zero (> 0)	N1 M
* G2167	Residual score for the neck impairment successfully calculated and the score was less than zero (< 0)	N1 M
* G2168	Services performed by a physical therapist assistant in the home health setting in the delivery of a safe and effective physical therapy maintenance program, each 15 minutes	B
* G2169	Services performed by an occupational therapist assistant in the home health setting in the delivery of a safe and effective occupational therapy maintenance program, each 15 minutes	B
* G2172	All inclusive payment for services related to highly coordinated and integrated opioid use disorder (oud) treatment services furnished for the demonstration project	A
* G2173	URI episodes where the patient had a comorbid condition during the 12 months prior to or on the episode date (e.g., tuberculosis, neutropenia, cystic fibrosis, chronic bronchitis, pulmonary edema, respiratory failure, rheumatoid lung disease)	M
* G2174	URI episodes when the patient is taking antibiotics (table 1) in the 30 days prior to the episode date	M
* G2175	Episodes where the patient had a comorbid condition during the 12 months prior to or on the episode date (e.g., tuberculosis, neutropenia, cystic fibrosis, chronic bronchitis, pulmonary edema, respiratory failure, rheumatoid lung disease)	M
* G2176	Outpatient, ED, or observation visits that result in an inpatient admission	M
* G2177	Acute bronchitis/bronchiolitis episodes when the patient had a new or refill prescription of antibiotics (table 1) in the 30 days prior to the episode date	M
* G2178	Clinician documented that patient was not an eligible candidate for lower extremity neurological exam measure, for example patient bilateral amputee; patient has condition that would not allow them to accurately respond to a neurological exam (dementia, Alzheimer's, etc.); patient has previously documented diabetic peripheral neuropathy with loss of protective sensation	M
* G2179	Clinician documented that patient had medical reason for not performing lower extremity neurological exam	M
* G2180	Clinician documented that patient was not an eligible candidate for evaluation of footwear as patient is bilateral lower extremity amputee	M
* G2181	BMI not documented due to medical reason or patient refusal of height or weight measurement	M
* G2182	Patient receiving first-time biologic and/or immune response modifier therapy	M
* G2183	Documentation patient unable to communicate and informant not available	M
* G2184	Patient does not have a caregiver	M

▶ New   ⟳ Revised   ✓ Reinstated   ~~deleted~~ Deleted   🚫 Not covered or valid by Medicare
Ⓢ Special coverage instructions   * Carrier discretion   Ⓑ Bill Part B MAC   Ⓑ Bill DME MAC

TEMPORARY PROCEDURES/PROFESSIONAL SERVICES

* **G2185** Documentation caregiver is trained and certified in dementia care M
* **G2186** Patient /caregiver dyad has been referred to appropriate resources and connection to those resources is confirmed M
* **G2187** Patients with clinical indications for imaging of the head: Head trauma M
* **G2188** Patients with clinical indications for imaging of the head: New or change in headache above 50 years of age M
* **G2189** Patients with clinical indications for imaging of the head: Abnormal neurologic exam M
* **G2190** Patients with clinical indications for imaging of the head: Headache radiating to the neck M
* **G2191** Patients with clinical indications for imaging of the head: Positional headaches M
* **G2192** Patients with clinical indications for imaging of the head: Temporal headaches in patients over 55 years of age M
* **G2193** Patients with clinical indications for imaging of the head: New onset headache in pre-school children or younger (<6 years of age) M
* **G2194** Patients with clinical indications for imaging of the head: New onset headache in pediatric patients with disabilities for which headache is a concern as inferred from behavior M
* **G2195** Patients with clinical indications for imaging of the head: Occipital headache in children M
* **G2196** Patient identified as an unhealthy alcohol user when screened for unhealthy alcohol use using a systematic screening method M
* **G2197** Patient screened for unhealthy alcohol use using a systematic screening method and not identified as an unhealthy alcohol user M
* **G2199** Patient not screened for unhealthy alcohol use using a systematic screening method M
* **G2200** Patient identified as an unhealthy alcohol user received brief counseling M
* **G2202** Patient did not receive brief counseling if identified as an unhealthy alcohol user M
* **G2204** Patients between 45 and 85 years of age who received a screening colonoscopy during the performance period M
* **G2205** Patients with pregnancy during adjuvant treatment course M
* **G2206** Patient received adjuvant treatment course including both chemotherapy and her 2-targeted therapy M
* **G2207** Reason for not administering adjuvant treatment course including both chemotherapy and her2-targeted therapy (e.g., poor performance status (ECOG 3-4; Karnofsky < 50), cardiac contraindications, insufficient renal function, insufficient hepatic function, other active or secondary cancer diagnoses, other medical contraindications, patients who died during initial treatment course or transferred during or after initial treatment course) M
* **G2208** Patient did not receive adjuvant treatment course including both chemotherapy and her 2-targeted therapy M
* **G2209** Patient refused to participate M
* **G2210** Residual score for the neck impairment not measured because the patient did not complete the neck fs prom at initial evaluation and/or near discharge, reason not given M
* **G2211** Visit complexity inherent to evaluation and management associated with medical care services that serve as the continuing focal point for all needed health care services and/or with medical care services that are part of ongoing care related to a patient's single, serious condition or a complex condition. (Add-on code, list separately in addition to office/outpatient evaluation and management visit, new or established) B
* **G2212** Prolonged office or other outpatient evaluation and management service(s) beyond the maximum required time of the primary procedure which has been selected using total time on the date of the primary service; each additional 15 minutes by the physician or qualified healthcare professional, with or without direct patient contact (list separately in addition to CPT codes 99205, 99215, 99483 for office or other outpatient evaluation and management services) (do not report G2212 on the same date of service as 99358, 99359, 99415, 99416). (Do not report G2212 for any time unit less than 15 minutes) N

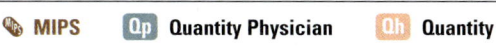 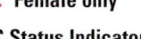

* **G2213** Initiation of medication for the treatment of opioid use disorder in the emergency department setting, including assessment, referral to ongoing care, and arranging access to supportive services (list separately in addition to code for primary procedure) **N**

* **G2214** Initial or subsequent psychiatric collaborative care management, first 30 minutes in a month of behavioral health care manager activities, in consultation with a psychiatric consultant, and directed by the treating physician or other qualified health care professional **S**

* **G2215** Take-home supply of nasal naloxone; 2-pack of 4mg per 0.1 ml nasal spray (provision of the services by a Medicare-enrolled opioid treatment program); list separately in addition to code for primary procedure **A**

* **G2216** Take-home supply of injectable naloxone (provision of the services by a Medicare-enrolled opioid treatment program); list separately in addition to code for primary procedure **A**

* **G2250** Remote assessment of recorded video and/or images submitted by an established patient (e.g., store and forward), including interpretation with follow-up with the patient within 24 business hours, not originating from a related service provided within the previous 7 days nor leading to a service or procedure within the next 24 hours or soonest available appointment **A**

* **G2251** Brief communication technology-based service, e.g., virtual check-in, by a qualified health care professional who cannot report Evaluation and Management services, provided to an established patient, not originating from a related service provided within the previous 7 days nor leading to a service or procedure within the next 24 hours or soonest available appointment; 5-10 minutes of clinical discussion **A**

* **G2252** Brief communication technology-based service, e.g., virtual check-in, by a physician or other qualified health care professional who can report Evaluation and Management services, provided to an established patient, not originating from a related e/m service provided within the previous 7 days nor leading to an e/m service or procedure within the next 24 hours or soonest available appointment; 11-20 minutes of medical discussion **A**

Pain Management

G3002 Chronic pain management and treatment, monthly bundle including, diagnosis; assessment and monitoring; administration of a validated pain rating scale or tool; the development, implementation, revision, and/or maintenance of a person-centered care plan that includes strengths, goals, clinical needs, and desired outcomes; overall treatment management; facilitation and coordination of any necessary behavioral health treatment; medication management; pain and health literacy counseling; any necessary chronic pain related crisis care; and ongoing communication and care coordination between relevant practitioners furnishing care, e.g. physical therapy and occupational therapy, complementary and integrative approaches, and community-based care, as appropriate. Required initial face-to-face visit at least 30 minutes provided by a physician or other qualified health professional; first 30 minutes personally provided by physician or other qualified health care professional, per calendar month. (When using G3002, 30 minutes must be met or exceeded.) **M**

G3003 Each additional 15 minutes of chronic pain management and treatment by a physician or other qualified health care professional, per calendar month. (List separately in addition to code for G3002. When using G3003, 15 minutes must be met or exceeded.) **M**

Specialty Set

* **G4000** Dermatology mips specialty set **M**
* **G4001** Diagnostic radiology mips specialty set **M**
* **G4002** Electrophysiology cardiac specialist mips specialty set **M**
* **G4003** Emergency medicine mips specialty set **M**
* **G4004** Endocrinology mips specialty set **M**
* **G4005** Family medicine mips specialty set **M**
* **G4006** Gastro-enterology mips specialty set **M**
* **G4007** General surgery mips specialty set **M**
* **G4008** Geriatrics mips specialty set **M**
* **G4009** Hospitalists mips specialty set **M**
* **G4010** Infectious disease mips specialty set **M**
* **G4011** Internal medicine mips specialty set **M**
* **G4012** Interventional radiology mips specialty set **M**

▶ New ↺ Revised ✓ Reinstated ~~deleted~~ Deleted ⊘ Not covered or valid by Medicare
◉ Special coverage instructions ✱ Carrier discretion Ⓑ Bill Part B MAC Ⓑ Bill DME MAC

TEMPORARY PROCEDURES/PROFESSIONAL SERVICES

* G4013 Mental/behavioral and psychiatry mips specialty set M
* G4014 Nephrology mips specialty set M
* G4015 Neurology mips specialty set M
* G4016 Neurosurgical mips specialty set M
* G4017 Nutrition/dietician mips specialty set M
* G4018 Obstetrics/gynecology mips specialty set M
* G4019 Oncology/hematology mips specialty set M
* G4020 Ophthalmology/optometry mips specialty set M
* G4021 Orthopedic surgery mips specialty set M
* G4022 Otolaryngology mips specialty set M
* G4023 Pathology mips specialty set M
* G4024 Pediatrics mips specialty set M
* G4025 Physical medicine mips specialty set M
* G4026 Physical therapy/occupational therapy mips specialty set M
* G4027 Plastic surgery mips specialty set M
* G4028 Podiatry mips specialty set M
* G4029 Preventive medicine mips specialty set M
* G4030 Pulmonology mips specialty set M
* G4031 Radiation oncology mips specialty set M
* G4032 Rheumatology mips specialty set M
* G4033 Skilled nursing facility mips specialty set M
* G4034 Speech language pathology mips specialty set M
* G4035 Thoracic surgery mips specialty set M
* G4036 Urgent care mips specialty set M
* G4037 Urology mips specialty set M
* G4038 Vascular surgery mips specialty set M

Guidance

* G6001 Ultrasonic guidance for placement of radiation therapy fields Qp Qh B
* G6002 Stereoscopic x-ray guidance for localization of target volume for the delivery of radiation therapy Qp Qh B

Radiation Treatment

* G6003 Radiation treatment delivery, single treatment area, single port or parallel opposed ports, simple blocks or no blocks: up to 5 mev Qp Qh B
* G6004 Radiation treatment delivery, single treatment area, single port or parallel opposed ports, simple blocks or no blocks: 6-10 mev Qp Qh B
* G6005 Radiation treatment delivery, single treatment area, single port or parallel opposed ports, simple blocks or no blocks: 11-19 mev Qp Qh B
* G6006 Radiation treatment delivery, single treatment area, single port or parallel opposed ports, simple blocks or no blocks: 20 mev or greater Qp Qh B
* G6007 Radiation treatment delivery, 2 separate treatment areas, 3 or more ports on a single treatment area, use of multiple blocks: up to 5 mev Qp Qh B
* G6008 Radiation treatment delivery, 2 separate treatment areas, 3 or more ports on a single treatment area, use of multiple blocks: 6-10 mev Qp Qh B
* G6009 Radiation treatment delivery, 2 separate treatment areas, 3 or more ports on a single treatment area, use of multiple blocks: 11-19 mev Qp Qh B
* G6010 Radiation treatment delivery, 2 separate treatment areas, 3 or more ports on a single treatment area, use of multiple blocks: 20 mev or greater Qp Qh B
* G6011 Radiation treatment delivery, 3 or more separate treatment areas, custom blocking, tangential ports, wedges, rotational beam, compensators, electron beam; up to 5 mev Qp Qh B
* G6012 Radiation treatment delivery, 3 or more separate treatment areas, custom blocking, tangential ports, wedges, rotational beam, compensators, electron beam; 6-10 mev Qp Qh B
* G6013 Radiation treatment delivery, 3 or more separate treatment areas, custom blocking, tangential ports, wedges, rotational beam, compensators, electron beam; 11-19 mev Qp Qh B
* G6014 Radiation treatment delivery, 3 or more separate treatment areas, custom blocking, tangential ports, wedges, rotational beam, compensators, electron beam; 20 mev or greater Qp Qh B
* G6015 Intensity modulated treatment delivery, single or multiple fields/arcs, via narrow spatially and temporally modulated beams, binary, dynamic MLC, per treatment session Qp Qh B
* G6016 Compensator-based beam modulation treatment delivery of inverse planned treatment using 3 or more high resolution (milled or cast) compensator, convergent beam modulated fields, per treatment session Qp Qh B

MIPS | Qp Quantity Physician | Qh Quantity Hospital | ♀ Female only
♂ Male only | A Age | DMEPOS | A2-Z3 ASC Payment Indicator | A-Y ASC Status Indicator | Coding Clinic

2026 HCPCS LEVEL II NATIONAL CODES

* **G6017** Intra-fraction localization and tracking of target or patient motion during delivery of radiation therapy (e.g., 3D positional tracking, gating, 3D surface tracking), each fraction of treatment ⓑ Qp Qh B

Quality Measures

* **G8395** Left ventricular ejection fraction (LVEF) >=40% or documentation as normal or mildly depressed left ventricular systolic function ⓑ M

* **G8396** Left ventricular ejection fraction (LVEF) not performed or documented ⓑ M

* **G8397** Dilated macular or fundus exam performed, including documentation of the presence or absence of macular edema and level of severity of retinopathy ⓑ M

* **G8399** Patient with documented results of a central dual-energy x-ray absorptiometry (DXA) ever being performed ⓑ M

* **G8400** Patient with central dual-energy x-ray absorptiometry (DXA) results not documented ⓑ M

* **G8404** Lower extremity neurological exam performed and documented ⓑ M

* **G8405** Lower extremity neurological exam not performed ⓑ M

* **G8410** Footwear evaluation performed and documented ⓑ M

* **G8415** Footwear evaluation was not performed ⓑ M

* **G8416** Clinician documented that patient was not an eligible candidate for footwear evaluation measure ⓑ M

* **G8417** BMI is documented above normal parameters and a follow-up plan is documented ⓑ M

* **G8418** BMI is documented below normal parameters and a follow-up plan is documented ⓑ M

* **G8419** BMI is documented outside normal parameters, no follow-up plan documented, no reason given ⓑ M

* **G8420** BMI is documented within normal parameters and no follow-up plan is required ⓑ M

* **G8421** BMI not documented and no reason is given ⓑ M

* **G8427** Eligible clinician attests to documenting in the medical record they obtained, updated, or reviewed the patient's current medications ⓑ M

* **G8428** Current list of medications not documented as obtained, updated, or reviewed by the eligible clinician, reason not given ⓑ M

* **G8430** Documentation of a medical reason(s) for not documenting, updating, or reviewing the patient's current medications list (e.g., patient is in an urgent or emergent medical situation) ⓑ M

* **G8431** Screening for depression is documented as being positive and a follow-up plan is documented ⓑ M

* **G8432** Depression screening not documented, reason not given ⓑ M

* **G8433** Screening for depression not completed, documented patient or medical reason ⓑ M

* **G8450** Beta-blocker therapy prescribed ⓑ M

* **G8451** Beta-blocker therapy for LVEF <40% not prescribed for reasons documented by the clinician (e.g., low blood pressure, fluid overload, asthma, patients recently treated with an intravenous positive inotropic agent, allergy, intolerance, other medical reasons, patient declined, other patient reasons) ⓑ M

* **G8452** Beta-blocker therapy not prescribed ⓑ M

* **G8465** High or very high risk of recurrence of prostate cancer ⓑ ♂ M

* **G8473** Angiotensin converting enzyme (ACE) inhibitor or angiotensin receptor blocker (ARB) therapy prescribed ⓑ M

* **G8474** Angiotensin converting enzyme (ACE) inhibitor or angiotensin receptor blocker (ARB) therapy not prescribed for reasons documented by the clinician (e.g., allergy, intolerance, pregnancy, renal failure due to ACE inhibitor, diseases of the aortic or mitral valve, other medical reasons) or (e.g., patient declined, other patient reasons) ⓑ M

* **G8475** Angiotensin converting enzyme (ACE) inhibitor or angiotensin receptor blocker (ARB) therapy not prescribed, reason not given ⓑ M

* **G8476** Most recent blood pressure has a systolic measurement of <140 mmHg and a diastolic measurement of <90 mmHg ⓑ M

* **G8477** Most recent blood pressure has a systolic measurement of >=140 mmHg and/or a diastolic measurement of >=90 mmHg ⓑ M

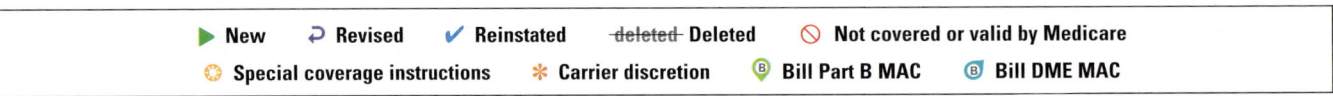

▶ New ↻ Revised ✓ Reinstated ~~deleted~~ Deleted ⊘ Not covered or valid by Medicare ◉ Special coverage instructions * Carrier discretion ⓑ Bill Part B MAC Ⓑ Bill DME MAC

TEMPORARY PROCEDURES/PROFESSIONAL SERVICES

* **G8478** Blood pressure measurement not performed or documented, reason not given ⓑ M

~~G8482 Influenza immunization administered or previously received~~

~~G8483 Influenza immunization was not administered for reasons documented by clinician (e.g., patient allergy or other medical reasons, patient declined or other patient reasons, vaccine not available or other system reasons)~~

~~G8484 Influenza immunization was not administered, reason not given~~

* **G8510** Screening for depression is documented as negative, a follow-up plan is not required ⓑ M

* **G8511** Screening for depression documented as positive, follow up plan not documented, reason not given ⓑ M

* **G8535** Elder maltreatment screen not documented; documentation that patient is not eligible for the elder maltreatment screen at the time of the encounter related to one of the following reasons: (1) patient refuses to participate in the screening and has reasonable decisional capacity for self-protection, or (2) patient is in an urgent or emergent situation where time is of the essence and to delay treatment to perform the screening would jeopardize the patient's health status ⓑ Ⓐ M

* **G8536** No documentation of an elder maltreatment screen, reason not given ⓑ Ⓐ M

* **G8539** Functional outcome assessment documented as positive using a standardized tool and a care plan based on identified deficiencies is documented within two days of the functional outcome assessment ⓑ M

* **G8540** Functional outcome assessment not documented as being performed, documentation the patient is not eligible for a functional outcome assessment using a standardized tool at the time of the encounter ⓑ M

* **G8541** Functional outcome assessment using a standardized tool not documented, reason not given ⓑ M

* **G8542** Functional outcome assessment using a standardized tool is documented; no functional deficiencies identified, care plan not required ⓑ M

* **G8543** Documentation of a positive functional outcome assessment using a standardized tool; care plan not documented within two days of assessment, reason not given ⓑ M

* **G8559** Patient referred to a physician (preferably a physician with training in disorders of the ear) for an otologic evaluation ⓑ M

* **G8560** Patient has a history of active drainage from the ear within the previous 90 days ⓑ M

* **G8561** Patient is not eligible for the referral for otologic evaluation for patients with a history of active drainage measure ⓑ M

* **G8562** Patient does not have a history of active drainage from the ear within the previous 90 days ⓑ M

* **G8563** Patient not referred to a physician (preferably a physician with training in disorders of the ear) for an otologic evaluation, reason not given ⓑ M

* **G8564** Patient was referred to a physician (preferably a physician with training in disorders of the ear) for an otologic evaluation, reason not specified ⓑ M

* **G8565** Verification and documentation of sudden or rapidly progressive hearing loss ⓑ M

* **G8566** Patient is not eligible for the "referral for otologic evaluation for sudden or rapidly progressive hearing loss" measure ⓑ M

* **G8567** Patient does not have verification and documentation of sudden or rapidly progressive hearing loss ⓑ M

* **G8568** Patient was not referred to a physician (preferably a physician with training in disorders of the ear) for an otologic evaluation, reason not given ⓑ M

* **G8569** Prolonged postoperative intubation (>24 hrs) required ⓑ M

* **G8570** Prolonged postoperative intubation (>24 hrs) not required ⓑ M

* **G8575** Developed postoperative renal failure or required dialysis ⓑ M

* **G8576** No postoperative renal failure/dialysis not required ⓑ M

↩ * **G8577** Re-exploration required due to mediastinal bleeding with or without tamponade, unplanned coronary artery intervention (native, vessel, graft, or both), valve disfunction, aortic reintervention, or other cardiac reason ⓑ M

↩ * **G8578** Re-exploration not required due to mediastinal bleeding with or without tamponade, unplanned coronary artery intervention (native, vessel, graft, or both), valve dysfunction, aortic reintervention, or other cardiac reason ⓑ M

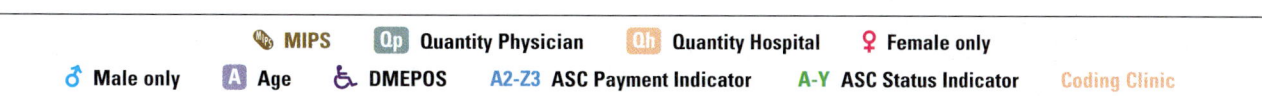

* G8598	Aspirin or another antiplatelet therapy used
* G8599	Aspirin or another antiplatelet therapy not used, reason not given
* G8600	IV thrombolytic therapy initiated within 4.5 hours (<= 270 minutes) of time last known well
* G8601	IV thrombolytic therapy not initiated within 4.5 hours (= 270 minutes) of time last known well for reasons documented by clinician (e.g. patient enrolled in clinical trial for stroke, patient admitted for elective carotid intervention
* G8602	IV thrombolytic therapy not initiated within 4.5 hours (= 270 minutes) of time last known well, reason not given
* G8633	Pharmacologic therapy (other than minerals/vitamins) for osteoporosis prescribed
* G8635	Pharmacologic therapy for osteoporosis was not prescribed, reason not given
* G8647	Residual score for the knee impairment successfully calculated and the score was equal to zero (0) or greater than zero (>0)
* G8648	Residual score for the knee impairment successfully calculated and the score was less than zero (<0)
* G8650	Residual scores for the knee impairment not measured because the patient did not complete the LEPT prom at initial evaluation and/or near discharge, reason not given
* G8651	Residual score for the hip impairment successfully calculated and the score was equal to zero (0) or greater than zero (>0)
* G8652	Residual score for the hip impairment successfully calculated and the score was less than zero (<0)
* G8654	Residual scores for the hip impairment not measured because the patient did not complete LEPT prom at initial evaluation and/or follow up status survey near discharge, reason not given
* G8655	Residual score for the foot or ankle impairment successfully calculated and the score was equal to zero (0) or greater than zero (>0)
* G8656	Residual score for the foot or ankle impairment successfully calculated and the score was less than zero (<0)
* G8658	Residual scores for the lower leg, foot or ankle impairment not measured because the patient did not complete LEPT prom at initial evaluation and/or follow up status survey near discharge, reason not given
* G8659	Residual score for the low back impairment successfully calculated and the score was equal to zero (0) or greater than zero (>0)
* G8660	Residual score for the low back impairment successfully calculated and the score was less than zero (<0)
* G8661	Risk-adjusted functional status change residual scores for the low back impairment not measured because the patient did not complete FOTO'S status survey near discharge, patient not appropriate
* G8662	Residual scores for the low back impairment not measured because the patient did not complete the low back FS prom at initial evaluation and/or near discharge, reason not given
* G8663	Residual score for the shoulder impairment successfully calculated and the score was equal to zero (0) or greater than zero (>0)
* G8664	Residual score for the shoulder impairment successfully calculated and the score was less than zero (<0)
* G8666	Residual scores for the shoulder impairment not measured because the patient did not complete the shoulder FS prom at initial evaluation and/or near discharge, reason not given
* G8667	Residual score for the elbow, wrist or hand impairment successfully calculated and the score was equal to zero (0) or greater than zero (>0)
* G8668	Residual score for the elbow, wrist or hand impairment successfully calculated and the score was less than zero (<0)
* G8670	Residual scores for the elbow, wrist or hand impairment not measured because the patient did not complete the the elbow/wrist/hand FS prom at initial evaluation near discharge, reason not given
↻ * G8694	Current or prior left ventriucular ejection fraction (LVEF) <=40% or documentation of moderate or severe LVSD
* G8708	Patient not prescribed antibiotic

▶ New ↻ Revised ✓ Reinstated deleted Deleted ⊘ Not covered or valid by Medicare ✦ Special coverage instructions * Carrier discretion Ⓑ Bill Part B MAC Ⓑ Bill DME MAC

TEMPORARY PROCEDURES/PROFESSIONAL SERVICES

* G8709 URI episodes when the patient had competing diagnoses on or three days after the episode date (e.g., intestinal infection, pertussis, bacterial infection, Lyme disease, otitis media, acute sinusitis, acute pharyngitis, acute tonsillitis, chronic sinusitis, infection of the pharynx/larynx/tonsils/adenoids, prostatitis, cellulitis, mastoiditis, or bone infections, acute lymphadenitis, impetigo, skin staph infections, pneumonia/gonococcal infections, venereal disease [syphilis, chlamydia, inflammatory diseases (female reproductive organs)], infections of the kidney, cystitis or UTI, and acne) M
* G8710 Patient prescribed antibiotic M
* G8711 Prescribed antibiotic on or within 3 days after the episode date M
* G8712 Antibiotic not prescribed or dispensed M
* G8721 PT category (primary tumor), PN category (regional lymph nodes), and histologic grade were documented in pathology report M
* G8722 Documentation of medical reason(s) for not including the PT category, the PN category or the histologic grade in the pathology report (e.g., re-excision without residual tumor; non-carcinomasanal canal) M
* G8723 Specimen site is other than anatomic location of primary tumor M
* G8724 PT category, PN category and histologic grade were not documented in the pathology report, reason not given M
* G8733 Elder maltreatment screen documented as positive and a follow-up plan is documented M
* G8734 Elder maltreatment screen documented as negative, follow-up is not required M
* G8735 Elder maltreatment screen documented as positive, follow-up plan not documented, reason not given M
* G8749 Absence of signs of melanoma (tenderness, jaundice, localized neurologic signs such as weakness, or any other sign suggesting systemic spread) or absence of symptoms of melanoma (cough, dyspnea, pain, paresthesia, or any other symptom suggesting the possibility of systemic spread of melanoma) M
* G8752 Most recent systolic blood pressure <140 mmhg M
* G8753 Most recent systolic blood pressure >=140 mmhg M
* G8754 Most recent diastolic blood pressure <90 mmhg M
* G8755 Most recent diastolic blood pressure >=90 mmhg M
* G8756 No documentation of blood pressure measurement, reason not given M
* G8783 Normal blood pressure reading documented, follow-up not required M
* G8785 Blood pressure reading not documented, reason not given M
* G8797 Specimen site other than anatomic location of esophagus M
* G8798 Specimen site other than anatomic location of prostate M
* G8806 Performance of trans-abdominal or trans-vaginal ultrasound and pregnancy location documented M
* G8807 Trans-abdominal or trans-vaginal ultrasound not performed for reasons documented by clinician (e.g., patient has a documented intrauterine pregnancy [IUP]) M
* G8808 Trans-abdominal or trans-vaginal ultrasound not performed, reason not given M
* G8815 Documented reason in the medical records for why the statin therapy was not prescribed (i.e., lower extremity bypass was for a patient with non-artherosclerotic disease) M
* G8816 Statin medication prescribed at discharge M
* G8817 Statin therapy not prescribed at discharge, reason not given M
* G8826 Patient discharged to home no later than post-operative day #2 following EVAR M
* G8833 Patient not discharged to home by post-operative day #2 following EVAR M
* G8834 Patient discharged to home no later than post-operative day #2 following CEA M
* G8838 Patient not discharged to home by post-operative day #2 following CEA M
* G8839 Sleep apnea symptoms assessed, including presence or absence of snoring and daytime sleepiness M

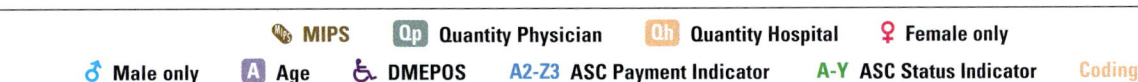

237

* G8840	Documentation of reason(s) for not documenting an assessment of sleep symptoms (e.g., patient didn't have initial daytime sleepiness, patient visited between initial testing and initiation of therapy) Ⓑ M
* G8841	Sleep apnea symptoms not assessed, reason not given Ⓑ M
↻ * G8842	Apnea Hypopnea Index (AHI), Respiratory Disturbance Index (RDI), or Respiratory Event Index (REI) documented or measured within 2 months after initial evaluation for suspected obstructive sleep apnea Ⓑ M
↻ * G8843	Documentation of reason(s) for not measuring an Apnea Hypopnea Index (AHI), a Respiratory Disturbance Index (RDI), or a Respiratory Event Index (REI) within 2 months after initial evaluation for suspected obstructive sleep apnea (e.g., medical, neurological, or psychiatric disease that prohibits successful completion of a sleep study, patients for whom a sleep study would present a bigger risk than benefit or would pose an undue burden, dementia, patients previously diagnosed with osa and severity assessed by another provider, patients who decline AHI/RDI/REI measurement, patients who had a financial reason for not completing testing, test was ordered but not completed, patients decline because their insurance [payer] does not cover the expense) Ⓑ M
↻ * G8844	Apnea Hypopnea Index (AHI), Respiratory Disturbance Index (RDI), or Respiratory Event Index (REI) not documented or measured within 2 months after initial evaluation for suspected obstructive sleep apnea, reason not given Ⓑ M
* G8845	Positive airway pressure therapy prescribed Ⓑ M
* G8846	Moderate or severe obstructive sleep apnea (Apnea Hypopnea Index (AHI) or Respiratory Disturbance Index (RDI) of 15 or greater) Ⓑ M
* G8849	Documentation of reason(s) for not prescribing positive airway pressure therapy (e.g., patient unable to tolerate, alternative therapies use, patient declined, financial, insurance coverage) Ⓑ M
* G8850	Positive airway pressure therapy not prescribed, reason not given Ⓑ M
* G8851	Adherence to therapy was assessed at least annually through an objective informatics system or through self-reporting (if objective reporting is not available, documented) Ⓑ M
* G8854	Documentation of reason(s) for not objectively reporting adherence to evidence-based therapy (e.g., patients who have been diagnosed with a terminal or advanced disease with an expected life span of less than 6 months, patients who decline therapy, patients who do not return for follow-up at least annually, patients unable to access/afford therapy, patient's insurance will not cover therapy) Ⓑ M
* G8855	Adherence to therapy was not assessed at least annually through an objective informatics system or through self-reporting (if objective reporting is not available) Ⓑ M
* G8856	Referral to a physician for an otologic evaluation performed Ⓑ M
* G8857	Patient is not eligible for the referral for otologic evaluation measure (e.g., patients who are already under the care of a physician for acute or chronic dizziness) Ⓑ M
* G8858	Referral to a physician for an otologic evaluation not performed, reason not given Ⓑ M
* G8863	Patients not assessed for risk of bone loss, reason not given Ⓑ M
* G8864	Pneumococcal vaccine administered or previously received Ⓑ M
* G8865	Documentation of medical reason(s) for not administering or previously receiving pneumococcal vaccine (e.g., patient allergic reaction, potential adverse drug reaction) Ⓑ M
* G8866	Documentation of patient reason(s) for not administering or previously receiving pneumococcal vaccine (e.g., patient refusal) Ⓑ M
* G8867	Pneumococcal vaccine not administered or previously received, reason not given Ⓑ M
* G8869	Patient has documented immunity to hepatitis B and initiating anti-TNF therapy Ⓑ M

▶ New ↻ Revised ✓ Reinstated ~~deleted~~ Deleted ⊘ Not covered or valid by Medicare ✻ Special coverage instructions * Carrier discretion Ⓑ Bill Part B MAC Ⓑ Bill DME MAC

TEMPORARY PROCEDURES/PROFESSIONAL SERVICES

* **G8875** Clinician diagnosed breast cancer preoperatively by a minimally invasive biopsy method ⓑ M
* **G8876** Documentation of reason(s) for not performing minimally invasive biopsy to diagnose breast cancer preoperatively (e.g., lesion too close to skin, implant, chest wall, etc., lesion could not be adequately visualized for needle biopsy, patient condition prevents needle biopsy [weight, breast thickness, etc.], duct excision without imaging abnormality, prophylactic mastectomy, reduction mammoplasty, excisional biopsy performed by another physician) ⓑ M
* **G8877** Clinician did not attempt to achieve the diagnosis of breast cancer preoperatively by a minimally invasive biopsy method, reason not given ⓑ M
* **G8878** Sentinel lymph node biopsy procedure performed ⓑ M
* **G8880** Documentation of reason(s) sentinel lymph node biopsy not performed (e.g., reasons could include but not limited to: non-invasive cancer, incidental discovery of breast cancer on prophylactic mastectomy, incidental discovery of breast cancer on reduction mammoplasty, pre-operative biopsy proven lymph node (LN) metastases, inflammatory carcinoma, stage 3 locally advanced cancer, recurrent invasive breast cancer, clinically node positive after neoadjuvant systemic therapy, patient refusal after informed consent; patient with significant age, comorbidities, or limited life expectancy and favorable tumor; adjuvant systemic therapy unlikely to change) ⓑ M
* **G8881** Stage of breast cancer is greater than T1N0M0 or T2N0M0 ⓑ M
* **G8882** Sentinel lymph node biopsy procedure not performed, reason not given ⓑ M
* **G8907** Patient documented not to have experienced any of the following events: a burn prior to discharge; a fall within the facility; wrong site/side/patient/procedure/implant event; or a hospital transfer or hospital admission upon discharge from the facility ⓑ M
* **G8908** Patient documented to have received a burn prior to discharge ⓑ M
* **G8909** Patient documented not to have received a burn prior to discharge ⓑ M
* **G8910** Patient documented to have experienced a fall within ASC ⓑ M
* **G8911** Patient documented not to have experienced a fall within ambulatory surgical center ⓑ M
* **G8912** Patient documented to have experienced a wrong site, wrong side, wrong patient, wrong procedure or wrong implant event ⓑ M
* **G8913** Patient documented not to have experienced a wrong site, wrong side, wrong patient, wrong procedure or wrong implant event ⓑ M
* **G8914** Patient documented to have experienced a hospital transfer or hospital admission upon discharge from ASC ⓑ M
* **G8915** Patient documented not to have experienced a hospital transfer or hospital admission upon discharge from ASC ⓑ M
* **G8916** Patient with preoperative order for IV antibiotic surgical site infection (SSI) prophylaxis, antibiotic initiated on time ⓑ M
* **G8917** Patient with preoperative order for IV antibiotic surgical site infection (SSI) prophylaxis, antibiotic not initiated on time ⓑ M
* **G8918** Patient without preoperative order for IV antibiotic surgical site infection (SSI) prophylaxis ⓑ M
* **G8923** Current or prior left ventricular ejection fraction (LVEF) <=40% or documentation of moderately or severely depressed left ventricular systolic function ⓑ M
* **G8924** Spirometry results documented (FEV1/FVC <70%) ⓑ M
* **G8934** Current or prior left ventricular ejection fraction (LVEF) <=40% or documentation of moderately or severely depressed left ventricular systolic function ⓑ M
* **G8935** Clinician prescribed angiotensin converting enzyme (ACE) inhibitor or angiotensin receptor blocker (ARB) therapy ⓑ M
* **G8936** Clinician documented that patient was not an eligible candidate for Angiotensin converting enzyme (ace) inhibitor or Angiotensin Receptor Blocker (ARB) therapy (eg, allergy, intolerance, pregnancy, renal failure due to ace inhibitor, diseases of the aortic or mitral valve, other medical reasons) or (eg, patient declined, other patient reasons) M

- * G8937 Clinician did not prescribe angiotensin converting enzyme (ACE) inhibitor or angiotensin receptor blocker (ARB) therapy, reason not given ⓑ M
- * G8939 Pain assessment documented as positive, follow-up plan not documented, documentation the patient is not eligible at the time of the encounter at the time of the encounter ⓑ M
- * G8942 Functional outcome assessment using a standardized tool is documented within the previous 30 days and care plan, based on identified deficiencies is documented within two days of the functional outcome assessment ⓑ M
- * G8944 AJCC melanoma cancer stage 0 through IIC melanoma ⓑ M
- * G8946 Minimally invasive biopsy method attempted but not diagnostic of breast cancer (e.g., high risk lesion of breast such as atypical ductal hyperplasia, lobular neoplasia, atypical lobular hyperplasia, lobular carcinoma in situ, atypical columnar hyperplasia, flat epithelial atypia, radial scar, complex sclerosing lesion, papillary lesion, or any lesion with spindle cells) ⓑ M
- * G8950 Elevated or hypertensive blood pressure reading documented, and the indicated follow-up documented ⓑ M
- * G8952 Elevated or hypertensive blood pressure reading documented, indicated follow-up not documented, reason not given ⓑ M
- * G8955 Most recent assessment of adequacy of volume management documented ⓑ M
- * G8956 Patient receiving maintenance hemodialysis in an outpatient dialysis facility ⓑ M
- * G8958 Assessment of adequacy of volume management not documented, reason not given ⓑ M
- * G8961 Cardiac stress imaging test primarily performed on low-risk surgery patient for preoperative evaluation within 30 days preceding this surgery ⓑ M
- * G8962 Cardiac stress imaging test performed on patient for any reason including those who did not have low risk surgery or test that was performed more than 30 days preceding low risk surgery ⓑ M
- G8965 Cardiac stress imaging test primarily performed on low CHD risk patient for initial detection and risk assessment
- G8966 Cardiac stress imaging test performed on symptomatic or higher than low CHD risk patient or for any reason other than initial detection and risk assessment
- * G8967 FDA-approved oral anticoagulant is prescribed ⓑ M
- * G8968 Documentation of medical reason(s) for not prescribing an FDA-approved anticoagulant (e.g., present or planned atrial appendage occlusion or ligation or patient being currently enrolled in a clinical trial related to AF/atrial flutter treatment) ⓑ M
- * G8969 Documentation of patient reason(s) for not prescribing an oral anticoagulant that is FDA approved for the prevention of thromboembolism (e.g., patient choice of having atrial appendage device placed) ⓑ M
- * G8970 No risk factors or one moderate risk factor for thromboembolism ⓑ M

Coordinated Care

- G9001 Coordinated care fee, initial rate ⓑ B
- G9002 Coordinated care fee, maintenance rate ⓑ B
- G9003 Coordinated care fee, risk adjusted high, initial ⓑ B
- G9004 Coordinated care fee, risk adjusted low, initial ⓑ B
- G9005 Coordinated care fee, risk adjusted maintenance ⓑ B
- G9006 Coordinated care fee, home monitoring ⓑ B
- G9007 Coordinated care fee, scheduled team conference ⓑ B
- G9008 Coordinated care fee, physician coordinated care oversight services ⓑ B
- G9009 Coordinated care fee, risk adjusted maintenance, level 3 ⓑ B
- G9010 Coordinated care fee, risk adjusted maintenance, level 4 ⓑ B
- G9011 Coordinated care fee, risk adjusted maintenance, level 5 ⓑ B
- G9012 Other specified case management services not elsewhere classified ⓑ B

Demonstration Project

- ⊘ G9013 ESRD demo basic bundle Level I ⓑ E1
- ⊘ G9014 ESRD demo expanded bundle including venous access and related services ⓑ E1

▶ New   ⤺ Revised   ✓ Reinstated   deleted Deleted   ⊘ Not covered or valid by Medicare
◎ Special coverage instructions   * Carrier discretion   ⓑ Bill Part B MAC   ⓑ Bill DME MAC

TEMPORARY PROCEDURES/PROFESSIONAL SERVICES

⊘ **G9016** Smoking cessation counseling, individual, in the absence of or in addition to any other evaluation and management service, per session (6-10 minutes) [demo project code only] ⓑ E1

~~**G9037** Interprofessional telephone/internet/electronic health record clinical question/request for specialty recommendations by a treating/requesting physician or other qualified health care professional for the care of the patient (i.e. not for professional education or scheduling) and may include subsequent follow up on the specialist's recommendations; 30 minutes~~

~~**G9038** Co-management services with the following elements: new diagnosis or acute exacerbation and stabilization of existing condition; condition which may benefit from joint care planning; condition for which specialist is taking a co-management role; condition expected to last at least 3 months; comprehensive care plan established, implemented, revised or monitored in partnership with co-managing clinicians; ongoing communication and care coordination between co-managing clinicians furnishing care~~

⊘ **G9050** Oncology; primary focus of visit; work-up, evaluation, or staging at the time of cancer diagnosis or recurrence (for use in a Medicare-approved demonstration project) ⓑ E1

⊘ **G9051** Oncology; primary focus of visit; treatment decision-making after disease is staged or restaged, discussion of treatment options, supervising/coordinating active cancer directed therapy or managing consequences of cancer directed therapy (for use in a Medicare-approved demonstration project) ⓑ E1

⊘ **G9052** Oncology; primary focus of visit; surveillance for disease recurrence for patient who has completed definitive cancer-directed therapy and currently lacks evidence of recurrent disease; cancer directed therapy might be considered in the future (for use in a Medicare-approved demonstration project) ⓑ E1

⊘ **G9053** Oncology; primary focus of visit; expectant management of patient with evidence of cancer for whom no cancer directed therapy is being administered or arranged at present; cancer directed therapy might be considered in the future (for use in a Medicare-approved demonstration project) ⓑ E1

⊘ **G9054** Oncology; primary focus of visit; supervising, coordinating or managing care of patient with terminal cancer or for whom other medical illness prevents further cancer treatment; includes symptom management, end-of-life care planning, management of palliative therapies (for use in a Medicare-approved demonstration project) ⓑ E1

⊘ **G9055** Oncology; primary focus of visit; other, unspecified service not otherwise listed (for use in a Medicare-approved demonstration project) ⓑ E1

⊘ **G9056** Oncology; practice guidelines; management adheres to guidelines (for use in a Medicare-approved demonstration project) ⓑ E1

⊘ **G9057** Oncology; practice guidelines; management differs from guidelines as a result of patient enrollment in an institutional review board approved clinical trial (for use in a Medicare-approved demonstration project) ⓑ E1

⊘ **G9058** Oncology; practice guidelines; management differs from guidelines because the treating physician disagrees with guideline recommendations (for use in a Medicare-approved demonstration project) ⓑ E1

⊘ **G9059** Oncology; practice guidelines; management differs from guidelines because the patient, after being offered treatment consistent with guidelines, has opted for alternative treatment or management, including no treatment (for use in a Medicare-approved demonstration project) ⓑ E1

⊘ **G9060** Oncology; practice guidelines; management differs from guidelines for reason(s) associated with patient comorbid illness or performance status not factored into guidelines (for use in a Medicare-approved demonstration project) ⓑ E1

⊘ **G9061** Oncology; practice guidelines; patient's condition not addressed by available guidelines (for use in a Medicare-approved demonstration project) ⓑ E1

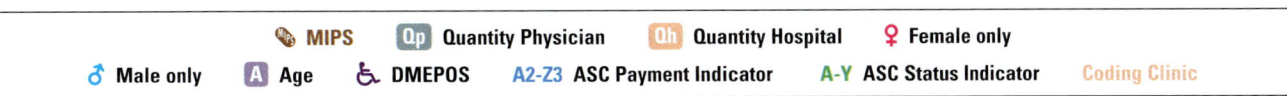

⊘ **G9062** Oncology; practice guidelines; management differs from guidelines for other reason(s) not listed (for use in a Medicare-approved demonstration project) Ⓑ E1

∗ **G9063** Oncology; disease status; limited to non-small cell lung cancer; extent of disease initially established as stage I (prior to neo-adjuvant therapy, if any) with no evidence of disease progression, recurrence, or metastases (for use in a Medicare-approved demonstration project) Ⓑ M

∗ **G9064** Oncology; disease status; limited to non-small cell lung cancer; extent of disease initially established as stage II (prior to neo-adjuvant therapy, if any) with no evidence of disease progression, recurrence, or metastases (for use in a Medicare-approved demonstration project) Ⓑ M

∗ **G9065** Oncology; disease status; limited to non-small cell lung cancer; extent of disease initially established as stage IIIA (prior to neo-adjuvant therapy, if any) with no evidence of disease progression, recurrence, or metastases (for use in a Medicare-approved demonstration project) Ⓑ M

∗ **G9066** Oncology; disease status; limited to non-small cell lung cancer; stage IIIB-IV at diagnosis, metastatic, locally recurrent, or progressive (for use in a Medicare-approved demonstration project) Ⓑ M

∗ **G9067** Oncology; disease status; limited to non-small cell lung cancer; extent of disease unknown, staging in progress, or not listed (for use in a Medicare-approved demonstration project) Ⓑ M

∗ **G9068** Oncology; disease status; limited to small cell and combined small cell/non-small cell; extent of disease initially established as limited with no evidence of disease progression, recurrence, or metastases (for use in a Medicare-approved demonstration project) Ⓑ M

∗ **G9069** Oncology; disease status; small cell lung cancer, limited to small cell and combined small cell/non-small cell; extensive stage at diagnosis, metastatic, locally recurrent, or progressive (for use in a Medicare-approved demonstration project) Ⓑ M

∗ **G9070** Oncology; disease status; small cell lung cancer, limited to small cell and combined small cell/non-small cell; extent of disease unknown, staging in progress, or not listed (for use in a Medicare-approved demonstration project) Ⓑ M

∗ **G9071** Oncology; disease status; invasive female breast cancer (does not include ductal carcinoma in situ); adenocarcinoma as predominant cell type; stage I or stage IIA-IIB; or T3, N1, M0; and ER and/or PR positive; with no evidence of disease progression, recurrence, or metastases (for use in a Medicare-approved demonstration project) Ⓑ ♀ M

∗ **G9072** Oncology; disease status; invasive female breast cancer (does not include ductal carcinoma in situ); adenocarcinoma as predominant cell type; stage I, or stage IIA-IIB; or T3, N1, M0; and ER and PR negative; with no evidence of disease progression, recurrence, or metastases (for use in a Medicare-approved demonstration project) Ⓑ ♀ M

∗ **G9073** Oncology; disease status; invasive female breast cancer (does not include ductal carcinoma in situ); adenocarcinoma as predominant cell type; stage IIIA-IIIB; and not T3, N1, M0; and ER and/or PR positive; with no evidence of disease progression, recurrence, or metastases (for use in a Medicare-approved demonstration project) Ⓑ ♀ M

∗ **G9074** Oncology; disease status; invasive female breast cancer (does not include ductal carcinoma in situ); adenocarcinoma as predominant cell type; stage IIIA-IIIB; and not T3, N1, M0; and ER and PR negative; with no evidence of disease progression, recurrence, or metastases (for use in a Medicare-approved demonstration project) Ⓑ ♀ M

∗ **G9075** Oncology; disease status; invasive female breast cancer (does not include ductal carcinoma in situ); adenocarcinoma as predominant cell type; M1 at diagnosis, metastatic, locally recurrent, or progressive (for use in a Medicare-approved demonstration project) Ⓑ ♀ M

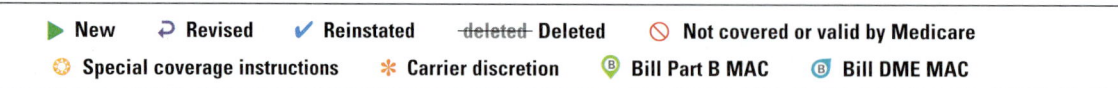

▶ New ⇄ Revised ✓ Reinstated ~~deleted~~ Deleted ⊘ Not covered or valid by Medicare ◐ Special coverage instructions ∗ Carrier discretion Ⓑ Bill Part B MAC Ⓑ Bill DME MAC

TEMPORARY PROCEDURES/PROFESSIONAL SERVICES

* **G9077** Oncology; disease status; prostate cancer, limited to adenocarcinoma as predominant cell type; T1-T2c and Gleason 2-7 and PSA < or equal to 20 at diagnosis with no evidence of disease progression, recurrence, or metastases (for use in a Medicare-approved demonstration project) ⓑ ♂ M

* **G9078** Oncology; disease status; prostate cancer, limited to adenocarcinoma as predominant cell type; T2 or T3a Gleason 8-10 or PSA >20 at diagnosis with no evidence of disease progression, recurrence, or metastases (for use in a Medicare-approved demonstration project) ⓑ ♂ M

* **G9079** Oncology; disease status; prostate cancer, limited to adenocarcinoma as predominant cell type; T3b-T4, any N; any T, N1 at diagnosis with no evidence of disease progression, recurrence, or metastases (for use in a Medicare-approved demonstration project) ⓑ ♂ M

* **G9080** Oncology; disease status; prostate cancer, limited to adenocarcinoma; after initial treatment with rising PSA or failure of PSA decline (for use in a Medicare-approved demonstration project) ⓑ ♂ M

* **G9083** Oncology; disease status; prostate cancer, limited to adenocarcinoma; extent of disease unknown, staging in progress, or not listed (for use in a Medicare-approved demonstration project) ⓑ ♂ M

* **G9084** Oncology; disease status; colon cancer, limited to invasive cancer, adenocarcinoma as predominant cell type; extent of disease initially established as T1-3, N0, M0 with no evidence of disease progression, recurrence, or metastases (for use in a Medicare-approved demonstration project) ⓑ M

* **G9085** Oncology; disease status; colon cancer, limited to invasive cancer, adenocarcinoma as predominant cell type; extent of disease initially established as T4, N0, M0 with no evidence of disease progression, recurrence, or metastases (for use in a Medicare-approved demonstration project) ⓑ M

* **G9086** Oncology; disease status; colon cancer, limited to invasive cancer, adenocarcinoma as predominant cell type; extent of disease initially established as T1-4, N1-2, M0 with no evidence of disease progression, recurrence, or metastases (for use in a Medicare-approved demonstration project) ⓑ M

* **G9087** Oncology; disease status; colon cancer, limited to invasive cancer, adenocarcinoma as predominant cell type; M1 at diagnosis, metastatic, locally recurrent, or progressive with current clinical, radiologic, or biochemical evidence of disease (for use in a Medicare-approved demonstration project) ⓑ M

* **G9088** Oncology; disease status; colon cancer, limited to invasive cancer, adenocarcinoma as predominant cell type; M1 at diagnosis, metastatic, locally recurrent, or progressive without current clinical, radiologic, or biochemical evidence of disease (for use in a Medicare-approved demonstration project) ⓑ M

* **G9089** Oncology; disease status; colon cancer, limited to invasive cancer, adenocarcinoma as predominant cell type; extent of disease unknown, staging in progress, or not listed (for use in a Medicare-approved demonstration project) ⓑ M

* **G9090** Oncology; disease status; rectal cancer, limited to invasive cancer, adenocarcinoma as predominant cell type; extent of disease initially established as T1-2, N0, M0 (prior to neo-adjuvant therapy, if any) with no evidence of disease progression, recurrence, or metastases (for use in a Medicare-approved demonstration project) ⓑ M

* **G9091** Oncology; disease status; rectal cancer, limited to invasive cancer, adenocarcinoma as predominant cell type; extent of disease initially established as T3, N0, M0 (prior to neo-adjuvant therapy, if any) with no evidence of disease progression, recurrence, or metastases (for use in a Medicare-approved demonstration project) ⓑ M

MIPS | Qp Quantity Physician | Qh Quantity Hospital | ♀ Female only
♂ Male only | A Age | & DMEPOS | A2-Z3 ASC Payment Indicator | A-Y ASC Status Indicator | Coding Clinic

* **G9092** Oncology; disease status; rectal cancer, limited to invasive cancer, adenocarcinoma as predominant cell type; extent of disease initially established as T1-3, N1-2, M0 (prior to neo-adjuvant therapy, if any) with no evidence of disease progression, recurrence or metastases (for use in a Medicare-approved demonstration project) Ⓑ M

* **G9093** Oncology; disease status; rectal cancer, limited to invasive cancer, adenocarcinoma as predominant cell type; extent of disease initially established as T4, any N, M0 (prior to neo-adjuvant therapy, if any) with no evidence of disease progression, recurrence, or metastases (for use in a Medicare-approved demonstration project) Ⓑ M

* **G9094** Oncology; disease status; rectal cancer, limited to invasive cancer, adenocarcinoma as predominant cell type; M1 at diagnosis, metastatic, locally recurrent, or progressive (for use in a Medicare-approved demonstration project) Ⓑ M

* **G9095** Oncology; disease status; rectal cancer, limited to invasive cancer, adenocarcinoma as predominant cell type; extent of disease unknown, staging in progress, or not listed (for use in a Medicare-approved demonstration project) Ⓑ M

* **G9096** Oncology; disease status; esophageal cancer, limited to adenocarcinoma or squamous cell carcinoma as predominant cell type; extent of disease initially established as T1-T3, N0-N1 or NX (prior to neo-adjuvant therapy, if any) with no evidence of disease progression, recurrence, or metastases (for use in a Medicare-approved demonstration project) Ⓑ M

* **G9097** Oncology; disease status; esophageal cancer, limited to adenocarcinoma or squamous cell carcinoma as predominant cell type; extent of disease initially established as T4, any N, M0 (prior to neo-adjuvant therapy, if any) with no evidence of disease progression, recurrence, or metastases (for use in a Medicare-approved demonstration project) Ⓑ M

* **G9098** Oncology; disease status; esophageal cancer, limited to adenocarcinoma or squamous cell carcinoma as predominant cell type; M1 at diagnosis, metastatic, locally recurrent, or progressive (for use in a Medicare-approved demonstration project) Ⓑ M

* **G9099** Oncology; disease status; esophageal cancer, limited to adenocarcinoma or squamous cell carcinoma as predominant cell type; extent of disease unknown, staging in progress, or not listed (for use in a Medicare-approved demonstration project) Ⓑ M

* **G9100** Oncology; disease status; gastric cancer, limited to adenocarcinoma as predominant cell type; post R0 resection (with or without neoadjuvant therapy) with no evidence of disease recurrence, progression, or metastases (for use in a Medicare-approved demonstration project) Ⓑ M

* **G9101** Oncology; disease status; gastric cancer, limited to adenocarcinoma as predominant cell type; post R1 or R2 resection (with or without neoadjuvant therapy) with no evidence of disease progression, or metastases (for use in a Medicare-approved demonstration project) Ⓑ M

* **G9102** Oncology; disease status; gastric cancer, limited to adenocarcinoma as predominant cell type; clinical or pathologic M0, unresectable with no evidence of disease progression, or metastases (for use in a Medicare-approved demonstration project) Ⓑ M

* **G9103** Oncology; disease status; gastric cancer, limited to adenocarcinoma as predominant cell type; clinical or pathologic M1 at diagnosis, metastatic, locally recurrent, or progressive (for use in a Medicare-approved demonstration project) Ⓑ M

* **G9104** Oncology; disease status; gastric cancer, limited to adenocarcinoma as predominant cell type; extent of disease unknown, staging in progress, or not listed (for use in a Medicare-approved demonstration project) Ⓑ M

* **G9105** Oncology; disease status; pancreatic cancer, limited to adenocarcinoma as predominant cell type; post R0 resection without evidence of disease progression, recurrence, or metastases (for use in a Medicare-approved demonstration project) Ⓑ M

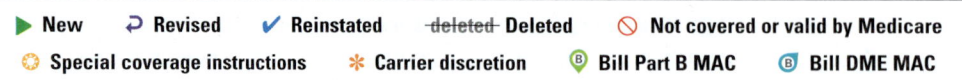

TEMPORARY PROCEDURES/PROFESSIONAL SERVICES

* **G9106** Oncology; disease status; pancreatic cancer, limited to adenocarcinoma; post R1 or R2 resection with no evidence of disease progression or metastases (for use in a Medicare-approved demonstration project) Ⓑ M

* **G9107** Oncology; disease status; pancreatic cancer, limited to adenocarcinoma; unresectable at diagnosis, M1 at diagnosis, metastatic, locally recurrent, or progressive (for use in a Medicare-approved demonstration project) Ⓑ M

* **G9108** Oncology; disease status; pancreatic cancer, limited to adenocarcinoma; extent of disease unknown, staging in progress, or not listed (for use in a Medicare-approved demonstration project) Ⓑ M

* **G9109** Oncology; disease status; head and neck cancer, limited to cancers of oral cavity, pharynx and larynx with squamous cell as predominant cell type; extent of disease initially established as T1-T2 and N0, M0 (prior to neo-adjuvant therapy, if any) with no evidence of disease progression, recurrence, or metastases (for use in a Medicare-approved demonstration project) Ⓑ M

* **G9110** Oncology; disease status; head and neck cancer, limited to cancers of oral cavity, pharynx, and larynx with squamous cell as predominant cell type; extent of disease initially established as T3-4 and/ or N1-3, M0 (prior to neo-adjuvant therapy, if any) with no evidence of disease progression, recurrence, or metastases (for use in a Medicare-approved demonstration project) Ⓑ M

* **G9111** Oncology; disease status; head and neck cancer, limited to cancers of oral cavity, pharynx and larynx with squamous cell as predominant cell type; M1 at diagnosis, metastatic, locally recurrent, or progressive (for use in a Medicare-approved demonstration project) Ⓑ M

* **G9112** Oncology; disease status; head and neck cancer, limited to cancers of oral cavity, pharynx and larynx with squamous cell as predominant cell type; extent of disease unknown, staging in progress, or not listed (for use in a Medicare-approved demonstration project) Ⓑ M

* **G9113** Oncology; disease status; ovarian cancer, limited to epithelial cancer; pathologic stage IA-B (grade 1) without evidence of disease progression, recurrence, or metastases (for use in a Medicare-approved demonstration project) Ⓑ ♀ M

* **G9114** Oncology; disease status; ovarian cancer, limited to epithelial cancer; pathologic stage IA-B (grade 2-3); or stage IC (all grades); or stage II; without evidence of disease progression, recurrence, or metastases (for use in a Medicare-approved demonstration project) Ⓑ ♀ M

* **G9115** Oncology; disease status; ovarian cancer, limited to epithelial cancer; pathologic stage III-IV; without evidence of progression, recurrence, or metastases (for use in a Medicare-approved demonstration project) Ⓑ ♀ M

* **G9116** Oncology; disease status; ovarian cancer, limited to epithelial cancer; evidence of disease progression, or recurrence and/or platinum resistance (for use in a Medicare-approved demonstration project) Ⓑ ♀ M

* **G9117** Oncology; disease status; ovarian cancer, limited to epithelial cancer; extent of disease unknown, staging in progress, or not listed (for use in a Medicare-approved demonstration project) Ⓑ ♀ M

* **G9123** Oncology; disease status; chronic myelogenous leukemia, limited to Philadelphia chromosome positive and/ or BCR-ABL positive; chronic phase not in hematologic, cytogenetic, or molecular remission (for use in a Medicare-approved demonstration project) Ⓑ M

* **G9124** Oncology; disease status; chronic myelogenous leukemia, limited to Philadelphia chromosome positive and/ or BCR-ABL positive; accelerated phase not in hematologic cytogenetic, or molecular remission (for use in a Medicare-approved demonstration project) Ⓑ M

* **G9125** Oncology; disease status; chronic myelogenous leukemia, limited to Philadelphia chromosome positive and/ or BCR-ABL positive; blast phase not in hematologic, cytogenetic, or molecular remission (for use in a Medicare-approved demonstration project) Ⓑ M

* **G9126** Oncology; disease status; chronic myelogenous leukemia, limited to Philadelphia chromosome positive and/or BCR-ABL positive; in hematologic, cytogenetic, or molecular remission (for use in a Medicare-approved demonstration project) Ⓑ   M

* **G9128** Oncology: disease status; limited to multiple myeloma, systemic disease; smouldering, stage I (for use in a Medicare-approved demonstration project) Ⓑ   M

* **G9129** Oncology; disease status; limited to multiple myeloma, systemic disease; stage II or higher (for use in a Medicare-approved demonstration project) Ⓑ   M

* **G9130** Oncology; disease status; limited to multiple myeloma, systemic disease; extent of disease unknown, staging in progress, or not listed (for use in a Medicare-approved demonstration project) Ⓑ   M

* **G9131** Oncology; disease status; invasive female breast cancer (does not include ductal carcinoma in situ); adenocarcinoma as predominant cell type; extent of disease unknown, staging in progress, or not listed (for use in a Medicare-approved demonstration project) Ⓑ ♀   M

* **G9132** Oncology; disease status; prostate cancer, limited to adenocarcinoma; hormone-refractory/androgen-independent (e.g., rising PSA on anti-androgen therapy or post-orchiectomy); clinical metastases (for use in a Medicare-approved demonstration project) Ⓑ ♂   M

* **G9133** Oncology; disease status; prostate cancer, limited to adenocarcinoma; hormone-responsive; clinical metastases or M1 at diagnosis (for use in a Medicare-approved demonstration project) Ⓑ ♂   M

* **G9134** Oncology; disease status; non-Hodgkin's lymphoma, any cellular classification; stage I, II at diagnosis, not relapsed, not refractory (for use in a Medicare-approved demonstration project) Ⓑ   M

* **G9135** Oncology; disease status; non-Hodgkin's lymphoma, any cellular classification; stage III, IV, not relapsed, not refractory (for use in a Medicare-approved demonstration project) Ⓑ   M

* **G9136** Oncology; disease status; non-Hodgkin's lymphoma, transformed from original cellular diagnosis to a second cellular classification (for use in a Medicare-approved demonstration project) Ⓑ   M

* **G9137** Oncology; disease status; non-Hodgkin's lymphoma, any cellular classification; relapsed/refractory (for use in a Medicare-approved demonstration project) Ⓑ   M

* **G9138** Oncology; disease status; non-Hodgkin's lymphoma, any cellular classification; diagnostic evaluation, stage not determined, evaluation of possible relapse or non-response to therapy, or not listed (for use in a Medicare-approved demonstration project) Ⓑ   M

* **G9139** Oncology; disease status; chronic myelogenous leukemia, limited to Philadelphia chromosome positive and/or BCR-ABL positive; extent of disease unknown, staging in progress, not listed (for use in a Medicare-approved demonstration project) Ⓑ   M

* **G9140** Frontier extended stay clinic demonstration; for a patient stay in a clinic approved for the CMS demonstration project; the following measures should be present: the stay must be equal to or greater than 4 hours; weather or other conditions must prevent transfer or the case falls into a category of monitoring and observation cases that are permitted by the rules of the demonstration; there is a maximum frontier extended stay clinic (FESC) visit of 48 hours, except in the case when weather or other conditions prevent transfer; payment is made on each period up to 4 hours, after the first 4 hours Ⓑ   A

Warfarin Responsiveness Testing

* **G9143** Warfarin responsiveness testing by genetic technique using any method, any number of specimen(s) Ⓑ Qp Qh   N

This would be a once-in-a-lifetime test unless there is a reason to believe that the patient's personal genetic characteristics would change over time. (https://www.cms.gov/ContractorLearningResources/downloads/JA6715.pdf)

Laboratory Certification: General immunology, Hematology

Coding Clinic: 2010, Q2, P10

▶ New   ↻ Revised   ✓ Reinstated   deleted Deleted   ⊘ Not covered or valid by Medicare
⊛ Special coverage instructions   ✱ Carrier discretion   Ⓑ Bill Part B MAC   Ⓑ Bill DME MAC

TEMPORARY PROCEDURES/PROFESSIONAL SERVICES

Outpatient IV Insulin Treatment

⊘ **G9147** Outpatient intravenous insulin treatment (OIVIT) either pulsatile or continuous, by any means, guided by the results of measurements for: respiratory quotient; and/or urine urea nitrogen (UUN); and/or arterial, venous or capillary glucose; and/or potassium concentration ⓑ　　　　　　E1

On December 23, 2009, CMS issued a national non-coverage decision on the use of OIVIT. CR 6775.

Not covered on Physician Fee Schedule

Coding Clinic: 2010, Q2, P10

Quality Assurance

* **G9148** National Committee for Quality Assurance - level 1 medical home ⓑ　M
* **G9149** National Committee for Quality Assurance - level 2 medical home ⓑ　M
* **G9150** National Committee for Quality Assurance - level 3 medical home ⓑ　M
* **G9151** MAPCP demonstration - state provided services ⓑ　M
* **G9152** MAPCP demonstration - community health teams ⓑ　M
* **G9153** MAPCP demonstration - physician incentive pool ⓑ　M

Wheelchair Evaluation

* **G9156** Evaluation for wheelchair requiring face to face visit with physician ⓑ Qp Qh　M

Cardiac Monitoring

* **G9157** Transesophageal doppler measurement of cardiac output (including probe placement, image acquisition, and interpretation per course of treatment) for monitoring purposes ⓑ Qp Qh　B

Bundled Payment Care Improvement

* **G9187** Bundled payments for care improvement initiative home visit for patient assessment performed by a qualified health care professional for individuals not considered homebound including, but not limited to, assessment of safety, falls, clinical status, fluid status, medication reconciliation/management, patient compliance with orders/plan of care, performance of activities of daily living, appropriateness of care setting; (for use only in the Medicare-approved bundled payments for care improvement initiative); may not be billed for a 30-day period covered by a transitional care management code ⓑ Qp Qh　E1

Quality Measures: Miscellaneous

* **G9188** Beta-blocker therapy not prescribed, reason not given ⓑ　M
* **G9189** Beta-blocker therapy prescribed or currently being taken ⓑ　M
* **G9190** Documentation of medical reason(s) for not prescribing beta-blocker therapy (e.g., allergy, intolerance, other medical reasons) ⓑ　M
* **G9191** Documentation of patient reason(s) for not prescribing beta-blocker therapy (e.g., patient declined, other patient reasons) ⓑ　M
* **G9212** DSM-IV-TM criteria for major depressive disorder documented at the initial evaluation ⓑ　M
* **G9213** DSM-IV-TR criteria for major depressive disorder not documented at the initial evaluation, reason not otherwise specified ⓑ　M
* **G9223** Pneumocystis jiroveci pneumonia prophylaxis prescribed within 3 months of low CD4+ cell count below 500 cells/mm3 or a CD4 percentage below 15% ⓑ　M
* **G9225** Foot exam was not performed, reason not given ⓑ　M
* **G9226** Foot examination performed (includes examination through visual inspection, sensory exam with 10-g monofilament plus testing any one of the following: vibration using 128-hz tuning fork, pinprick sensation, ankle reflexes, or vibration perception threshold, and pulse exam; report when all of the 3 components are completed) ⓑ　M

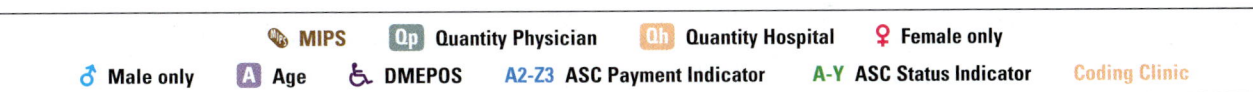

MIPS　　Qp Quantity Physician　　Qh Quantity Hospital　　♀ Female only
♂ Male only　　A Age　　DMEPOS　　A2-Z3 ASC Payment Indicator　　A-Y ASC Status Indicator　　Coding Clinic

2026 HCPCS LEVEL II NATIONAL CODES

* **G9227** Functional outcome assessment documented, care plan not documented, documentation the patient is not eligible for a care plan at the time of the encounter ⒷⓂ
* **G9228** Chlamydia, gonorrhea and syphilis screening results documented (report when results are present for all of the 3 screenings) ⒷⓂ
* **G9230** Chlamydia, gonorrhea, and syphilis not screened, reason not given ⒷⓂ
* **G9231** Documentation of end stage renal disease (ESRD), dialysis, renal transplant before or during the measurement period or pregnancy during the measurement period ⒷⓂ
* **G9242** Documentation of viral load equal to or greater than 200 copies/ml or viral load not performed ⒷⓂ
* **G9243** Documentation of viral load less than 200 copies/ml ⒷⓂ
⇄ * **G9246** Patient did not have two eligible encounters at least 90 days apart or one eligible encounter and one HIV viral load test at least 90 days apart ⒷⓂ
⇄ * **G9247** Patient had two eligible encounters at least 90 days apart or one eligible encounter and one HIV viral load test at least 90 days apart ⒷⓂ
⇄ * **G9254** Documentation of patient discharged to home later than post-operative day 2 following CEA or CAS ⒷⓂ
⇄ * **G9255** Documentation of patient discharged to home no later than post operative day 2 following CEA or CAS ⒷⓂ
* **G9273** Blood pressure has a systolic value of <140 and a diastolic value of <90 ⒷⓂ
* **G9274** Blood pressure has a systolic value of = 140 and a diastolic value of = 90 or systolic value <140 and diastolic value = 90 or systolic value = 140 and diastolic value <90 ⒷⓂ
* **G9275** Documentation that patient is a current non-tobacco user ⒷⓂ
* **G9276** Documentation that patient is a current tobacco user ⒷⓂ
* **G9277** Documentation that the patient is on daily aspirin or anti-platelet or has documentation of a valid contraindication or exception to aspirin/anti-platelet; contraindications/exceptions include anti-coagulant use, allergy to aspirin or anti-platelets, history of gastrointestinal bleed and bleeding disorder; additionally, the following exceptions documented by the physician as a reason for not taking daily aspirin or anti-platelet are acceptable (use of non-steroidal anti-inflammatory agents, documented risk for drug interaction, uncontrolled hypertension defined as >180 systolic or >110 diastolic or gastroesophageal reflux) ⒷⓂ
* **G9278** Documentation that the patient is not on daily aspirin or anti-platelet regimen ⒷⓂ
* **G9279** Pneumococcal screening performed and documentation of vaccination received prior to discharge ⒷⓂ
* **G9280** Pneumococcal vaccination not administered prior to discharge, reason not specified ⒷⓂ
* **G9281** Screening performed and documentation that vaccination not indicated/patient refusal ⒷⓂ
* **G9282** Documentation of medical reason(s) for not reporting the histological type or NSCLC-NOS classification with an explanation (e.g., biopsy taken for other purposes in a patient with a history of non-small cell lung cancer or other documented medical reasons) ⒷⓂ
* **G9283** Non-small-cell lung cancer biopsy and cytology specimen report documents classification into specific histologic type or classified as NSCLC-NOS with an explanation ⒷⓂ
* **G9284** Non-small-cell lung cancer biopsy and cytology specimen report does not document classification into specific histologic type or classified as NSCLC-NOS with an explanation ⒷⓂ
* **G9285** Specimen site other than anatomic location of lung or is not classified as non-small-cell lung cancer ⒷⓂ
* **G9286** Antibiotic regimen prescribed within 10 days after onset of symptoms ⒷⓂ
* **G9287** Antibiotic regimen not prescribed within 10 days after onset of symptoms ⒷⓂ

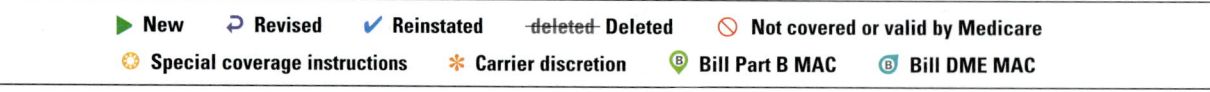

* G9288	Documentation of medical reason(s) for not reporting the histological type or NSCLC-NOS classification with an explanation (e.g., a solitary fibrous tumor in a person with a history of non-small cell carcinoma or other documented medical reasons) ⓑ M
* G9289	Non-small cell lung cancer biopsy and cytology specimen report documents classification into specific histologic type or classified as NSCLC-NOS with an explanation ⓑ M
* G9290	Non-small cell lung cancer biopsy and cytology specimen report does not document classification into specific histologic type or classified as NSCLC-NOS with an explanation ⓑ M
* G9291	Specimen site other than anatomic location of lung, is not classified as non-small-cell lung cancer or classified as NSCLC-NOS ⓑ M
* G9292	Documentation of medical reason(s) for not reporting PT category and a statement on thickness and ulceration and for PT1, mitotic rate (e.g., negative skin biopsies in a patient with a history of melanoma or other documented medical reasons) ⓑ M
* G9293	Pathology report does not include the PT category and a statement on thickness and ulceration and for PT1, mitotic rate ⓑ M
* G9294	Pathology report includes the PT category and a statement on thickness and ulceration and for PT1, mitotic rate ⓑ M
* G9295	Specimen site other than anatomic cutaneous location ⓑ M
🌀 * G9296	Patients with documented shared decision-making including discussion of conservative (non-surgical) therapy (e.g., NSAIDs, analgesics, weight loss, exercise, injections) prior to the procedure ⓑ M
🌀 * G9297	Shared decision-making including discussion of conservative (non-surgical) therapy (e.g., NSAIDs, analgesics, weight loss, exercise, injections) prior to the procedure not documented, reason not given M
🌀 * G9298	Patients who are evaluated for venous thromboembolic and cardiovascular risk factors within 30 days prior to the procedure (e.g., history of DVT, PE, MI, arrhythmia and stroke) ⓑ M
🌀 * G9299	Patients who are not evaluated for venous thromboembolic and cardiovascular risk factors within 30 days prior to the procedure (e.g., history of DVT, PE, MI, arrhythmia and stroke, reason not given) ⓑ M
🌀 * G9305	Intervention for presence of leak of endoluminal contents through an anastomosis not required ⓑ M
🌀 * G9306	Intervention for presence of leak of endoluminal contents through an anastomosis required ⓑ M
🌀 * G9307	No return to the operating room for a surgical procedure, for complications of the principal operative procedure, within 30 days of the principal operative procedure ⓑ M
🌀 * G9308	Unplanned return to the operating room for a surgical procedure, for complications of the principal operative procedure, within 30 days of the principal operative procedure ⓑ M
🌀 * G9309	No unplanned hospital readmission within 30 days of principal procedure ⓑ M
🌀 * G9310	Unplanned hospital readmission within 30 days of principal procedure ⓑ M
🌀 * G9311	No surgical site infection ⓑ M
🌀 * G9312	Surgical site infection ⓑ M
🌀 * G9313	Amoxicillin, with or without clavulanate, not prescribed as first line antibiotic at the time of diagnosis for documented reason ⓑ M
🌀 * G9314	Amoxicillin, with or without clavulanate, not prescribed as first line antibiotic at the time of diagnosis, reason not given ⓑ M
🌀 * G9315	Amoxicillin, with or without clavulanate, prescribed as a first line antibiotic at the time of diagnosis ⓑ M
🌀 * G9316	Documentation of patient-specific risk assessment with a risk calculator based on multi-institutional clinical data, the specific risk calculator used, and communication of risk assessment from risk calculator with the patient or family ⓑ M
🌀 * G9317	Documentation of patient-specific risk assessment with a risk calculator based on multi-institutional clinical data, the specific risk calculator used, and communication of risk assessment from risk calculator with the patient or family not completed ⓑ M
🌀 * G9318	Imaging study named according to standardized nomenclature ⓑ M

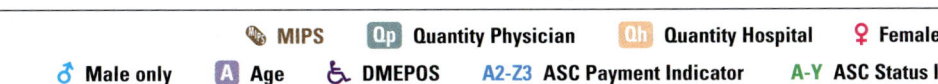

* G9319	Imaging study not named according to standardized nomenclature, reason not given Ⓑ M
↻ * G9321	Count of previous CT (any type of CT) and cardiac nuclear medicine (myocardial perfusion or infarct avid imaging) studies documented in the 12-month period prior to the current study Ⓑ M
↻ * G9322	Count of previous CT and cardiac nuclear medicine (myocardial perfusion or infarct avid imaging) studies not documented in the 12-month period prior to the current study, reason not given Ⓑ M
* G9341	Search conducted for prior patient CT studies completed at non-affiliated external healthcare facilities or entities within the past 12-months and are available through a secure, authorized, media-free, shared archive prior to an imaging study being performed Ⓑ M
* G9342	Search not conducted prior to an imaging study being performed for prior patient CT studies completed at non-affiliated external healthcare facilities or entities within the past 12-months and are available through a secure, authorized, media-free, shared archive, reason not given Ⓑ M
* G9344	Due to system reasons search not conducted for DICOM format images for prior patient CT imaging studies completed at non-affiliated external healthcare facilities or entities within the past 12 months that are available through a secure, authorized, media-free, shared archive (e.g., non-affiliated external healthcare facilities or entities does not have archival abilities through a shared archival system) Ⓑ M
* G9345	Follow-up recommendations documented according to recommended guidelines for incidentally detected pulmonary nodules (e.g., follow-up CT imaging studies needed or that no follow-up is needed) based at a minimum on nodule size and patient risk factors Ⓑ M
* G9347	Follow-up recommendations not documented according to recommended guidelines for incidentally detected pulmonary nodules, reason not given Ⓑ M
* G9351	More than one CT scan of the paranasal sinuses ordered or received within 90 days after diagnosis Ⓑ M
* G9352	More than one CT scan of the paranasal sinuses ordered or received within 90 days after the date of diagnosis, reason not given Ⓑ M
* G9353	More than one CT scan of the paranasal sinuses ordered or received within 90 days after the date of diagnosis for documented reasons (e.g., patients with complications, second CT obtained prior to surgery, other medical reasons) Ⓑ M
* G9354	One CT scan or no CT scan of the paranasal sinuses ordered within 90 days after the date of diagnosis Ⓑ M
* G9355	Elective delivery (without medical indication) by c-section, or early induction not performed (less than 39 weeks gestation) Ⓑ M
* G9356	Elective delivery (without medical indication) by c-section, or early induction performed (less than 39 weeks gestation) Ⓑ M
* G9357	Post-partum screenings, evaluations and education performed Ⓑ M
* G9358	Post-partum screenings, evaluations and education not performed Ⓑ M
* G9361	Medical indication for induction [delivery by cesarean birth or induction of labor (<39 weeks of gestation)] [documentation of reason(s) for elective delivery (e.g., hemorrhage and placental complications, hypertension, preeclampsia and eclampsia, rupture of membranes-premature or prolonged, maternal conditions complicating pregnancy/delivery, fetal conditions complicating pregnancy/delivery, late pregnancy, prior uterine surgery, or participation in clinical trial)] Ⓑ M
* G9364	Sinusitis caused by, or presumed to be caused by, bacterial infection Ⓑ M
* G9367	At least two orders for high-risk medications from the same drug class ordered Ⓑ M
* G9368	At least two orders for high-risk medications from the same drug class not ordered Ⓑ M
* G9380	Patient offered assistance with end of life issues or existing end of life plan was not reviewed or updated during the measurement period Ⓑ M
* G9382	Patient not offered assistance with end of life issues or existing end of life plan was reviewed or updated during the measurement period Ⓑ M

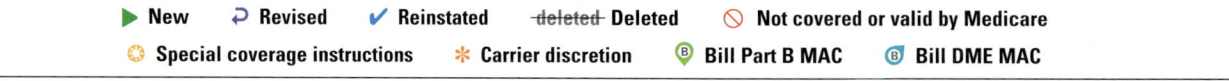

▶ New ↻ Revised ✓ Reinstated ~~deleted~~ Deleted ⊘ Not covered or valid by Medicare
◎ Special coverage instructions * Carrier discretion Ⓑ Bill Part B MAC Ⓓ Bill DME MAC

TEMPORARY PROCEDURES/PROFESSIONAL SERVICES

* **G9383** Patient received screening for HCV infection within the 12 month reporting period ⓑ M
* **G9384** Documentation of medical reason(s) for not receiving annual screening for HCV infection (e.g., decompensated cirrhosis indicating advanced disease [i.e., ascites, esophageal variceal bleeding, hepatic encephalopathy], hepatocellular carcinoma, waitlist for organ transplant, limited life expectancy, other medical reasons) ⓑ M
* **G9385** Documentation of patient reason(s) for not receiving annual screening for HCV infection (e.g., patient declined, other patient reasons) ⓑ M
* **G9386** Screening for HCV infection not received within the 12 month reporting period, reason not given ⓑ M
* **G9393** Patient with an initial PHQ-9 score greater than nine who achieves remission at 12 months as demonstrated by a 12 month (+/- 30 days) PHQ-9 score of less than five ⓑ M
* **G9394** Patient who had a diagnosis of bipolar disorder or personality disorder, death, permanent nursing home resident or receiving hospice or palliative care any time during the measurement or assessment period ⓑ M
* **G9395** Patient with an initial PHQ-9 score greater than nine who did not achieve remission at 12 months as demonstrated by a 12 month (+/- 30 days) PHQ-9 score greater than or equal to five ⓑ M
* **G9396** Patient with an initial PHQ-9 score greater than nine who was not assessed for remission at 12 months (+/- 30 days) ⓑ M
* ~~G9402~~ ~~Patient received follow up within 30 days after discharge~~
* ~~G9403~~ ~~Clinician documented reason patient was not able to complete 30 day follow up from acute inpatient setting discharge (e.g., patient death prior to follow-up visit, patient non-compliant for visit follow up)~~
* ~~G9404~~ ~~Patient did not receive follow-up within 30 days after discharge~~
* ~~G9405~~ ~~Patient received follow-up within 7 days after discharge~~
* ~~G9406~~ ~~Clinician documented reason patient was not able to complete 7 day follow up from acute inpatient setting discharge (i.e patient death prior to follow-up visit, patient non-compliance for visit follow up)~~
* ~~G9407~~ ~~Patient did not receive follow up within 7 days after discharge~~
* **G9408** Patients with cardiac tamponade and/or pericardiocentesis occurring within 30 days ⓑ M
* **G9409** Patients without cardiac tamponade and/or pericardiocentesis occurring within 30 days ⓑ M
* **G9410** Patient admitted within 180 days, status post CIED implantation, replacement, or revision with an infection requiring device removal or surgical revision ⓑ M
* **G9411** Patient not admitted within 180 days, status post CIED implantation, replacement, or revision with an infection requiring device removal or surgical revision ⓑ M
* **G9412** Patient admitted within 180 days, status post CIED implantation, replacement, or revision with an infection requiring device removal or surgical revision ⓑ M
* **G9413** Patient not admitted within 180 days, status post CIED implantation, replacement, or revision with an infection requiring device removal or surgical revision ⓑ M
* **G9414** Patient had one dose of meningococcal vaccine (serogroups a, c, w, y) on or between the patient's 11th and 13th birthdays ⓑ M
* **G9415** Patient did not have one dose of meningococcal (serogroups a, c, w, y) vaccine on or between the patient's 11th and 13th birthdays ⓑ M
* **G9416** Patient had one tetanus, diphtheria toxoids and acellular pertussis vaccine (Tdap) or one tetanus, diphtheria toxoids vaccine (Td) on or between the patient's 10th and 13th birthdays ⓑ M
* **G9417** Patient did not have one tetanus, diphtheria toxoids and acellular pertussis vaccine (Tdap) on or between the patient's 10th and 13th birthdays ⓑ M

| MIPS | Qp Quantity Physician | Qh Quantity Hospital | ♀ Female only |
| ♂ Male only | Ⓐ Age | DMEPOS | A2-Z3 ASC Payment Indicator | A-Y ASC Status Indicator | Coding Clinic |

* **G9418** Primary non-small cell lung cancer lung biopsy and cytology specimen report documents classification into specific histologic type following IASLC guidance or classified as NSCLC-NOS with an explanation ⓑ M

* **G9419** Documentation of medical reason(s) for not including the histological type or NSCLC-NOS classification with an explanation (e.g., specimen insufficient or non-diagnostic, specimen does not contain cancer, other documented medical reasons) ⓑ M

* **G9420** Specimen site other than anatomic location of lung or is not classified as primary non-small cell lung cancer ⓑ M

* **G9421** Primary non-small cell lung cancer biopsy and cytology specimen report does not document classification into specific histologic type or histologic type does not follow IASLC guidance or is classified as NSCLC-NOS but without an explanation ⓑ M

* **G9422** Primary lung carcinoma resection report documents pT category, pN category and for non-small cell lung cancer, histologic type (e.g., squamous cell carcinoma, adenocarcinoma and not NSCLC-NOS) ⓑ M

* **G9423** Documentation of medical reason for not including pT category, pN category and histologic type [for patient with appropriate exclusion criteria (e.g., metastatic disease, benign tumors, malignant tumors other than carcinomas, inadequate surgical specimens)] ⓑ M

* **G9424** Specimen site other than anatomic location of lung, or classified as NSCLC-NOS ⓑ M

* **G9425** Primary lung carcinoma resection report does not document pT category, pN category and for non-small cell lung cancer, histologic type (e.g., squamous cell carcinoma, adenocarcinoma) ⓑ M

* **G9426** Improvement in median time from ED arrival to initial ED oral or parenteral pain medication administration performed for ED admitted patients ⓑ M

* **G9427** Improvement in median time from ED arrival to initial ED oral or parenteral pain medication administration not performed for ED admitted patients ⓑ M

* **G9428** Pathology report includes the pT category, thickness, ulceration and mitotic rate, peripheral and deep margin status and presence or absence of microsatellitosis for invasive tumors ⓑ M

* **G9429** Documentation of medical reason(s) for not including pT category, thickness, ulceration and mitotic rate, peripheral and deep margin status and presence or absence of microsatellitosis for invasive tumors (e.g., negative skin biopsies in a patient with a history of melanoma or other documented medical reasons) ⓑ M

* **G9430** Specimen site other than anatomic cutaneous location ⓑ M

* **G9431** Pathology report does not include the pT category, thickness, ulceration and mitotic rate, peripheral and deep margin status and presence or absence of microsatellitosis for invasive tumors ⓑ M

* **G9432** Asthma well-controlled based on the ACT, C-ACT, ACQ, or ATAQ score and results documented ⓑ M

* **G9434** Asthma not well-controlled based on the ACT, C-ACT, ACQ, or ATAQ score, or specified asthma control tool not used, reason not given ⓑ M

* **G9452** Documentation of medical reason(s) for not receiving HCV antibody test due to limited life expectancy ⓑ M

* **G9455** Patient underwent abdominal imaging with ultrasound, contrast enhanced CT or contrast MRI for HCC ⓑ M

* **G9456** Documentation of medical or patient reason(s) for not ordering or performing screening for HCC. medical reason: comorbid medical conditions with expected survival <5 years, hepatic decompensation and not a candidate for liver transplantation, or other medical reasons; patient reasons: patient declined or other patient reasons (e.g., cost of tests, time related to accessing testing equipment) ⓑ M

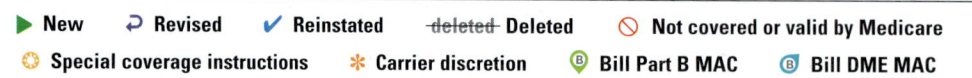

▶ New ⤾ Revised ✓ Reinstated ~~deleted~~ Deleted ⊘ Not covered or valid by Medicare
⊛ Special coverage instructions * Carrier discretion ⓑ Bill Part B MAC ⓑ Bill DME MAC

TEMPORARY PROCEDURES/PROFESSIONAL SERVICES

* **G9457** Patient did not undergo abdominal imaging and did not have a documented reason for not undergoing abdominal imaging in the submission period ⓑ M

~~G9458 Patient documented as tobacco user and received tobacco cessation intervention (must include at least one of the following: advice given to quit smoking or tobacco use, counseling on the benefits of quitting smoking or tobacco use, assistance with or referral to external smoking or tobacco cessation support programs, or current enrollment in smoking or tobacco use cessation program) if identified as a tobacco user~~

~~G9459 Currently a tobacco non-user~~

~~G9460 Tobacco assessment or tobacco cessation intervention not performed, reason not given~~

* **G9468** Patient not receiving corticosteroids greater than or equal to 10 mg/day of prednisone equivalents for 60 or greater consecutive days or a single prescription equating to 600 mg prednisone or greater for all fills ⓑ M

* **G9470** Patients not receiving corticosteroids greater than or equal to 10 mg/day of prednisone equivalents for 60 or greater consecutive days or a single prescription equating to 600 mg prednisone or greater for all fills ⓑ M

* **G9471** Within the past 2 years, central dual-energy x-ray absorptiometry (DXA) not ordered or documented ⓑ M

* **G9473** Services performed by chaplain in the hospice setting, each 15 minutes ⓑ B

* **G9474** Services performed by dietary counselor in the hospice setting, each 15 minutes ⓑ B

* **G9475** Services performed by other counselor in the hospice setting, each 15 minutes ⓑ B

* **G9476** Services performed by volunteer in the hospice setting, each 15 minutes ⓑ B

* **G9477** Services performed by care coordinator in the hospice setting, each 15 minutes ⓑ B

* **G9478** Services performed by other qualified therapist in the hospice setting, each 15 minutes ⓑ B

* **G9479** Services performed by qualified pharmacist in the hospice setting, each 15 minutes ⓑ B

* **G9480** Admission to Medicare Care Choice Model program (MCCM) ⓑ Qp Qh B

* **G9481** Remote in-home visit for the evaluation and management of a new patient for use only in the Medicare-approved comprehensive care for joint replacement model, which requires these 3 key components: a problem focused history; a problem focused examination; and straightforward medical decision making, furnished in real time using interactive audio and video technology. Counseling and coordination of care with other physicians, other qualified health care professionals or agencies are provided consistent with the nature of the problem(s) and the needs of the patient or the family or both. Usually, the presenting problem(s) are self limited or minor. Typically, 10 minutes are spent with the patient or family or both via real time, audio and video intercommunications technology ⓑ B

* **G9482** Remote in-home visit for the evaluation and management of a new patient for use only in the Medicare-approved comprehensive care for joint replacement model, which requires these 3 key components: an expanded problem focused history; an expanded problem focused examination; straightforward medical decision making, furnished in real time using interactive audio and video technology. Counseling and coordination of care with other physicians, other qualified health care professionals or agencies are provided consistent with the nature of the problem(s) and the needs of the patient or the family or both. Usually, the presenting problem(s) are of low to moderate severity. Typically, 20 minutes are spent with the patient or family or both via real time, audio and video intercommunications technology ⓑ B

 MIPS   Qp Quantity Physician   Qh Quantity Hospital   ♀ Female only
♂ Male only   A Age   ♿ DMEPOS   A2-Z3 ASC Payment Indicator   A-Y ASC Status Indicator   Coding Clinic

* **G9483** Remote in-home visit for the evaluation and management of a new patient for use only in the Medicare-approved comprehensive care for joint replacement model, which requires these 3 key components: a detailed history; a detailed examination; medical decision making of low complexity, furnished in real time using interactive audio and video technology. Counseling and coordination of care with other physicians, other qualified health care professionals or agencies are provided consistent with the nature of the problem(s) and the needs of the patient or the family or both. Usually, the presenting problem(s) are of moderate severity. Typically, 30 minutes are spent with the patient or family or both via real time, audio and video intercommunications technology Ⓑ B

* **G9484** Remote in-home visit for the evaluation and management of a new patient for use only in the Medicare-approved comprehensive care for joint replacement model, which requires these 3 key components: a comprehensive history; a comprehensive examination; medical decision making of moderate complexity, furnished in real time using interactive audio and video technology. Counseling and coordination of care with other physicians, other qualified health care professionals or agencies are provided consistent with the nature of the problem(s) and the needs of the patient or the family or both. Usually, the presenting problem(s) are of moderate to high severity. Typically, 45 minutes are spent with the patient or family or both via real time, audio and video intercommunications technology Ⓑ B

* **G9485** Remote in-home visit for the evaluation and management of a new patient for use only in the Medicare-approved comprehensive care for joint replacement model, which requires these 3 key components: a comprehensive history; a comprehensive examination; medical decision making of high complexity, furnished in real time using interactive audio and video technology. Counseling and coordination of care with other physicians, other qualified health care professionals or agencies are provided consistent with the nature of the problem(s) and the needs of the patient or the family or both. Usually, the presenting problem(s) are of moderate to high severity. Typically, 60 minutes are spent with the patient or family or both via real time, audio and video intercommunications technology Ⓑ B

* **G9486** Remote in-home visit for the evaluation and management of an established patient for use only in the Medicare-approved comprehensive care for joint replacement model, which requires at least 2 of the following 3 key components: a problem focused history; a problem focused examination; straightforward medical decision making, furnished in real time using interactive audio and video technology. Counseling and coordination of care with other physicians, other qualified health care professionals or agencies are provided consistent with the nature of the problem(s) and the needs of the patient or the family or both. Usually, the presenting problem(s) are self limited or minor. Typically, 10 minutes are spent with the patient or family or both via real time, audio and video intercommunications technology Ⓑ B

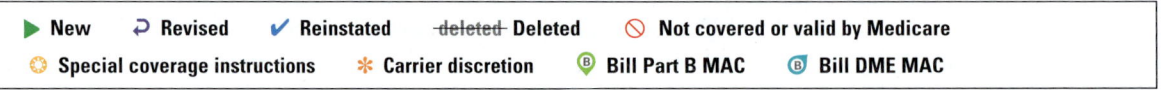

TEMPORARY PROCEDURES/PROFESSIONAL SERVICES

* **G9487** Remote in-home visit for the evaluation and management of an established patient for use only in the Medicare-approved comprehensive care for joint replacement model, which requires at least 2 of the following 3 key components: an expanded problem focused history; an expanded problem focused examination; medical decision making of low complexity, furnished in real time using interactive audio and video technology. Counseling and coordination of care with other physicians, other qualified health care professionals or agencies are provided consistent with the nature of the problem(s) and the needs of the patient or the family or both. Usually, the presenting problem(s) are of low to moderate severity. Typically, 15 minutes are spent with the patient or family or both via real time, audio and video intercommunications technology ⓑ **B**

* **G9488** Remote in-home visit for the evaluation and management of an established patient for use only in the Medicare-approved comprehensive care for joint replacement model, which requires at least 2 of the following 3 key components: a detailed history; a detailed examination; medical decision making of moderate complexity, furnished in real time using interactive audio and video technology. Counseling and coordination of care with other physicians, other qualified health care professionals or agencies are provided consistent with the nature of the problem(s) and the needs of the patient or the family or both. Usually, the presenting problem(s) are of moderate to high severity. Typically, 25 minutes are spent with the patient or family or both via real time, audio and video intercommunications technology ⓑ **B**

* **G9489** Remote in-home visit for the evaluation and management of an established patient for use only in the Medicare-approved comprehensive care for joint replacement model, which requires at least 2 of the following 3 key components: a comprehensive history; a comprehensive examination; medical decision making of high complexity, furnished in real time using interactive audio and video technology. Counseling and coordination of care with other physicians, other qualified health care professionals or agencies are provided consistent with the nature of the problem(s) and the needs of the patient or the family or both. Usually, the presenting problem(s) are of moderate to high severity. Typically, 40 minutes are spent with the patient or family or both via real time, audio and video intercommunications technology ⓑ **B**

* **G9490** Comprehensive care for joint replacement model, home visit for patient assessment performed by clinical staff for an individual not considered homebound, including, but not necessarily limited to patient assessment of clinical status, safety/fall prevention, functional status/ambulation, medication reconciliation/management, compliance with orders/plan of care, performance of activities of daily living, and ensuring beneficiary connections to community and other services. (for use only in the Medicare-approved CJR model); may not be billed for a 30 day period covered by a transitional care management code ⓑ **B**

* **G9497** Received instruction from the anesthesiologist or proxy prior to the day of surgery to abstain from smoking on the day of surgery ⓑ **M**

* **G9498** Antibiotic regimen prescribed ⓑ **M**

* **G9500** Radiation exposure indices documented in final report for procedure using fluoroscopy ⓑ **M**

* **G9501** Radiation exposure indices not documented in final report for procedure using fluoroscopy, reason not given ⓑ **M**

* **G9502** Documentation of medical reason for not performing foot exam (i.e., patients who have had either a bilateral amputation above or below the knee, or both a left and right amputation above or below the knee before or during the measurement period) ⓑ **M**

 MIPS   Qp Quantity Physician   Qh Quantity Hospital   ♀ Female only
♂ Male only   A Age   ♿ DMEPOS   A2-Z3 ASC Payment Indicator   A-Y ASC Status Indicator   Coding Clinic

* G9504	Documented reason for not assessing Hepatitis B virus (HBV) status (e.g. patient not initiating anti-TNF therapy, patient declined) prior to initiating anti-TNF therapy ⒷM
* G9505	Antibiotic regimen prescribed within 10 days after onset of symptoms for documented medical reason ⒷM
* G9507	Documentation that the patient is on a statin medication or has documentation of a valid contraindication or exception to statin medications; contraindications/exceptions that can be defined by diagnosis codes include pregnancy during the measurement period, active liver disease, rhabdomyolysis, end stage renal disease on dialysis and heart failure; provider documented contraindications/exceptions include breastfeeding during the measurement period, woman of child-bearing age not actively taking birth control, allergy to statin, drug interaction (HIV protease inhibitors, nefazodone, cyclosporine, gemfibrozil, and danazol) and intolerance (with supporting documentation of trying a statin at least once within the last 5 years or diagnosis codes for myositis or toxic myopathy related to drugs) ⒷM
* G9508	Documentation that the patient is not on a statin medication ⒷM
* G9509	Adult patients 18 years of age or older with major depression or dysthymia who reached remission at 12 months as demonstrated by a 12 month (+/-60 days) PHQ-9 or PHQ-9m score of less than 5 ⒷM
* G9510	Adult patients 18 years of age or older with major depression or dysthymia who did not reach remission at twelve months as demonstrated by a twelve month (+/-60 days) PHQ-9 or PHQ-9m score of less than 5. Either PHQ-9 or PHQ-9m score was not assessed or is greater than or equal to 5 ⒷM
* G9511	Index event date PHQ-9 score greater than 9 documented during the 12 month denominator identification period ⒷM
* G9512	Individual had a PDC of 0.8 or greater ⒷM
* G9513	Individual did not have a PDC of 0.8 or greater ⒷM
* G9514	Patient required a return to the operating room within 90 days of surgery ⒷM
* G9515	Patient did not require a return to the operating room within 90 days of surgery ⒷM
* G9516	Patient achieved an improvement in visual acuity, from their preoperative level, within 90 days of surgery ⒷM
* G9517	Patient did not achieve an improvement in visual acuity, from their preoperative level, within 90 days of surgery, reason not given ⒷM
* G9518	Documentation of active injection drug use ⒷM
* G9519	Patient achieves final refraction (spherical equivalent) +/-1.0 diopters of their planned refraction within 90 days of surgery ⒷM
* G9520	Patient does not achieve final refraction (spherical equivalent) +/-1.0 diopters of their planned refraction within 90 days of surgery ⒷM
* G9521	Total number of emergency department visits and inpatient hospitalizations less than two in the past 12 months ⒷM
* G9522	Total number of emergency department visits and inpatient hospitalizations equal to or greater than two in the past 12 months or patient not screened, reason not given ⒷM
* G9529	Patient with minor blunt head trauma had an appropriate indication(s) for a head CT ⒷM
* G9530	Patient presented within a minor blunt head trauma and had a head CT ordered for trauma by an emergency care provider ⒷM
* G9531	Patient has documentation of ventricular shunt, brain tumor, multisystem trauma, or is currently taking an antiplatelet medication including: abciximab, anagrelide, cangrelor, cilostazol, clopidogrel, dipyridamole, eptifibatide, prasugrel, ticlopidine, ticagrelor, tirofiban, or vorapaxar ⒷM
* G9533	Patient with minor blunt head trauma did not have an appropriate indication(s) for a head CT ⒷM
* G9537	Imaging needed as part of a clinical trial; or other clinician ordered the study ⒷM
* G9539	Intent for potential removal at time of placement ⒷM
* G9540	Patient alive 3 months post procedure ⒷM
* G9541	Filter removed within 3 months of placement ⒷM

▶ New ↻ Revised ✓ Reinstated ̶d̶e̶l̶e̶t̶e̶d̶ Deleted ⊘ Not covered or valid by Medicare ⓒ Special coverage instructions * Carrier discretion Ⓑ Bill Part B MAC Ⓑ Bill DME MAC

TEMPORARY PROCEDURES/PROFESSIONAL SERVICES

* **G9542** Documented re-assessment for the appropriateness of filter removal within 3 months of placement ⓑ M
* **G9543** Documentation of at least two attempts to reach the patient to arrange a clinical re-assessment for the appropriateness of filter removal within 3 months of placement ⓑ M
* **G9544** Patients that do not have the filter removed, documented re-assessment for the appropriateness of filter removal, or documentation of at least two attempts to reach the patient to arrange a clinical re-assessment for the appropriateness of filter removal within 3 months of placement ⓑ M
* **G9547** Cystic renal lesion that is simple appearing (Bosniak I or II), or adrenal lesion less than or equal to 1.0 cm or adrenal lesion greater than 1.0 cm but less than or equal to 4.0 cm classified as likely benign by unenhanced CT or washout protocol CT, or MRI with in- and opposed-phase sequences or other equivalent institutional imaging protocols ⓑ M
* **G9548** Final reports for imaging studies stating no follow-up imaging is recommended ⓑ M
* **G9549** Documentation of medical reason(s) that follow-up imaging is indicated (e.g., patient has lymphadenopathy, signs of metastasis or an active diagnosis or history of cancer, and other medical reason(s)) ⓑ M
* **G9550** Final reports for imaging studies with follow-up imaging recommended, or final reports that do not include a specific recommendation of no follow-up ⓑ M
* **G9551** Final reports for imaging studies without an incidentally found lesion noted ⓑ M
* **G9552** Incidental thyroid nodule <1.0 cm noted in report ⓑ M
* **G9553** Prior thyroid disease diagnosis ⓑ M
* **G9554** Final reports for CT, CTA, MRI or MRA of the chest or neck with follow-up imaging recommended ⓑ M
* **G9555** Documentation of medical reason(s) for recommending follow up imaging (e.g., patient has multiple endocrine neoplasia, patient has cervical lymphadenopathy, other medical reason(s)) ⓑ M
* **G9556** Final reports for CT, CTA, MRI or MRA of the chest or neck with follow-up imaging not recommended ⓑ M
* **G9557** Final reports for CT, CTA, MRI or MRA studies of the chest or neck without an incidentally found thyroid nodule <1.0 cm noted or no nodule found ⓑ M
* **G9580** Door to puncture time of 90 minutes or less ⓑ M
* **G9582** Door to puncture time of greater than 90 minutes, no reason given ⓑ M
* **G9593** Pediatric patient with minor blunt head trauma classified as low risk according to the pecarn Prediction Rules ⓑ A M
* **G9594** Patient presented with a minor blunt head trauma and had a head CT ordered for trauma by an emergency care provider ⓑ M
* **G9595** Patient has documentation of ventricular shunt, brain tumor, or coagulopathy ⓑ M
* **G9597** Pediatric patient with minor blunt head trauma not classified as low risk according to the pecarn Prediction Rules ⓑ A M
* **G9598** Aortic aneurysm 5.5-5.9 cm maximum diameter on centerline formatted CT or minor diameter on axial formatted CT ⓑ M
* **G9599** Aortic aneurysm 6.0 cm or greater maximum diameter on centerline formatted CT or minor diameter on axial formatted CT ⓑ M
* **G9603** Patient survey score improved from baseline following treatment ⓑ M
* **G9604** Patient survey results not available ⓑ M
* **G9605** Patient survey score did not improve from baseline following treatment ⓑ M
* **G9606** Intraoperative cystoscopy performed to evaluate for lower tract injury ⓑ M
* **G9607** Documented medical reasons for not performing intraoperative cystoscopy (e.g., urethral pathology precluding cystoscopy, any patient who has a congenital or acquired absence of the urethra) or in the case of patient death ⓑ M
* **G9608** Intraoperative cystoscopy not performed to evaluate for lower tract injury ⓑ M
* **G9609** Documentation of an order for anti-platelet agents ⓑ M
* **G9610** Documentation of medical reason(s) in the patient's record for not ordering anti-platelet agents ⓑ M

✱ G9611	Order for anti-platelet agents was not documented in the patient's record, reason not given ⒷM
✱ G9621	Patient identified as an unhealthy alcohol user when screened for unhealthy alcohol use using a systematic screening method and received brief counseling ⒷM
✱ G9622	Patient not identified as an unhealthy alcohol user when screened for unhealthy alcohol use using a systematic screening method ⒷM
✱ G9624	Patient not screened for unhealthy alcohol use using a systematic screening method or patient did not receive brief counseling if identified as an unhealthy alcohol user ⒷM
✱ G9625	Patient sustained bladder injury at the time of surgery or discovered subsequently up to 30 days post-surgery ⒷM
✱ G9626	Documented medical reason for not reporting bladder injury (e.g., gynecologic or other pelvic malignancy documented, concurrent surgery involving bladder pathology, injury that occurs during urinary incontinence procedure, patient death from non-medical causes not related to surgery, patient died during procedure without evidence of bladder injury) ⒷM
✱ G9627	Patient did not sustain bladder injury at the time of surgery nor discovered subsequently up to 30 days post-surgery ⒷM
✱ G9628	Patient sustained bowel injury at the time of surgery or discovered subsequently up to 30 days post-surgery ⒷM
✱ G9629	Documented medical reasons for not reporting bowel injury (e.g., gynecologic or other pelvic malignancy documented, planned (e.g., not due to an unexpected bowel injury) resection and/or re-anastomosis of bowel, or patient death from non-medical causes not related to surgery, patient died during procedure without evidence of bowel injury) ⒷM
✱ G9630	Patient did not sustain a bowel injury at the time of surgery nor discovered subsequently up to 30 days post-surgery ⒷM
✱ G9637	At least two orders for the same high-risk medications ⒷM
✱ G9638	At least two orders for the same high-risk medications not ordered ⒷM
✱ G9642	Current smoker (e.g., cigarette, cigar, pipe, e-cigarette or marijuana) ⒷM
✱ G9643	Elective surgery ⒷM
✱ G9644	Patients who abstained from smoking prior to anesthesia on the day of surgery or procedure ⒷM
✱ G9645	Patients who did not abstain from smoking prior to anesthesia on the day of surgery or procedure ⒷM
✱ G9646	Patients with 90 day MRS score of 0 to 2 ⒷM
✱ G9648	Patients with 90 day MRS score greater than 2 ⒷM
✱ G9649	Psoriasis assessment tool documented meeting any one of the specified benchmarks (e.g., PGA; 5-point or 6-point scale), body surface area (BSA), psoriasis area and severity index (PASI) and/or dermatology life quality index) (DLQI)) ⒷM
✱ G9651	Psoriasis assessment tool documented not meeting any one of the specified benchmarks (e.g., (pga; 5-point or 6-point scale), body surface area (bsa), psoriasis area and severity index (pasi) and/or dermatology life quality index) (dlqi)) or psoriasis assessment tool not documented ⒷM
✱ G9654	Monitored anesthesia care (mac) ⒷM
✱ G9655	A transfer of care protocol or handoff tool/checklist that includes the required key handoff elements is used ⒷM
✱ G9656	Patient transferred directly from anesthetizing location to PACU or other non-ICU location ⒷM
✱ G9658	A transfer of care protocol or handoff tool/checklist that includes the required key handoff elements is not used ⒷM
↻ ✱ G9659	Patients greater than or equal to 86 years of age who underwent a screening colonoscopy and did not have a history of colorectal cancer or other valid medical reason for the colonoscopy, including: iron deficiency anemia, lower gastrointestinal bleeding, familial adenomatous polyposis, Lynch syndrome (i.e., hereditary non-polyposis colorectal cancer), inflammatory bowel disease (i.e., Crohn's disease or ulcerative colitis), abnormal finding of gastrointestinal tract, or changes in bowel habits ⒷM

▶ New ↻ Revised ✔ Reinstated ~~deleted~~ Deleted ⊘ Not covered or valid by Medicare ⓢ Special coverage instructions ✱ Carrier discretion Ⓑ Bill Part B MAC Ⓑ Bill DME MAC

TEMPORARY PROCEDURES/PROFESSIONAL SERVICES

* **G9660** Documentation of medical reason(s) for a colonoscopy performed on a patient greater than or equal to 86 years of age (e.g., iron deficiency anemia, lower gastrointestinal bleeding, familial history of adenomatous polyposis, Lynch syndrome (i.e., hereditary non-polyposis colorectal cancer), inflammatory bowel disease (i.e., Crohn's disease or ulcerative colitis), abnormal finding of gastrointestinal tract, or changes in bowel habits) Ⓑ **M**

* **G9661** Patients greater than or equal to 86 years of age who received a colonoscopy for an assessment of signs/symptoms of GI tract illness, and/or because the patient meets high risk criteria, and/or to follow-up on previously diagnosed advance lesions Ⓑ **M**

* **G9662** Previously diagnosed or have a diagnosis of clinical ASCVD, including ASCVD procedure Ⓑ **M**

* **G9663** Any ldl-c laboratory test result >=190 mg/dL Ⓑ **M**

* **G9664** Patients who are currently statin therapy users or received an order (prescription) for statin therapy Ⓑ **M**

* **G9665** Patients who are not currently statin therapy users or did not receive an order (prescription) for statin therapy Ⓑ **M**

* **G9674** Patients with clinical ascvd diagnosis Ⓑ **M**

* **G9675** Patients who have ever had a fasting or direct laboratory result of ldl-c = 190 mg/dl Ⓑ **M**

* **G9676** Patients aged 40 to 75 years at the beginning of the measurement period with type 1 or type 2 diabetes and with an ldl-c result of 70-189 mg/dl recorded as the highest fasting or direct laboratory test result in the measurement year or during the two years prior to the beginning of the measurement period Ⓑ **M**

* **G9679** This code is for onsite acute care treatment of a nursing facility resident with pneumonia; may only be billed once per day per beneficiary Ⓑ **B**

* **G9680** This code is for onsite acute care treatment of a nursing facility resident with CHF; may only be billed once per day per beneficiary Ⓑ **B**

* **G9681** This code is for onsite acute care treatment of a resident with COPD or asthma; may only be billed once per day per beneficiary Ⓑ **B**

* **G9682** This code is for the onsite acute care treatment a nursing facility resident with a skin infection; may only be billed once per day per beneficiary Ⓑ **B**

* **G9683** Facility service(s) for the onsite acute care treatment of a nursing facility resident with fluid or electrolyte disorder. (May only be billed once per day per beneficiary). This service is for a demonstration project. Ⓑ **B**

* **G9684** This code is for the onsite acute care treatment of a nursing facility resident for a UTI; may only be billed once per day per beneficiary Ⓑ **B**

* **G9685** Physician service or other qualified health care professional for the evaluation and management of a beneficiary's acute change in condition in a nursing facility. This service is for a demonstration project. Ⓑ **M**

* **G9687** Hospice services provided to patient any time during the measurement period Ⓑ **M**

* **G9688** Patients using hospice services any time during the measurement period Ⓑ **M**

* **G9689** Patient admitted for performance of elective carotid intervention Ⓑ **M**

* **G9690** Patient receiving hospice services any time during the measurement period Ⓑ **M**

* **G9691** Patient had hospice services any time during the measurement period Ⓑ **M**

* **G9692** Hospice services received by patient any time during the measurement period Ⓑ **M**

* **G9693** Patient use of hospice services any time during the measurement period Ⓑ **M**

* **G9694** Hospice services utilized by patient any time during the measurement period Ⓑ **M**

* **G9695** Long-acting inhaled bronchodilator prescribed Ⓑ **M**

* **G9696** Documentation of medical reason(s) for not prescribing a long-acting inhaled bronchodilator (e.g., patient intolerance or history of side effects) Ⓑ **M**

* **G9698** Documentation of system reason(s) for not prescribing a long-acting inhaled bronchodilator (e.g., cost of treatment or lack of insurance) Ⓑ **M**

* **G9699** Long-acting inhaled bronchodilator not prescribed, reason not otherwise specified Ⓑ **M**

MIPS Qp Quantity Physician Qh Quantity Hospital ♀ Female only
♂ Male only A Age ♿ DMEPOS A2-Z3 ASC Payment Indicator A-Y ASC Status Indicator Coding Clinic

* G9700	Patients who use hospice services any time during the measurement period ⒷⒷ	M
* G9702	Patients who use hospice services any time during the measurement period Ⓑ	M
* G9703	Episodes where the patient is taking antibiotics (table 1) in the 30 days prior to the episode date Ⓑ	M
* G9704	AJCC breast cancer stage I: T1 mic or T1a documented Ⓑ	M
* G9705	AJCC breast cancer stage I: T1b (tumor >0.5 cm but <=1 cm in greatest dimension) documented Ⓑ	M
* G9706	Low (or very low) risk of recurrence, prostate cancer Ⓑ	M
~~G9707~~	~~Patient received hospice services any time during the measurement period~~	
* G9708	Women who had a bilateral mastectomy or who have a history of a bilateral mastectomy or for whom there is evidence of a right and a left unilateral mastectomy Ⓑ	M
* G9709	Hospice services used by patient any time during the measurement period Ⓑ	M
* G9710	Patient was provided hospice services any time during the measurement period Ⓑ	M
* G9711	Patients with a diagnosis or past history of total colectomy or colorectal cancer Ⓑ	M
* G9712	Documentation of medical reason(s) for prescribing or dispensing antibiotic (e.g., intestinal infection, pertussis, bacterial infection, Lyme disease, otitis media, acute sinusitis, acute pharyngitis, acute tonsillitis, chronic sinusitis, infection of the pharynx/larynx/tonsils/adenoids, prostatitis, cellulitis/ mastoiditis/bone infections, acute lymphadenitis, impetigo, skin staph infections, pneumonia, gonococcal infections/venereal disease/syphilis, chlamydia, inflammatory diseases, female reproductive organs), infections of the kidney, cystitis/UTI, acne, HIV disease/asymptomatic HIV, cystic fibrosis, disorders of the immune system, malignancy neoplasms, chronic bronchitis, emphysema, bronchiectasis, extrinsic allergic alveolitis, chronic airway obstruction, chronic obstructive asthma, pneumoconiosis and other lung disease due to external agents, other diseases of the respiratory system, and tuberculosis Ⓑ	M
* G9713	Patients who use hospice services any time during the measurement period Ⓑ	M
* G9714	Patient is using hospice services any time during the measurement period Ⓑ	M
* G9716	BMI is documented as being outside of normal parameters, follow-up plan is not completed for documented medical reason Ⓑ	M
* G9717	Documentation stating the patient has had a diagnosis of bipolar disorder Ⓑ	M
* G9719	Patient is not ambulatory, bed ridden, immobile, confined to chair, wheelchair bound, dependent on helper pushing wheelchair, independent in wheelchair or minimal help in wheelchair Ⓑ	M
* G9720	Hospice services for patient occurred any time during the measurement period Ⓑ	M
* G9721	Patient not ambulatory, bed ridden, immobile, confined to chair, wheelchair bound, dependent on helper pushing wheelchair, independent in wheelchair or minimal help in wheelchair Ⓑ	M
* G9722	Documented history of renal failure or baseline serum creatinine > = 4.0 mg/dl; renal transplant recipients are not considered to have preoperative renal failure, unless, since transplantation the CR has been or is 4.0 or higher Ⓑ	M
* G9723	Hospice services for patient received any time during the measurement period Ⓑ	M
* G9724	Patients who had documentation of use of anticoagulant medications overlapping the measurement year Ⓑ	M
* G9726	Patient refused to participate Ⓑ	M
* G9727	Patient unable to complete the LEPF prom at initial evaluation and/or discharge due to blindness, illiteracy, severe mental incapacity or language incompatibility and an adequate proxy is not available Ⓑ	M
* G9728	Patient refused to participate Ⓑ	M
* G9729	Patient unable to complete the LEPF prom at initial evaluation and/or discharge due to blindness, illiteracy, severe mental incapacity or language incompatibility and an adequate proxy is not available Ⓑ	M
* G9730	Patient refused to participate Ⓑ	M

▶ New ↻ Revised ✓ Reinstated ~~deleted~~ Deleted ⊘ Not covered or valid by Medicare
✪ Special coverage instructions * Carrier discretion Ⓑ Bill Part B MAC Ⓑ Bill DME MAC

TEMPORARY PROCEDURES/PROFESSIONAL SERVICES

* G9731 — Patient unable to complete the LEPF prom at initial evaluation and/or discharge due to blindness, illiteracy, severe mental incapacity or language incompatibility and an adequate proxy is not available ⓑ M
* G9732 — Patient refused to participate ⓑ M
* G9733 — Patient unable to complete the low back FS prom at initial evaluation and/or discharge due to blindness, illiteracy, severe mental incapacity or language incompatibility and an adequate proxy is not available ⓑ M
* G9734 — Patient refused to participate ⓑ M
* G9735 — Patient unable to complete the shoulder FS prom at initial evaluation and/or discharge due to blindness, illiteracy, severe mental incapacity or language incompatibility and an adequate proxy is not available ⓑ M
* G9736 — Patient refused to participate ⓑ M
* G9737 — Patient unable to complete the elbow/wrist/hand FS prom at initial evaluation and/or discharge due to blindness, illiteracy, severe mental incapacity or language incompatibility and an adequate proxy is not available ⓑ M
* G9740 — Hospice services given to patient any time during the measurement period ⓑ M
* G9741 — Patients who use hospice services any time during the measurement period ⓑ M
* G9744 — Patient not eligible due to active diagnosis of hypertension ⓑ M
* G9745 — Documented reason for not screening or recommending a follow-up for high blood pressure ⓑ M
* G9746 — Patient has mitral stenosis or prosthetic heart valves or patient has transient or reversible cause of AF (e.g., pneumonia, hyperthyroidism, pregnancy, cardiac surgery) ⓑ M
* ~~G9751 — Patient died at any time during the 24-month measurement period~~
* G9752 — Emergency surgery ⓑ M
* G9753 — Documentation of medical reason for not conducting a search for DICOM format images for prior patient CT imaging studies completed at non-affiliated external healthcare facilities or entities within the past 12 months that are available through a secure, authorized, media-free, shared archive (e.g., trauma, acute myocardial infarction, stroke, aortic aneurysm where time is of the essence) ⓑ M
* G9754 — A finding of an incidental pulmonary nodule ⓑ M
* G9755 — Documentation of medical reason(s) for not including a recommended interval and modality for follow-up or for no follow-up, and source of recommendations (e.g., patients with unexplained fever, immunocompromised patients who are at risk for infection) ⓑ M
* G9756 — Surgical procedures that included the use of silicone oil ⓑ M
* G9757 — Surgical procedures that included the use of silicone oil ⓑ M
* G9758 — Patient in hospice at any time during the measurement period ⓑ M
* ~~G9760 — Patients who use hospice services any time during the measurement period~~
* G9761 — Patients who use hospice services any time during the measurement period ⓑ M
* G9762 — Patient had at least two HPV vaccines (with at least 146 days between the two) or three HPV vaccines on or between the patient's 9th and 13th birthdays ⓑ M
* G9763 — Patient did not have at least two HPV vaccines (with at least 146 days between the two) or three HPV vaccines on or between the patient's 9th and 13th birthdays ⓑ M
* G9764 — Patient has been treated with systemic medication for psoriasis vulgaris ⓑ M
* G9765 — Documentation that the patient declined change in medication or alternative therapies were unavailable, has documented contraindications, or has not been treated with systemic for at least six consecutive months (e.g., experienced adverse effects or lack of efficacy with all other therapy options) in order to achieve better disease control as measured by PGA, BSA, PASI, or DLQI ⓑ M
* G9766 — Patients who are transferred from one institution to another with a known diagnosis of CVA for endovascular stroke treatment ⓑ M
* G9767 — Hospitalized patients with newly diagnosed CVA considered for endovascular stroke treatment ⓑ M
* G9768 — Patients who utilize hospice services any time during the measurement period ⓑ M

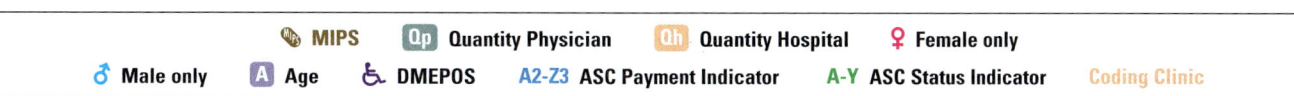

* G9769	Patient had a bone mineral density test in the past two years or received osteoporosis medication or therapy in the past 12 months Ⓑ Ⓜ
* G9770	Peripheral nerve block (PNB) Ⓑ Ⓜ
* G9771	At least 1 body temperature measurement equal to or greater than 35.5 degrees Celsius (or 95.9 degrees Fahrenheit) achieved within the 30 minutes immediately before or 15 minutes immediately after anesthesia end time Ⓑ Ⓜ
* G9772	Documentation of medical reason(s) for not achieving at least 1 body temperature measurement equal to or greater than 35.5 degrees Celsius (or 95.9 degrees Fahrenheit) within the 30 minutes immediately before or 15 minutes immediately after anesthesia end time (e.g., emergency cases, intentional hypothermia, etc.) Ⓑ Ⓜ
* G9773	At least 1 body temperature measurement equal to or greater than 35.5 degrees Celsius (or 95.9 degrees Fahrenheit) not achieved within the 30 minutes immediately before or 15 minutes immediately after anesthesia end time, reason not given Ⓑ Ⓜ
* G9775	Patient received at least 2 prophylactic pharmacologic anti-emetic agents of different classes preoperatively and/or intraoperatively Ⓑ Ⓜ
* G9776	Documentation of medical reason for not receiving at least 2 prophylactic pharmacologic anti-emetic agents of different classes preoperatively and/or intraoperatively (e.g., intolerance or other medical reason) Ⓑ Ⓜ
* G9777	Patient did not receive at least 2 prophylactic pharmacologic anti-emetic agents of different classes preoperatively and/or intraoperatively Ⓑ Ⓜ
* G9779	Patients who are breastfeeding at any time during the performance period Ⓑ Ⓜ
* G9780	Patients who have a diagnosis of rhabdomyolysis at any time during the performance period Ⓑ Ⓜ
* G9781	Documentation of medical reason(s) for not currently being a statin therapy user or receiving an order (prescription) for statin therapy (e.g., patients with statin-associated muscle symptoms, patients who are receiving palliative care or hospice care, patients with active liver disease or hepatic disease or insufficiency, and patients with end stage renal disease [ESRD]) Ⓑ Ⓜ
* G9782	History of or active diagnosis of familial hypercholesterolemia Ⓑ Ⓜ
* G9784	Pathologists/dermatopathologists providing a second opinion on a biopsy Ⓑ Ⓜ
* G9785	Pathology report diagnosing cutaneous basal cell carcinoma, squamous cell carcinoma, or melanoma (to include in situ disease) sent from the pathologist/dermatopathologist to the biopsying clinician for review within 7 days from the time when the tissue specimen was received by the pathologist Ⓑ Ⓜ
* G9786	Pathology report diagnosing cutaneous basal cell carcinoma, squamous cell carcinoma, or melanoma (to include in situ disease) was not sent from the pathologist/dermatopathologist to the biopsying clinician for review within 7 days from the time when the tissue specimen was received by the pathologist Ⓑ Ⓜ
* G9787	Patient alive as of the last day of the measurement year Ⓑ Ⓜ
* G9788	Most recent bp is less than or equal to 140/90 mm hg Ⓑ Ⓜ
* G9789	Blood pressure recorded during inpatient stays, emergency room visits, urgent care visits Ⓑ Ⓜ
* G9790	Most recent BP is greater than 140/90 mm hg, or blood pressure not documented Ⓑ Ⓜ
* G9791	Most recent tobacco status is tobacco free Ⓑ Ⓜ
* G9792	Most recent tobacco status is not tobacco free Ⓑ Ⓜ
* G9793	Patient is currently on a daily aspirin or other antiplatelet Ⓑ Ⓜ
* G9794	Documentation of medical reason(s) for not on a daily aspirin or other antiplatelet (e.g., history of gastrointestinal bleed, intra-cranial bleed, idiopathic thrombocytopenic purpura (ITP), gastric bypass or documentation of active anticoagulant use during the measurement period) Ⓑ Ⓜ
* G9795	Patient is not currently on a daily aspirin or other antiplatelet Ⓑ Ⓜ
* G9796	Patient is currently on a statin therapy Ⓑ Ⓜ
* G9797	Patient is not on a statin therapy Ⓑ Ⓜ
* G9805	Patients who use hospice services any time during the measurement period Ⓑ Ⓜ
* G9806	Patients who received cervical cytology or an HPV test Ⓑ Ⓜ

▶ New   ↻ Revised   ✔ Reinstated   ~~deleted~~ Deleted   🚫 Not covered or valid by Medicare
⊛ Special coverage instructions   * Carrier discretion   Ⓑ Bill Part B MAC   Ⓑ Bill DME MAC

TEMPORARY PROCEDURES/PROFESSIONAL SERVICES

* **G9807** Patients who did not receive cervical cytology or an HPV test ⓑ M
* **G9812** Patient died including all deaths occurring during the hospitalization in which the operation was performed, even if after 30 days, and those deaths occurring after discharge from the hospital, but within 30 days of the procedure ⓑ M
* **G9813** Patient did not die within 30 days of the procedure or during the index hospitalization ⓑ M
* **G9818** Documentation of sexual activity ⓑ M
* **G9819** Patients who use hospice services any time during the measurement period ⓑ M
* **G9820** Documentation of a chlamydia screening test with proper follow-up ⓑ M
* **G9821** No documentation of a chlamydia screening test with proper follow-up ⓑ M
* **G9822** Patient who had an endometrial ablation procedure during the year prior to the index date (exclusive of the index date) ⓑ M
* **G9823** Endometrial sampling or hysteroscopy with biopsy and results documented during the 12 months prior to the index date (exclusive of the index date) of the endometrial ablation ⓑ M
* **G9824** Endometrial sampling or hysteroscopy with biopsy and results not documented during the 12 months prior to the index date (exclusive of the index date) of the endometrial ablation ⓑ M
* **G9830** HER-2/neu positive ⓑ M
* **G9831** AJCC stage at breast cancer diagnosis = II or III ⓑ M
* **G9832** AJCC stage at breast cancer diagnosis = I (Ia or Ib) and T-stage at breast cancer diagnosis does not equal = T1, T1a, T1b ⓑ M
* **G9838** Patient has metastatic disease at diagnosis ⓑ M
* **G9839** Anti-EGFR monoclonal antibody therapy ⓑ M
* **G9840** Ras (KRas and NRas) gene mutation testing performed before initiation of anti-EGFR MoAb ⓑ M
* **G9841** Ras (KRas and NRas) gene mutation testing not performed before initiation of anti-EGFR MoAb ⓑ M
* **G9842** Patient has metastatic disease at diagnosis ⓑ M
* **G9843** Ras (KRas and NRas) gene mutation ⓑ M
* **G9844** Patient did not receive anti-EGFR monoclonal antibody therapy ⓑ M
* **G9845** Patient received anti-EGFR monoclonal antibody therapy ⓑ M
* **G9846** Patients who died from cancer ⓑ M
* **G9847** Patient received systemic cancer-directed therapy in the last 14 days of life ⓑ M
* **G9848** Patient did not receive systemic cancer-directed therapy in the last 14 days of life ⓑ M
* **G9858** Patient enrolled in hospice ⓑ M
* **G9859** Patients who died from cancer ⓑ M
* **G9860** Patient spent less than three days in hospice care ⓑ M
* **G9861** Patient spent greater than or equal to three days in hospice care ⓑ M
* **G9862** Documentation of medical reason(s) for not recommending at least a 10 year follow-up interval (e.g., inadequate prep, familial or personal history of colonic polyps, patient had no adenoma and age is = 66 years old, or life expectancy <10 years old, other medical reasons) ⓑ M
* **G9868** Receipt and analysis of remote, asynchronous images for dermatologic and/or ophthalmologic evaluation, for use only in a medicare-approved CMMI model, less than 10 minutes B
* **G9869** Receipt and analysis of remote, asynchronous images for dermatologic and/or ophthalmologic evaluation, for use only in a medicare-approved CMMI model, 10-20 minutes B
* **G9870** Receipt and analysis of remote, asynchronous images for dermatologic and/or ophthalmologic evaluation, for use only in a medicare-approved CMMI model, more than 20 minutes B
* **G9873** First Medicare diabetes prevention program (MDPP) core session was attended by an MDPP beneficiary under the MDPP expanded model (EM). A core session is an MDPP service that: (1) is furnished by an MDPP supplier during months 1 through 6 of the MDPP services period; (2) is approximately 1 hour in length; and (3) adheres to a CDC-approved DPP curriculum for core sessions. M
* **G9874** Four total Medicare diabetes prevention program (MDPP) core sessions were attended by an MDPP beneficiary under the mdpp expanded model (EM). A core session is an MDPP service that: (1) is furnished by an MDPP supplier during months 1 through 6 of the MDPP services period; (2) is approximately 1 hour in length; and (3) adheres to a CDC-approved DPP curriculum for core sessions. M

| MIPS | Qp Quantity Physician | Qh Quantity Hospital | ♀ Female only |
| ♂ Male only | A Age | ♿ DMEPOS | A2-Z3 ASC Payment Indicator | A-Y ASC Status Indicator | Coding Clinic |

* **G9875** Nine total Medicare diabetes prevention program (MDPP) core sessions were attended by an MDPP beneficiary under the MDPP expanded model (EM). A core session is an MDPP service that: (1) is furnished by an MDPP supplier during months 1 through 6 of the MDPP services period; (2) is approximately 1 hour in length; and (3) adheres to a CDC-approved DPP curriculum for core sessions. M

* **G9876** Two Medicare diabetes prevention program (MDPP) core maintenance sessions (MS) were attended by an MDPP beneficiary in months (mo) 7-9 under the mdpp expanded model (EM). A core maintenance session is an MDPP service that: (1) is furnished by an MDPP supplier during months 7 through 12 of the MDPP services period; (2) is approximately 1 hour in length; and (3) adheres to a CDC-approved DPP curriculum for maintenance sessions. The beneficiary did not achieve at least 5% weight loss (WL) from his/her baseline weight, as measured by at least one in-person weight measurement at a core maintenance session in months 7-9. M

* **G9877** Two Medicare diabetes prevention program (MDPP) core maintenance sessions (MS) were attended by an MDPP beneficiary in months (mo) 10-12 under the MDPP expanded model (EM). A core maintenance session is an MDPP service that: (1) is furnished by an MDPP supplier during months 7 through 12 of the MDPP services period; (2) is approximately 1 hour in length; and (3) adheres to a CDC-approved DPP curriculum for maintenance sessions. The beneficiary did not achieve at least 5% weight loss (WL) from his/her baseline weight, as measured by at least one in-person weight measurement at a core maintenance session in months 10-12. M

* **G9878** Two Medicare diabetes prevention program (MDPP) core maintenance sessions (MS) were attended by an MDPP beneficiary in months (mo) 7-9 under the MDPP expanded model (EM). A core maintenance session is an MDPP service that: (1) is furnished by an MDPP supplier during months 7 through 12 of the MDPP services period; (2) is approximately 1 hour in length; and (3) adheres to a CDC-approved DPP curriculum for maintenance sessions. The beneficiary achieved at least 5% weight loss (WL) from his/her baseline weight, as measured by at least one in-person weight measurement at a core maintenance session in months 7-9. M

* **G9879** Two Medicare diabetes prevention program (MDPP) core maintenance sessions (MS) were attended by an MDPP beneficiary in months (mo) 10-12 under the MDPP expanded model (EM). A core maintenance session is an MDPP service that: (1) is furnished by an MDPP supplier during months 7 through 12 of the MDPP services period; (2) is approximately 1 hour in length; and (3) adheres to a CDC-approved DPP curriculum for maintenance sessions. The beneficiary achieved at least 5% weight loss (WL) from his/her baseline weight, as measured by at least one in-person weight measurement at a core maintenance session in months 10-12. M

* **G9880** The MDPP beneficiary achieved at least 5% weight loss (WL) from his/her baseline weight in months (mo) 1-12 of the MDPP services period under the MDPP expanded model (EM). This is a one-time payment available when a beneficiary first achieves at least 5% weight loss from baseline as measured by an in-person weight measurement at a core session or core maintenance session. M

* **G9881** The MDPP beneficiary achieved at least 9% weight loss (WL) from his/her baseline weight in months (mo) 1-24 under the MDPP expanded model (EM). This is a one-time payment available when a beneficiary first achieves at least 9% weight loss from baseline as measured by an in-person weight measurement at a core session, core maintenance session, or ongoing maintenance session. M

TEMPORARY PROCEDURES/PROFESSIONAL SERVICES

* **G9882** Two Medicare diabetes prevention program (MDPP) ongoing maintenance sessions (MS) were attended by an MDPP beneficiary in months (mo) 13-15 under the MDPP expanded model (EM). An ongoing maintenance session is an MDPP service that: (1) is furnished by an MDPP supplier during months 13 through 24 of the MDPP services period; (2) is approximately 1 hour in length; and (3) adheres to a CDC-approved DPP curriculum for maintenance sessions. The beneficiary maintained at least 5% weight loss (WL) from his/her baseline weight, as measured by at least one in-person weight measurement at an ongoing maintenance session in months 13-15. M

* **G9883** Two Medicare diabetes prevention program (MDPP) ongoing maintenance sessions (MS) were attended by an MDPP beneficiary in months (mo) 16-18 under the MDPP expanded model (EM). An ongoing maintenance session is an MDPP service that: (1) is furnished by an MDPP supplier during months 13 through 24 of the MDPP services period; (2) is approximately 1 hour in length; and (3) adheres to a CDC-approved DPP curriculum for maintenance sessions. The beneficiary maintained at least 5% weight loss (WL) from his/her baseline weight, as measured by at least one in-person weight measurement at an ongoing maintenance session in months 16-18. M

* **G9884** Two Medicare diabetes prevention program (MDPP) ongoing maintenance sessions (MS) were attended by an MDPP beneficiary in months (mo) 19-21 under the MDPP expanded model (EM). An ongoing maintenance session is an MDPP service that: (1) is furnished by an MDPP supplier during months 13 through 24 of the MDPP services period; (2) is approximately 1 hour in length; and (3) adheres to a CDC-approved DPP curriculum for maintenance sessions. The beneficiary maintained at least 5% weight loss (WL) from his/her baseline weight, as measured by at least one in-person weight measurement at an ongoing maintenance session in months 19-21. M

* **G9885** Two Medicare diabetes prevention program (MDPP) ongoing maintenance sessions (MS) were attended by an MDPP beneficiary in months (mo) 22-24 under the MDPP expanded model (EM). An ongoing maintenance session is an MDPP service that: (1) is furnished by an MDPP supplier during months 13 through 24 of the MDPP services period; (2) is approximately 1 hour in length; and (3) adheres to a CDC-approved DPP curriculum for maintenance sessions. The beneficiary maintained at least 5% weight loss (WL) from his/her baseline weight, as measured by at least one in-person weight measurement at an ongoing maintenance session in months 22-24. M

* **G9886** Behavioral counseling for diabetes prevention, in-person, group, 60 minutes M

* **G9887** Behavioral counseling for diabetes prevention, distance learning, 60 minutes M

* **G9888** Maintenance 5% wl from baseline weight in months 7-12 M

NOTE: The following codes do not imply that codes in other sections are necessarily covered.

Quality Measures: Miscellaneous

* **G9890** Bridge payment: a one-time payment for the first Medicare diabetes prevention program (MDPP) core session, core maintenance session, or ongoing maintenance session furnished by an MDPP supplier to an MDPP beneficiary during months 1-24 of the MDPP expanded model (EM) who has previously received MDPP services from a different MDPP supplier under the MDPP expanded model. A supplier may only receive one bridge payment per MDPP beneficiary. B M

* **G9891** MDPP session reported as a line-item on a claim for a payable MDPP expanded model (EM) HCPCS code for a session furnished by the billing supplier under the MDPP expanded model and counting toward achievement of the attendance performance goal for the payable MDPP expanded model HCPCS code (this code is for reporting purposes only) B M

~~G9892~~	~~Documentation of patient reason(s) for not performing a dilated macular examination~~
~~G9893~~	~~Dilated macular exam was not performed, reason not otherwise specified~~
* G9894	Androgen deprivation therapy prescribed/administered in combination with external beam radiotherapy to the prostate Ⓑ M
* G9895	Documentation of medical reason(s) for not prescribing/administering androgen deprivation therapy in combination with external beam radiotherapy to the prostate (e.g., salvage therapy) Ⓑ M
* G9896	Documentation of patient reason(s) for not prescribing/administering androgen deprivation therapy in combination with external beam radiotherapy to the prostate Ⓑ M
* G9897	Patients who were not prescribed/administered androgen deprivation therapy in combination with external beam radiotherapy to the prostate, reason not given Ⓑ M
* G9898	Patient age 66 or older in institutional special needs plans (SNP) or residing in long-term care with pos code 32, 33, 34, 54, or 56 for more than 90 consecutive days during the measurement period Ⓑ M
* G9899	Screening, diagnostic, film, digital or digital breast tomosynthesis (3D) mammography results documented and reviewed Ⓑ M
* G9900	Screening, diagnostic, film, digital or digital breast tomosynthesis (3D) mammography results were not documented and reviewed, reason not otherwise specified Ⓑ M
* G9901	Patient age 66 or older in institutional special needs plans (SNP) or residing in long-term care with pos code 32, 33, 34, 54, or 56 for more than 90 consecutive days during the measurement period Ⓑ M
* G9902	Patient screened for tobacco use and identified as a tobacco user Ⓑ M
* G9903	Patient screened for tobacco use and identified as a tobacco non-user Ⓑ M
* G9905	Patient not screened for tobacco use Ⓑ M
* G9906	Patient identified as a tobacco user received tobacco cessation intervention during the measurement period or in the six months prior to the measurement period (counseling and/or pharmacotherapy) Ⓑ M
* G9908	Patient identified as tobacco user did not receive tobacco cessation intervention during the measurement period or in the six months prior to the measurement period (counseling and/or pharmacotherapy) Ⓑ M
* G9910	Patients age 66 or older in institutional special needs plans (SNP) or residing in long-term care with pos code 32, 33, 34, 54, or 56 for more than 90 consecutive days during the measurement period Ⓑ M
* G9911	Clinically node negative (t1n0m0 or t2n0m0) invasive breast cancer before or after neoadjuvant systemic therapy Ⓑ M
* G9912	Hepatitis B virus (HBV) status assessed and results interpreted prior to initiating anti-TNF (tumor necrosis factor) therapy Ⓑ M
* G9913	Hepatitis B virus (HBV) status not assessed and results interpreted prior to initiating anti-TNF (tumor necrosis factor) therapy, reason not otherwise specified Ⓑ M
* G9914	Patient initiated an anti-TNF agent Ⓑ M
* G9915	No record of HBV results documented Ⓑ M
* G9916	Functional status performed once in the last 12 months Ⓑ M
* G9917	Documentation of advanced stage dementia and caregiver knowledge is limited Ⓑ M
* G9918	Functional status not performed, reason not otherwise specified Ⓑ M
* G9919	Screening performed and positive and provision of recommendations Ⓑ D
* G9920	Screening performed and negative Ⓑ M
~~G9921~~	~~No screening performed, partial screening performed or positive screen without recommendations and reason is not given or otherwise specified~~
* G9922	Safety concerns screen provided and if positive then documented mitigation recommendations Ⓑ M
* G9923	Safety concerns screen provided and negative Ⓑ M
* G9925	Safety concerns screening not provided, reason not otherwise specified Ⓑ M
* G9926	Safety concerns screening positive screen is without provision of mitigation recommendations, including but not limited to referral to other resources Ⓑ M

TEMPORARY PROCEDURES/PROFESSIONAL SERVICES

* **G9928** FDA-approved anticoagulant not prescribed, reason not given ⓑ M
* **G9929** Patient with transient or reversible cause of AF (e.g., pneumonia, hyperthyroidism, pregnancy, cardiac surgery) ⓑ M
* **G9930** Patients who are receiving comfort care only ⓑ M
* **G9931** Documentation of CHA2DS2-VASc risk score of 0 or 1 for men; or 0, 1, or 2 for women ⓑ M
* **G9938** Patients aged 66 or older in institutional special needs plans (SNP) or residing in long-term care with POS code 32, 33, 34, 54, or 56 for more than 90 consecutive days during the six months prior to the measurement period through December 31 of the measurement period ⓑ M
* **G9939** Pathologist/dermatopathologist is the same clinician who performed the biopsy ⓑ M
* **G9940** Documentation of medical reason(s) for not on a statin (e.g., pregnancy, in vitro fertilization, clomiphene rx, ESRD, cirrhosis, muscular pain and disease during the measurement period or prior year) ⓑ M
* **G9943** Back pain was not measured by the visual analog scale (VAS) or numeric pain scale at three months (6-20 weeks) postoperatively ⓑ M
* **G9945** Patient had cancer, acute fracture or infection related to the lumbar spine or patient had neuromuscular, idiopathic or congenital lumbar scoliosis ⓑ M
* **G9946** Back pain was not measured by the visual analog scale (VAS) or numeric pain scale at one year (9 to 15 months) postoperatively ⓑ M
* **G9949** Leg pain was not measured by the visual analog scale (VAS) or numeric pain scale at three months (6 to 20 weeks) postoperatively ⓑ M
* **G9954** Patient exhibits 2 or more risk factors for post-operative vomiting ⓑ M
* **G9955** Cases in which an inhalational anesthetic is used only for induction ⓑ M
* **G9956** Patient received combination therapy consisting of at least two prophylactic pharmacologic anti-emetic agents of different classes preoperatively and/or intraoperatively ⓑ M
* **G9957** Documentation of medical reason for not receiving combination therapy consisting of at least two prophylactic pharmacologic anti-emetic agents of different classes preoperatively and/or intraoperatively (e.g., intolerance or other medical reason) ⓑ M
* **G9958** Patient did not receive combination therapy consisting of at least two prophylactic pharmacologic anti-emetic agents of different classes preoperatively and/or intraoperatively ⓑ M
* **G9959** Systemic antimicrobials not prescribed ⓑ M
* **G9960** Documentation of medical reason(s) for prescribing systemic antimicrobials ⓑ M
* **G9961** Systemic antimicrobials prescribed ⓑ M
* **G9962** Embolization endpoints are documented separately for each embolized vessel and ovarian artery angiography or embolization performed in the presence of variant uterine artery anatomy ⓑ M
* **G9963** Embolization endpoints are not documented separately for each embolized vessel or ovarian artery angiography or embolization not performed in the presence of variant uterine artery anatomy ⓑ M
* **G9964** Patient received at least one well-child visit with a PCP during the performance period ⓑ M
* **G9965** Patient did not receive at least one well-child visit with a PCP during the performance period ⓑ M
* **G9968** Patient was referred to another clinician or specialist during the performance period ⓑ M
* **G9969** Clinician who referred the patient to another clinician received a report from the provider to whom the patient was referred ⓑ M
* **G9970** Clinician who referred the patient to another clinician did not receive a report from the provider to whom the patient was referred ⓑ M
* ~~G9974~~ ~~Dilated macular exam performed, including documentation of the presence or absence of macular thickening or geographic atrophy or hemorrhage and the level of macular degeneration severity~~
* ~~G9975~~ ~~Documentation of medical reason(s) for not performing a dilated macular examination~~

 MIPS 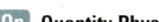 Quantity Physician   Quantity Hospital ♀ Female only ♂ Male only   Age ♿ DMEPOS A2-Z3 ASC Payment Indicator A-Y ASC Status Indicator Coding Clinic

267

* **G9976** Documentation of patient reason(s) for not performing a dilated macular examination ⓑ M

* **G9977** Dilated macular exam was not performed, reason not otherwise specified ⓑ M

* **G9978** Remote in-home visit for the evaluation and management of a new patient for use only in a Medicare-approved bundled payments for care improvement advanced (BCPI advanced) model episode of care, which requires these 3 key components: a problem focused history; a problem focused examination; and straightforward medical decision making, furnished in real time using interactive audio and video technology. Counseling and coordination of care with other physicians, other qualified health care professionals or agencies are provided consistent with the nature of the problem(s) and the needs of the patient or the family or both. Usually, the presenting problem(s) are self limited or minor. Typically, 10 minutes are spent with the patient or family or both via real time, audio and video intercommunications technology. ⓑ B

* **G9979** Remote in-home visit for the evaluation and management of a new patient for use only in a Medicare-approved bundled payments for care improvement advanced (BCPI advanced) model episode of care, which requires these 3 key components: an expanded problem focused history; an expanded problem focused examination; straightforward medical decision making, furnished in real time using interactive audio and video technology. Counseling and coordination of care with other physicians, other qualified health care professionals or agencies are provided consistent with the nature of the problem(s) and the needs of the patient or the family or both. Usually, the presenting problem(s) are of low to moderate severity. Typically, 20 minutes are spent with the patient or family or both via real time, audio and video intercommunications technology. ⓑ B

* **G9980** Remote in-home visit for the evaluation and management of a new patient for use only in a Medicare-approved bundled payments for care improvement advanced (BCPI advanced) model episode of care, which requires these 3 key components: a detailed history; a detailed examination; medical decision making of low complexity, furnished in real time using interactive audio and video technology. Counseling and coordination of care with other physicians, other qualified health care professionals or agencies are provided consistent with the nature of the problem(s) and the needs of the patient or the family or both. Usually, the presenting problem(s) are of moderate severity. Typically, 30 minutes are spent with the patient or family or both via real time, audio and video intercommunications technology. ⓑ B

* **G9981** Remote in-home visit for the evaluation and management of a new patient for use only in a Medicare-approved bundled payments for care improvement advanced (BCPI advanced) model episode of care, which requires these 3 key components: a comprehensive history; a comprehensive examination; medical decision making of moderate complexity, furnished in real time using interactive audio and video technology. Counseling and coordination of care with other physicians, other qualified health care professionals or agencies are provided consistent with the nature of the problem(s) and the needs of the patient or the family or both. Usually, the presenting problem(s) are of moderate to high severity. Typically, 45 minutes are spent with the patient or family or both via real time, audio and video intercommunications technology. ⓑ B

TEMPORARY PROCEDURES/PROFESSIONAL SERVICES

* **G9982** Remote in-home visit for the evaluation and management of a new patient for use only in a Medicare-approved bundled payments for care improvement advanced (BCPI advanced) model episode of care, which requires these 3 key components: a comprehensive history; a comprehensive examination; medical decision making of high complexity, furnished in real time using interactive audio and video technology. Counseling and coordination of care with other physicians, other qualified health care professionals or agencies are provided consistent with the nature of the problem(s) and the needs of the patient or the family or both. Usually, the presenting problem(s) are of moderate to high severity. Typically, 60 minutes are spent with the patient or family or both via real time, audio and video intercommunications technology. ⓑ B

* **G9983** Remote in-home visit for the evaluation and management of an established patient for use only in a Medicare-approved bundled payments for care improvement advanced (BCPI advanced) model episode of care, which requires at least 2 of the following 3 key components: a problem focused history; a problem focused examination; straightforward medical decision making, furnished in real time using interactive audio and video technology. Counseling and coordination of care with other physicians, other qualified health care professionals or agencies are provided consistent with the nature of the problem(s) and the needs of the patient or the family or both. Usually, the presenting problem(s) are self limited or minor. Typically, 10 minutes are spent with the patient or family or both via real time, audio and video intercommunications technology. ⓑ B

* **G9984** Remote in-home visit for the evaluation and management of an established patient for use only in a Medicare-approved bundled payments for care improvement advanced (BCPI advanced) model episode of care, which requires at least 2 of the following 3 key components: an expanded problem focused history; an expanded problem focused examination; medical decision making of low complexity, furnished in real time using interactive audio and video technology. Counseling and coordination of care with other physicians, other qualified health care professionals or agencies are provided consistent with the nature of the problem(s) and the needs of the patient or the family or both. Usually, the presenting problem(s) are of low to moderate severity. Typically, 15 minutes are spent with the patient or family or both via real time, audio and video intercommunications technology. ⓑ B

* **G9985** Remote in-home visit for the evaluation and management of an established patient for use only in a Medicare-approved bundled payments for care improvement advanced (BCPI advanced) model episode of care, which requires at least 2 of the following 3 key components: a detailed history; a detailed examination; medical decision making of moderate complexity, furnished in real time using interactive audio and video technology. Counseling and coordination of care with other physicians, other qualified health care professionals or agencies are provided consistent with the nature of the problem(s) and the needs of the patient or the family or both. Usually, the presenting problem(s) are of moderate to high severity. Typically, 25 minutes are spent with the patient or family or both via real time, audio and video intercommunications technology. ⓑ B

* **G9986** Remote in-home visit for the evaluation and management of an established patient for use only in a Medicare-approved bundled payments for care improvement advanced (BCPI advanced) model episode of care, which requires at least 2 of the following 3 key components: a comprehensive history; a comprehensive examination; medical decision making of high complexity, furnished in real time using interactive audio and video technology. Counseling and coordination of care with other physicians, other qualified health care professionals or agencies are provided consistent with the nature of the problem(s) and the needs of the patient or the family or both. Usually, the presenting problem(s) are of moderate to high severity. Typically, 40 minutes are spent with the patient or family or both via real time, audio and video intercommunications technology. Ⓑ B

* **G9987** Bundled payments for care improvement advanced (BCPI advanced) model home visit for patient assessment performed by clinical staff for an individual not considered homebound, including, but not necessarily limited to patient assessment of clinical status, safety/fall prevention, functional status/ambulation, medication reconciliation/management, compliance with orders/plan of care, performance of activities of daily living, and ensuring beneficiary connections to community and other services; for use only for a BCPI advanced model episode of care; may not be billed for a 30-day period covered by a transitional care management code. Ⓑ B

* **G9988** Palliative care services provided to patient any time during the measurement period Ⓑ M

~~G9990~~ ~~Patient did not receive any pneumococcal conjugate or polysaccharide vaccine on or after their 19th birthday and before the end of the measurement period~~

~~G9991~~ ~~Patient received any pneumococcal conjugate or polysaccharide vaccine on or after their 19th birthday and before the end of the measurement period~~

* **G9992** Palliative care services used by patient any time during the measurement period M

* **G9993** Patient was provided palliative care services any time during the measurement period M

* **G9994** Patient is using palliative care services any time during the measurement period M

* **G9996** Documentation stating the patient has received or is currently receiving palliative or hospice care M

* **G9997** Documentation of patient pregnancy anytime during the measurement period prior to and including the current encounter M

* **G9998** Documentation of medical reason(s) for an interval of less than 3 years since the last colonoscopy (e.g., last colonoscopy incomplete, last colonoscopy had inadequate prep, piecemeal removal of adenomas, or sessile serrated polyps > 20 mm in size, last colonoscopy found greater than 10 adenomas, lower gastrointestinal bleeding, or patient at high risk for colon cancer due to underlying medical history [Crohn's disease, ulcerative colitis, personal or family history of colon cancer, hereditary colorectal cancer syndromes]) M

↻ * **G9999** Documentation of system reason(s) for an interval of less than 3 years since the last colonoscopy (e.g., unable to locate previous colonoscopy report, patient cannot provide precise date or details from previous colonoscopy, previous colonoscopy report was incomplete) Ⓑ M

▶ New   ↻ Revised   ✓ Reinstated   ~~deleted~~ Deleted   ⊘ Not covered or valid by Medicare
◉ Special coverage instructions   * Carrier discretion   Ⓑ Bill Part B MAC   Ⓑ Bill DME MAC

BEHAVIORAL HEALTH AND/OR SUBSTANCE ABUSE TREATMENT SERVICES (H0001-H9999)

NOTE: Used by Medicaid state agencies because no national code exists to meet the reporting needs of these agencies.

⊘ H0001	Alcohol and/or drug assessment
⊘ H0002	Behavioral health screening to determine eligibility for admission to treatment program
⊘ H0003	Alcohol and/or drug screening; laboratory analysis of specimens for presence of alcohol and/or drugs
⊘ H0004	Behavioral health counseling and therapy, per 15 minutes
⊘ H0005	Alcohol and/or drug services; group counseling by a clinician
⊘ H0006	Alcohol and/or drug services; case management
⊘ H0007	Alcohol and/or drug services; crisis intervention (outpatient)
⊘ H0008	Alcohol and/or drug services; sub-acute detoxification (hospital inpatient)
⊘ H0009	Alcohol and/or drug services; acute detoxification (hospital inpatient)
⊘ H0010	Alcohol and/or drug services; sub-acute detoxification (residential addiction program inpatient)
⊘ H0011	Alcohol and/or drug services; acute detoxification (residential addiction program inpatient)
⊘ H0012	Alcohol and/or drug services; sub-acute detoxification (residential addiction program outpatient)
⊘ H0013	Alcohol and/or drug services; acute detoxification (residential addiction program outpatient)
⊘ H0014	Alcohol and/or drug services; ambulatory detoxification
⊘ H0015	Alcohol and/or drug services; intensive outpatient (treatment program that operates at least 3 hours/day and at least 3 days/week and is based on an individualized treatment plan), including assessment, counseling; crisis intervention, and activity therapies or education
⊘ H0016	Alcohol and/or drug services; medical/somatic (medical intervention in ambulatory setting)
⊘ H0017	Behavioral health; residential (hospital residential treatment program), without room and board, per diem
⊘ H0018	Behavioral health; short-term residential (non-hospital residential treatment program), without room and board, per diem
⊘ H0019	Behavioral health; long-term residential (non-medical, non-acute care in a residential treatment program where stay is typically longer than 30 days), without room and board, per diem
⊘ H0020	Alcohol and/or drug services; methadone administration and/or service (provision of the drug by a licensed program)
⊘ H0021	Alcohol and/or drug training service (for staff and personnel not employed by providers)
⊘ H0022	Alcohol and/or drug intervention service (planned facilitation)
⊘ H0023	Behavioral health outreach service (planned approach to reach a targeted population)
⊘ H0024	Behavioral health prevention information dissemination service (one-way direct or non-direct contact with service audiences to affect knowledge and attitude)
⊘ H0025	Behavioral health prevention education service (delivery of services with target population to affect knowledge, attitude and/or behavior)
⊘ H0026	Alcohol and/or drug prevention process service, community-based (delivery of services to develop skills of impactors)
⊘ H0027	Alcohol and/or drug prevention environmental service (broad range of external activities geared toward modifying systems in order to mainstream prevention through policy and law)
⊘ H0028	Alcohol and/or drug prevention problem identification and referral service (e.g., student assistance and employee assistance programs), does not include assessment
⊘ H0029	Alcohol and/or drug prevention alternatives service (services for populations that exclude alcohol and other drug use, e.g., alcohol-free social events)
⊘ H0030	Behavioral health hotline service
⊘ H0031	Mental health assessment, by non-physician
⊘ H0032	Mental health service plan development by non-physician
⊘ H0033	Oral medication administration, direct observation
⊘ H0034	Medication training and support, per 15 minutes
⊘ H0035	Mental health partial hospitalization, treatment, less than 24 hours

| MIPS | **Qp** Quantity Physician | **Qh** Quantity Hospital | ♀ Female only |
| ♂ Male only | **A** Age | & DMEPOS | A2-Z3 ASC Payment Indicator | A-Y ASC Status Indicator | Coding Clinic |

🪙⊘	**H0036**	Community psychiatric supportive treatment, face-to-face, per 15 minutes		
🪙⊘	**H0037**	Community psychiatric supportive treatment program, per diem		
⊘	**H0038**	Self-help/peer services, per 15 minutes		
🪙⊘	**H0039**	Assertive community treatment, face-to-face, per 15 minutes		
🪙⊘	**H0040**	Assertive community treatment program, per diem		
⊘	**H0041**	Foster care, child, non-therapeutic, per diem Ⓐ		
⊘	**H0042**	Foster care, child, non-therapeutic, per month Ⓐ		
⊘	**H0043**	Supported housing, per diem		
⊘	**H0044**	Supported housing, per month		
⊘	**H0045**	Respite care services, not in the home, per diem		
⊘	**H0046**	Mental health services, not otherwise specified		
⊘	**H0047**	Alcohol and/or other drug abuse services, not otherwise specified		
⊘	**H0048**	Alcohol and/or other drug testing: collection and handling only, specimens other than blood		
⊘	**H0049**	Alcohol and/or drug screening		
⊘	**H0050**	Alcohol and/or drug services, brief intervention, per 15 minutes		
⊘	**H0051**	Traditional healing service		
▶⊘	**H0052**	Missing and murdered indigenous persons (MMIP) mental health and clinical care		
▶⊘	**H0053**	Historical trauma (HT) mental health and clinical care for indigenous persons		
⊘	**H1000**	Prenatal care, at-risk assessment ♀		
⊘	**H1001**	Prenatal care, at-risk enhanced service; antepartum management ♀		
⊘	**H1002**	Prenatal care, at-risk enhanced service; care coordination ♀		
⊘	**H1003**	Prenatal care, at-risk enhanced service; education ♀		
⊘	**H1004**	Prenatal care, at-risk enhanced service; follow-up home visit ♀		
⊘	**H1005**	Prenatal care, at-risk enhanced service package (includes H1001-H1004) ♀		
⊘	**H1010**	Non-medical family planning education, per session		
⊘	**H1011**	Family assessment by licensed behavioral health professional for state defined purposes		
🪙⊘	**H2000**	Comprehensive multidisciplinary evaluation		
🪙⊘	**H2001**	Rehabilitation program, per 1/2 day		
🪙⊘	**H2010**	Comprehensive medication services, per 15 minutes		
🪙⊘	**H2011**	Crisis intervention service, per 15 minutes		
🪙⊘	**H2012**	Behavioral health day treatment, per hour		
🪙⊘	**H2013**	Psychiatric health facility service, per diem		
🪙⊘	**H2014**	Skills training and development, per 15 minutes		
🪙⊘	**H2015**	Comprehensive community support services, per 15 minutes		
🪙⊘	**H2016**	Comprehensive community support services, per diem		
🪙⊘	**H2017**	Psychosocial rehabilitation services, per 15 minutes		
🪙⊘	**H2018**	Psychosocial rehabilitation services, per diem		
🪙⊘	**H2019**	Therapeutic behavioral services, per 15 minutes		
🪙⊘	**H2020**	Therapeutic behavioral services, per diem		
⊘	**H2021**	Community-based wrap-around services, per 15 minutes		
⊘	**H2022**	Community-based wrap-around services, per diem		
⊘	**H2023**	Supported employment, per 15 minutes		
⊘	**H2024**	Supported employment, per diem		
⊘	**H2025**	Ongoing support to maintain employment, per 15 minutes		
⊘	**H2026**	Ongoing support to maintain employment, per diem		
⊘	**H2027**	Psychoeducational service, per 15 minutes		
⊘	**H2028**	Sexual offender treatment service, per 15 minutes		
⊘	**H2029**	Sexual offender treatment service, per diem		
⊘	**H2030**	Mental health clubhouse services, per 15 minutes		
⊘	**H2031**	Mental health clubhouse services, per diem		
⊘	**H2032**	Activity therapy, per 15 minutes		
⊘	**H2033**	Multisystemic therapy for juveniles, per 15 minutes Ⓐ		
⊘	**H2034**	Alcohol and/or drug abuse halfway house services, per diem		
⊘	**H2035**	Alcohol and/or other drug treatment program, per hour		
⊘	**H2036**	Alcohol and/or other drug treatment program, per diem		
⊘	**H2037**	Developmental delay prevention activities, dependent child of client, per 15 minutes Ⓐ		
⊘	**H2040**	Coordinated specialty care, team-based, for first episode psychosis, per month		
⊘	**H2041**	Coordinated specialty care, team-based, for first episode psychosis, per encounter		

▶ New　↻ Revised　✓ Reinstated　~~deleted~~ Deleted　⊘ Not covered or valid by Medicare
✹ Special coverage instructions　✱ Carrier discretion　Ⓑ Bill Part B MAC　Ⓑ Bill DME MAC

DRUGS OTHER THAN CHEMOTHERAPY DRUGS (J0100-J8999)

Injection

○ **J0120** Injection, tetracycline, up to 250 mg ⓑ Ⓑ Qp Qh N1 N
Other: Achromycin
IOM: 100-02, 15, 50

✳ **J0121** Injection, omadacycline, 1 mg ⓑ Ⓑ K2 K
Other: Nuzyra

✳ **J0122** Injection, eravacycline, 1 mg ⓑ Ⓑ K2 N
Other: Xerava

✳ **J0129** Injection, abatacept, 10 mg (Code may be used for Medicare when drug administered under the direct supervision of a physician, not for use when drug is self-administered) ⓑ Ⓑ Qp Qh K2 K
Other: Orencia

○ **J0130** Injection, abciximab, 10 mg ⓑ Ⓑ Qp Qh N1 N
Other: ReoPro
IOM: 100-02, 15, 50

✳ **J0131** Injection, acetaminophen, not otherwise specified, 10 mg ⓑ Ⓑ Qp Qh N1 N
Other: Acetaminophen
Coding Clinic: 2012, Q1, P9

✳ **J0132** Injection, acetylcysteine, 100 mg ⓑ Ⓑ Qp Qh N1 N
Other: Acetadote, Acettylcysteine

✳ **J0133** Injection, acyclovir, 5 mg ⓑ Ⓑ Qp Qh N1 N

J0134 Injection, acetaminophen (fresenius kabi), not therapeutically equivalent to J0131, 10 mg ⓑ Ⓑ N
Other: Acetaminophen

~~J0135~~ ~~Injection, adalimumab, 20 mg~~

✳ **J0136** Injection, acetaminophen (b braun), not therapeutically equivalent to J0131, 10 mg ⓑ Ⓑ N
Other: Acetaminophen

✳ **J0137** Injection, acetaminophen (hikma), not therapeutically equivalent to J0131, 10 mg ⓑ Ⓑ N

✳ **J0138** Injection, acetaminophen 10 mg and ibuprofen 3 mg ⓑ Ⓑ N

✳ **J0139** Injection, adalimumab, 1 mg ⓑ Ⓑ K

○ **J0153** Injection, adenosine, 1 mg (not to be used to report any adenosine phosphate compounds) ⓑ Ⓑ Qp Qh N1 N

▶ **J0163** Injection, epinephrine in sodium chloride (endo), 0.1 mg N1 N

▶ **J0164** Injection, epinephrine in sodium chloride (baxter), 0.1 mg N1 N

▶ **J0165** Injection, epinephrine, not otherwise specified, 0.1 mg N1 N

▶ **J0166** Injection, epinephrine (bpi), not therapeutically equivalent to J0165, 0.1 mg N1 N

▶ **J0167** Injection, epinephrine (hospira), not therapeutically equivalent to J0165, 0.1 mg N1 N

▶ **J0168** Injection, epinephrine (international medication systems), not therapeutically equivalent to J0165, 0.1 mg N1 N

▶ **J0169** Injection, epinephrine (adrenalin), not therapeutically equivalent to J0165, 0.1 mg N1 N

~~J0171~~ ~~Injection, adrenalin, epinephrine, 0.1 mg~~

J0172 Injection, aducanumab-avwa, 2 mg ⓑ Ⓑ K2 K

~~J0173~~ ~~Injection, epinephrine (belcher), not therapeutically equivalent to J0171, 0.1 mg~~

J0174 Injection, lecanemab-irmb, 1 mg ⓑ Ⓑ G
Other: Leqembi

J0175 Injection, donanemab-azbt, 2 mg ⓑ Ⓑ G

J0177 Injection, aflibercept hd, 1 mg ⓑ Ⓑ G

✳ **J0178** Injection, aflibercept, 1 mg ⓑ Ⓑ Qp Qh K2 K
Other: Eylea

✳ **J0179** Injection, brolucizumab-dbll, 1 mg ⓑ Ⓑ K2 K
Other: Beovu

✳ **J0180** Injection, agalsidase beta, 1 mg ⓑ Ⓑ Qp Qh K2 K
Other: Fabrazyme
IOM: 100-02, 15, 50

J0184 Injection, amisulpride, 1 mg ⓑ Ⓑ G

✳ **J0185** Injection, aprepitant, 1 mg ⓑ Ⓑ K
Other: Emend, Comvanti

○ **J0190** Injection, biperiden lactate, per 5 mg ⓑ Ⓑ Qp Qh E2
Other: Akineton
IOM: 100-02, 15, 50

○ **J0200** Injection, alatrofloxacin mesylate, 100 mg ⓑ Ⓑ Qp Qh E2
Other: Trovan
IOM: 100-02, 15, 50

| 🪙 MIPS | Qp Quantity Physician | Qh Quantity Hospital | ♀ Female only |
| ♂ Male only | Ⓐ Age | ♿ DMEPOS | A2-Z3 ASC Payment Indicator | A-Y ASC Status Indicator | Coding Clinic |

273

✱ **J0202**	Injection, alemtuzumab, 1 mg ⓑ Ⓑ Qp Qh	K2 K	⊛ **J0256**	Injection, alpha 1-proteinase inhibitor (human), not otherwise specified, 10 mg ⓑ Ⓑ Qp Qh	K2 K
	Other: Lemtrada			Other: Zemaira	
⊛ **J0205**	Injection, alglucerase, per 10 units ⓑ Ⓑ Qp Qh	E2		IOM: 100-02, 15, 50	
	Other: Ceredase			Coding Clinic: 2012, Q1, P9	
	IOM: 100-02, 15, 50		⊛ **J0257**	Injection, alpha 1 proteinase inhibitor (human), (glassia), 10 mg ⓑ Ⓑ Qp Qh	K2 K
⊛ **J0206**	Injection, allopurinol sodium, 1 mg ⓑ Ⓑ	K		IOM: 100-02, 15, 50	
✱⊛ **J0207**	Injection, amifostine, 500 mg ⓑ Ⓑ Qp Qh	K2 E2		Coding Clinic: 2012, Q1, P8	
	Other: Ethyol		⊛ **J0270**	Injection, alprostadil, per 1.25 mcg (Code may be used for Medicare when drug administered under the direct supervision of a physician, not for use when drug is self-administered) ⓑ Ⓑ Qp Qh	B
	IOM: 100-02, 15, 50				
⊛ **J0208**	Injection, sodium thiosulfate (pedmark), 100 mg ⓑ Ⓑ	G		Other: Caverject, Prostaglandin E1, Prostin VR Pediatric	
⊛ **J0209**	Injection, sodium thiosulfate (hope), 100 mg ⓑ Ⓑ	N		IOM: 100-02, 15, 50	
⊛ **J0210**	Injection, methyldopate HCL, up to 250 mg ⓑ Ⓑ Qp Qh	N1 E2	⊛ **J0275**	Alprostadil urethral suppository (Code may be used for Medicare when drug administered under the direct supervision of a physician, not for use when drug is self-administered) ⓑ Ⓑ Qp Qh	B
	Other: Aldomet				
	IOM: 100-02, 15, 50			Other: Muse	
⊛ **J0211**	Injection, sodium nitrite 3 mg and sodium thiosulfate 125 mg (nithiodote) ⓑ Ⓑ	K		IOM: 100-02, 15, 50	
✱ **J0215**	Injection, alefacept, 0.5 mg ⓑ Ⓑ Qp Qh	E2	✱ **J0278**	Injection, amikacin sulfate, 100 mg ⓑ Ⓑ Qp Qh	N1 N
J0216	Injection, alfentanil hydrochloride, 500 mcg ⓑ Ⓑ	N	⊛ **J0280**	Injection, aminophylline, up to 250 mg ⓑ Ⓑ Qp Qh	N1 N
J0217	Injection, velmanase alfa-tycv, 1 mg ⓑ Ⓑ	G		IOM: 100-02, 15, 50	
	Other: Lamzede		▶ ⊛ **J0281**	Injection, aminocaproic acid, 1 gram ⓑ Ⓑ Qp Qh	N1 N
J0218	Injection, olipudase alfa-rpcp, 1 mg ⓑ Ⓑ	G	⊛ **J0282**	Injection, amiodarone hydrochloride, 30 mg ⓑ Ⓑ Qp Qh	N1 N
	Other: Xenpozyme			Other: Cordarone	
✱ **J0220**	Injection, alglucosidase alfa, not otherwise specified, 10 mg ⓑ Ⓑ Qp Qh	K2 N		IOM: 100-02, 15, 50	
			J0283	Injection, amiodarone hydrochloride (nexterone), 30 mg ⓑ Ⓑ	E2
	Coding Clinic: 2013, Q2, P5; 2012, Q1, P9		⊛ **J0285**	Injection, amphotericin B, 50 mg ⓑ Ⓑ Qp Qh	N1 N
✱ **J0221**	Injection, alglucosidase alfa, (lumizyme), 10 mg ⓑ Ⓑ Qp Qh	K2 K		Other: ABLC, Amphocin, Fungizone	
	Other: Lumizyme			IOM: 100-02, 15, 50	
	Coding Clinic: 2013, Q2, P5		⊛ **J0287**	Injection, amphotericin B lipid complex, 10 mg ⓑ Ⓑ Qp Qh	K2 K
✱ **J0222**	Injection, patisiran, 0.1 mg ⓑ Ⓑ	K2 K		IOM: 100-02, 15, 50	
	Other: Onpattro		⊛ **J0288**	Injection, amphotericin B cholesteryl sulfate complex, 10 mg ⓑ Ⓑ Qp Qh	E2
✱ **J0223**	Injection, givosiran, 0.5 mg ⓑ Ⓑ	K2 K			
	Other: Givlaari			IOM: 100-02, 15, 50	
✱ **J0224**	Injection, lumasiran, 0.5 mg ⓑ Ⓑ	K2 K			
	Other: Oxlumo				
J0225	Injection, vutrisiran, 1 mg ⓑ Ⓑ	K2 G			
	Other: Amvuttra				

▶ New ↻ Revised ✓ Reinstated ~~deleted~~ Deleted ⊘ Not covered or valid by Medicare
⊛ Special coverage instructions ✱ Carrier discretion ⓑ Bill Part B MAC Ⓑ Bill DME MAC

DRUGS OTHER THAN CHEMOTHERAPY DRUGS

⊛ J0289	Injection, amphotericin B liposome, 10 mg ⓑ Ⓑ Qp Qh	K2 K
	Other: AmBisome, Amphotericin B Liposome	
	IOM: 100-02, 15, 50	
⊛ J0290	Injection, ampicillin sodium, 500 mg ⓑ Qp Qh	N1 N
	Other: Omnipen-N, Polycillin-N, Totacillin-N	
	IOM: 100-02, 15, 50	
✱ J0291	Injection, plazomicin, 5 mg ⓑ Ⓑ	K2 K
	Other: Zemdri	
⊛ J0295	Injection, ampicillin sodium/sulbactam sodium, per 1.5 gm ⓑ Ⓑ Qp Qh	N1 N
	Other: Omnipen-N, Polycillin-N, Totacillin-N, Unasyn	
	IOM: 100-02, 15, 50	
⊛ J0300	Injection, amobarbital, up to 125 mg ⓑ Ⓑ Qp Qh	K2 N
	Other: Amytal	
	IOM: 100-02, 15, 50	
⊛ J0330	Injection, succinylcholine chloride, up to 20 mg ⓑ Ⓑ Qp Qh	N1 N
	Other: Anectine, Quelicin, Surostrin	
	IOM: 100-02, 15, 50	
✱ J0348	Injection, anidulafungin, 1 mg ⓑ Qp Qh	N1 N
	Other: Eraxis	
J0349	Injection, rezafungin, 1 mg ⓑ Ⓑ	G
⊛ J0350	Injection, anistreplase, per 30 units ⓑ Ⓑ Qp Qh	E2
	Other: Eminase	
	IOM: 100-02, 15, 50	
▶ J0458	Injection, aztreonam/avibactam, 7.5 mg/2.5 mg (10 mg)	G
⊛ J0360	Injection, hydralazine hydrochloride, up to 20 mg ⓑ Ⓑ Qp Qh	N1 N
	Other: Apresoline	
	IOM: 100-02, 15, 50	
▶ J0462	Injection, atropine sulfate, not therapeutically equivalent to J0461, 0.01 mg	N1 N
✱ J0364	Injection, apomorphine hydrochloride, 1 mg ⓑ Ⓑ Qp Qh	E2
⊛ J0365	Injection, aprotinin, 10,000 KIU ⓑ Ⓑ Qp Qh	E2
	IOM: 100-02, 15, 50	
⊛ J0380	Injection, metaraminol bitartrate, per 10 mg ⓑ Ⓑ Qp Qh	N1 E2
	Other: Aramine	
	IOM: 100-02, 15, 50	
⊛ J0390	Injection, chloroquine hydrochloride, up to 250 mg ⓑ Ⓑ Qp Qh	N1 N
	Benefit only for diagnosed malaria or amebiasis	
	Other: Aralen	
	IOM: 100-02, 15, 50	
J0391	Injection, artesunate, 1 mg ⓑ Ⓑ	K
⊛ J0395	Injection, arbutamine HCL, 1 mg ⓑ Ⓑ Qp Qh	E2
	IOM: 100-02, 15, 50	
✱ J0400	Injection, aripiprazole, intramuscular, 0.25 mg ⓑ Ⓑ Qp Qh	K2 N
✱ J0401	Injection, aripiprazole, (abilify mairntena), 1 mg ⓑ Ⓑ Qp Qh	K2 K
	Other: Abilify Maintena	
J0402	Injection, aripiprazole (abilify asimtufii), 1 mg ⓑ Ⓑ	G
	Other: Abilify Maintena	
⊛ J0456	Injection, azithromycin, 500 mg ⓑ Ⓑ Qp Qh	N1 N
	Other: Zithromax	
	IOM: 100-02, 15, 50	
J0457	Injection, aztreonam ⓑ Ⓑ	E2
⊛ J0461	Injection, atropine sulfate, 0.01 mg ⓑ Ⓑ Qp Qh	N1 N
	IOM: 100-02, 15, 50	
⊛ J0470	Injection, dimercaprol, per 100 mg ⓑ Ⓑ Qp Qh	K2 N
	Other: BAL In Oil	
	IOM: 100-02, 15, 50	
⊛ J0475	Injection, baclofen, 10 mg ⓑ Ⓑ Qp Qh	K2 K
	Other: Gablofen, Lioresal	
	IOM: 100-02, 15, 50	
⊛ J0476	Injection, baclofen 50 mcg for intrathecal trial ⓑ Ⓑ Qp Qh	K2 N
	Other: Gablofen, Lioresal	
	IOM: 100-02, 15, 50	
⊛ J0480	Injection, basiliximab, 20 mg ⓑ Ⓑ Qp Qh	K2 K
	Other: Simulect	
	IOM: 100-02, 15, 50	
✱ J0485	Injection, belatacept, 1 mg ⓑ Ⓑ Qp Qh	K2 K
	Other: Nulojix	
✱ J0490	Injection, belimumab, 10 mg ⓑ Ⓑ Qp Qh	K2 K
	Other: Benlysta	
	Coding Clinic: 2012, Q1, P9	

🏵 MIPS	Qp Quantity Physician	Qh Quantity Hospital	♀ Female only
♂ Male only	Ⓐ Age	♿ DMEPOS	A2-Z3 ASC Payment Indicator	A-Y ASC Status Indicator	Coding Clinic

Code	Description	Status
⊚ **J0500**	Injection, dicyclomine HCL, up to 20 mg ⓑ Ⓑ Qp Qh	N1 N
	Other: Antispas, Bentyl, Dibent, Dilomine, Di-Spaz, Neoquess, Or-Tyl, Spasmoject	
	IOM: 100-02, 15, 50	
⊚ **J0515**	Injection, benztropine mesylate, per 1 mg ⓑ Ⓑ Qp Qh	N1 N
	Other: Cogentin	
	IOM: 100-02, 15, 50	
✱ **J0517**	Injection, benralizumab, 1 mg ⓑ Ⓑ	K
	Other: Fasenra	
⊚ **J0520**	Injection, bethanechol chloride, myotonachol or urecholine, up to 5 mg ⓑ Ⓑ Qp Qh	E2
	IOM: 100-02, 15, 50	
▶ **J0525**	Injection, cefotetan disodium, 10 mg	N1 N
✱ **J0558**	Injection, penicillin G benzathine and penicillin G procaine, 100,000 units ⓑ Ⓑ Qp Qh	N1 K
	Other: Bicillin C-R	
	Coding Clinic: 2011, Q1, P8	
⊚ **J0561**	Injection, penicillin G benzathine, 100,000 units ⓑ Ⓑ Qp Qh	K2 K
	Other: Bicillin L-A, Permapen	
	IOM: 100-02, 15, 50	
	Coding Clinic: 2013, Q2, P3; 2011, Q1, P8	
✱ **J0565**	Injection, bezlotoxumab, 10 mg ⓑ Ⓑ	K2 K
✱ **J0567**	Injection, cerliponase alfa, 1 mg ⓑ Ⓑ	
	Other: Brineura	
	~~J0570~~ ~~Buprenorphine implant, 74.2 mg~~	
⊚ **J0571**	Buprenorphine, oral, 1 mg ⓑ Ⓑ Qp Qh	E1
⊚ **J0572**	Buprenorphine/naloxone, oral, less than or equal to 3 mg buprenorphine ⓑ Ⓑ Qp Qh	E1
⊚ **J0573**	Buprenorphine/naloxone, oral, greater than 3 mg, but less than or equal to 6 mg buprenorphine ⓑ Ⓑ Qp Qh	E1
⊚ **J0574**	Buprenorphine/naloxone, oral, greater than 6 mg, but less than or equal to 10 mg buprenorphine ⓑ Ⓑ Qp Qh	E1
⊚ **J0575**	Buprenorphine/naloxone, oral, greater than 10 mg buprenorphine ⓑ Ⓑ Qp Qh	E1
J0577	Injection, buprenorphine extended-release (brixadi), less than or equal to 7 days of therapy ⓑ Ⓑ	G
J0578	Injection, buprenorphine extended-release (brixadi), greater than 7 days and up to 28 days of therapy ⓑ Ⓑ	G
▶ **J0582**	Injection, bivalirudin (endo), not therapeutically equivalent to J0583, 1 mg	N1 N
✱ **J0583**	Injection, bivalirudin, 1 mg ⓑ Ⓑ Qp Qh	N1 N
	Other: Angiomax	
✱ **J0584**	Injection, burosumab-twza 1 mg ⓑ Ⓑ	K
	Other: Crysvita	
⊚ **J0585**	Injection, onabotulinumtoxinA, 1 unit ⓑ Ⓑ Qp Qh	K2 K
	Other: Botox, Botox Cosmetic, Oculinum	
	IOM: 100-02, 15, 50	
✱ **J0586**	Injection, abobotulinumtoxinA, 5 units ⓑ Ⓑ Qp Qh	K2 K
⊚ **J0587**	Injection, rimabotulinumtoxinB, 100 units ⓑ Ⓑ Qp Qh	K2 K
	Other: Myobloc, Nplate	
	IOM: 100-02, 15, 50	
✱ **J0588**	Injection, incobotulinumtoxin A, 1 unit ⓑ Ⓑ Qp Qh	K2 K
	Other: Xeomin	
	Coding Clinic: 2012, Q1, P9	
J0589	Injection, daxibotulinumtoxina-lanm, 1 unit ⓑ Ⓑ	G
✱ **J0591**	Injection, deoxycholic acid, 1 mg ⓑ	E1
✱ **J0592**	Injection, buprenorphine hydrochloride, 0.1 mg ⓑ Ⓑ Qp Qh	N1 N
	Other: Buprenex	
	IOM: 100-02, 15, 50	
✱ **J0593**	Injection, lanadelumab-flyo, 1 mg (Code may be used for Medicare when drug administered under direct supervision of a physician, not for use when drug is self-administered) ⓑ Ⓑ	K2 E2
✱ **J0594**	Injection, busulfan, 1 mg ⓑ Ⓑ Qp Qh	K2 K
	Other: Myleran	
✱ **J0595**	Injection, butorphanol tartrate, 1 mg ⓑ Ⓑ Qp Qh	N1 N
✱ **J0596**	Injection, C1 esterase inhibitor (recombinant), ruconest, 10 units ⓑ Ⓑ Qp Qh	K2 K
✱ **J0597**	Injection, C-1 esterase inhibitor (human), Berinert, 10 units ⓑ Ⓑ Qp Qh	K2 K
	Coding Clinic: 2011, Q1, P7	
✱ **J0598**	Injection, C1 esterase inhibitor (human), cinryze, 10 units ⓑ Ⓑ Qp Qh	K2 K

▶ New ↻ Revised ✓ Reinstated ~~deleted~~ Deleted ⊘ Not covered or valid by Medicare
⊚ Special coverage instructions ✱ Carrier discretion ⓑ Bill Part B MAC Ⓑ Bill DME MAC

DRUGS OTHER THAN CHEMOTHERAPY DRUGS

* **J0599** Injection, c-1 esterase inhibitor (human), (haegarda), 10 units ⓑ ⓑ E2
  Other: Berinert

* **J0600** Injection, edetate calcium disodium, up to 1000 mg ⓑ ⓑ Qp Qh K2 K
  IOM: 100-02, 15, 50

▶ **J0601** Sevelamer carbonate (renvela or therapeutically equivalent), oral, 20 mg (for ESRD on dialysis) B

▶ **J0602** Sevelamer carbonate (renvela or therapeutically equivalent), oral, powder, 20 mg (for ESRD on dialysis) B

▶ **J0603** Sevelamer hydrochloride (renagel or therapeutically equivalent), oral, 20 mg (for ESRD on dialysis) B

J0604 Cinacalcet, oral, 1 mg, (for ESRD on dialysis) B

▶ **J0605** Sucroferric oxyhydroxide, oral, 5 mg (for ESRD on dialysis) B

J0606 Injection, etelcalcetide, 0.1 mg ⓑ ⓑ K2 K

▶ **J0607** Lanthanum carbonate, oral, 5 mg (for ESRD on dialysis) B

▶ **J0608** Lanthanum carbonate, oral, powder, 5 mg, not therapeutically equivalent to J0607 (for ESRD on dialysis) B

▶ **J0609** Ferric citrate, oral, 3 mg ferric iron, (for ESRD on dialysis) B

J0612 Injection, calcium gluconate not otherwise specified, per 10 mg ⓑ ⓑ

J0613 Injection, calcium gluconate (wg critical care), not therapeutically equivalent to J0612, per 10 mg ⓑ ⓑ

▶ **J0614** Injection, treosulfan, 50 mg G

▶ **J0615** Calcium acetate, oral, 23 mg (for ESRD on dialysis) B

▶ **J0616** Injection, metoprolol tartrate, 1 mg N

▶ **J0618** Injection, calcium chloride, 2 mg N

J0620 Injection, calcium glycerophosphate and calcium lactate, per 10 ml ⓑ ⓑ Qp Qh N1 N
  Other: Calphosan
  MCM: 2049
  IOM: 100-02, 15, 50

J0630 Injection, calcitonin (salmon), up to 400 units ⓑ ⓑ Qp Qh K2 K
  Other: Calcimar, Calcitonin-salmon, Miacalcin
  IOM: 100-02, 15, 50

J0636 Injection, calcitriol, 0.1 mcg ⓑ ⓑ Qp Qh N1 N
  Non-dialysis use
  Other: Calcijex
  IOM: 100-02, 15, 50

* **J0637** Injection, caspofungin acetate, 5 mg ⓑ ⓑ Qp Qh K2 N
  Other: Cancidas, Caspofungin

* **J0638** Injection, canakinumab, 1 mg ⓑ ⓑ Qp Qh K2 K
  Other: Ilaris

J0640 Injection, leucovorin, calcium, per 50 mg ⓑ ⓑ Qp Qh N1 N
  Other: Wellcovorin
  IOM: 100-02, 15, 50
  Coding Clinic: 2009, Q1, P10

J0641 Injection, levoleucovorin, not otherwise specified, 0.5 mg ⓑ ⓑ Qp Qh K2 N
  Part of treatment regimen for osteosarcoma

* **J0642** Injection, levoleucovorin, (khapzory), 0.5 mg ⓑ ⓑ K2 N

J0650 Injection, levothyroxine sodium, not otherwise specified, 10 mcg ⓑ ⓑ

J0651 Injection, levothyroxine sodium (fresenius kabi), not therapeutically equivalent to J0650, 10 mcg ⓑ ⓑ

J0652 Injection, levothyroxine sodium (hikma), not therapeutically equivalent to J0650, 10 mcg ⓑ ⓑ

J0665 Injection, bupivicaine, not otherwise specified, 0.5 mg ⓑ ⓑ

▶ **J0666** Injection, bupivacaine liposome, 1 mg K1

▶ **J0668** Instillation, bupivacaine and meloxicam, 1 mg/0.03 mg K1

J0670 Injection, mepivacaine HCL, per 10 ml ⓑ ⓑ Qp Qh N1 N
  Other: Carbocaine, Isocaine HCl, Polocaine
  IOM: 100-02, 15, 50

▶ **J0675** Injection, carboprost tromethamine, 0.1 mg K

▶ **J0681** Injection, ceftobiprole medocaril sodium, 3 mg G

J0687 Injection, cefazolin sodium (wg critical care), not therapeutically equivalent to J0690, 500 mg ⓑ ⓑ K

J0688 Injection, cefazolin sodium (hikma), not therapeutically equivalent to J0690, 500 mg ⓑ ⓑ K

J0689 Injection, cefazolin sodium (baxter), not therapeutically equivalent to J0690, 500 mg ⓑ ⓑ N

J0690 Injection, cefezolin sodium, 500 mg ⓑ ⓑ Qp Qh N1 N
  Other: Ancef, Kefzol, Zolicef
  IOM: 100-02, 15, 50

* **J0691** Injection, lefamulin, 1 mg ⓑ ⓑ K2 N

* **J0692** Injection, cefepime 500 mg ⓑ ⓑ Qp Qh N1 N
  Other: Maxipime

MIPS | Qp Quantity Physician | Qh Quantity Hospital | ♀ Female only
♂ Male only | A Age | ♿ DMEPOS | A2-Z3 ASC Payment Indicator | A-Y ASC Status Indicator | Coding Clinic

✺ **J0694**	Injection, cefoxitin sodium, 1 gm ⓑ Ⓑ Qp Qh N1 N

Other: Mefoxin

IOM: 100-02, 15, 50,

Cross Reference Q0090

✳ **J0695** Injection, ceftolozane 50 mg and tazobactam 25 mg ⓑ Ⓑ Qp Qh   K2 K

Other: Zerbaxa

✺ **J0696** Injection, ceftriaxone sodium, per 250 mg ⓑ Ⓑ Qp Qh   N1 N

Other: Rocephin

IOM: 100-02, 15, 50

✺ **J0697** Injection, sterile cefuroxime sodium, per 750 mg ⓑ Ⓑ Qp Qh   N1 N

Other: Kefurox, Zinacef

IOM: 100-02, 15, 50

✺ **J0698** Injection, cefotaxime sodium, per gm ⓑ Ⓑ Qp Qh   N1 N

Other: Claforan

IOM: 100-02, 15, 50

✺ **J0699** Injection, cefiderocol, 10 mg ⓑ Ⓑ   K

J0701 Injection, cefepime hydrochloride (baxter), not therapeutically equivalent to maxipime, 500 mg ⓑ Ⓑ   N

✺ **J0702** Injection, betamethasone acetate 3 mg and betamethasone sodium phosphate 3 mg ⓑ Ⓑ Qp Qh   N1 N

Other: Betameth, Celestone Soluspan, Selestoject

IOM: 100-02, 15, 50

Coding Clinic: 2024, Q3, P24; 2018, Q4, P6

J0703 Injection, cefepime hydrochloride (b braun), not therapeutically equivalent to maxipime, 500 mg ⓑ Ⓑ   N

✳ **J0706** Injection, caffeine citrate, 5 mg ⓑ Ⓑ Qp Qh   N1 N

Other: Cafcit, Cipro IV, Ciprofloxacin

✺ **J0710** Injection, cephapirin sodium, up to 1 gm ⓑ Ⓑ Qp Qh   E2

Other: Cefadyl

IOM: 100-02, 15, 50

✳ **J0712** Injection, ceftaroline fosamil, 10 mg ⓑ Ⓑ Qp Qh   K2 K

Other: Teflaro

Coding Clinic: 2012, Q1, P9

✺ **J0713** Injection, ceftazidime, per 500 mg ⓑ Ⓑ Qp Qh   N1 N

Other: Fortaz, Tazicef

IOM: 100-02, 15, 50

✳ **J0714** Injection, ceftazidime and avibactam, 0.5 g/0.125 g ⓑ Ⓑ Qp Qh   K2 K

✺ **J0715** Injection, ceftizoxime sodium, per 500 mg ⓑ Ⓑ Qp Qh   N1 E2

IOM: 100-02, 15, 50

✳ **J0716** Injection, centruroides immune F(ab)2, up to 120 milligrams ⓑ Ⓑ Qp Qh   K2 K

Other: Anascorp

✳ **J0717** Injection, certolizumab pegol, 1 mg (Code may be used for Medicare when drug administered under the direct supervision of a physician, not for use when drug is self-administered) ⓑ Ⓑ Qp Qh   K2 K

Other: Cimzia

✺ **J0720** Injection, chloramphenicol sodium succinate, up to 1 gm ⓑ Ⓑ Qp Qh   N1 N

Other: Chloromycetin Sodium Succinate

IOM: 100-02, 15, 50

✺ **J0725** Injection, chorionic gonadotropin, per 1,000 USP units ⓑ Ⓑ Qp Qh   N1 N

Other: A.P.L., Chorex-5, Chorex-10, Chorignon, Choron-10, Chorionic Gonadotropin, Choron 10, Corgonject-5, Follutein, Glukor, Gonic, Novarel, Pregnyl, Profasi HP

IOM: 100-02, 15, 50

✺ **J0735** Injection, clonidine hydrochloride (HCL), 1 mg ⓑ Ⓑ Qp Qh   N1 N

Other: Duraclon

IOM: 100-02, 15, 50

J0736 Injection, clindamycin phosphate, 300 mg ⓑ Ⓑ   N

J0737 Injection, clindamycin phosphate (baxter), not therapeutically equivalent to J0736, 300 mg ⓑ Ⓑ   N

▶ **J0738** Injection, lenacapavir, 1 mg, FDA approved prescription, only for use as HIV pre-exposure prophylaxis (not for use as treatment for HIV)   K

J0739 Injection, cabotegravir, 1 mg ⓑ Ⓑ   K

✺ **J0740** Injection, cidofovir, 375 mg ⓑ Ⓑ Qp Qh   K2 K

Other: Vistide

IOM: 100-02, 15, 50

✺ **J0741** Injection, cabotegravir and rilpivirine, 2mg/3mg ⓑ Ⓑ   K2 K

✺ **J0742** Injection, imipenem 4 mg, cilastatin 4 mg and relebactam 2 mg ⓑ Ⓑ   K2 K

✺ **J0743** Injection, cilastatin sodium; imipenem, per 250 mg ⓑ Ⓑ Qp Qh   N1 N

Other: Primaxin

IOM: 100-02, 15, 50

▶ New   ⤺ Revised   ✓ Reinstated   ~~deleted~~ Deleted   ⊘ Not covered or valid by Medicare   ⦿ Special coverage instructions   ✳ Carrier discretion   ⓑ Bill Part B MAC   Ⓑ Bill DME MAC

DRUGS OTHER THAN CHEMOTHERAPY DRUGS

Code	Description	Indicators
✱ J0744	Injection, ciprofloxacin for intravenous infusion, 200 mg ⓑ Ⓑ Qp Qh	N1 N
⊛ J0745	Injection, codeine phosphate, per 30 mg ⓑ Ⓑ Qp Qh	N1 N
	IOM: 100-02, 15, 50	
J0750	Emtricitabine 200mg and tenofovir disoproxil fumarate 300mg, oral, FDA approved prescription, only for use as HIV pre-exposure prophylaxis (not for use as treatment of HIV) ⓑ Ⓑ	K
J0751	Emtricitabine 200mg and tenofovir alafenamide 25mg, oral, FDA approved prescription, only for use as HIV pre-exposure prophylaxis (not for use as treatment of HIV) ⓑ Ⓑ	K
▶ J0752	Oral, lenacapavir, 300 mg, FDA approved prescription, only for use as HIV pre-exposure prophylaxis (not for use as treatment for HIV)	K
▶ J0759	Injection, clevidipine butyrate, 1 mg	K
J0770	Injection, colistimethate sodium, up to 150 mg ⓑ Ⓑ Qp Qh	N1 N
	Other: Coly-Mycin M	
	IOM: 100-02, 15, 50	
✱ J0775	Injection, collagenase, clostridium histolyticum, 0.01 mg ⓑ Ⓑ Qp Qh	K2 K
	Other: Xiaflex	
	Coding Clinic: 2011, Q1, P7	
⊛ J0780	Injection, prochlorperazine, up to 10 mg ⓑ Ⓑ Qp Qh	N1 N
	Other: Compa-Z, Compazine, Cotranzine, Ultrazine-10	
	IOM: 100-02, 15, 50	
⊛ J0791	Injection, crizanlizumab-tmca, 5 mg ⓑ Ⓑ	K2 K
⊛ J0795	Injection, corticorelin ovine triflutate, 1 mcg ⓑ Ⓑ Qp Qh	K2 E2
	Other: Acthrel	
	IOM: 100-02, 15, 50	
J0799	FDA approved prescription drug, only for use as HIV pre-exposure prophylaxis (not for use as treatment of HIV), not otherwise classified ⓑ Ⓑ	A
⊛ J0801	Injection, corticotropin (acthar gel), up to 40 units ⓑ Ⓑ	K2 N
⊛ J0802	Injection, corticotropin (ani), up to 40 units ⓑ Ⓑ	K2 N
✱ J0834	Injection, cosyntropin, 0.25 mg ⓑ Ⓑ Qp Qh	N1 N
✱ J0840	Injection, crotalidae polyvalent immune fab (ovine), up to 1 gram ⓑ Ⓑ Qp Qh	K2 K
	Other: Crofab	
	Coding Clinic: 2012, Q1, P9	
✱ J0841	Injection, crotalidae immune f(ab')2 (equine), 120 mg ⓑ Ⓑ	K
	Other: Anavip	
⊛ J0850	Injection, cytomegalovirus immune globulin intravenous (human), per vial ⓑ Ⓑ Qp Qh	K2 K
	Prophylaxis to prevent cytomegalovirus disease associated with transplantation of kidney, lung, liver, pancreas, and heart.	
	Other: Cytogam	
	IOM: 100-02, 15, 50	
▶ J0870	Injection, imetelstat, 1 mg	K
J0872	Injection, daptomycin (xellia), unrefrigerated, not therapeutically equivalent to J0878 or J0873, 1 mg ⓑ Ⓑ	K
J0873	Injection, daptomycin (xellia), not therapeutically equivalent to J0878 or J0872, 1 mg ⓑ Ⓑ	K
J0874	Injection, daptomycin (baxter), not therapeutically equivalent to J0878, 1 mg ⓑ Ⓑ	E2
✱ J0875	Injection, dalbavancin, 5 mg ⓑ Ⓑ Qp Qh	K2 K
	Other: Dalvance	
J0877	Injection, daptomycin (hospira), not therapeutically equivalent to J0878, 1 mg ⓑ Ⓑ Qp Qh	N
✱ J0878	Injection, daptomycin, 1 mg ⓑ Ⓑ Qp Qh	K2 N
	Other: Cubicin	
J0879	Injection, difelikefalin, 0.1 mcg, (for ESRD on dialysis) ⓑ Qp Qh	K2 K
⊛ J0881	Injection, darbepoetin alfa, 1 mcg (non-ESRD use) ⓑ Ⓑ Qp Qh	K2 K
	Other: Aranesp	
⊛ J0882	Injection, darbepoetin alfa, 1 mcg (for ESRD on dialysis) ⓑ Ⓑ Qp Qh	K2 K
	Other: Aranesp	
	IOM: 100-02, 6, 10; 100-04, 4, 240	
⊛ J0883	Injection, argatroban, 1 mg (for non-ESRD use) ⓑ Ⓑ Qp Qh	K2 K
	IOM: 100-02, 15, 50	
⊛ J0884	Injection, argatroban, 1 mg (for ESRD on dialysis) ⓑ Ⓑ Qp Qh	K2 K
	IOM: 100-02, 15, 50	
⊛ J0885	Injection, epoetin alfa, (for non-ESRD use), 1000 units ⓑ Ⓑ Qp Qh	K2 N
	Other: Epogen, Procrit	
	IOM: 100-02, 15, 50	
	Coding Clinic: 2006, Q2, P5	

🝉 MIPS Qp Quantity Physician Qh Quantity Hospital ♀ Female only
♂ Male only   Ⓐ Age   ♿ DMEPOS   A2-Z3 ASC Payment Indicator   A-Y ASC Status Indicator   Coding Clinic

2026 HCPCS LEVEL II NATIONAL CODES

✺ **J0887**	Injection, epoetin beta, 1 mcg, (for ESRD on dialysis) ⓑ Ⓑ Qp Qh N1 N
	Other: Mircera
✺ **J0888**	Injection, epoetin beta, 1 mcg, (for non-ESRD use) ⓑ Ⓑ Qp Qh K2 K
	Other: Mircera
J0889	Daprodustat, oral, 1 mg, (for ESRD on dialysis) ⓑ Ⓑ Qp Qh E2
✱ **J0890**	Injection, peginesatide, 0.1 mg (for ESRD on dialysis) ⓑ Ⓑ Qp Qh E1
	Other: Omontys
J0891	Injection, argatroban (accord), not therapeutically equivalent to J0883, 1 mg (for non-ESRD use) ⓑ Ⓑ Qp Qh K2 N
J0892	Injection, argatroban (accord), not therapeutically equivalent to J0884, 1 mg (for ESRD on dialysis) ⓑ Ⓑ Qp Qh K2 K
J0893	Injection, decitabine (sun pharma), not therapeutically equivalent to J0894, 1 mg ⓑ Ⓑ Qp Qh N
✱ **J0894**	Injection, decitabine, 1 mg ⓑ Ⓑ Qp Qh K2 N
	Indicated for treatment of myelodysplastic syndromes (MDS)
	Other: Dacogen
✺ **J0895**	Injection, deferoxamine mesylate, 500 mg ⓑ Ⓑ Qp Qh N1 N
	Other: Desferal, Desferal mesylate
	IOM: 100-02, 15, 50,
	Cross Reference Q0087
✺ **J0896**	Injection, luspatercept-aamt, 0.25 mg ⓑ Ⓑ K2 K
✱ **J0897**	Injection, denosumab, 1 mg ⓑ Ⓑ Qp Qh K2 K
	Other: Prolia, Xgeva
	Coding Clinic: 2016, Q1, P5; 2012, Q1, P9
J0898	Injection, argatroban (auromedics), not therapeutically equivalent to J0883, 1 mg (for non-ESRD use) ⓑ Ⓑ K2 K
J0899	Injection, argatroban (auromedics), not therapeutically equivalent to J0884, 1 mg (for ESRD on dialysis) ⓑ Ⓑ K2 N
▶ **J0901**	Vadadustat, oral, 1 mg (for ESRD on dialysis) B
J0911	Instillation, taurolidine 1.35 mg and heparin sodium 100 units (central venous catheter lock for adult patients receiving chronic hemodialysis) G
✺ **J0945**	Injection, brompheniramine maleate, per 10 mg ⓑ Ⓑ Qp Qh N1 E2
	Other: Codimal-A, Cophene-B, Dehist, Histaject, Nasahist B, ND Stat, Oraminic II, Sinusol-B
	IOM: 100-02, 15, 50
✺ **J1000**	Injection, depo-estradiol cypionate, up to 5 mg ⓑ Ⓑ Qp Qh N1 N
	Other: DepGynogen, Depogen, Dura-Estrin, Estra-D, Estro-Cyp, Estroject LA, Estronol-LA
	IOM: 100-02, 15, 50
J1010	Injection, methylprednisolone acetate, 1 mg ⓑ Ⓑ K
✺ **J1040**	Injection, methylprednisolone acetate, 80 mg ⓑ Ⓑ Qp Qh N1 N
	Other: DepMedalone, Depoject, Depo-Medrol, Depopred, D-Med 80, Duralone, Medralone, M-Prednisol, Rep-Pred
	IOM: 100-02, 15, 50
	Coding Clinic: 2018, Q4, P6
✱ **J1050**	Injection, medroxyprogesterone acetate, 1 mg ⓑ Ⓑ Qp Qh N1 N
	Other: Depo-Provera Contraceptive
✺ **J1071**	Injection, testosterone cypionate, 1 mg Qp Qh N1 N
	Other: Andro-Cyp, Andro/Fem, Andronaq-LA, Andronate, De-Comberol, DepAndro, DepAndrogyn, Depotest, Depo-Testadiol, Depo-Testosterone, Depotestrogen, Duratest, Duratestrin, Menoject LA, Testa-C, Testadiate-Depo, Testaject-LA, Test-Estro Cypionates, Testoject-LA
	Coding Clinic: 2015, Q2, P7
▶ **J1072**	Injection, testosterone cypionate (azmiro), 1 mg N1 N
~~J1094~~	~~Injection, dexamethasone acetate, 1 mg~~
✺ **J1095**	Injection, dexamethasone 9% ⓑ N
✱ **J1096**	Dexamethasone, lacrimal ophthalmic insert, 0.1 mg ⓑ K2 K1
✱ **J1097**	Phenylephrine 10.16 mg/ml and ketorolac 2.88 mg/ml ophthalmic irrigation solution, 1 ml ⓑ K2 K1
✺ **J1100**	Injection, dexamethasone sodium phosphate, 1 mg ⓑ Ⓑ Qp Qh N1 N
	Other: Dalalone, Decadron Phosphate, Decaject, Dexacen-4, Dexone, Hexadrol Phosphate, Solurex
	IOM: 100-02, 15, 50
J1105	Dexmedetomidine, oral, 1 mcg ⓑ Ⓑ K

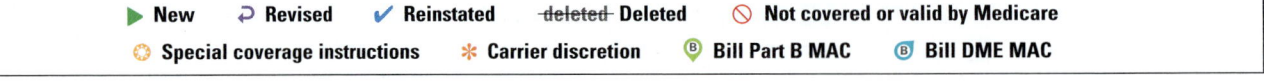

▶ New   ⟳ Revised   ✓ Reinstated   ~~deleted~~ Deleted   ⊘ Not covered or valid by Medicare
✺ Special coverage instructions   ✱ Carrier discretion   ⓑ Bill Part B MAC   Ⓑ Bill DME MAC

DRUGS OTHER THAN CHEMOTHERAPY DRUGS

- ✺ **J1110** Injection, dihydroergotamine mesylate, per 1 mg K2 N
  Other: D.H.E. 45
  IOM: 100-02, 15, 50

- ✺ **J1120** Injection, acetazolamide sodium, up to 500 mg N1 N
  Other: Diamox
  IOM: 100-02, 15, 50

- ✱ **J1130** Injection, diclofenac sodium, 0.5 mg K2 N
  Coding Clinic: 2017, Q1, P9

- ✺ **J1160** Injection, digoxin, up to 0.5 mg N1 N
  Other: Lanoxin
  IOM: 100-02, 15, 50

- ✺ **J1162** Injection, digoxin immune Fab (ovine), per vial K2 K
  Other: DigiFab
  IOM: 100-02, 15, 50

- ▶ ✺ **J1163** Injection, diltiazem hydrochloride, 0.5 mg N1 N

- ✺ **J1165** Injection, phenytoin sodium, per 50 mg N1 N
  Other: Dilantin
  IOM: 100-02, 15, 50

- ✺ **J1171** Injection, hydromorphone, 0.1 mg K2 K

- ✺ **J1180** Injection, dyphylline, up to 500 mg E2
  Other: Dilor, Lufyllin
  IOM: 100-02, 15, 50

- ✺ **J1190** Injection, dexrazoxane hydrochloride, per 250 mg K2 K
  Other: Totect, Zinecard
  IOM: 100-02, 15, 50

- ✺ **J1200** Injection, diphenhydramine HCL, up to 50 mg N1 N
  Other: Bena-D, Benadryl, Benahist, Ben-Allergin, Benoject, Chlorothiazide sodium, Dihydrex, Diphenacen-50, Hyrexin-50, Nordryl, Wehdryl
  IOM: 100-02, 15, 50

- ✺ **J1201** Injection, cetirizine hydrochloride, 0.5 mg K2 K

- **J1202** Miglustat, oral, 65 mg E2

- **J1203** Injection, cipaglucosidase alfa-atga, 5 mg N

- ✺ **J1205** Injection, chlorothiazide sodium, per 500 mg N1 N
  Other: Diuril
  IOM: 100-02, 15, 50

- ✺ **J1212** Injection, DMSO, dimethyl sulfoxide, 50%, 50 ml K2 K
  Other: Rimso-50
  IOM: 100-02, 15, 50; 100-03, 4, 230.12

- ✺ **J1230** Injection, methadone HCL, up to 10 mg N1 N
  Other: Dolophine HCl
  MCM: 2049
  IOM: 100-02, 15, 50

- ✺ **J1240** Injection, dimenhydrinate, up to 50 mg N1 N
  Other: Dinate, Dommanate, Dramamine, Dramanate, Dramilin, Dramocen, Dramoject, Dymenate, Hydrate, Marmine, Wehamine
  IOM: 100-02, 15, 50

- ✺ **J1245** Injection, dipyridamole, per 10 mg N1 N
  Other: Persantine
  IOM: 100-04, 15, 50; 100-04, 12, 30.6

- ✺ **J1250** Injection, dobutamine HCL, per 250 mg N1 N
  Other: Dobutrex
  IOM: 100-02, 15, 50

- ✺ **J1260** Injection, dolasetron mesylate, 10 mg N1 N
  Other: Anzemet
  IOM: 100-02, 15, 50

- ✱ **J1265** Injection, dopamine HCL, 40 mg N1 N

- ✱ **J1267** Injection, doripenem, 10 mg N1 E2
  Other: Donbax, Doribax

- ✱ **J1270** Injection, doxercalciferol, 1 mcg N1 N
  Other: Hectorol

- ▶ **J1271** Injection, doxycycline hyclate, 1 mg N1 N

- ✱ **J1290** Injection, ecallantide, 1 mg K2 K
  Other: Kalbitor
  Coding Clinic: 2011, Q1, P7

- ▶ **J1299** Injection, eculizumab, 2 mg K2 K

- ~~J1300~~ ~~Injection, eculizumab, 10 mg~~

- ✱ **J1301** Injection, edaravone, 1 mg K
  Other: Radicava

- **J1302** Injection, sutimlimab-jome, 10 mg K2 G

- ✱ **J1303** Injection, ravulizumab-cwvz, 10 mg K2 K

J1304	Injection, tofersen, 1 mg ⓑ ⓑ	G
✱ J1305	Injection, evinacumab-dgnb, 5mg ⓑ ⓑ	K2 K
J1306	Injection, inclisiran, 1 mg ⓑ ⓑ	K2 G
▶ J1307	Injection, crovalimab-akkz, 10 mg	K
▶ J1308	Injection, famotidine, 0.25 mg	N
⊛ J1320	Injection, amitriptyline HCL, up to 20 mg ⓑ ⓑ Qp Qh	N1 N
	Other: Elavil, Enovil	
	IOM: 100-02, 15, 50	
✱ J1322	Injection, elosulfase alfa, 1 mg ⓑ ⓑ Qp Qh	K2 K
J1323	Injection, elranatamab-bcmm, 1 mg ⓑ ⓑ	G
✱ J1324	Injection, enfuvirtide, 1 mg ⓑ ⓑ Qp Qh	E2
⊛ J1325	Injection, epoprostenol, 0.5 mg ⓑ ⓑ Qp Qh	N1 N
	Other: Flolan, Veletri	
	IOM: 100-02, 15, 50	
▶ J1326	Injection, zolbetuximab-clzb, 2 mg	G
⊛ J1327	Injection, eptifibatide, 5 mg ⓑ ⓑ Qp Qh	K2 N
	Other: Integrilin	
	IOM: 100-02, 15, 50	
⊛ J1330	Injection, ergonovine maleate, up to 0.2 mg ⓑ ⓑ Qp Qh	N1 E2
	Benefit limited to obstetrical diagnosis	
	IOM: 100-02, 15, 50	
✱ J1335	Injection, ertapenem sodium, 500 mg ⓑ ⓑ Qp Qh	N1 N
	Other: Invanz	
⊛ J1364	Injection, erythromycin lactobionate, per 500 mg ⓑ ⓑ Qp Qh	K2 N
	IOM: 100-02, 15, 50	
▶ J1370	Injection, esomeprazole sodium, 1 mg	N1 N
⊛ J1380	Injection, estradiol valerate, up to 10 mg ⓑ ⓑ Qp Qh	N1 N
	Other: Delestrogen, Dioval, Duragen, Estra-L, Gynogen L.A., L.A.E. 20, Valergen	
	IOM: 100-02, 15, 50	
	Coding Clinic: 2011, Q1, P8	
⊛ J1410	Injection, estrogen conjugated, per 25 mg ⓑ ⓑ Qp Qh	K2 K
	Other: Premarin	
	IOM: 100-02, 15, 50	
J1411	Injection, etranacogene dezaparvovec-drlb, per therapeutic dose ⓑ ⓑ	G
J1412	Injection, valoctocogene roxaparvovec-rvox, per ml, containing nominal 2×10^{13} vector genomes ⓑ ⓑ	G
J1413	Injection, delandistrogene moxeparvovec-rokl, per therapeutic dose ⓑ ⓑ	G
▶ J1414	Injection, fidanacogene elaparvovec-dzkt	E1
	Other: Beqvez	
✱ J1426	Injection, casimersen, 10 mg ⓑ ⓑ	K2 E2
✱ J1427	Injection, viltolarsen, 10 mg ⓑ ⓑ	K2 N
✱ J1428	Injection, eteplirsen, 10 mg ⓑ ⓑ	K2 E2
✱ J1429	Injection, golodirsen, 10 mg ⓑ ⓑ	K2 N
⊛ J1430	Injection, ethanolamine oleate, 100 mg ⓑ ⓑ Qp Qh	K2 K
	Other: Ethamolin	
	IOM: 100-02, 15, 50	
J1434	Injection, fosaprepitant (focinvez), 1 mg ⓑ	G
⊛ J1435	Injection, estrone, per 1 mg ⓑ ⓑ Qp Qh	E2
	Other: Estronol, Kestrone 5, Theelin Aqueous	
	IOM: 100-02, 15, 50	
⊛ J1436	Injection, etidronate disodium, per 300 mg ⓑ ⓑ Qp Qh	E1
	Other: Didronel	
	IOM: 100-02, 15, 50	
⊛ J1437	Injection, ferric derisomaltose, 10 mg ⓑ ⓑ	K2 K
⊛ J1438	Injection, etanercept, 25 mg (Code may be used for Medicare when drug administered under the direct supervision of a physician, not for use when drug is self-administered) ⓑ ⓑ Qp Qh	K2 K
	Other: Enbrel	
	IOM: 100-02, 15, 50	
✱ J1439	Injection, ferric carboxymaltose, 1 mg ⓑ ⓑ Qp Qh	K2 K
	Other: Injectafer	
J1440	Fecal microbiota, live - jslm, 1 ml ⓑ	G
⊛ J1442	Injection, filgrastim (G-CSF), excludes biosimilars, 1 mcg ⓑ ⓑ Qp Qh	K2 K
	Other: Neupogen	
✱ J1443	Injection, ferric pyrophosphate citrate solution (triferic), 0.1 mg of iron ⓑ Qp Qh	N1 E2
⊛ J1444	Injection, ferric pyrophosphate citrate powder, 0.1 mg of iron ⓑ ⓑ	E2
⊛ J1445	Injection, ferric pyrophosphate citrate solution (triferic avnu), 0.1 mg of iron ⓑ	K2 E2
⊛ J1447	Injection, TBO-filgrastim, 1 mcg ⓑ ⓑ Qp Qh	K2 K
	Other: GRANIX	
	IOM: 100-02, 15, 50	

▶ New   ⟲ Revised   ✓ Reinstated   ~~deleted~~ Deleted   ⊘ Not covered or valid by Medicare
⊛ Special coverage instructions   ✱ Carrier discretion   ⓑ Bill Part B MAC   ⓑ Bill DME MAC

DRUGS OTHER THAN CHEMOTHERAPY DRUGS

⊛ J1448	Injection, trilaciclib, 1 mg ⓑ ⓑ	K2 K
J1449	Injection, eflapegrastim-xnst, 0.1 mg ⓑ ⓑ	G
⊛ J1450	Injection, fluconazole, 200 mg ⓑ ⓑ Qp Qh	N1 N

Other: Diflucan

IOM: 100-02, 15, 50

⊛ J1451	Injection, fomepizole, 15 mg ⓑ ⓑ Qp Qh	K2 K

IOM: 100-02, 15, 50

⊛ J1452	Injection, fomivirsen sodium, intraocular, 1.65 mg ⓑ ⓑ Qp Qh	E2

IOM: 100-02, 15, 50

✱ J1453	Injection, fosaprepitant, 1 mg ⓑ ⓑ Qp Qh	K2 N

Prevents chemotherapy-induced nausea and vomiting

Other: Emend

✱ J1454	Injection, fosnetupitant 235 mg and palonosetron 0.25 mg ⓑ ⓑ	K

Other: Akynzeo and Aloxi

⊛ J1455	Injection, foscarnet sodium, per 1000 mg ⓑ ⓑ Qp Qh	K2 K

Other: Foscavir

IOM: 100-02, 15, 50

J1456	Injection, fosaprepitant (teva), not therapeutically equivalent to J1453, 1 mg ⓑ ⓑ	K
✱ J1457	Injection, gallium nitrate, 1 mg ⓑ ⓑ Qp Qh	E2
✱ J1458	Injection, galsulfase, 1 mg ⓑ ⓑ Qp Qh	K2 N

Other: Naglazyme

✱ J1459	Injection, immune globulin (Privigen), intravenous, non-lyophilized (e.g., liquid), 500 mg ⓑ ⓑ Qp Qh	K2 K
⊛ J1460	Injection, gamma globulin, intramuscular, 1 cc ⓑ ⓑ Qp Qh	K2 K

Other: Gammar, GamaSTAN

IOM: 100-02, 15, 50

Coding Clinic: 2011, Q1, P8

J1551	Injection, immune globulin (cutaquig), 100 mg ⓑ ⓑ	K2 N
▶ J1552	Injection, (alyglo), 500 mg	K
✱ J1554	Injection, immune globulin (asceniv), 500 mg ⓑ	K2 K
✱ J1555	Injection, immune globulin (cuvitru), 100 mg ⓑ ⓑ	K2 K
✱ J1556	Injection, immune globulin (Bivigam), 500 mg ⓑ ⓑ Qp Qh	K2 N
✱ J1557	Injection, immune globulin, (gammaplex), intravenous, non-lyophilized (e.g., liquid), 500 mg ⓑ ⓑ Qp Qh	K2 K

Coding Clinic: 2012, Q1, P9

✱ J1558	Injection, immune globulin (xembify), 100 mg ⓑ ⓑ	K2 K
✱ J1559	Injection, immune globulin (hizentra), 100 mg ⓑ ⓑ Qp Qh	K2 K

Coding Clinic: 2011, Q1, P6

⊛ J1560	Injection, gamma globulin, intramuscular, over 10 cc ⓑ ⓑ Qp Qh	K2 K

Other: Gammar, GamaSTAN

IOM: 100-02, 15, 50

⊛ J1561	Injection, immune globulin, (Gamunex-C/Gammaked), non-lyophilized (e.g., liquid), 500 mg ⓑ ⓑ Qp Qh	K2 K

IOM: 100-02, 15, 50

Coding Clinic: 2012, Q1, P9

✱ J1562	Injection, immune globulin (Vivaglobin), 100 mg ⓑ ⓑ Qp Qh	E2
⊛ J1566	Injection, immune globulin, intravenous, lyophilized (e.g., powder), not otherwise specified, 500 mg ⓑ ⓑ Qp Qh	K2 K

Other: Carimune, Gammagard S/D, Polygam

IOM: 100-02, 15, 50

✱ J1568	Injection, immune globulin, (Octagam), intravenous, non-lyophilized (e.g., liquid), 500 mg ⓑ ⓑ Qp Qh	K2 K
⊛ J1569	Injection, immune globulin, (Gammagard Liquid), non-lyophilized (e.g., liquid), 500 mg ⓑ ⓑ Qp Qh	K2 K

IOM: 100-02, 15, 50

⊛ J1570	Injection, ganciclovir sodium, 500 mg ⓑ ⓑ Qp Qh	N1 N

Other: Cytovene

IOM: 100-02, 15, 50

⊛ J1571	Injection, hepatitis B immune globulin (HepaGam B), intramuscular, 0.5 ml ⓑ ⓑ Qp Qh	K2 K

IOM: 100-02, 15, 50

Coding Clinic: 2008, Q3, P7-8

⊛ J1572	Injection, immune globulin, (flebogamma/flebogamma DIF) intravenous, non-lyophilized (e.g., liquid), 500 mg ⓑ ⓑ Qp Qh	K2 K

IOM: 100-02, 15, 50

✱ J1573	Injection, hepatitis B immune globulin (HepaGam B), intravenous, 0.5 ml ⓑ ⓑ Qp Qh	K2 K

Coding Clinic: 2008, Q3, P8

MIPS | Qp Quantity Physician | Qh Quantity Hospital | ♀ Female only
♂ Male only | Ⓐ Age | ♿ DMEPOS | A2-Z3 ASC Payment Indicator | A-Y ASC Status Indicator | Coding Clinic

J1574	Injection, ganciclovir sodium (exela), not therapeutically equivalent to J1570, 500 mg	N
* J1575	Injection, immune globulin/hyaluronidase (HYQVIA), 100 mg immunoglobulin	K2 K
J1576	Injection, immune globulin (panzyga), intravenous, non-lyophilized (e.g., liquid), 500 mg	
J1580	Injection, Garamycin, gentamicin, up to 80 mg	N1 N
	Other: Gentamicin Sulfate, Jenamicin	
	IOM: 100-02, 15, 50	
J1595	Injection, glatiramer acetate, 20 mg	K2 K
	Other: Copaxone	
	IOM: 100-02, 15, 50	
J1596	Injection, glycopyrrolate, 0.1 mg	
J1597	Injection, glycopyrrolate (glyrx-pf), 0.1 mg	
J1598	Injection, glycopyrrolate (fresenius kabi), not therapeutically equivalent to J1596, 0.1 mg	
* J1599	Injection, immune globulin, intravenous, non-lyophilized (e.g., liquid), not otherwise specified, 500 mg	N1 N
	Coding Clinic: 2011, P1, Q6	
J1600	Injection, gold sodium thiomalate, up to 50 mg	E2
	Other: Myochrysine	
	IOM: 100-02, 15, 50	
* J1602	Injection, golimumab, 1 mg for intravenous use	K2 K
	Other: Simponi Aria	
J1610	Injection, glucagon hydrochloride, per 1 mg	K2 K
	Other: GlucaGen, Glucagon Emergency	
	IOM: 100-02, 15, 50	
J1611	Injection, glucagon hydrochloride (fresenius kabi), not therapeutically equivalent to J1610, per 1 mg	K2 K
▶ J1612	Injection, glucagon (gvoke), 0.01 mg	K
J1620	Injection, gonadorelin hydrochloride, per 100 mcg	E2
	Other: Factrel	
	IOM: 100-02, 15, 50	
J1626	Injection, granisetron hydrochloride, 100 mcg	N1 N
	Other: Kytril	
	IOM: 100-02, 15, 50	
* J1627	Injection, granisetron, extended-release, 0.1 mg	K2 K
* J1628	Injection, guselkumab, 1 mg	K
	Other: Tremfya	
J1630	Injection, haloperidol, up to 5 mg	N1 N
	Other: Haldol, Haloperidol Lactate	
	IOM: 100-02, 15, 50	
J1631	Injection, haloperidol decanoate, per 50 mg	N1 N
	IOM: 100-02, 15, 50	
J1632	Injection, brexanolone, 1 mg	K2 N
J1640	Injection, hemin, 1 mg	K2 K
	Other: Panhematin	
	IOM: 100-02, 15, 50	
J1642	Injection, heparin sodium (heparin lock flush), per 10 units	N1 N
	Other: Hep-Lock U/P, Vasceze	
	IOM: 100-02, 15, 50	
J1643	Injection, heparin sodium (pfizer), not therapeutically equivalent to J1644, per 1000 units	N
J1644	Injection, heparin sodium, per 1000 units	N1 N
	Other: Heparin Sodium (Porcine), Liquaemin Sodium	
	IOM: 100-02, 15, 50	
J1645	Injection, dalteparin sodium, per 2500 IU	N1 N
	Other: Fragmin	
	IOM: 100-02, 15, 50	
* J1650	Injection, enoxaparin sodium, 10 mg	N1 N
	Other: Lovenox	
J1652	Injection, fondaparinux sodium, 0.5 mg	N1 N
	Other: Arixtra	
	IOM: 100-02, 15, 50	
* J1655	Injection, tinzaparin sodium, 1000 IU	N1 E2
	Other: Innohep	
J1670	Injection, tetanus immune globulin, human, up to 250 units	K2 K
	Indicated for transient protection against tetanus post-exposure to tetanus (Z23).	
	Other: Hyper-Tet	
	IOM: 100-02, 15, 50	
J1675	Injection, histrelin acetate, 10 mcg	B
	IOM: 100-02, 15, 50	

▶ New ⮂ Revised ✔ Reinstated ~~deleted~~ Deleted ⊘ Not covered or valid by Medicare ⊛ Special coverage instructions * Carrier discretion Ⓑ Bill Part B MAC Ⓑ Bill DME MAC

DRUGS OTHER THAN CHEMOTHERAPY DRUGS

✺ J1700	Injection, hydrocortisone acetate, up to 25 mg ⓑ Ⓑ Qp Qh	N1 N
	Other: Hydrocortone Acetate	
	IOM: 100-02, 15, 50	
✺ J1710	Injection, hydrocortisone sodium phosphate, up to 50 mg ⓑ Ⓑ Qp Qh	N1 E2
	Other: A-hydroCort, Hydrocortone phosphate, Solu-Cortef	
	IOM: 100-02, 15, 50	
✺ J1720	Injection, hydrocortisone sodium succinate, up to 100 mg ⓑ Ⓑ Qp Qh	N1 N
	Other: A-HydroCort, Solu-Cortef	
	IOM: 100-02, 15, 50	
✱ J1726	Injection, hydroxyprogesterone caproate (makena), 10 mg ⓑ Ⓑ	K2 K
✱ J1729	Injection, hydroxyprogesterone caproate, not otherwise specified, 10 mg ⓑ Ⓑ	N1 N
✺ J1730	Injection, diazoxide, up to 300 mg ⓑ Ⓑ Qp Qh	E2
	Other: Hyperstat	
	IOM: 100-02, 15, 50	
✱ J1738	Injection, meloxicam, 1 mg ⓑ Ⓑ	K2 N
✱ J1740	Injection, ibandronate sodium, 1 mg ⓑ Ⓑ Qp Qh	K2 N
	Other: Boniva	
✱ J1741	Injection, ibuprofen, 100 mg ⓑ Ⓑ Qp Qh	N1 N
	Other: Caldolor	
✺ J1742	Injection, ibutilide fumarate, 1 mg ⓑ Ⓑ Qp Qh	K2 K
	Other: Corvert	
	IOM: 100-02, 15, 50	
✱ J1743	Injection, idursulfase, 1 mg ⓑ Ⓑ Qp Qh	K2 K
	Other: Elaprase	
✱ J1744	Injection, icatibant, 1 mg ⓑ Ⓑ Qp Qh	K2 K
	Other: Firazyr	
✺ J1745	Injection, infliximab, excludes biosimilar, 10 mg ⓑ Ⓑ Qp Qh	K2 K
	Report total number of 10 mg increments administered	
	For biosimilar, Inflectra, report Q5102	
	Other: Remicade	
	IOM: 100-02, 15, 50	
✱ J1746	Injection, ibalizumab-uiyk, 10 mg ⓑ Ⓑ	K
	Other: Trogarzo	
J1747	Injection, spesolimab-sbzo, 1 mg ⓑ Ⓑ	G
J1748	Injection, infliximab-dyyb (zymfentra), 10 mg ⓑ Ⓑ	N1 N
J1749	Injection, iloprost, 0.1 mcg ⓑ Ⓑ	N1 E2
✺ J1750	Injection, iron dextran, 50 mg ⓑ Ⓑ Qp Qh	K2 K
	Other: Dexferrum, Imferon, Infed	
	IOM: 100-02, 15, 50	
✱ J1756	Injection, iron sucrose, 1 mg ⓑ Ⓑ Qp Qh	N1 N
	Other: Venofer	
✺ J1786	Injection, imiglucerase, 10 units ⓑ Ⓑ Qp Qh	K2 K
	Other: Cerezyme	
	IOM: 100-02, 15, 50	
	Coding Clinic: 2011, Q1, P8	
✺ J1790	Injection, droperidol, up to 5 mg ⓑ Ⓑ Qp Qh	N1 N
	Other: Inapsine	
	IOM: 100-02, 15, 50	
✺ J1800	Injection, propranolol HCL, up to 1 mg ⓑ Ⓑ Qp Qh	N1 N
	Other: Inderal	
	IOM: 100-02, 15, 50	
J1805	Injection, esmolol hydrochloride, 10 mg ⓑ Ⓑ	N
J1806	Injection, esmolol hydrochloride (wg critical care), not therapeutically equivalent to J1805, 10 mg ⓑ Ⓑ	N
▶ J1807	Injection, ethacrynate sodium, 1 mg	K
▶ J1808	Folic acid, 0.1 mg	N
▶ J1809	Injection, fosdenopterin, 0.1 mg	K
~~J1810~~	~~Injection, droperidol and fentanyl citrate, up to 2 ml ampule~~	
J1811	Insulin (fiasp) for administration through dme (i.e., insulin pump) per 50 units ⓑ Ⓑ	K
J1812	Insulin (fiasp), per 5 units ⓑ Ⓑ	N
J1813	Insulin (lyumjev) for administration through dme (i.e., insulin pump) per 50 units ⓑ Ⓑ	N
J1814	Insulin (lyumjev), per 5 units ⓑ Ⓑ	E2
✺ J1815	Injection, insulin, per 5 units ⓑ Ⓑ Qp Qh	N1 N
	Other: Humalog, Humulin, Lantus, Novolin, Novolog	
	IOM: 100-02, 15, 50; 100-03, 4, 280.14	
✱ J1817	Insulin for administration through DME (i.e., insulin pump) per 50 units ⓑ Ⓑ Qp Qh	N1 N
	Other: Apidra Solostar, Insulin Lispro, Humalog, Humulin, Novolin, Novolog	

	ⓑ MIPS	Qp Quantity Physician	Qh Quantity Hospital	♀ Female only
♂ Male only	Ⓐ Age	♿ DMEPOS	A2-Z3 ASC Payment Indicator	A-Y ASC Status Indicator	Coding Clinic

Code	Description	Status
✱ J1823	Injection, inebilizumab-cdon, 1 mg ⑧ ⑧	K2 K
✱ J1826	Injection, interferon beta-1a, 30 mcg ⑧ ⑧	K2 K
	Other: Avonex	
	Coding Clinic: 2011, Q2, P9; Q1, P8	
⊛ J1830	Injection, interferon beta-1b, 0.25 mg (Code may be used for Medicare when drug administered under the direct supervision of a physician, not for use when drug is self-administered) ⑧ ⑧ Qp Qh	K2 E2
	Other: Betaseron	
	IOM: 100-02, 15, 50	
✱ J1833	Injection, isavuconazonium, 1 mg ⑧ ⑧ Qp Qh	K2 K
▶ J1834	Injection, isoniazid, 1 mg	K
✱ J1835	Injection, itraconazole, 50 mg ⑧ ⑧ Qp Qh	E2
	Other: Sporanox	
J1836	Injection, metronidazole, 10 mg ⑧ ⑧	N
⊛ J1885	Injection, ketorolac tromethamine, per 15 mg ⑧ ⑧ Qp Qh	N1 K1
	Other: Toradol	
	IOM: 100-02, 15, 50	
~~J1890~~	~~Injection, cephalothin sodium, up to 1 gram~~	
J1920	Injection, labetalol hydrochloride, 5 mg ⑧ ⑧	N
J1921	Injection, labetalol hydrochloride (hikma), not therapeutically equivalent to J1920, 5 mg ⑧ ⑧	N
✱ J1930	Injection, lanreotide, 1 mg ⑧ ⑧ Qp Qh	K2 K
	Treats acromegaly and symptoms caused by neuroendocrine tumors	
	Other: Somatuline Depot	
✱ J1931	Injection, laronidase, 0.1 mg ⑧ ⑧ Qp Qh	K2 K
	Other: Aldurazyme	
J1932	Injection, lanreotide, (cipla), 1 mg ⑧ ⑧	K2 G
▶ J1938	Furosemide, 1 mg	N
J1939	Injection, bumetanide, 0.5 mg ⑧ ⑧	K
~~J1940~~	~~Injection, furosemide, up to 20 mg~~	
J1941	Injection, furosemide (furoscix), 20 mg ⑧ ⑧	E1
✱ J1943	Injection, aripiprazole lauroxil, (aristada initio) 1 mg ⑧ ⑧	K2 K
✱ J1944	Injection, aripiprazole lauroxil, (aristada), 1 mg ⑧ ⑧	K2 K
⊛ J1945	Injection, lepirudin, 50 mg ⑧ ⑧ Qp Qh	E2
	IOM: 100-02, 15, 50	
⊛ J1950	Injection, leuprolide acetate (for depot suspension), per 3.75 mg ⑧ ⑧ Qp Qh	K2 K
	Other: Lupron, Lupron Depot, Lupron Depot-Ped	
	IOM: 100-02, 15, 50	
	Coding Clinic: 2019, Q2, P11-12	
✱ J1951	Injection, leuprolide acetate for depot suspension (fensolvi), 0.25 mg ⑧ ⑧	K2 K
✱ J1952	Leuprolide injectable, camcevi, 1 mg ⑧ ⑧	K5 G
✱ J1953	Injection, levetiracetam, 10 mg ⑧ ⑧ Qp Qh	N1 N
	Other: Keppra	
↻ J1954	Injection, leuprolide acetate for depot suspension (lutrate depot), 7.5 mg ⑧ ⑧	G
⊛ J1955	Injection, levocarnitine, per 1 gm ⑧ ⑧ Qp Qh	B
	Other: Carnitor	
	IOM: 100-02, 15, 50	
⊛ J1956	Injection, levofloxacin, 250 mg ⑧ ⑧ Qp Qh	N1 N
	Other: Levaquin	
	IOM: 100-02, 15, 50	
⊛ J1960	Injection, levorphanol tartrate, up to 2 mg ⑧ ⑧ Qp Qh	N1 E2
	Other: Levo-Dromoran	
	MCM: 2049	
	IOM: 100-02, 15, 50	
↻ J1961	Injection, lenacapavir (only for use as HIV treatment), 1 mg ⑧ ⑧	G
⊛ J1980	Injection, hyoscyamine sulfate, up to 0.25 mg ⑧ ⑧ Qp Qh	N1 N
	Other: Levsin	
	IOM: 100-02, 15, 50	
⊛ J1990	Injection, chlordiazepoxide HCL, up to 100 mg ⑧ ⑧ Qp Qh	N1 E2
	Other: Librium	
	IOM: 100-02, 15, 50	
J2002	Injection, lidocaine hcl in 5% dextrose, 1 mg ⑧ ⑧ Qp Qh	K2 K
	Coding Clinic: 2024, Q4, P30	
J2003	Injection, lidocaine hydrochloride, 1 mg ⑧ ⑧ Qp Qh	N1 N

▶ New   ↻ Revised   ✓ Reinstated   ~~deleted~~ Deleted   ⊘ Not covered or valid by Medicare
⊛ Special coverage instructions   ✱ Carrier discretion   ⑧ Bill Part B MAC   ⑧ Bill DME MAC

DRUGS OTHER THAN CHEMOTHERAPY DRUGS

J2004	Injection, lidocaine hcl with epinephrine, 1 mg ⓑ Ⓑ Qp Qh	N1 N
	Coding Clinic: 2024, Q4, P30	
✺ J2010	Injection, lincomycin HCL, up to 300 mg ⓑ Ⓑ Qp Qh	N1 N
	Other: Lincocin	
	IOM: 100-02, 15, 50	
✱ J2020	Injection, linezolid, 200 mg ⓑ Ⓑ Qp Qh	N1 N
	Other: Zyvox	
J2021	Injection, linezolid (hospira), not therapeutically equivalent to J2020, 200 mg ⓑ Ⓑ	N
✺ J2060	Injection, lorazepam, 2 mg ⓑ Ⓑ Qp Qh	N1 N
	Other: Ativan	
	IOM: 100-02, 15, 50	
✱ J2062	Loxapine for inhalation, 1 mg ⓑ Ⓑ	E2
	Other: Adasuve	
~~J2150~~	~~Injection, mannitol, 25% in 50 ml~~	
▶ ✱ J2151	Injection, mannitol, 250 mg ⓑ Ⓑ Qp Qh	N1 N
✱ J2170	Injection, mecasermin, 1 mg ⓑ Ⓑ Qp Qh	N1 N
	Other: Increlex	
✺ J2175	Injection, meperidine hydrochloride, per 100 mg ⓑ Ⓑ Qp Qh	N1 N
	Other: Demerol	
	IOM: 100-02, 15, 50	
✺ J2180	Injection, meperidine and promethazine HCL, up to 50 mg ⓑ Ⓑ Qp Qh	N1 N
	Other: Mepergan	
	IOM: 100-02, 15, 50	
✱ J2182	Injection, mepolizumab, 1 mg ⓑ Ⓑ Qp Qh	K2 K
J2183	Injection, meropenem (wg critical care), not therapeutically equivalent to J2185, 100 mg ⓑ Ⓑ	K
J2184	Injection, meropenem (b. braun), not therapeutically equivalent to J2185, 100 mg ⓑ Ⓑ	N
✱ J2185	Injection, meropenem, 100 mg ⓑ Ⓑ Qp Qh	N1 N
	Other: Merrem	
✱ J2186	Inj., meropenem, vaborbactam ⓑ Ⓑ	K
	Other: Vabomere	
	Medicare Statute 1833(t)	
✺ J2210	Injection, methylergonovine maleate, up to 0.2 mg ⓑ Ⓑ Qp Qh	N1 N
	Benefit limited to obstetrical diagnoses for prevention and control of post-partum hemorrhage	
	Other: Methergine	
	IOM: 100-02, 15, 50	
✱ J2212	Injection, methylnaltrexone, 0.1 mg ⓑ Ⓑ Qp Qh	N1 N
	Other: Relistor	
✱ J2246	Injection, micafungin in sodium (baxter), not therapeutically equivalent to J2248, 1 mg ⓑ Ⓑ	K5 E2
✱ J2247	Injection, micafungin sodium (par pharm) not therapeutically equivalent to J2248, 1 mg ⓑ Ⓑ	N1 N
✱ J2248	Injection, micafungin sodium, 1 mg ⓑ Ⓑ Qp Qh	N1 N
	Other: Mycamine	
✱ J2249	Injection, remimazolam, 1 mg ⓑ Ⓑ	N1 N
✺ J2250	Injection, midazolam hydrochloride, per 1 mg ⓑ Ⓑ Qp Qh	N1 N
	Other: Versed	
	IOM: 100-02, 15, 50	
✺ J2251	Injection, midazolam in 0.9% sodium chloride, intravenous, not therapeutically equivalent to J2250, per 1 mg ⓑ Ⓑ	N
✺ J2252	Injection, midazolam in 0.8% sodium chloride, intravenous, not therapeutically equivalent to J2250, 1 mg ⓑ Ⓑ	N
✺ J2253	Injection, midazolam (seizalam), 1 mg ⓑ Ⓑ	N
✺ J2260	Injection, milrinone lactate, 5 mg ⓑ Ⓑ Qp Qh	N1 N
	Other: Primacor	
	IOM: 100-02, 15, 50	
✱ J2265	Injection, minocycline hydrochloride, 1 mg ⓑ Ⓑ Qp Qh	K2 K
	Other: Minocine	
J2267	Injection, mirikizumab-mrkz, 1 mg ⓑ Ⓑ Qp Qh	K2 G
✺ J2270	Injection, morphine sulfate, up to 10 mg ⓑ Ⓑ Qp Qh	N1 N
	Other: Astramorph PF, Duramorph	
	IOM: 100-02, 15, 50	
	Coding Clinic: 2013, Q2, P4	
✺ J2272	Injection, morphine sulfate (fresenius kabi), not therapeutically equivalent to J2270, up to 10 mg ⓑ Ⓑ	N

 MIPS   Qp Quantity Physician   Qh Quantity Hospital   ♀ Female only
♂ Male only   Ⓐ Age   DMEPOS   A2-Z3 ASC Payment Indicator   A-Y ASC Status Indicator   Coding Clinic

287

Code	Description	Indicator
◉ J2274	Injection, morphine sulfate, preservative-free for epidural or intrathecal use, 10 mg ⑬ ⑬ Qp Qh	N1 N
	Other: Duramorph, Infumorph	
	IOM: 100-03, 4, 280.1; 100-02, 15, 50	
J2277	Injection, motixafortide, 0.25 mg ⑬ ⑬	K2 G
◉ J2278	Injection, ziconotide, 1 mcg ⑬ ⑬ Qp Qh	K2 K
	Other: Prialt	
✻ J2280	Injection, moxifloxacin, 100 mg ⑬ ⑬ Qp Qh	N1 N
	Other: Avelox	
◉ J2281	Injection, moxifloxacin (fresenius kabi), not therapeutically equivalent to J2280, 100 mg ⑬ ⑬	N1 N
▶ ◉ J2290	Injection, nafcillin sodium, 20 mg ⑬ ⑬ Qp Qh	N1 N
▶ ◉ J2291	Injection, nafcillin sodium (baxter), 20 mg ⑬ ⑬ Qp Qh	N1 N
◉ J2300	Injection, nalbuphine hydrochloride, per 10 mg ⑬ ⑬ Qp Qh	N1 N
	Other: Nubain	
	IOM: 100-02, 15, 50	
J2305	Injection, nitroglycerin, 5 mg ⑬ ⑬	
~~J2310~~	~~Injection, naloxone hydrochloride, per 1 mg~~	
~~J2311~~	~~Injection, naloxone hydrochloride (zimhi), 1 mg~~	
▶ ◉ J2312	Injection, naloxone hydrochloride, not otherwise specified, 0.01 mg	N1 N
▶ ◉ J2313	Injection, naloxone hydrochloride (zimhi), 0.01 mg	N1 N
✻ J2315	Injection, naltrexone, depot form, 1 mg ⑬ ⑬ Qp Qh	K2 K
	Other: Vivitrol	
◉ J2320	Injection, nandrolone decanoate, up to 50 mg ⑬ ⑬ Qp Qh	K2 N
	Other: Anabolin LA 100, Androlone, Deca-Durabolin, Decolone, Hybolin Decanoate, Nandrobolic LA, Neo-Durabolic	
	IOM: 100-02, 15, 50	
	Coding Clinic: 2011, Q1, P8	
✻ J2323	Injection, natalizumab, 1 mg ⑬ ⑬ Qp Qh	K2 K
	Other: Tysabri	
◉ J2325	Injection, nesiritide, 0.1 mg ⑬ ⑬ Qp Qh	K2 E1
	Other: Natrecor	
	IOM: 100-02, 15, 50	
✻ J2326	Injection, nusinersen, 0.1 mg ⑬ ⑬	K2 K
	Coding Clinic: 2021, Q1, P11; 2020, Q1, P11	
J2327	Injection, risankizumab-rzaa, intravenous, 1 mg ⑬ ⑬	K2 G
J2329	Injection, ublituximab-xiiy, 1 mg ⑬ ⑬	G
✻ J2350	Injection, ocrelizumab, 1 mg ⑬ ⑬	K2 K
▶ ✻ J2351	Injection, ocrelizumab, 1 mg and hyaluronidase-ocsq ⑬ ⑬	K2 K
✻ J2353	Injection, octreotide, depot form for intramuscular injection, 1 mg ⑬ ⑬ Qp Qh	K2 K
	Other: Sandostatin LAR Depot	
✻ J2354	Injection, octreotide, non-depot form for subcutaneous or intravenous injection, 25 mcg ⑬ ⑬ Qp Qh	N1 N
	Other: Sandostatin LAR Depot	
◉ J2355	Injection, oprelvekin, 5 mg ⑬ ⑬ Qp Qh	K2 E2
	Other: Neumega	
	IOM: 100-02, 15, 50	
J2356	Injection, tezepelumab-ekko, 1 mg ⑬ ⑬	K2 G
✻ J2357	Injection, omalizumab, 5 mg ⑬ ⑬ Qp Qh	K2 K
	Other: Xolair	
✻ J2358	Injection, olanzapine, long-acting, 1 mg ⑬ ⑬ Qp Qh	N1 K
	Other: Zyprexa Relprevv	
	Coding Clinic: 2011, Q1, P6	
J2359	Injection, olanzapine, 0.5 mg ⑬ ⑬	N
◉ J2360	Injection, orphenadrine citrate, up to 60 mg ⑬ ⑬ Qp Qh	N1 N
	Other: Antiflex, Banflex, Flexoject, Flexon, K-Flex, Myolin, Neocyten, Norflex, O-Flex, Orphenate	
	IOM: 100-02, 15, 50	
J2371	Injection, phenylephrine hydrochloride, 20 mcg ⑬ ⑬	N
J2372	Injection, phenylephrine hydrochloride (biorphen), 20 mcg ⑬ ⑬	N
J2373	Injection, phenylephrine hydrochloride (immphentiv), 20 mcg ⑬ ⑬	
J2401	Injection, chloroprocaine hydrochloride, per 1 mg ⑬ ⑬	N
J2402	Injection, chloroprocaine hydrochloride (clorotekal), per 1 mg ⑬ ⑬	E2
J2403	Chloroprocaine hcl ophthalmic, 3% gel, 1 mg ⑬ ⑬	G
J2404	Injection, nicardipine, 0.1 mg ⑬ ⑬	N
◉ J2406	Injection, oritavancin (kimyrsa), 10 mg ⑬ ⑬	K2 K

▶ New ⤶ Revised ✓ Reinstated ~~deleted~~ Deleted ⊘ Not covered or valid by Medicare
◉ Special coverage instructions ✻ Carrier discretion ⑬ Bill Part B MAC ⑬ Bill DME MAC

DRUGS OTHER THAN CHEMOTHERAPY DRUGS

☼ **J2407** Injection, oritavancin (orbactiv), 10 mg ⓑ Ⓑ Qp Qh K2 K
Other: Orbactiv
IOM: 100-02, 15, 50

☼ **J2410** Injection, oxymorphone HCL, up to 1 mg ⓑ Ⓑ Qp Qh N1 E2
Other: Numorphan, Opana
IOM: 100-02, 15, 50

✱ **J2425** Injection, palifermin, 50 mcg ⓑ Ⓑ Qp Qh K2 K
Other: Kepivance

✱ **J2426** Injection, paliperidone palmitate extended release, (invega sustenna) 1 mg ⓑ Ⓑ Qp Qh K2 K
Other: Invega Sustenna
Coding Clinic: 2011, Q1, P7

J2427 Injection, paliperidone palmitate extended release (invega hafyera, or invega trinza), 1 mg ⓑ Ⓑ K

▶ **J2428** Injection, paliperidone palmitate extended release (erzofri), 1 mg K

☼ **J2430** Injection, pamidronate disodium, per 30 mg ⓑ Ⓑ Qp Qh N1 N
Other: Aredia
IOM: 100-02, 15, 50

☼ **J2440** Injection, papaverine HCL, up to 60 mg ⓑ Ⓑ Qp Qh N1 N
IOM: 100-02, 15, 50

☼ **J2460** Injection, oxytetracycline HCL, up to 50 mg ⓑ Ⓑ Qp Qh E2
Other: Terramycin IM
IOM: 100-02, 15, 50

↻ **J2468** Injection, palonosetron hydrochloride (posfrea), 25 mcg ⓑ Ⓑ G

✱ **J2469** Injection, palonosetron HCL, 25 mcg ⓑ Ⓑ Qp Qh K2 G

Example: 0.25 mgm dose = 10 units
Example of use is acute, delayed, nausea and vomiting due to chemotherapy

Other: Aloxi

J2470 Injection, pantoprazole sodium, 40 mg ⓑ Ⓑ N

J2471 Injection, pantoprazole (hikma), not therapeutically equivalent to J2470, 40 mg ⓑ Ⓑ N

▶ **J2472** Injection, pantoprazole sodium in sodium chloride (baxter), 40 mg ⓑ Ⓑ N

☼ **J2501** Injection, paricalcitol, 1 mcg ⓑ Ⓑ Qp Qh N1 N
Other: Zemplar
IOM: 100-02, 15, 50

✱ **J2502** Injection, pasireotide long acting, 1 mg ⓑ Ⓑ Qp Qh K2 K
Other: Signifor LAR

~~J2503~~ ~~Injection, pegaptanib sodium, 0.3 mg~~

☼ **J2504** Injection, pegademase bovine, 25 IU ⓑ Ⓑ Qp Qh K2 E2
Other: Adagen
IOM: 100-02, 15, 50

✱ **J2506** Injection, pegfilgrastim, excludes biosimilar, 0.5 mg ⓑ Ⓑ K2 K

✱ **J2507** Injection, pegloticase, 1 mg ⓑ Ⓑ Qp Qh K2 K
Other: Krystexxa
Coding Clinic: 2012, Q1, P9

J2508 Injection, pegunigalsidase alfa-iwxj, 1 mg ⓑ Ⓑ G
Other: Elfabrio

☼ **J2510** Injection, penicillin G procaine, aqueous, up to 600,000 units ⓑ Ⓑ Qp Qh N1 K
Other: Crysticillin, Duracillin AS, Pfizerpen AS, Wycillin
IOM: 100-02, 15, 50

☼ **J2513** Injection, pentastarch, 10% solution, 100 ml ⓑ Ⓑ Qp Qh E2
IOM: 100-02, 15, 50

☼ **J2515** Injection, pentobarbital sodium, per 50 mg ⓑ Ⓑ Qp Qh K2 N
Other: Nembutal sodium solution
IOM: 100-02, 15, 50

☼ **J2540** Injection, penicillin G potassium, up to 600,000 units ⓑ Ⓑ Qp Qh N1 N
Other: Pfizerpen-G
IOM: 100-02, 15, 50

☼ **J2543** Injection, piperacillin sodium/tazobactam sodium, 1 gram/0.125 grams (1.125 grams) ⓑ Ⓑ Qp Qh N1 N
Other: Zosyn
IOM: 100-02, 15, 50

☼ **J2545** Pentamidine isethionate, inhalation solution, FDA-approved final product, non-compounded, administered through DME, unit dose form, per 300 mg ⓑ Ⓑ Qp Qh B
Other: Nebupent

MIPS | Qp Quantity Physician | Qh Quantity Hospital | ♀ Female only
♂ Male only | A Age | ♿ DMEPOS | A2-Z3 ASC Payment Indicator | A-Y ASC Status Indicator | Coding Clinic

2026 HCPCS LEVEL II NATIONAL CODES

* **J2547** Injection, peramivir, 1 mg ⒷⒷ Qp Qh — K2 K
* **J2550** Injection, promethazine HCL, up to 50 mg ⒷⒷ Qp Qh — N1 N

    Administration of phenergan suppository considered part of E/M encounter

    Other: Anergan, Phenazine, Phenergan, Prorex, Prothazine, V-Gan

    IOM: 100-02, 15, 50

* **J2560** Injection, phenobarbital sodium, up to 120 mg ⒷⒷ Qp Qh — N1 N

    Other: Luminal Sodium

    IOM: 100-02, 15, 50

* **J2561** Injection, phenobarbital sodium (sezaby), 1 mg ⒷⒷ — K
* **J2562** Injection, plerixafor, 1 mg ⒷⒷ Qp Qh — K2 K

    FDA approved for non-Hodgkin lymphoma and multiple myeloma in 2008.

    Other: Mozobil

* **J2590** Injection, oxytocin, up to 10 units ⒷⒷ Qp Qh — N1 N

    Other: Pitocin, Syntocinon

    IOM: 100-02, 15, 50

* **J2597** Injection, desmopressin acetate, per 1 mcg ⒷⒷ Qp Qh — K2 K

    Other: DDAVP

    IOM: 100-02, 15, 50

* **J2598** Injection, vasopressin, 1 unit ⒷⒷ — K2 N
* **J2599** Injection, vasopressin (american regent), not therapeutically equivalent to J2598, 1 unit ⒷⒷ — K2 N
* **J2601** Injection, vasopressin (baxter), 1 unit ⒷⒷ — G
* **J2650** Injection, prednisolone acetate, up to 1 ml ⒷⒷ Qp Qh — N1 E2

    Other: Key-Pred, Predalone, Predcor, Predicort, Predoject

    IOM: 100-02, 15, 50

* **J2670** Injection, tolazoline HCL, up to 25 mg ⒷⒷ Qp Qh — N1 E2

    Other: Priscoline HCl

    IOM: 100-02, 15, 50

* **J2675** Injection, progesterone, per 50 mg ⒷⒷ Qp Qh — N1 N

    Other: Gesterol 50, Progestaject

    IOM: 100-02, 15, 50

* **J2679** Injection, fluphenazine hcl, 1.25 mg ⒷⒷ — N1 K
* **J2680** Injection, fluphenazine decanoate, up to 25 mg ⒷⒷ Qp Qh — N1 N

    Other: Prolixin Decanoate

    MCM: 2049

    IOM: 100-02, 15, 50

* **J2690** Injection, procainamide HCL, up to 1 gm ⒷⒷ Qp Qh ♀ — N1 K

    Benefit limited to obstetrical diagnoses

    Other: Pronestyl, Prostaphlin

    IOM: 100-02, 15, 50

* **J2700** Injection, oxacillin sodium, up to 250 mg ⒷⒷ Qp Qh — N1 N

    Other: Bactocill

    IOM: 100-02, 15, 50

* **J2704** Injection, propofol, 10 mg ⒷⒷ Qp Qh — N1 N

    Other: Diprivan

* **J2710** Injection, neostigmine methylsulfate, up to 0.5 mg ⒷⒷ Qp Qh — N1 N

    Other: Prostigmin

    IOM: 100-02, 15, 50

* **J2720** Injection, protamine sulfate, per 10 mg ⒷⒷ Qp Qh — N1 N

    IOM: 100-02, 15, 50

* **J2724** Injection, protein C concentrate, intravenous, human, 10 IU ⒷⒷ Qp Qh — K2 K

    Other: Ceprotin

* **J2725** Injection, protirelin, per 250 mcg ⒷⒷ Qp Qh — E2

    Other: Relefact TRH, Thypinone

    IOM: 100-02, 15, 50

* **J2730** Injection, pralidoxime chloride, up to 1 gm ⒷⒷ Qp Qh — N1 N

    Other: Protopam Chloride

    IOM: 100-02, 15, 50

* **J2760** Injection, phentolamine mesylate, up to 5 mg ⒷⒷ Qp Qh — K2 K

    Other: Regitine

    IOM: 100-02, 15, 50

* **J2765** Injection, metoclopramide HCL, up to 10 mg ⒷⒷ Qp Qh — N1 N

    Other: Reglan

    IOM: 100-02, 15, 50

* **J2770** Injection, quinupristin/dalfopristin, 500 mg (150/350) ⒷⒷ Qp Qh — K2 K

    Other: Synercid

    IOM: 100-02, 15, 50

* **J2777** Injection, faricimab-svoa, 0.1 mg — K2 G

▶ New ↻ Revised ✓ Reinstated ~~deleted~~ Deleted ⊘ Not covered or valid by Medicare ⊕ Special coverage instructions ✱ Carrier discretion Ⓑ Bill Part B MAC Ⓑ Bill DME MAC

DRUGS OTHER THAN CHEMOTHERAPY DRUGS

* **J2778** Injection, ranibizumab, 0.1 mg — K2 K

  May be reported for exudative senile macular degeneration (wet AMD) with 67028 (RT or LT)

  Other: Lucentis

J2779 Injection, ranibizumab, via intravitreal implant (susvimo), 0.1 mg — K2 G

J2781 Injection, pegcetacoplan, intravitreal, 1 mg — G

J2782 Injection, avacincaptad pegol, 0.1 mg — G

* **J2783** Injection, rasburicase, 0.5 mg — K2 K

  Other: Elitek

* **J2785** Injection, regadenoson, 0.1 mg — N1 N

  One billing unit equal to 0.1 mg of regadenoson

  Other: Lexiscan

* **J2786** Injection, reslizumab, 1 mg — K2 K

  Coding Clinic: 2016, Q4, P9

* **J2787** Riboflavin 5'-phosphate, ophthalmic solution, up to 3 mL — N

  Other: Photrexa Viscous

○ **J2788** Injection, Rho D immune globulin, human, minidose, 50 mcg (250 IU) — N1 N

  Other: HypRho-D, MicRhoGAM, Rhesonativ, RhoGam

  IOM: 100-02, 15, 50

○ **J2790** Injection, Rho D immune globulin, human, full dose, 300 mcg (1500 IU) — N1 N

  Administered to pregnant female to prevent hemolistic disease of newborn. Report 90384 to private payer

  Other: Gamulin Rh, Hyperrho S/D, HypRho-D, Rhesonativ, RhoGAM

  IOM: 100-02, 15, 50

○ **J2791** Injection, Rho(D) immune globulin (human), (Rhophylac), intramuscular or intravenous, 100 IU — N1 N

  Agent must be billed per 100 IU in both physician office and hospital outpatient settings

  Other: HypRho-D

  IOM: 100-02, 15, 50

○ **J2792** Injection, Rho D immune globulin intravenous, human, solvent detergent, 100 IU — K2 K

  Other: Gamulin Rh, Hyperrho S/D, WinRHo-SDF

  IOM: 100-02, 15, 50

○ **J2793** Injection, rilonacept, 1 mg — K2 E2

  Other: Arcalyst

  IOM: 100-02, 15, 50

* **J2794** Injection, risperidone (risperdal consta), 0.5 mg — K2 K

  Other: Risperdal Costa

* **J2795** Injection, ropivacaine hydrochloride, 1 mg — N1 N

  Other: Naropin

~~J2796~~ ~~Injection, romiplostim, 10 mcg~~

○ **J2797** Injection, rolapitant, 0.5 mg — E1

  Other: Varubi

* **J2798** Injection, risperidone, (perseris), 0.5 mg — K2 E1

J2799 Injection, risperidone (uzedy), 1 mg — G

○ **J2800** Injection, methocarbamol, up to 10 ml — N1 N

  Other: Robaxin

J2801 Injection, risperidone (rykindo), 0.5 mg — K

▶ * **J2802** Injection, romplostim, 10 mcg — K

▶ * **J2804** Injection, rifampin, 1 mg — N1 N

* **J2805** Injection, sincalide, 5 mcg — N1 N

  Other: Kinevac

~~J2806~~ ~~Injection, sincalide (maia), not therapeutically equivalent to J2805, 5 mcg~~

○ **J2810** Injection, theophylline, per 40 mg — N1 E2

  IOM: 100-02, 15, 50

○ **J2820** Injection, sargramostim (GM-CSF), 50 mcg — K2 K

  Other: Leukine, Prokine

  IOM: 100-02, 15, 50

* **J2840** Injection, sebelipase alfa, 1 mg — K2 K

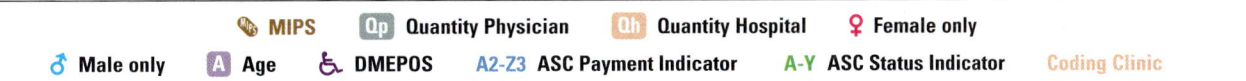

2026 HCPCS LEVEL II NATIONAL CODES

⊕ **J2850** Injection, secretin, synthetic, human, 1 mcg ⓑ Ⓑ Qp Qh   K2 K

Other: Chirhostim

IOM: 100-02, 15, 50

✱ **J2860** Injection, siltuximab, 10 mg ⓑ Ⓑ Qp Qh   K2 K

▶ **J2865** Injection, sulfamethoxazole 5 mg and trimethoprim 1 mg   N

⊕ **J2910** Injection, aurothioglucose, up to 50 mg ⓑ Ⓑ Qp Qh   E2

Other: Solganal

IOM: 100-02, 15, 50

⊕ **J2916** Injection, sodium ferric gluconate complex in sucrose injection, 12.5 mg ⓑ Ⓑ Qp Qh   N1 N

Other: Ferrlecit, Nulecit

IOM: 100-02, 15, 50

J2919 Injection, methylprednisolone sodium succinate, 5 mg ⓑ Ⓑ   N1 K

⊕ **J2940** Injection, somatrem, 1 mg ⓑ Ⓑ Qp Qh   E2

IOM: 100-02, 15, 50,

Medicare Statute 1861s2b

⊕ **J2941** Injection, somatropin, 1 mg ⓑ Ⓑ Qp Qh   K2 K

Other: Genotropin, Humatrope, Nutropin, Omnitrope, Saizen, Serostim, Zorbtive

IOM: 100-02, 15, 50,

Medicare Statute 1861s2b

⊕ **J2950** Injection, promazine HCL, up to 25 mg ⓑ Ⓑ Qp Qh   N1 N

Other: Prozine-50, Sparine

IOM: 100-02, 15, 50

⊕ **J2993** Injection, reteplase, 18.1 mg ⓑ Ⓑ Qp Qh   K2 K

Other: Retavase

IOM: 100-02, 15, 50

⊕ **J2995** Injection, streptokinase, per 250,000 IU ⓑ Ⓑ Qp Qh   N1 E2

Bill 1 unit for each 250,000 IU

Other: Kabikinase, Streptase

IOM: 100-02, 15, 50

⊕ **J2997** Injection, alteplase recombinant, 1 mg ⓑ Ⓑ Qp Qh   K2 K

Thrombolytic agent, treatment of occluded catheters. Bill units of 1 mg administered.

Other: Activase, Cathflo Activase

IOM: 100-02, 15, 50

Coding Clinic: 2014, Q1, P4

⊕ **J2998** Injection, plasminogen, human-tvmh, 1 mg ⓑ Ⓑ   K2 G

⊕ **J3000** Injection, streptomycin, up to 1 gm ⓑ Ⓑ Qp Qh   N1 N

IOM: 100-02, 15, 50

⊕ **J3010** Injection, fentanyl citrate, 0.1 mg ⓑ Ⓑ Qp Qh   N1 N

Other: Sublimaze

IOM: 100-02, 15, 50

⊕ **J3030** Injection, sumatriptan succinate, 6 mg (Code may be used for Medicare when drug administered under the direct supervision of a physician, not for use when drug is self-administered) ⓑ Ⓑ Qp Qh   N1 N

Other: Imitrex, Sumarel Dosepro

IOM: 100-02, 15, 150

✱ **J3031** Injection, fremanezumab-vfrm, 1 mg (Code may be used for Medicare when drug administered under the direct supervision of a physician, not for use when drug is self-administered) ⓑ Ⓑ   K2 N

✱ **J3032** Injection, eptinezumab-jjmr, 1 mg ⓑ Ⓑ   K2 K

J3055 Injection, talquetamab-tgvs, 0.25 mg ⓑ Ⓑ   G

✱ **J3060** Injection, taliglucerase alfa, 10 units ⓑ Ⓑ Qp Qh   K2 K

Other: Elelyso

⊕ **J3070** Injection, pentazocine, 30 mg ⓑ Ⓑ Qp Qh   K2 N

Other: Talwin

IOM: 100-02, 15, 50

✱ **J3090** Injection, tedizolid phosphate, 1 mg ⓑ Ⓑ Qp Qh   K2 K

Other: Sivextro

✱ **J3095** Injection, televancin, 10 mg ⓑ Ⓑ Qp Qh   K2 K

Prescribed for the treatment of adults with complicated skin and skin structure infections (cSSSI) of the following Gram-positive microorganisms: Staphylococcus aureus; Streptococcus pyogenes, Streptococcus agalactiae, Streptococcus anginosusgroup. Separately payable under the ASC payment system.

Other: Vibativ

Coding Clinic: 2011, Q1, P7

✱ **J3101** Injection, tenecteplase, 1 mg ⓑ Ⓑ Qp Qh   K2 K

Other: TNKase

▶ New	⤺ Revised	✓ Reinstated	deleted Deleted	⊘ Not covered or valid by Medicare
⊕ Special coverage instructions		✱ Carrier discretion	ⓑ Bill Part B MAC	Ⓑ Bill DME MAC

DRUGS OTHER THAN CHEMOTHERAPY DRUGS

✸ **J3105** Injection, terbutaline sulfate, up to 1 mg ⓑ Ⓑ Qp Qh   N1 N

Other: Brethine

IOM: 100-02, 15, 50

✸ **J3110** Injection, teriparatide, 10 mcg Ⓑ Ⓑ Qp Qh   B

* **J3111** Injection, romosozumab-aqqg, 1 mg   K2 K

✸ **J3121** Injection, testosterone enanthate, 1 mg ⓑ Ⓑ Qp Qh   N1 N

Other: Andrest 90-4, Andro L.A. 200, Andro-Estro 90-4, Androgyn L.A, Andropository 100, Andryl 200, Deladumone, Deladumone OB, Delatest, Delatestadiol, Delatestryl, Ditate-DS, Dua-Gen L.A., Duoval P.A., Durathate-200, Estra-Testrin, Everone, TEEV, Testadiate, Testone LA, Testradiol 90/4, Testrin PA, Valertest

✸ **J3145** Injection, testosterone undecanoate, 1 mg ⓑ Ⓑ Qp Qh   K2 K

✸ **J3230** Injection, chlorpromazine HCL, up to 50 mg ⓑ Ⓑ Qp Qh   N1 N

Other: Ormazine, Thorazine

IOM: 100-02, 15, 50

✸ **J3240** Injection, thyrotropin alfa, 0.9 mg provided in 1.1 mg vial ⓑ Ⓑ Qp Qh   K2 K

Other: Thyrogen

IOM: 100-02, 15, 50

* **J3241** Injection, teprotumumab-trbw, 10 mg Ⓑ Ⓑ   K2 K

* **J3243** Injection, tigecycline, 1 mg ⓑ Qp Qh   K2 N

J3244 Injection, tigecycline (accord), not therapeutically equivalent to J3243, 1 mg ⓑ Ⓑ   N

* **J3245** Injection, tildrakizumab, 1 mg Ⓑ Ⓑ   K

Other: Ilumya

* **J3246** Injection, tirofiban HCL, 0.25 mg ⓑ Ⓑ Qp Qh   K2 N

Other: Aggrastat

J3247 Injection, secukinumab, intravenous, 1 mg Ⓑ Ⓑ   G

✸ **J3250** Injection, trimethobenzamide HCL, up to 200 mg ⓑ Ⓑ Qp Qh   N1 N

Other: Arrestin, Ticon, Tigan, Tiject 20

IOM: 100-02, 15, 50

✸ **J3260** Injection, tobramycin sulfate, up to 80 mg ⓑ Ⓑ Qp Qh   N1 N

Other: Nebcin

IOM: 100-02, 15, 50

* **J3262** Injection, tocilizumab, 1 mg ⓑ Ⓑ Qp Qh   K2 K

Indicated for the treatment of adult patients with moderately to severely active rheumatoid arthritis (RA) who have had an inadequate response to one or more tumor necrosis factor (TNF) antagonist therapies.

Other: Actemra

Coding Clinic: 2011, Q1, P7

J3263 Injection, toripalimab-tpzi, 1 mg Ⓑ Ⓑ   G

✸ **J3265** Injection, torsemide, 10 mg/ml ⓑ Ⓑ Qp Qh   N1 E2

Other: Demadex

IOM: 100-02, 15, 50

✸ **J3280** Injection, thiethylperazine maleate, up to 10 mg ⓑ Ⓑ Qp Qh   E2

Other: Norzine, Torecan

IOM: 100-02, 15, 50

* **J3285** Injection, treprostinil, 1 mg ⓑ Ⓑ Qp Qh   K2 K

Other: Remodulin

▶ **J3290** Injection, tranexamic acid, 5 mg   E1

J3299 Injection, triamcinolone acetonide (xipere), 1 mg Ⓑ   G

✸ **J3300** Injection, triamcinolone acetonide, preservative free, 1 mg ⓑ Ⓑ Qp Qh   K2 N

Other: Cenacort A-40, Kenaject-40, Kenalog, Triam-A, Triesence, Tri-Kort, Trilog

✸ **J3301** Injection, triamcinolone acetonide, not otherwise specified, 10 mg ⓑ Ⓑ Qp Qh   N1 N

Other: Cenacort A-40, Kenaject-40, Kenalog, Triam A, Triesence, Tri-Kort, Trilog

IOM: 100-02, 15, 50

Coding Clinic: 2024, Q1, P26; 2018, Q4, P7; 2013, Q2, P4

✸ **J3302** Injection, triamcinolone diacetate, per 5 mg ⓑ Ⓑ Qp Qh   N1 N

Other: Amcort, Aristocort, Cenacort Forte, Trilone

IOM: 100-02, 15, 50

✸ **J3303** Injection, triamcinolone hexacetonide, per 5 mg ⓑ Ⓑ Qp Qh   N1 N

Other: Aristospan

IOM: 100-02, 15, 50

🖐 MIPS	Qp Quantity Physician	Qh Quantity Hospital	♀ Female only
♂ Male only	Ⓐ Age	♿ DMEPOS	A2-Z3 ASC Payment Indicator	A-Y ASC Status Indicator	Coding Clinic

2026 HCPCS LEVEL II NATIONAL CODES

○ **J3304** Injection, triamcinolone acetonide, preservative-free, extended-release, microsphere formulation, 1 mg Ⓑ Ⓑ K

Other: Zilretta

○ **J3305** Injection, trimetrexate glucuronate, per 25 mg Ⓑ Ⓑ Qp Qh E2

Other: NeuTrexin

IOM: 100-02, 15, 50

○ **J3310** Injection, perphenazine, up to 5 mg Ⓑ Ⓑ Qp Qh N1 E2

Other: Trilafon

IOM: 100-02, 15, 50

○ **J3315** Injection, triptorelin pamoate, 3.75 mg Ⓑ Ⓑ Qp Qh K2 K

Other: Trelstar

IOM: 100-02, 15, 50

○ **J3316** Injection, triptorelin, extended-release, 3.75 mg Ⓑ Ⓑ K

Other: Trelstar, Trelstar Depot, Trelstar LA

○ **J3320** Injection, spectinomycin dihydrochloride, up to 2 gm Ⓑ Ⓑ Qp Qh E2

Other: Trobicin

IOM: 100-02, 15, 50

○ **J3350** Injection, urea, up to 40 gm Ⓑ Ⓑ Qp Qh N1 E2

Other: Ureaphil

IOM: 100-02, 15, 50

○ **J3355** Injection, urofollitropin, 75 IU Ⓑ Ⓑ Qp Qh E2

Other: Bravelle, Metrodin

IOM: 100-02, 15, 50

✱ **J3357** Ustekinumab, for subcutaneous injection, 1 mg Ⓑ Ⓑ Qp Qh K2 K

Other: Stelara

Coding Clinic: 2017, Q1, P3; 2016, Q4, P10; 2011, Q1, P7

✱ **J3358** Ustekinumab, for intravenous injection, 1 mg K2 K

Cross Reference Q9989

○ **J3360** Injection, diazepam, up to 5 mg Ⓑ Ⓑ Qp Qh N1 N

Other: Valium, Zetran

IOM: 100-02, 15, 50

Coding Clinic: 2007, Q2, P6-7

○ **J3364** Injection, urokinase, 5000 IU vial Ⓑ Ⓑ Qp Qh N1 E2

Other: Abbokinase

IOM: 100-02, 15, 50

○ **J3365** Injection, IV, urokinase, 250,000 IU vial Ⓑ Ⓑ Qp Qh E2

Other: Abbokinase

IOM: 100-02, 15, 50,

Cross Reference Q0089

~~J3370~~ ~~Injection, vancomycin HCL, 500 mg~~

~~J3371~~ ~~Injection, vancomycin hcl (mylan), not therapeutically equivalent to J3370, 500 mg~~

~~J3372~~ ~~Injection, vancomycin hcl (xellia), not therapeutically equivalent to J3370, 500 mg~~

▶ **J3373** Injection, vancomycin hydrochloride, 10 mg N1 N

▶ **J3374** Injection, vancomycin hydrochloride (mylan) not therapeutically equivalent to J3373, 10 mg N1 N

▶ **J3375** Injection, vancomycin hydrochloride (xellia), not therapeutically equivalent to J3373, 10 mg N1 N

○ **J3380** Injection, vedolizumab, intravenous, 1 mg Ⓑ Ⓑ Qp Qh K2 K

Other: Entyvio

✱ **J3385** Injection, velaglucerase alfa, 100 units Ⓑ Ⓑ Qp Qh K2 K

Enzyme replacement therapy in Gaucher Disease that results from a specific enzyme deficiency in the body, caused by a genetic mutation received from both parents. Type 1 is the most prevalent Ashkenazi Jewish genetic disease, occurring in one in every 1,000.

Other: VPRIV

Coding Clinic: 2011, Q1, P7

▶ **J3391** Injection, atidarsagene autotemcel, per treatment K

▶ **J3392** Injection, exagamglogen autotemcel, per treatment K

J3393 Injection, betibeglogene autotemcel, per treatment Ⓑ Ⓑ

J3394 Injection, lovotibeglogene autotemcel, per treatment Ⓑ

○ **J3396** Injection, verteporfin, 0.1 mg Ⓑ Ⓑ Qp Qh K2 K

Other: Visudyne

IOM: 100-03, 1, 80.2; 100-03, 1, 80.3

✱ **J3397** Injection, vestronidase alfa-vjbk, 1 mg Ⓑ Ⓑ E2

Other: Mepsevii

✱ **J3398** Injection, voretigene neparvovec-rzyl, 1 billion vector genomes Ⓑ Ⓑ K

Other: Luxturna

▶ New ⤷ Revised ✓ Reinstated ~~deleted~~ Deleted ⊘ Not covered or valid by Medicare
○ Special coverage instructions ✱ Carrier discretion Ⓑ Bill Part B MAC Ⓑ Bill DME MAC

DRUGS OTHER THAN CHEMOTHERAPY DRUGS

✱ J3399	Injection, onasemnogene abeparvovec-xioi, per treatment, up to 5x10^15 vector genomes	K
⊛ J3400	Injection, triflupromazine HCL, up to 20 mg	E2
	Other: Vesprin	
	IOM: 100-02, 15, 50	
J3401	Beremagene geperpavec-svdt for topical administration, containing nominal 5 x 10^9 pfu/ml vector genomes, per 0.1 ml	G
	Other: Vyjuvek	
▶ J3402	Injection, remestemcel-l-rknd, per therapeutic dose	N1 N
▶ J3403	Revakinagene taroretcel-lwey, per implant	N1 N
⊛ J3410	Injection, hydroxyzine HCL, up to 25 mg	N1 N
	Other: Hyzine-50, Vistaject 25, Vistaril	
	IOM: 100-02, 15, 50	
✱ J3411	Injection, thiamine HCL, 100 mg	N1 N
✱ J3415	Injection, pyridoxine HCL, 100 mg	N1 N
⊛ J3420	Injection, vitamin B-12 cyanocobalamin, up to 1000 mcg	N1 N
	Medicare carriers may have local coverage decisions regarding vitamin B12 injections that provide reimbursement only for patients with certain types of anemia and other conditions.	
	Other: Berubigen, Betalin 12, Cobex, Redisol, Rubramin PC, Sytobex	
	IOM: 100-02, 15, 50; 100-03, 2, 150.6	
J3424	Injection, hydroxocobalamin, intravenous, 25 mg	K
J3425	Injection, hydroxocobalamin, intramuscular, 10 mcg	K
⊛ J3430	Injection, phytonadione (vitamin K), per 1 mg	N1 N
	Other: AquaMephyton, Konakion, Menadione, Synkavite, Vitamin K1	
	IOM: 100-02, 15, 50	
⊛ J3465	Injection, voriconazole, 10 mg	K2 N
	Other: VFEND	
	IOM: 100-02, 15, 50	
⊛ J3470	Injection, hyaluronidase, up to 150 units	N1 N
	Other: Amphadase, Wydase	
	IOM: 100-02, 15, 50	
⊛ J3471	Injection, hyaluronidase, ovine, preservative free, per 1 USP unit (up to 999 USP units)	N1 N
	Other: Vitrase	
⊛ J3472	Injection, hyaluronidase, ovine, preservative free, per 1000 USP units	N1 N
⊛ J3473	Injection, hyaluronidase, recombinant, 1 USP unit	N1 N
	Other: Hylenex	
	IOM: 100-02, 15, 50	
⊛ J3475	Injection, magnesium sulfate, per 500 mg	N1 N
	IOM: 100-02, 15, 50	
⊛ J3480	Injection, potassium chloride, per 2 meq	N1 N
	IOM: 100-02, 15, 50	
⊛ J3485	Injection, zidovudine, 10 mg	N1 N
	Other: Retrovir	
	IOM: 100-02, 15, 50	
✱ J3486	Injection, ziprasidone mesylate, 10 mg	N1 N
	Other: Geodon	
✱ J3489	Injection, zoledronic acid, 1 mg	N1 N
	Other: Reclast, Zometa	
⊛ J3490	Unclassified drugs	N1 N
	Bill on paper. Bill one unit. Identify drug and total dosage in "Remarks" field.	
	Other: Acthib, Aminocaproic Acid, Baciim, Bacitracin, Benzocaine, Bumetanide, Bupivacaine, Cefotetan, Ciprofloxacin, Cleocin Phosphate, Clindamycin, Cortisone Acetate Micronized, Definity, Diprivan, Doxy, Engerix-B, Ethanolamine, Famotidine, Ganirelix, Gonal-F, Hyaluronic Acid, Marcaine, Metronidazole, Nafcillin, Naltrexone, Ovidrel, Pegasys, Peg-Intron, Penicillin G Sodium, Propofol, Protonix, Recombivax, Rifadin, Rifampin, Sensorcaine-MPF, Smz-TMP, Sufentanil Citrate, Testopel Pellets, Testosterone, Treanda, Valcyte, Veritas Collagen Matrix	
	IOM: 100-02, 15, 50	
	Coding Clinic: 2024, Q4, P30; 2017, Q1, P1-3, P8; 2014, Q2, P6; 2013, Q2, P3-4	
⊘ J3520	Edetate disodium, per 150 mg	E1
	Other: Chealamide, Disotate, Endrate ethylenediamine-tetra-acetic	
	IOM: 100-03, 1, 20.21; 100-03, 1, 20.22	

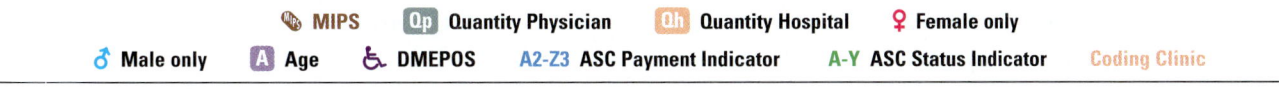

Code	Description	Status
⊘ **J3530**	Nasal vaccine inhalation	N1 N
	IOM: 100-02, 15, 50	
⊘ **J3535**	Drug administered through a metered dose inhaler	E1
	Other: Ipratropium bromide	
	IOM: 100-02, 15, 50	
⊘ **J3570**	Laetrile, amygdalin, vitamin B-17	E1
	IOM: 100-03, 1, 30.7	
* **J3590**	Unclassified biologics	N1 N
	Bill on paper. Bill one unit. Identify drug and total dosage in "Remarks" field.	
	Coding Clinic: 2017, Q1, P1-3; 2016, Q4, P10	
* **J3591**	Unclassified drug or biological used for ESRD on dialysis	B
⊘ **J7030**	Infusion, normal saline solution, 1000 cc	N1 N
	Other: Sodium Chloride	
	IOM: 100-02, 15, 50	
⊘ **J7040**	Infusion, normal saline solution, sterile (500 ml = 1 unit)	N1 N
	Other: Sodium Chloride	
	IOM: 100-02, 15, 50	
⊘ **J7042**	5% dextrose/normal saline (500 ml = 1 unit)	N1 N
	Other: Dextrose-Nacl	
	IOM: 100-02, 15, 50	
⊘ **J7050**	Infusion, normal saline solution, 250 cc	N1 N
	Other: Sodium Chloride	
	IOM: 100-02, 15, 50	
⊘ **J7060**	5% dextrose/water (500 ml = 1 unit)	N1 N
	IOM: 100-02, 15, 50	
⊘ **J7070**	Infusion, D 5 W, 1000 cc	N1 N
	Other: Dextrose	
	IOM: 100-02, 15, 50	
⊘ **J7100**	Infusion, dextran 40, 500 ml	N1 N
	Other: Gentran, LMD, Rheomacrodex	
	IOM: 100-02, 15, 50	
⊘ **J7110**	Infusion, dextran 75, 500 ml	N1 N
	Other: Gentran 75	
	IOM: 100-02, 15, 50	
⊘ **J7120**	Ringer's lactate infusion, up to 1000 cc	N1 N
	Replacement fluid or electrolytes.	
	Other: Potassium Chloride	
	IOM: 100-02, 15, 50	
⊘ **J7121**	5% dextrose in lactated ringers infusion, up to 1000 cc	N1 N
	IOM: 100-02, 15, 50	
⊘ **J7131**	Hypertonic saline solution, 1 ml	N1 N
	IOM: 100-02, 15, 50	
	Coding Clinic: 2012, Q1, P9	

Clotting Factors

Code	Description	Status
J7165	Injection, prothrombin complex concentrate, human-lans, per i.u. of Factor IX activity	G
* **J7168**	Prothrombin complex concentrate (human), kcentra, per i.u. of Factor IX activity	K2 K
* **J7169**	Injection, coagulation Factor XA (recombinant), inactivated-zhzo (andexxa), 10 mg	K2 K
* **J7170**	Injection, emicizumab-kxwh, 0.5 mg	K
	Other: Hemlibra	
J7171	Injection, adamts13, recombinant-krhn, 10 iu	G
▶ * **J7172**	Injection, marstacimab-hncq, 0.5 mg	G
▶ * **J7173**	Injection, concizumab-mtci, 0.5 mg	K
▶ * **J7174**	Injection, fitusiran, 0.04 mg	G
* **J7175**	Injection, Factor X, (human), 1 IU	K2 K
	Coding Clinic: 2017, Q1, P9	
* **J7177**	Injection, human fibrinogen concentrate (fibryga), 1 mg	K
* **J7178**	Injection, human fibrinogen concentrate, not otherwise specified, 1 mg	K2 K
	Other: Riastap	
⊘ **J7179**	Injection, von Willebrand factor (recombinant), (vonvendi), 1 IU VWF:RCo	K2 K
	Coding Clinic: 2017, Q1, P9	
* **J7180**	Injection, factor XIII (antihemophilic factor, human), 1 IU	K2 K
	Other: Corifact	
	Coding Clinic: 2012, Q1, P8	
* **J7181**	Injection, factor XIII a-subunit, (recombinant), per IU	K2 K

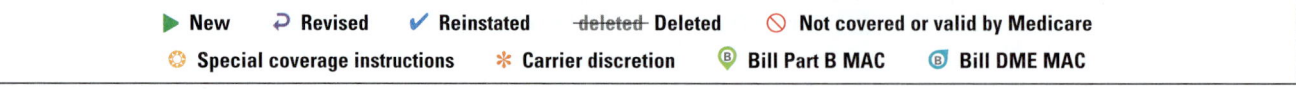

▶ New   ↻ Revised   ✓ Reinstated   ~~deleted~~ Deleted   ⊘ Not covered or valid by Medicare   ⊛ Special coverage instructions   * Carrier discretion   Ⓑ Bill Part B MAC   Ⓓ Bill DME MAC

DRUGS OTHER THAN CHEMOTHERAPY DRUGS

* **J7182** Injection, factor VIII, (antihemophilic factor, recombinant), (novoeight), per IU Qp Qh K2 K

* **J7183** Injection, von Willebrand factor complex (human), wilate, 1 IU VWF:RCo Qp Qh K2 K

  IOM: 100-02, 15, 50

  Coding Clinic: 2012, Q1, P9

* **J7185** Injection, Factor VIII (antihemophilic factor, recombinant) (Xyntha), per IU Qp Qh K2 K

* **J7186** Injection, anti-hemophilic factor VIII/von Willebrand factor complex (human), per factor VIII IU Qp Qh K2 K

  Other: Alphanate

  IOM: 100-02, 15, 50

* **J7187** Injection, von Willebrand factor complex (HUMATE-P), per IU VWF:RCo Qp Qh K2 K

  Other: Humate-P Low Dilutent

  IOM: 100-02, 15, 50

* **J7188** Injection, factor VIII (antihemophilic factor, recombinant), (obizur), per IU Qp Qh K2 K

  IOM: 100-02, 15, 50

* **J7189** Factor VIIa (anti-hemophilic factor, recombinant), (novoseven rt), per 1 mcg Qp Qh K2 K

  Other: NovoSeven

  IOM: 100-02, 15, 50

* **J7190** Factor VIII anti-hemophilic factor, human, per IU Qp Qh K2 K

  Other: Alphanate/von Willebrand factor complex, Hemofil M, Koate DVI, Koate-HP, Kogenate, Monoclate-P, Recombinate

  IOM: 100-02, 15, 50

* **J7191** Factor VIII, anti-hemophilic factor (porcine), per IU Qp Qh E2

  Other: Hyate:C, Koate-HP, Kogenate, Monoclate-P, Recombinate

  IOM: 100-02, 15, 50

* **J7192** Factor VIII (anti-hemophilic factor, recombinant) per IU, not otherwise specified Qp Qh K2 K

  Other: Advate, Helixate FS, Kogenate FS, Koate-HP, Recombinate, Xyntha

  IOM: 100-02, 15, 50

* **J7193** Factor IX (anti-hemophilic factor, purified, non-recombinant) per IU Qp Qh K2 K

  Other: AlphaNine SD, Mononine, Proplex

  IOM: 100-02, 15, 50

* **J7194** Factor IX, complex, per IU Qp Qh K2 K

  Other: Bebulin, Konyne-80, Profilnine Heat-treated, Profilnine SD, Proplex SX-T, Proplex T

  IOM: 100-02, 15, 50

* **J7195** Injection, Factor IX (anti-hemophilic factor, recombinant) per IU, not otherwise specified Qp Qh K2 K

  Other: Benefix, Profiline, Proplex T

  IOM: 100-02, 15, 50

* **J7196** Injection, antithrombin recombinant, 50 IU Qp Qh E2

  Other: ATryn, Feiba VH Immuno

  Coding Clinic: 2011, Q1, P6

* **J7197** Anti-thrombin III (human), per IU Qp Qh K2 K

  Other: Thrombate III

  IOM: 100-02, 15, 50

* **J7198** Anti-inhibitor, per IU Qp Qh K2 K

  Diagnosis examples: D66 Congenital Factor VIII disorder; D67 Congenital Factor IX disorder; D68.0 VonWillebrand's disease

  Other: Autoplex T, Feiba NF, Hemophilia clotting factors

  IOM: 100-02, 15, 50; 100-03, 2, 110.3

* **J7199** Hemophilia clotting factor, not otherwise classified B

  Other: Autoplex T

  IOM: 100-02, 15, 50; 100-03, 2, 110.3

* **J7200** Injection, factor IX, (antihemophilic factor, recombinant), rixubis, per IU Qp Qh K2 N

  IOM: 100-02, 15, 50

* **J7201** Injection, factor IX, fc fusion protein (recombinant), alprolix, 1 IU Qp Qh K2 K

  IOM: 100-02, 15, 50

* **J7202** Injection, Factor IX, albumin fusion protein, (recombinant), idelvion, 1 IU Qp Qh K2 K

  Coding Clinic: 2016, Q4, P9

* **J7203** Injection Factor IX, (antihemophilic factor, recombinant), glycopegylated, (rebinyn), 1 iu K

  Other: Profilnine SD, Bebulin VH, Bebulin, Proplex T

* **J7204** Injection, Factor VIII, antihemophilic factor (recombinant), (esperoct), glycopegylated-exei, per iu K2 K

MIPS | Qp Quantity Physician | Qh Quantity Hospital | ♀ Female only
♂ Male only | A Age | DMEPOS | A2-Z3 ASC Payment Indicator | A-Y ASC Status Indicator | Coding Clinic

	J7205	Injection, Factor VIII Fc fusion protein (recombinant), per IU ⓑ Qp Qh　K2 K
		Other: Eloctate
	J7207	Injection, Factor VIII, (antihemophilic factor, recombinant), PEGylated, 1 IU Qp Qh　K2 K
		Other: Adynovate
	J7208	Injection, Factor VIII, (antihemophilic factor, recombinant), pegylated-aucl, (jivi), 1 i.u.　K2 K
*	J7209	Injection, Factor VIII, (antihemophilic factor, recombinant), (Nuwiq), 1 IU Qp Qh　K2 K
*	J7210	Injection, Factor VIII, (antihemophilic factor, recombinant), (afstyla), 1 i.u. ⓑ　K2 K
*	J7211	Injection, Factor VIII, (antihemophilic factor, recombinant), (kovaltry), 1 i.u. ⓑ　K2 K
	J7212	Factor VIIA (antihemophilic factor, recombinant)-jncw (sevenfact), 1 mcg　K2 N
	J7213	Injection, coagulation Factor IX (recombinant), ixinity, 1 IU　K
	J7214	Injection, Factor VIII/von willebrand factor complex, recombinant (altuviiio), per factor VIII IU　G

Contraceptives

	J7294	Segesterone acetate and ethinyl estradiol 0.15mg, 0.013mg per 24 hours; yearly vaginal system, each　E1
	J7295	Ethinyl estradiol and etonogestrel 0.015mg, 0.12mg per 24 hours; monthly vaginal ring, each　E1
	J7296	Levonorgestrel-releasing intrauterine contraceptive system (Kyleena), 19.5 mg ♀　E1
		Medicare Statute 1862(a)(1)
		Cross Reference Q9984
	J7297	Levonorgestrel-releasing intrauterine contraceptive system (Liletta), 52 mg ⓑ Qp Qh ♀　E1
		Medicare Statute 1862(a)(1)
	J7298	Levonorgestrel-releasing intrauterine contraceptive system (Mirena), 52 mg Qp Qh ♀　E1
		Medicare Statute 1862(a)(1)
		Coding Clinic: 2023, Q1, P21
⤺	J7300	Intrauterine copper contraceptive (paragard) ⓑ ♀　E1
		Report IUD insertion with 58300. Bill usual and customary charge.
		Other: Paragard T 380 A
		Medicare Statute 1862a1
	J7301	Levonorgestrel-releasing intrauterine contraceptive system (Skyla), 13.5 mg ⓑ Qp Qh ♀　E1
		Medicare Statute 1862(a)(1)
	J7304	Contraceptive supply, hormone containing patch, each ⓑ ♀　E1
		Only billed by Family Planning Clinics
		Medicare Statute 1862.1
	J7306	Levonorgestrel (contraceptive) implant system, including implants and supplies ⓑ ♀　E1
	J7307	Etonogestrel (contraceptive) implant system, including implant and supplies ⓑ ♀　E1

Aminolevulinic Acid HCL

*	J7308	Aminolevulinic acid HCL for topical administration, 20%, single unit dosage form (354 mg) ⓑ Qp Qh　K2 K
		Other: Levulan Kerastick
	J7309	Methyl aminolevulinate (MAL) for topical administration, 16.8%, 1 gram ⓑ Qp Qh　N1 E2
		Other: Metvixia
		Coding Clinic: 2011, Q1, P6

Ganciclovir

	J7310	Ganciclovir, 4.5 mg, long-acting implant ⓑ Qp Qh　E2
		IOM: 100-02, 15, 50

Ophthalmic Drugs

*	J7311	Injection, fluocinolone acetonide, intravitreal implant (retisert), 0.01 mg ⓑ Qp Qh　K2 K
		Treatment of chronic noninfectious posterior segment uveitis
		Other: Retisert
*	J7312	Injection, dexamethasone, intravitreal implant, 0.1 mg ⓑ Qp Qh　K2 K
		To bill for Ozurdex services submit the following codes: J7312 and 67028 with the modifier -22 (for the increased work difficulty and increased risk). Indicated for the treatment of macular edema occurring after branch retinal vein occlusion (BRVO) or central retinal vein occlusion (CRVO) and non-infectious uveitis affecting the posterior segment of the eye.
		Other: Ozurdex
		Coding Clinic: 2011, Q1, P7

▶ New　↻ Revised　✓ Reinstated　deleted Deleted　⊘ Not covered or valid by Medicare
✤ Special coverage instructions　* Carrier discretion　ⓑ Bill Part B MAC　Ⓓ Bill DME MAC

DRUGS OTHER THAN CHEMOTHERAPY DRUGS

* **J7313** Injection, fluocinolone acetonide, intravitreal implant (iluvien), 0.01 mg ⓑ Qp Qh — K2 K
   Other: Iluvien

* **J7314** Injection, fluocinolone acetonide, intravitreal implant (yutiq), 0.01 mg — K2 K

* **J7315** Mitomycin, ophthalmic, 0.2 mg ⓑ Qp Qh — N1 N
   Other: Mitosol, Mutamycin
   Coding Clinic: 2016, Q4, P8; 2014, Q2, P6

* **J7316** Injection, ocriplasmin, 0.125 mg ⓑ Qp Qh — K2 N
   Other: Jetrea

Hyaluronan

* **J7318** Hyaluronan or derivative, durolane, for intra-articular injection, 1 mg ⓑ — K
   Other: Morisu

* **J7320** Hyaluronan or derivitive, genvisc 850, for intra-articular injection, 1 mg ⓑ Qp Qh — K2 K

* **J7321** Hyaluronan or derivative, Hyalgan, Supartz or Visco-3, for intra-articular injection, per dose ⓑ Qp Qh — K2 N

   Therapeutic goal is to restore visco-elasticity of synovial hyaluronan, thereby decreasing pain, improving mobility and restoring natural protective functions of hyaluronan in joint

* **J7322** Hyaluronan or derivative, hymovis, for intra-articular injection, 1 mg ⓑ Qp Qh — K2 K

* **J7323** Hyaluronan or derivative, Euflexxa, for intra-articular injection, per dose ⓑ Qp Qh — K2 K

* **J7324** Hyaluronan or derivative, Orthovisc, for intra-articular injection, per dose ⓑ Qp Qh — K2 K

* **J7325** Hyaluronan or derivative, Synvisc or Synvisc-One, for intra-articular injection, 1 mg ⓑ Qp Qh — K2 K

* **J7326** Hyaluronan or derivative, Gel-One, for intra-articular injection, per dose ⓑ Qp Qh — K2 K
   Coding Clinic: 2012, Q1, P8

* **J7327** Hyaluronan or derivative, monovisc, for intra-articular injection, per dose ⓑ Qp Qh — K2 K

* **J7328** Hyaluronan or derivative, gelsyn-3, for intra-articular injection, 0.1 mg ⓑ Qp Qh — K2 N

* **J7329** Hyaluronan or derivative, trivisc, for intra-articular injection, 1 mg ⓑ — K

Miscellaneous Drugs

* **J7330** Autologous cultured chondrocytes, implant ⓑ Qp Qh — B
   Other: Carticel
   Coding Clinic: 2010, Q4, P3

* **J7331** Hyaluronan or derivative, synojoynt, for intra-articular injection, 1 mg ⓑ — N

* **J7332** Hyaluronan or derivative, triluron, for intra-articular injection, 1 mg ⓑ — K

* **J7336** Capsaicin 8% patch, per square centimeter ⓑ Qp Qh — K2 K
   Other: Qutenza

* **J7340** Carbidopa 5 mg/levodopa 20 mg enteral suspension, 100 ml ⓑ ⓑ Qp Qh — K2 K
   Other: Duopa

* **J7342** Instillation, ciprofloxacin otic suspension, 6 mg ⓑ Qp Qh — K2 N

○ **J7345** Aminolevulinic acid HCL for topical administration, 10% gel, 10 mg ⓑ — K2 K

* **J7351** Injection, bimatoprost, intracameral implant, 1 mcg — K2 K

* **J7352** Afamelanotide implant, 1 mg — K2 G

   J7353 Anacaulase-bcdb, 8.8% gel, 1 gram — G

   J7354 Cantharidin for topical administration, 0.7%, single unit dose applicator (3.2 mg) — G

   J7355 Injection, travoprost, intracameral implant, 1 mcg — G

▶ * **J7356** Foscarbidopa 0.25 mg/Foslevodopa 5 mg ⓑ ⓑ Qp Qh — N1 N

* **J7402** Mometasone furoate sinus implant, (sinuva), 10 mcg — K2 K

Immunosuppressive Drugs (Includes Non-injectibles)

○ **J7500** Azathioprine, oral, 50 mg ⓑ ⓑ Qp Qh — N1 N
   Other: Azasan, Imuran
   IOM: 100-02, 15, 50

○ **J7501** Azathioprine, parenteral, 100 mg ⓑ ⓑ Qp Qh — K2 K
   Other: Imuran
   IOM: 100-02, 15, 50

○ **J7502** Cyclosporine, oral, 100 mg ⓑ ⓑ Qp Qh — N1 N
   Other: Gengraf, Neoral, Sandimmune
   IOM: 100-02, 15, 50

○ **J7503** Tacrolimus, extended release, (Envarsus XR), oral, 0.25 mg ⓑ ⓑ Qp Qh — K2 N
   IOM: 100-02, 15, 50

 MIPS   Qp Quantity Physician   Qh Quantity Hospital   ♀ Female only
♂ Male only   A Age   ♿ DMEPOS   A2-Z3 ASC Payment Indicator   A-Y ASC Status Indicator   Coding Clinic

- **J7504** Lymphocyte immune globulin, antithymocyte globulin, equine, parenteral, 250 mg ⓑ Ⓑ Qp Qh K2 K
  Other: Atgam
  IOM: 100-02, 15, 50; 100-03, 2, 110.3

- **J7505** Muromonab-CD3, parenteral, 5 mg ⓑ Ⓑ Qp Qh K2 E2
  Other: Monoclonal antibodies (parenteral)
  IOM: 100-02, 15, 50

- **J7507** Tacrolimus, immediate release, oral, 1 mg ⓑ Ⓑ Qp Qh N1 N
  Other: Prograf
  IOM: 100-02, 15, 50

- **J7508** Tacrolimus, extended release, (Astagraf XL), oral, 0.1 mg ⓑ Ⓑ Qp Qh N1 N
  IOM: 100-02, 15, 50

- **J7509** Methylprednisolone oral, per 4 mg ⓑ Ⓑ Qp Qh N1 N
  Other: Medrol
  IOM: 100-02, 15, 50

- **J7510** Prednisolone oral, per 5 mg ⓑ Ⓑ Qp Qh N1 N
  Other: Delta-Cortef, Flo-Pred, Orapred
  IOM: 100-02, 15, 50

- ✱ **J7511** Lymphocyte immune globulin, antithymocyte globulin, rabbit, parenteral, 25 mg ⓑ Ⓑ Qp Qh K2 K
  Other: Thymoglobulin

- **J7512** Prednisone, immediate release or delayed release, oral, 1 mg ⓑ Ⓑ Qp Qh N1 N
  Other: Cyclosporine
  IOM: 100-02, 15, 50

- **J7513** Daclizumab, parenteral, 25 mg ⓑ Ⓑ Qp Qh E2
  Other: Zenapax
  IOM: 100-02, 15, 50

- ▶ ✱ **J7514** Injection, mycophenolate mofetil (myhibbin), oral, 100 mg ⓑ Ⓑ Qp Qh N1 N

- ✱ **J7515** Cyclosporine, oral, 25 mg ⓑ Ⓑ Qp Qh N1 N
  Other: Gengraf, Neoral, Sandimmune

- ✱ **J7516** Injection, cyclosporin, parenteral, 250 mg ⓑ Ⓑ Qp Qh N1 N
  Other: Sandimmune

- ✱ **J7517** Mycophenolate mofetil, oral, 250 mg ⓑ Ⓑ Qp Qh N1 N
  Other: CellCept

- **J7518** Mycophenolic acid, oral, 180 mg ⓑ Ⓑ Qp Qh N1 N
  Other: Myfortic
  IOM: 100-04, 4, 240; 100-4, 17, 80.3.1

- **J7519** Injection, mycophenolate mofetil, 10 mg ⓑ Ⓑ N1 N

- **J7520** Sirolimus, oral, 1 mg ⓑ Ⓑ Qp Qh N1 N
  Other: Rapamune
  IOM: 100-02, 15, 50

- ▶ ✱ **J7521** Tacrolimus, granules, oral suspension, 0.1 mg ⓑ Ⓑ Qp Qh N

- **J7525** Tacrolimus, parenteral, 5 mg ⓑ Ⓑ Qp Qh K2 K
  Other: Prograf
  IOM: 100-02, 15, 50

- **J7527** Everolimus, oral, 0.25 mg ⓑ Ⓑ Qp Qh N1 N
  Other: Zortress
  IOM: 100-02, 15, 50

- **J7599** Immunosuppressive drug, not otherwise classified ⓑ Ⓑ N1 N
  Bill on paper. Bill one unit. Identify drug and total dosage in "Remarks" field.
  IOM: 100-02, 15, 50

Inhalation Solutions

- ▶ ✱ **J7601** Ensifentrine, inhalation suspension, FDA approved final product, non-compounded, administered through DME, unit dose form, 3 mg ⓑ Ⓑ Qp Qh B

- ✱ **J7604** Acetylcysteine, inhalation solution, compounded product, administered through DME, unit dose form, per gram ⓑ Ⓑ Qp Qh M
  Other: Mucomyst (unit dose form), Mucosol

- ✱ **J7605** Arformoterol, inhalation solution, FDA approved final product, non-compounded, administered through DME, unit dose form, 15 mcg ⓑ Ⓑ Qp Qh M
  Maintenance treatment of bronchoconstriction in patients with chronic obstructive pulmonary disease (COPD).
  Other: Brovana

- ✱ **J7606** Formoterol fumarate, inhalation solution, FDA approved final product, non-compounded, administered through DME, unit dose form, 20 mcg ⓑ Ⓑ Qp Qh M
  Other: Perforomist

- ✱ **J7607** Levalbuterol, inhalation solution, compounded product, administered through DME, concentrated form, 0.5 mg ⓑ Ⓑ Qp Qh M

▶ New ⤺ Revised ✔ Reinstated ~~deleted~~ Deleted ⊘ Not covered or valid by Medicare
✪ Special coverage instructions ✱ Carrier discretion Ⓑ Bill Part B MAC ⓑ Bill DME MAC

DRUGS OTHER THAN CHEMOTHERAPY DRUGS

○ **J7608** Acetylcysteine, inhalation solution, FDA-approved final product, non-compounded, administered through DME, unit dose form, per gram ⓑ Ⓑ Qp Qh M

Other: Mucomyst, Mucosol

✱ **J7609** Albuterol, inhalation solution, compounded product, administered through DME, unit dose, 1 mg ⓑ Ⓑ Qp Qh M

Patient's home, medications—such as albuterol when administered through a nebulizer—are considered DME and are payable under Part B.

Other: Proventil, Ventolin, Xopenex

✱ **J7610** Albuterol, inhalation solution, compounded product, administered through DME, concentrated form, 1 mg ⓑ Ⓑ Qp Qh M

Other: Proventil, Ventolin, Xopenex

○ **J7611** Albuterol, inhalation solution, FDA-approved final product, non-compounded, administered through DME, concentrated form, 1 mg ⓑ Ⓑ Qp Qh M

Report once for each milligram administered. For example, 2 mg of concentrated albuterol (usually diluted with saline), reported with J7611×2.

Other: Proventil, Ventolin, Xopenex

○ **J7612** Levalbuterol, inhalation solution, FDA-approved final product, non-compounded, administered through DME, concentrated form, 0.5 mg ⓑ Ⓑ Qp Qh M

Other: Xopenex

○ **J7613** Albuterol, inhalation solution, FDA-approved final product, non-compounded, administered through DME, unit dose, 1 mg ⓑ Ⓑ Qp Qh M

Other: Accuneb, Proventil, Ventolin, Xopenex

○ **J7614** Levalbuterol, inhalation solution, FDA-approved final product, non-compounded, administered through DME, unit dose, 0.5 mg ⓑ Ⓑ Qp Qh M

Other: Xopenex

✱ **J7615** Levalbuterol, inhalation solution, compounded product, administered through DME, unit dose, 0.5 mg ⓑ Ⓑ Qp Qh M

○ **J7620** Albuterol, up to 2.5 mg and ipratropium bromide, up to 0.5 mg, FDA-approved final product, non-compounded, administered through DME ⓑ Ⓑ Qp Qh M

Other: DuoNeb

✱ **J7622** Beclomethasone, inhalation solution, compounded product, administered through DME, unit dose form, per mg ⓑ Ⓑ Qp Qh M

✱ **J7624** Betamethasone, inhalation solution, compounded product, administered through DME, unit dose form, per mg ⓑ Ⓑ Qp Qh M

✱ **J7626** Budesonide inhalation solution, FDA-approved final product, non-compounded, administered through DME, unit dose form, up to 0.5 mg ⓑ Ⓑ Qp Qh M

Other: Pulmicort

✱ **J7627** Budesonide, inhalation solution, compounded product, administered through DME, unit dose form, up to 0.5 mg ⓑ Ⓑ Qp Qh M

Other: Pulmicort Respules

○ **J7628** Bitolterol mesylate, inhalation solution, compounded product, administered through DME, concentrated form, per milligram ⓑ Ⓑ Qp Qh M

Other: Tornalate

○ **J7629** Bitolterol mesylate, inhalation solution, compounded product, administered through DME, unit dose form, per milligram ⓑ Ⓑ Qp Qh M

Other: Tornalate

○ **J7631** Cromolyn sodium, inhalation solution, FDA-approved final product, non-compounded, administered through DME, unit dose form, per 10 mg ⓑ Ⓑ Qp Qh M

Other: Intal

✱ **J7632** Cromolyn sodium, inhalation solution, compounded product, administered through DME, unit dose form, per 10 mg ⓑ Ⓑ Qp Qh M

Other: Intal

✱ **J7633** Budesonide, inhalation solution, FDA-approved final product, non-compounded, administered through DME, concentrated form, per 0.25 mg ⓑ Ⓑ Qp Qh M

Other: Pulmicort Respules

| ♦ MIPS | Qp Quantity Physician | Qh Quantity Hospital | ♀ Female only |
| ♂ Male only | A Age | ♿ DMEPOS | A2-Z3 ASC Payment Indicator | A-Y ASC Status Indicator | Coding Clinic |

* **J7634** Budesonide, inhalation solution, compounded product, administered through DME, concentrated form, per 0.25 mg Ⓑ Ⓑ Qp Qh M

　　Other: Pulmicort Respules

⊛ **J7635** Atropine, inhalation solution, compounded product, administered through DME, concentrated form, per milligram Ⓑ Ⓑ Qp Qh M

⊛ **J7636** Atropine, inhalation solution, compounded product, administered through DME, unit dose form, per milligram Ⓑ Ⓑ Qp Qh M

⊛ **J7637** Dexamethasone, inhalation solution, compounded product, administered through DME, concentrated form, per milligram Ⓑ Ⓑ Qp Qh M

⊛ **J7638** Dexamethasone, inhalation solution, compounded product, administered through DME, unit dose form, per milligram Ⓑ Ⓑ Qp Qh M

⊛ **J7639** Dornase alfa, inhalation solution, FDA-approved final product, non-compounded, administered through DME, unit dose form, per milligram Ⓑ Ⓑ Qp Qh M

　　Other: Pulmozyme

* **J7640** Formoterol, inhalation solution, compounded product, administered through DME, unit dose form, 12 mcg Ⓑ Ⓑ Qp Qh E1

* **J7641** Flunisolide, inhalation solution, compounded product, administered through DME, unit dose, per milligram Ⓑ Ⓑ Qp Qh M

⊛ **J7642** Glycopyrrolate, inhalation solution, compounded product, administered through DME, concentrated form, per milligram Ⓑ Ⓑ Qp Qh M

⊛ **J7643** Glycopyrrolate, inhalation solution, compounded product, administered through DME, unit dose form, per milligram Ⓑ Ⓑ Qp Qh M

⊛ **J7644** Ipratropium bromide, inhalation solution, FDA-approved final product, non-compounded, administered through DME, unit dose form, per milligram Ⓑ Ⓑ Qp Qh M

　　Other: Atrovent

* **J7645** Ipratropium bromide, inhalation solution, compounded product, administered through DME, unit dose form, per milligram Ⓑ Ⓑ Qp Qh M

　　Other: Atrovent

* **J7647** Isoetharine HCL, inhalation solution, compounded product, administered through DME, concentrated form, per milligram Ⓑ Ⓑ Qp Qh M

　　Other: Bronkosol

⊛ **J7648** Isoetharine HCL, inhalation solution, FDA-approved final product, non-compounded, administered through DME, concentrated form, per milligram Ⓑ Ⓑ Qp Qh M

　　Other: Bronkosol

⊛ **J7649** Isoetharine HCL, inhalation solution, FDA-approved final product, non-compounded, administered through DME, unit dose form, per milligram Ⓑ Ⓑ Qp Qh M

　　Other: Bronkosol

* **J7650** Isoetharine HCL, inhalation solution, compounded product, administered through DME, unit dose form, per milligram Ⓑ Ⓑ Qp Qh M

　　Other: Bronkosol

* **J7657** Isoproterenol HCL, inhalation solution, compounded product, administered through DME, concentrated form, per milligram Ⓑ Ⓑ Qp Qh M

　　Other: Isuprel

⊛ **J7658** Isoproterenol HCL inhalation solution, FDA-approved final product, non-compounded, administered through DME, concentrated form, per milligram Ⓑ Ⓑ Qp Qh M

　　Other: Isuprel

⊛ **J7659** Isoproterenol HCL, inhalation solution, FDA-approved final product, non-compounded, administered through DME, unit dose form, per milligram Ⓑ Ⓑ Qp Qh M

　　Other: Isuprel

* **J7660** Isoproterenol HCL, inhalation solution, compounded product, administered through DME, unit dose form, per milligram Ⓑ Ⓑ Qp Qh M

　　Other: Isuprel

* **J7665** Mannitol, administered through an inhaler, 5 mg Ⓑ Ⓑ Qp Qh N1 N

　　Other: Aridol

* **J7667** Metaproterenol sulfate, inhalation solution, compounded product, concentrated form, per 10 mg Ⓑ Ⓑ Qp Qh M

　　Other: Alupent, Metaprel

▶ New　↺ Revised　✓ Reinstated　~~deleted~~ Deleted　⊘ Not covered or valid by Medicare　⊛ Special coverage instructions　* Carrier discretion　Ⓑ Bill Part B MAC　Ⓑ Bill DME MAC

DRUGS OTHER THAN CHEMOTHERAPY DRUGS

- ⊛ **J7668** Metaproterenol sulfate, inhalation solution, FDA-approved final product, non-compounded, administered through DME, concentrated form, per 10 mg ⓑ Ⓑ Qp Qh M

  Other: Alupent, Metaprel

- ⊛ **J7669** Metaproterenol sulfate, inhalation solution, FDA-approved final product, non-compounded, administered through DME, unit dose form, per 10 mg ⓑ Ⓑ Qp Qh M

  Other: Alupent, Metaprel

- ✱ **J7670** Metaproterenol sulfate, inhalation solution, compounded product, administered through DME, unit dose form, per 10 mg ⓑ Ⓑ Qp Qh M

  Other: Alupent, Metaprel

- ✱ **J7674** Methacholine chloride administered as inhalation solution through a nebulizer, per 1 mg ⓑ Ⓑ Qp Qh N1 N

  Other: Provocholine

- ✱ **J7676** Pentamidine isethionate, inhalation solution, compounded product, administered through DME, unit dose form, per 300 mg ⓑ Ⓑ Qp Qh M

  Other: NebuPent, Pentam

- ✱ **J7677** Revefenacin inhalation solution, FDA-approved final product, non-compounded, administered through DME, 1 mcg ⓑ Ⓑ M

- ⊛ **J7680** Terbutaline sulfate, inhalation solution, compounded product, administered through DME, concentrated form, per milligram ⓑ Ⓑ Qp Qh M

  Other: Brethine

- ⊛ **J7681** Terbutaline sulfate, inhalation solution, compounded product, administered through DME, unit dose form, per milligram ⓑ Ⓑ Qp Qh M

  Other: Brethine

- ⊛ **J7682** Tobramycin, inhalation solution, FDA-approved final product, non-compounded unit dose form, administered through DME, per 300 mg ⓑ Ⓑ Qp Qh M

  Other: Bethkis, Kitabis PAK, Tobi

- ⊛ **J7683** Triamcinolone, inhalation solution, compounded product, administered through DME, concentrated form, per milligram ⓑ Ⓑ Qp Qh M

- ⊛ **J7684** Triamcinolone, inhalation solution, compounded product, administered through DME, unit dose form, per milligram ⓑ Ⓑ Qp Qh M

  Other: Triamcinolone acetonide

- ✱ **J7685** Tobramycin, inhalation solution, compounded product, administered through DME, unit dose form, per 300 mg ⓑ Ⓑ Qp Qh M

  Other: Tobi

- ✱ **J7686** Treprostinil, inhalation solution, FDA-approved final product, non-compounded, administered through DME, unit dose form, 1.74 mg ⓑ Ⓑ Qp Qh M

  Other: Tyvaso

Not Otherwise Classified/Specified

- ⊛ **J7699** NOC drugs, inhalation solution administered through DME ⓑ Ⓑ M

  Other: Gentamicin Sulfate

- ⊛ **J7799** NOC drugs, other than inhalation drugs, administered through DME ⓑ Ⓑ N1 N

  Bill on paper. Bill one unit and identify drug and total dosage in the "Remark" field.

  Other: Cuvitru, Epinephrine, Mannitol, Osmitrol, Phenylephrine, Resectisol, Sodium chloride

  IOM: 100-02, 15, 110.3

- ⊛ **J7999** Compounded drug, not otherwise classified ⓑ Ⓑ N1 N

  Coding Clinic: 2017, Q1, P1-2; 2016, Q4, P8

- ⊛ **J8498** Antiemetic drug, rectal/suppository, not otherwise specified Ⓑ B

  Other: Compazine, Compro, Phenadoz, Phenergan, Prochlorperazine, Promethazine, Promethegan

  Medicare Statute 1861(s)2t

- ⊘ **J8499** Prescription drug, oral, non chemotherapeutic, NOS Ⓑ E1

  Other: Acyclovir, Calcitrol, Cromolyn Sodium, OFEV, Valganciclovir HCL, Zovirax

  IOM: 100-02, 15, 50

  Coding Clinic: 2013, Q2, P4

Oral Anti-Cancer Drugs

- ⊛ **J8501** Aprepitant, oral, 5 mg ⓑ Qp Qh K2 N

  Other: Emend

- ⊛ **J8510** Busulfan; oral, 2 mg Ⓑ Qp Qh N1 K

  Other: Myleran

  IOM: 100-02, 15, 50; 100-04, 4, 240; 100-04, 17, 80.1.1

MIPS | Qp Quantity Physician | Qh Quantity Hospital | ♀ Female only
♂ Male only | A Age | ♿ DMEPOS | A2-Z3 ASC Payment Indicator | A-Y ASC Status Indicator | Coding Clinic

303

2026 HCPCS LEVEL II NATIONAL CODES

⊘ **J8515** Cabergoline, oral, 0.25 mg Ⓑ   E1
     IOM: 100-02, 15, 50; 100-04, 4, 240

✺ **J8522** Capecitabine, oral, 50 mg Ⓑ   K

✺ **J8530** Cyclophosphamide; oral, 25 mg Ⓑ Qp Qh   N1 N
     Other: Cytoxan
     IOM: 100-02, 15, 50; 100-04, 4, 240; 100-04, 17, 80.1.1

✺ **J8540** Dexamethasone, oral, 0.25 mg Ⓑ Qp Qh   N1 N
     Other: Decadron, Dexone, Dexpak, Locort
     Medicare Statute 1861(s)2t

✺ **J8541** Dexamethasone (hemady), oral, 0.25 mg Ⓑ   N

✺ **J8560** Etoposide; oral, 50 mg Ⓑ Qp Qh   K2 N
     Other: VePesid
     IOM: 100-02, 15, 50; 100-04, 4, 230.1; 100-04, 4, 240; 100-04, 17, 80.1.1

✱ **J8562** Fludarabine phosphate, oral, 10 mg Ⓑ Qp Qh   E2
     Other: Fludara, Oforta
     Coding Clinic: 2011, Q1, P9

✺ **J8565** Gefitinib, oral, 250 mg Ⓑ   E2
     Other: Iressa

✺ **J8597** Antiemetic drug, oral, not otherwise specified Ⓑ   N1 N
     Medicare Statute 1861(s)2t

✺ **J8600** Melphalan; oral, 2 mg Ⓑ Qp Qh   N1 E2
     Other: Alkeran
     IOM: 100-02, 15, 50; 100-04, 4, 240; 100-04, 17, 80.1.1

✺ **J8610** Methotrexate; oral, 2.5 mg Ⓑ Qp Qh   N1 N
     Other: Rheumatrex, Trexall
     IOM: 100-02, 15, 50; 100-04, 4, 240; 100-04, 17, 80.1.1

     J8611 Methotrexate (jylamvo), oral, 2.5 mg

     J8612 Methotrexate (xatmep), oral, 2.5 mg

✱ **J8650** Nabilone, oral, 1 mg Ⓑ Qp Qh   E2

✺ **J8655** Netupitant 300 mg and palonosetron 0.5 mg, oral Ⓑ Qp Qh   K2 K
     Other: Akynzeo
     Coding Clinic: 2015, Q4, P4

✺ **J8670** Rolapitant, oral, 1 mg Qp Qh   K2 K
     Other: Varubi

✺ **J8700** Temozolomide, oral, 5 mg Ⓑ Qp Qh   N1 N
     Other: Temodar
     IOM: 100-02, 15, 50; 100-04, 4, 240

✱ **J8705** Topotecan, oral, 0.25 mg Ⓑ Qp Qh   K2 N
     Treatment for ovarian and lung cancers, etc. Report J9350 (Topotecan, 4 mg) for intravenous version
     Other: Hycamtin

✺ **J8999** Prescription drug, oral, chemotherapeutic, NOS Ⓑ   B
     Other: Anastrozole, Arimidex, Aromasin, Droxia, Erivedge, Flutamide, Gleevec, Hydrea, Hydroxyurea, Leukeran, Matulane, Megestrol Acetate, Mercaptopurine, Nolvadex, Tamoxifen Citrate
     IOM: 100-02, 15, 50; 100-04, 4, 250; 100-04, 17, 80.1.1; 100-04, 17, 80.1.2

CHEMOTHERAPY DRUGS (J9000-J9999)

NOTE: These codes cover the cost of the chemotherapy drug only, not to include the administration

✺ **J9000** Injection, doxorubicin hydrochloride, 10 mg Ⓑ Ⓑ Qp Qh   N1 N
     Other: Adriamycin, Rubex
     IOM: 100-02, 15, 50
     Coding Clinic: 2007, Q4, P5

▶ **J9011** Injection, datopotamab deruxtecan-dlnk, 1 mg   G

✺ **J9015** Injection, aldesleukin, per single use vial Ⓑ Ⓑ Qp Qh   K2 K
     Other: Proleukin
     IOM: 100-02, 15, 50

✱ **J9017** Injection, arsenic trioxide, 1 mg Ⓑ Qp Qh   K2 K
     Other: Trisenox

✺ **J9019** Injection, asparaginase (Erwinaze), 1,000 IU Ⓑ Qp Qh   K2 E2
     IOM: 100-02, 15, 50

✺ **J9020** Injection, asparaginase, not otherwise specified 10,000 units Ⓑ Ⓑ Qp Qh   N1 E2
     IOM: 100-02, 15, 50

     J9021 Injection, asparaginase, recombinant, (rylaze), 0.1 mg Ⓑ   K2 K

✱ **J9022** Injection, atezolizumab, 10 mg Ⓑ   K2 K

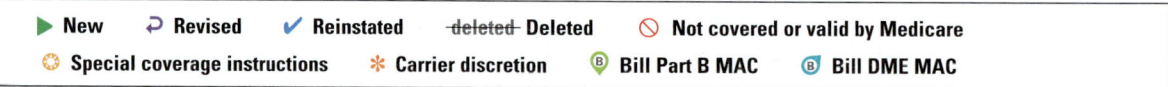

▶ New   ⟲ Revised   ✓ Reinstated   ~~deleted~~ Deleted   ⊘ Not covered or valid by Medicare
✺ Special coverage instructions   ✱ Carrier discretion   Ⓑ Bill Part B MAC   Ⓑ Bill DME MAC

CHEMOTHERAPY DRUGS

✱ **J9023**	Injection, avelumab, 10 mg ⓑ Ⓑ	K2 K
▶ ✱ **J9024**	Injection, atezolizumab, 5 mg and hyaluronidase-tqjs	K2 K
✱ **J9025**	Injection, azacitidine, 1 mg ⓑ Ⓑ Qp Qh	K2 N
▶ ✱ **J9026**	Injection, tarlatamab-dlle, 1 mg	G
✱ **J9027**	Injection, clofarabine, 1 mg ⓑ Ⓑ Qp Qh	K2 K
	Other: Clolar	
▶ **J9028**	Injection, nogapendekin alfa inbakicept-pmln, for intravesical use, 1 mcg	G
J9029	Intravesical instillation, nadofaragene firadenovec-vncg, per therapeutic dose ⓑ Ⓑ	G
⊙ **J9030**	BCG live intravesical instillation, 1 mg ⓑ Ⓑ	K2 N
✱ **J9032**	Injection, belinostat, 10 mg ⓑ Ⓑ Qp Qh	K2 K
	Other: Beleodaq	
↪ ✱ **J9033**	Injection, bendamustine hydrochloride, 1 mg ⓑ Ⓑ Qp Qh	K2 K
	Treatment for form of non-Hodgkin's lymphoma; standard administration time is as an intravenous infusion over 30 minutes	
	Other: Treanda	
✱ **J9034**	Injection, bendamustine HCL (bendeka), 1 mg Qp Qh	K2 K
	Coding Clinic: 2017, Q1, P10	
✱ **J9035**	Injection, bevacizumab, 10 mg ⓑ Ⓑ Qp Qh	K2 K
	For malignant neoplasm of breast, considered J9207.	
	Other: Avastin	
	Coding Clinic: 2013, Q3, P9, Q2, P8	
✱ **J9036**	Injection, bendamustine hydrochloride, (belrapzo/bendamustine), 1 mg ⓑ Ⓑ	K2 K
~~J9037~~	~~Injection, belantamab mafodontin-blmf, 0.5 mg~~	
▶ **J9038**	Injection, axatilimab-csfr, 0.1 mg	G
✱ **J9039**	Injection, blinatumomab, 1 mcg ⓑ Ⓑ Qp Qh	K2 K
	Other: Blincyto	
⊙ **J9040**	Injection, bleomycin sulfate, 15 units ⓑ Ⓑ Qp Qh	N1 N
	Other: Blenoxane	
	IOM: 100-02, 15, 50	
✱ **J9041**	Injection, bortezomib, 0.1 mg ⓑ Ⓑ Qp Qh	K2 N
	Other: Velcade	
✱ **J9042**	Injection, brentuximab vedotin, 1 mg ⓑ Ⓑ Qp Qh	K2 K
	Other: Adcetris	
✱ **J9043**	Injection, cabazitaxel, 1 mg ⓑ Ⓑ Qp Qh	K2 K
	Other: Jevtana	
	Coding Clinic: 2012, Q1, P9	
⊙ **J9045**	Injection, carboplatin, 50 mg ⓑ Ⓑ Qp Qh	N1 N
	Other: Paraplatin	
	IOM: 100-02, 15, 50	
J9046	Injection, bortezomib (Dr. Reddy's), not therapeutically equivalent to J9041, 0.1 mg ⓑ Ⓑ	K2 K
✱ **J9047**	Injection, carfilzomib, 1 mg ⓑ Ⓑ Qp Qh	K2 K
	Other: Kyprolis	
J9048	Injection, bortezomib (fresenius kabi), not therapeutically equivalent to J9041, 0.1 mg ⓑ Ⓑ	K2 K
J9049	Injection, bortezomib (hospira), not therapeutically equivalent to J9041, 0.1 mg ⓑ Ⓑ	K2 N
⊙ **J9050**	Injection, carmustine, 100 mg ⓑ Ⓑ Qp Qh	K2 K
	Other: BiCNU	
	IOM: 100-02, 15, 50	
J9051	Injection, bortezomib (maia), not therapeutically equivalent to J9041, 0.1 mg ⓑ Ⓑ	K2 K
J9052	Injection, carmustine (accord), not therapeutically equivalent to J9050, 100 mg ⓑ Ⓑ	K2 K
▶ **J9054**	Injection, bortezomib (boruzu), 0.1 mg	G
✱ **J9055**	Injection, cetuximab, 10 mg ⓑ Ⓑ Qp Qh	K2 K
	Other: Erbitux	
J9056	Injection, bendamustine hydrochloride (vivimusta), 1 mg ⓑ Ⓑ	
✱ **J9057**	Injection, copanlisib, 1 mg ⓑ Ⓑ	K
	Other: Aliqopa	
~~J9058~~	~~Injection, bendamustine hydrochloride (apotex), 1 mg~~	
~~J9059~~	~~Injection, bendamustine hydrochloride (baxter), 1 mg~~	

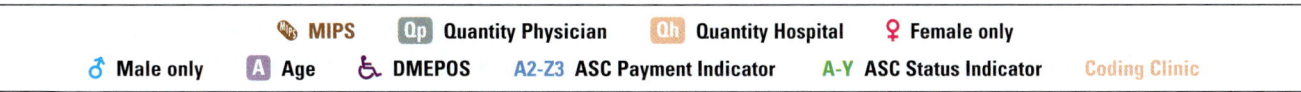

 MIPS   Qp Quantity Physician   Qh Quantity Hospital   ♀ Female only
♂ Male only   A Age   ♿ DMEPOS   A2-Z3 ASC Payment Indicator   A-Y ASC Status Indicator   *Coding Clinic*

Code	Description	Status
✺ **J9060**	Injection, cisplatin, powder or solution, 10 mg ⓑ Ⓑ Qp Qh	N1 N
	Other: Plantinol AQ	
	IOM: 100-02, 15, 50	
	Coding Clinic: 2013, Q2, P6; 2011, Q1, P8	
✱ **J9061**	Injection, amivantamab-vmjw, 2 mg ⓑ Ⓑ	K2 K
J9063	Injection, mirvetuximab soravtansine-gynx, 1 mg ⓑ Ⓑ	G
J9064	Injection, cabazitaxel (sandoz), not therapeutically equivalent to J9043, 1 mg ⓑ Ⓑ	K2 E2
✺ **J9065**	Injection, cladribine, per 1 mg ⓑ Ⓑ Qp Qh	K2 K
	Other: Leustatin	
	IOM: 100-02, 15, 50	
⟲ **J9072**	Injection, cyclophosphamide, (frindovyx), 5 mg ⓑ Ⓑ	
⟲ **J9073**	Injection, cyclophosphamide (Dr. Reddy's), 5 mg ⓑ Ⓑ	K
J9074	Injection, cyclophosphamide (sandoz), 5 mg ⓑ Ⓑ	K
J9075	Injection, cyclophosphamide, not otherwise specified, 5 mg ⓑ Ⓑ	K
▶ **J9076**	Injection, cyclophosphamide, (baxter), 5 mg ⓑ Ⓑ	K
✱ **J9098**	Injection, cytarabine liposome, 10 mg ⓑ Ⓑ Qp Qh	K2 E2
	Other: DepoCyt	
✺ **J9100**	Injection, cytarabine, 100 mg ⓑ Ⓑ Qp Qh	N1 N
	Other: Cytosar-U	
	IOM: 100-02, 15, 50	
	Coding Clinic: 2011, Q1, P9	
✱ **J9118**	Injection, calaspargase pegol-mknl, 10 units ⓑ	E2
✱ **J9119**	Injection, cemiplimab-rwlc, 1 mg ⓑ Ⓑ	K2 K
✺ **J9120**	Injection, dactinomycin, 0.5 mg ⓑ Ⓑ Qp Qh	K2 K
	Other: Cosmegen	
	IOM: 100-02, 15, 50	
✺ **J9130**	Dacarbazine, 100 mg ⓑ Ⓑ Qp Qh	N1 N
	Other: DTIC-Dome	
	IOM: 100-02, 15, 50	
	Coding Clinic: 2011, Q1, P9	
✺ **J9144**	Injection, daratumumab, 10 mg and hyaluronidase-fihj ⓑ Ⓑ	K2 K
✺ **J9145**	Injection, daratumumab, 10 mg Qp Qh	K2 K
	Other: Darzalex	
	IOM: 100-02, 15, 50	
✺ **J9150**	Injection, daunorubicin, 10 mg ⓑ Ⓑ Qp Qh	K2 K
	Other: Cerubidine	
	IOM: 100-02, 15, 50	
✺ **J9151**	Injection, daunorubicin citrate, liposomal formulation, 10 mg ⓑ Ⓑ Qp Qh	E2
	Other: Daunoxome	
	IOM: 100-02, 15, 50	
✱ **J9153**	njection, liposomal, 1 mg daunorubicin and 2.27 mg cytarabine ⓑ	K
	Other: Vyxeos	
✱ **J9155**	Injection, degarelix, 1 mg ⓑ Qp Qh	K2 K
	Report 1 unit for every 1 mg.	
	Other: Firmagon	
▶ **J9161**	Injection, denileukin diftitox-cxdl, 1 mcg	E2
✺ **J9165**	Injection, diethylstilbestrol diphosphate, 250 mg ⓑ Ⓑ Qp Qh	E2
	Other: Stilphostrol	
	IOM: 100-02, 15, 50	
✺ **J9171**	Injection, docetaxel, 1 mg ⓑ Ⓑ Qp Qh	K2 N
	Report 1 unit for every 1 mg.	
	Other: Docefrez, Taxotere	
	IOM: 100-02, 15, 50	
	Coding Clinic: 2012, Q1, P9	
J9172	Injection, docetaxel (docivyx), 1 mg ⓑ Ⓑ	G
✱ **J9173**	Injection, durvalumab, 10 mg ⓑ Ⓑ	K
	Other: Imfinzi	
▶ **J9174**	Docetaxel (beizray), 1 mg	G
✺ **J9175**	Injection, Elliott's B solution, 1 ml ⓑ Ⓑ Qp Qh	N1 N
	IOM: 100-02, 15, 50	
✱ **J9176**	Injection, elotuzumab, 1 mg Qp Qh	K2 K
	Other: Empliciti	
✱ **J9177**	Injection, enfortumab vedotin-ejfv, 0.25 mg ⓑ Ⓑ	K2 K
✱ **J9178**	Injection, epirubicin HCL, 2 mg ⓑ Ⓑ Qp Qh	N1 N
	Other: Ellence	

▶ New ⟲ Revised ✓ Reinstated ~~deleted~~ Deleted ⊘ Not covered or valid by Medicare
✺ Special coverage instructions ✱ Carrier discretion Ⓑ Bill Part B MAC Ⓑ Bill DME MAC

CHEMOTHERAPY DRUGS

* **J9179** Injection, eribulin mesylate, 0.1 mg ⓑ Qp Qh — K2 K
  Other: Halaven

○ **J9181** Injection, etoposide, 10 mg ⓑ ⓑ Qp Qh — N1 N
  Other: Etopophos, Toposar

○ **J9185** Injection, fludarabine phosphate, 50 mg ⓑ ⓑ Qp Qh — K2 K
  Other: Fludara
  IOM: 100-02, 15, 50

○ **J9190** Injection, fluorouracil, 500 mg ⓑ ⓑ Qp Qh — N1 N
  Other: Adrucil
  IOM: 100-02, 15, 50

J9196 Injection, gemcitabine hydrochloride (accord), not therapeutically equivalent to J9201, 200 mg ⓑ ⓑ — N1 N

○ **J9198** Injection, gemcitabine hydrochloride, (infugem), 100 mg ⓑ ⓑ — K2 K

○ **J9200** Injection, floxuridine, 500 mg ⓑ ⓑ Qp Qh — N1 K
  Other: FUDR
  IOM: 100-02, 15, 50

○ **J9201** Injection, gemcitabine hydrochloride, not otherwise specified, 200 mg ⓑ ⓑ Qp Qh — N1 N
  Other: Gemzar
  IOM: 100-02, 15, 50

○ **J9202** Goserelin acetate implant, per 3.6 mg ⓑ ⓑ Qp Qh — K2 K
  Other: Zoladex
  IOM: 100-02, 15, 50

* **J9203** Injection, gemtuzumab ozogamicin, 0.1 mg ⓑ ⓑ — K2 K

* **J9204** Injection, mogamulizumab-kpkc, 1 mg ⓑ ⓑ — K2 K

○ **J9205** Injection, irinotecan liposome, 1 mg Qp Qh — K2 K
  Other: ONIVYDE
  IOM: 100-02, 15, 50

○ **J9206** Injection, irinotecan, 20 mg ⓑ ⓑ Qp Qh — N1 N
  Other: Camptosar
  IOM: 100-02, 15, 50

* **J9207** Injection, ixabepilone, 1 mg ⓑ ⓑ Qp Qh — K2 K
  Other: Ixempra Kit

○ **J9208** Injection, ifosfamide, 1 gm ⓑ ⓑ Qp Qh — N1 N
  Other: Ifex
  IOM: 100-02, 15, 50

○ **J9209** Injection, mesna, 200 mg ⓑ ⓑ Qp Qh — N1 N
  Other: Mesnex
  IOM: 100-02, 15, 50

* **J9210** Injection, emapalumab-lzsg, 1 mg ⓑ ⓑ — K2 K

○ **J9211** Injection, idarubicin hydrochloride, 5 mg ⓑ ⓑ Qp Qh — K2 N
  Other: Idamycin PFS
  IOM: 100-02, 15, 50

○ **J9212** Injection, interferon alfacon-1, recombinant, 1 mcg ⓑ ⓑ Qp Qh — N1 E2
  Other: Amgen, Infergen
  IOM: 100-02, 15, 50

○ **J9213** Injection, interferon, alfa-2a, recombinant, 3 million units ⓑ ⓑ Qp Qh — N1 E2
  Other: Roferon-A
  IOM: 100-02, 15, 50

○ **J9214** Injection, interferon, alfa-2b, recombinant, 1 million units ⓑ ⓑ Qp Qh — K2 N
  Other: Intron-A
  IOM: 100-02, 15, 50

○ **J9215** Injection, interferon, alfa-n3 (human leukocyte derived), 250,000 IU ⓑ ⓑ Qp Qh — E2
  Other: Alferon N
  IOM: 100-02, 15, 50

○ **J9216** Injection, interferon, gamma-1B, 3 million units ⓑ ⓑ Qp Qh — K2 E2
  Other: Actimmune
  IOM: 100-02, 15, 50

○ **J9217** Leuprolide acetate (for depot suspension), 7.5 mg ⓑ ⓑ Qp Qh — K2 K
  Other: Eligard, Lupron Depot
  IOM: 100-02, 15, 50
  Coding Clinic: 2019, Q2, P11; 2015, Q3, P3

○ **J9218** Leuprolide acetate, per 1 mg ⓑ ⓑ Qp Qh — K2 N
  Other: Lupron
  IOM: 100-02, 15, 50
  Coding Clinic: 2019, Q2, P11; 2015, Q3, P3

○ **J9219** Leuprolide acetate implant, 65 mg ⓑ ⓑ Qp Qh — E2
  Other: Viadur
  IOM: 100-02, 15, 50

 MIPS   Qp Quantity Physician   Qh Quantity Hospital   ♀ Female only
♂ Male only   A Age   ♿ DMEPOS   A2-Z3 ASC Payment Indicator   A-Y ASC Status Indicator   Coding Clinic

Code	Description	Status
▶ ⊛ J9220	Indigotindisulfonate sodium, 1 mg ⒷⒷ	G
⊛ J9223	Injection, lurbinectedin, 0.1 mg Ⓑ	K2 K
⊛ J9225	Histrelin implant (Vantas), 50 mg ⒷⒷ Qp Qh	K2 N
	IOM: 100-02, 15, 50	
⊛ J9226	Histrelin implant (Supprelin LA), 50 mg ⒷⒷ Qp Qh	K2 K
	Other: Vantas	
	IOM: 100-02, 15, 50	
⊛ J9227	Injection, isatuximab-irfc, 10 mg ⒷⒷ	K2 K
* J9228	Injection, ipilimumab, 1 mg ⒷⒷ Qp Qh	K2 K
	Other: Yervoy	
	Coding Clinic: 2012, Q1, P9	
* J9229	Injection, inotuzumab ozogamicin, 0.1 mg ⒷⒷ	K
	Other: Besponsa	
⊛ J9230	Injection, mechlorethamine hydrochloride, (nitrogen mustard), 10 mg ⒷⒷ Qp Qh	K2 N
	Other: Mustargen	
	IOM: 100-02, 15, 50	
⊛ J9245	Injection, melphalan hydrochloride, not otherwise specified, 50 mg ⒷⒷ Qp Qh	K2 K
⊛ J9246	Injection, melphalan (evomela), 1 mg ⒷⒷ	K2 K
	Other: Alkeran, Evomela	
	IOM: 100-02, 15, 50	
~~J9247~~	~~Injection, melphalan flufenamide, 1 mg~~	
⊛ J9248	Injection, melphalan (hepzato), 1 mg ⒷⒷ	K2 G
⊛ J9249	Injection, melphalan (apotex), 1 mg ⒷⒷ	K2 E2
	Coding Clinic: 2025, Q3, P16	
J9255	Injection, methotrexate (accord), not therapeutically equivalent to J9260, 50 mg ⒷⒷ	E2
~~J9259~~	~~Injection, paclitaxel protein-bound particles (american regent), not therapeutically equivalent to J9264, 1 mg~~	
⊛ J9260	Injection, methotrexate sodium, 50 mg ⒷⒷ Qp Qh	N1 N
	Other: Folex	
	IOM: 100-02, 15, 50	
* J9261	Injection, nelarabine, 50 mg Ⓑ Qp Qh	K2 K
	Other: Arranon	
* J9262	Injection, omacetaxine mepesuccinate, 0.01 mg ⒷⒷ Qp Qh	K2 K
	Other: Synribo	
* J9263	Injection, oxaliplatin, 0.5 mg ⒷⒷ Qp Qh	N1 N
	Eloxatin, platinum-based anticancer drug that destroys cancer cells	
	Other: Eloxatin	
	Coding Clinic: 2009, Q1, P10	
* J9264	Injection, paclitaxel protein-bound particles, 1 mg ⒷⒷ	K2 K
	Other: Abraxane	
⊛ J9266	Injection, pegaspargase, per single dose vial ⒷⒷ Qp Qh	K2 K
	Other: Oncaspar	
	IOM: 100-02, 15, 50	
⊛ J9267	Injection, paclitaxel, 1 mg ⒷⒷ Qp Qh	N1 N
	Other: Taxol	
⊛ J9268	Injection, pentostatin, 10 mg ⒷⒷ Qp Qh	K2 K
	Other: Nipent	
	IOM: 100-02, 15, 50	
* J9269	Injection, tagraxofusp-erzs, 10 mcg	K2 K
⊛ J9270	Injection, plicamycin, 2.5 mg ⒷⒷ Qp Qh	N1 E2
	Other: Mithracin	
	IOM: 100-02, 15, 50	
* J9271	Injection, pembrolizumab, 1 mg ⒷⒷ Qp Qh	K2 K
	Other: Keytruda	
J9272	Injection, dostarlimab-gxly, 10 mg ⒷⒷ	K2 K
J9274	Injection, tebentafusp-tebn, 1 mcg Ⓑ	K2 G
▶ J9275	Cosibelimab-ipdl, 2 mg	E2
▶ J9276	Zanidatamab-hrii, 2 mg	G
⊛ J9280	Injection, mitomycin, 5 mg ⒷⒷ Qp Qh	K2 K
	Other: Mitosol, Mutamycin	
	IOM: 100-02, 15, 50	
	Coding Clinic: 2016, Q4, P8; 2014, Q2, P6; 2011, Q1, P9	
⊛ J9281	Mitomycin pyelocalyceal instillation, 1 mg Ⓑ	K2 K

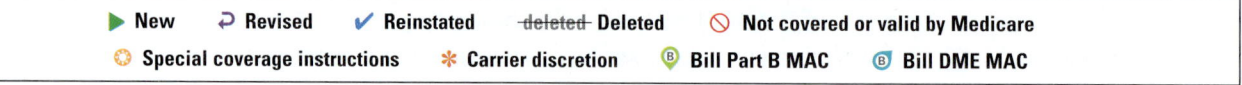

▶ New   ↻ Revised   ✓ Reinstated   ~~deleted~~ Deleted   ⊘ Not covered or valid by Medicare
⊛ Special coverage instructions   * Carrier discretion   Ⓑ Bill Part B MAC   Ⓑ Bill DME MAC

CHEMOTHERAPY DRUGS

✴ **J9285**	Injection, olaratumab, 10 mg Ⓑ Ⓑ	K2 E2
J9286	Injection, glofitamab-gxbm, 2.5 mg Ⓑ Ⓑ	G
▶ ✴ **J9289**	Nivolumab, 2 mg and hyaluronidase-nvhy Ⓑ Ⓑ	G
▶ ✴ **J9292**	Injection, pemetrexed (dipotassium), 10 mg Ⓑ Ⓑ	G
✴ **J9293**	Injection, mitoxantrone hydrochloride, per 5 mg Ⓑ Qp Qh	K2 K
	Other: Novantrone	
	IOM: 100-02, 15, 50	
J9294	Injection, pemetrexed (hospira), not therapeutically equivalent to J9305, 10 mg Ⓑ Ⓑ	K2 K
✴ **J9295**	Injection, necitumumab, 1 mg Ⓑ Ⓑ Qp Qh	K2 K
	Other: Portrazza	
J9296	Injection, pemetrexed (accord), not therapeutically equivalent to J9305, 10 mg Ⓑ Ⓑ	K2 K
J9297	Injection, pemetrexed (sandoz), not therapeutically equivalent to J9305, 10 mg Ⓑ Ⓑ	K2 N
J9298	Injection, nivolumab and relatlimab-rmbw, 3 mg/1 mg Ⓑ Ⓑ	K2 G
✴ **J9299**	Injection, nivolumab, 1 mg Ⓑ Ⓑ Qp Qh	K2 K
	Other: Opdivo	
✴ **J9301**	Injection, obinutuzumab, 10 mg Ⓑ Ⓑ Qp Qh	K2 K
	Other: Gazyva	
✴ **J9302**	Injection, ofatumumab, 10 mg Ⓑ Ⓑ Qp Qh	K2 K
	Other: Arzerra	
	Coding Clinic: 2011, Q1, P7	
✴ **J9303**	Injection, panitumumab, not otherwise specified, 10 mg Ⓑ Ⓑ Qp Qh	K2 K
	Other: Vectibix	
✴ **J9304**	Injection, pemetrexed (pemfexy), 10 mg Ⓑ Ⓑ	K5 G
✴ **J9305**	Injection, pemetrexed, 10 mg Ⓑ Ⓑ Qp Qh	K2 K
	Other: Alimta	
✴ **J9306**	Injection, pertuzumab, 1 mg Ⓑ Ⓑ Qp Qh	K2 K
	Other: Perjeta	
✴ **J9307**	Injection, pralatrexate, 1 mg Ⓑ Ⓑ Qp Qh	K2 K
	Other: Folotyn	
	Coding Clinic: 2011, Q1, P7	
✴ **J9308**	Injection, ramucirumab, 5 mg Ⓑ Ⓑ Qp Qh	K2 K
	Other: Cyramza	
✴ **J9309**	Injection, polatuzumab vedotin-piiq, 1 mg Ⓑ Ⓑ	K2 K
✴ **J9311**	Injection, rituximab 10 mg and hyaluronidase Ⓑ Ⓑ	K
	Other: Rituxan	
✴ **J9312**	Injection, rituximab, 10 mg Ⓑ Ⓑ	K
	Other: Rituxan	
✴ **J9313**	Injection, moxetumomab pasudotox-tdfk, 0.01 mg Ⓑ Ⓑ	K2 K
J9314	Injection, pemetrexed (teva), not therapeutically equivalent to J9305, 10 mg Ⓑ Ⓑ	K2 K
✴ **J9316**	Injection, pertuzumab, trastuzumab, and hyaluronidase-zzxf, per 10 mg Ⓑ Ⓑ	K2 K
✴ **J9317**	Injection, sacituzumab govitecan-hziy, 2.5 mg Ⓑ Ⓑ	K2 K
✴ **J9318**	Injection, romidepsin, non-lyophilized, 0.1 mg Ⓑ Ⓑ	K2 K
✴ **J9319**	Injection, romidepsin, lyophilized, 0.1 mg Ⓑ Ⓑ	K2 K
✴ **J9320**	Injection, streptozocin, 1 gram Ⓑ Ⓑ Qp Qh	K2 N
	Other: Zanosar	
	IOM: 100-02, 15, 50	
J9321	Injection, epcoritamab-bysp, 0.16 mg Ⓑ Ⓑ	G
J9322	Injection, pemetrexed (bluepoint), not therapeutically equivalent to J9305, 10 mg Ⓑ Ⓑ	K2 E2
J9323	Injection, pemetrexed ditromethamine, 10 mg Ⓑ	K
J9324	Injection, pemetrexed (pemrydi rtu), 10 mg Ⓑ Ⓑ	G
✴ **J9325**	Injection, talimogene laherparepvec, per 1 million plaque forming units Qp Qh	K2 K
	Other: Imlygic	
	Coding Clinic: 2019, Q2, P12	
✴ **J9328**	Injection, temozolomide, 1 mg Ⓑ Ⓑ Qp Qh	K2 K
	Intravenous formulation, not for oral administration	
	Other: Temodar	
J9329	Injection, tislelizumab-jsgr, 1 mg Ⓑ Ⓑ	G

Code	Description	Status
* J9330	Injection, temsirolimus, 1 mg	K2 K
	Treatment for advanced renal cell carcinoma; standard administration is intravenous infusion greater than 30-60 minutes	
	Other: Torisel	
J9331	Injection, sirolimus protein-bound particles, 1 mg	K2 G
J9332	Injection, efgartigimod alfa-fcab, 2mg	K2 G
J9333	Injection, rozanolixizumab-noli, 1 mg	G
J9334	Injection, efgartigimod alfa, 2 mg and hyaluronidase-qvfc	K
~~J9340~~	~~Injection, thiotepa, 15 mg~~	
▶ J9341	Thiotepa (tepylute), 1 mg	E2
▶ J9342	Thiotepa, not otherwise specified, 1 mg	K
J9345	Injection, retifanlimab-dlwr, 1 mg	G
J9347	Injection, tremelimumab-actl, 1 mg	G
* J9348	Injection, naxitamab-gqgk, 1 mg	K2 K
* J9349	Injection, tafasitamab-cxix, 2 mg	K2 K
J9350	Injection, mosunetuzumab-axgb, 1 mg	G
* J9351	Injection, topotecan, 0.1 mg	N1 N
	Other: Hycamtin	
	Coding Clinic: 2011, Q1, P9	
* J9352	Injection, trabectedin, 0.1 mg	K2 K
	Other: Yondelis	
* J9353	Injection, margetuximab-cmkb, 5 mg	K2 K
* J9354	Injection, ado-trastuzumab emtansine, 1 mg	K2 K
	Other: Kadcyla	
* J9355	Injection, trastuzumab, excludes biosimilar, 10 mg	K2 K
	Other: Herceptin	
* J9356	Injection, trastuzumab, 10 mg and hyaluronidase-oysk	K2 K
J9357	Injection, valrubicin, intravesical, 200 mg	K2 K
	Other: Valstar	
	IOM: 100-02, 15, 50	
J9358	Injection, fam-trastuzumab deruxtecan-nxki, 1 mg	K2 K
J9360	Injection, vinblastine sulfate, 1 mg	N1 K
	Other: Alkaban-AQ, Velban, Velsar	
	IOM: 100-02, 15, 50	
J9361	Injection, efbemalenograstim alfa-vuxw, 0.5 mg	E2
J9370	Vincristine sulfate, 1 mg	N1 N
	Other: Oncovin, Vincasar PFS	
	IOM: 100-02, 15, 50	
	Coding Clinic: 2011, Q1, P9	
J9376	Injection, pozelimab-bbfg, 1 mg	E2
J9380	Injection, teclistamab-cqyv, 0.5 mg	G
J9381	Injection, teplizumab-mzwv, 5 mcg	G
▶ J9382	Zenocutuzumab-zbco, 1 mg	G
J9390	Injection, vinorelbine tartrate, 10 mg	N1 N
	Other: Navelbine	
	IOM: 100-02, 15, 50	
J9393	Injection, fulvestrant (teva), not therapeutically equivalent to J9395, 25 mg	K2 K
J9394	Injection, fulvestrant (fresenius kabi) not therapeutically equivalent to J9395, 25 mg	K2 K
* J9395	Injection, fulvestrant, 25 mg	K2 K
	Other: Faslodex	
* J9400	Injection, ziv-aflibercept, 1 mg	K2 K
	Other: Zaltrap	
J9600	Injection, porfimer sodium, 75 mg	K2 K
	Other: Photofrin	
	IOM: 100-02, 15, 50	
J9999	Not otherwise classified, antineoplastic drugs	N1 N
	Bill on paper, bill one unit, and identify drug and total dosage in "Remarks" field. Include invoice of cost or NDC number in "Remarks" field.	
	Other: Imlygic, Yondelis	
	IOM: 100-02, 15, 50; 100-03, 2, 110.2	
	Coding Clinic: 2017, Q1, P3; 2013, Q2, P3	

▶ New ↻ Revised ✓ Reinstated ~~deleted~~ Deleted ⊘ Not covered or valid by Medicare
◯ Special coverage instructions * Carrier discretion Ⓑ Bill Part B MAC Ⓑ Bill DME MAC

TEMPORARY CODES ASSIGNED TO DME REGIONAL CARRIERS (K0000-K9999)

NOTE: This section contains national codes assigned by CMS on a temporary basis and for the exclusive use of the durable medical equipment regional carriers (DMERC).

Wheelchairs and Accessories

* **K0001** Standard wheelchair Y
  Capped rental

* **K0002** Standard hemi (low seat) wheelchair Y
  Capped rental

* **K0003** Lightweight wheelchair Y
  Capped rental

* **K0004** High strength, lightweight wheelchair Y
  Capped rental

* **K0005** Ultralightweight wheelchair Y
  Capped rental. Inexpensive and routinely purchased DME

* **K0006** Heavy duty wheelchair Y
  Capped rental

* **K0007** Extra heavy duty wheelchair Y
  Capped rental

○ **K0008** Custom manual wheelchair/base Y

* **K0009** Other manual wheelchair/base Y
  Not otherwise classified

* **K0010** Standard - weight frame motorized/power wheelchair Y
  Capped rental. Codes K0010-K0014 are not for manual wheelchairs with add-on power packs. Use the appropriate code for the manual wheelchair base provided (K0001-K0009) and code K0460.

* **K0011** Standard - weight frame motorized/power wheelchair with programmable control parameters for speed adjustment, tremor dampening, acceleration control and braking Y
  Capped rental. A patient who requires a power wheelchair usually is totally nonambulatory and has severe weakness of the upper extremities due to a neurologic or muscular disease/condition.

* **K0012** Lightweight portable motorized/power wheelchair Y
  Capped rental

○ **K0013** Custom motorized/power wheelchair base Y

* **K0014** Other motorized/power wheelchair base Y
  Capped rental

* **K0015** Detachable, non-adjustable height armrest, replacement only, each Y
  Inexpensive and routinely purchased DME

* **K0017** Detachable, adjustable height armrest, base, replacement only, each Y
  Inexpensive and routinely purchased DME

* **K0018** Detachable, adjustable height armrest, upper portion, replacement only, each Y
  Inexpensive and routinely purchased DME

* **K0019** Arm pad, replacement only, each Y
  Inexpensive and routinely purchased DME

* **K0020** Fixed, adjustable height armrest, pair Y
  Inexpensive and routinely purchased DME

* **K0037** High mount flip-up footrest, each Y
  Inexpensive and routinely purchased DME

* **K0038** Leg strap, each Y
  Inexpensive and routinely purchased DME

* **K0039** Leg strap, H style, each Y
  Inexpensive and routinely purchased DME

* **K0040** Adjustable angle footplate, each Y
  Inexpensive and routinely purchased DME

* **K0041** Large size footplate, each Y
  Inexpensive and routinely purchased DME

* **K0042** Standard size footplate, replacement only, each Y
  Inexpensive and routinely purchased DME

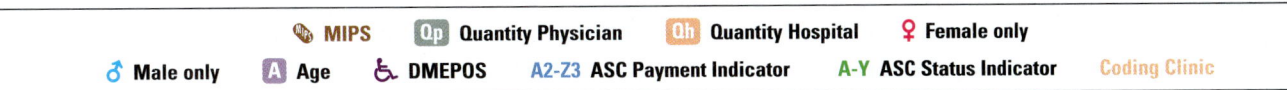

* **K0043** Footrest, lower extension tube, replacement only, each ⓑ Qp Qh ♿ Y
Inexpensive and routinely purchased DME

* **K0044** Footrest, upper hanger bracket, replacement only, each ⓑ Qp Qh ♿ Y
Inexpensive and routinely purchased DME

* **K0045** Footrest, complete assembly, replacement only, each ⓑ Qp Qh ♿ Y
Inexpensive and routinely purchased DME

* **K0046** Elevating legrest, lower extension tube, replacement only, each ⓑ Qp Qh ♿ Y
Inexpensive and routinely purchased DME

* **K0047** Elevating legrest, upper hanger bracket, replacement only, each ⓑ Qp Qh ♿ Y
Inexpensive and routinely purchased DME

* **K0050** Ratchet assembly, replacement only ⓑ Qp Qh ♿ Y
Inexpensive and routinely purchased DME

* **K0051** Cam release assembly, footrest or legrests, replacement only, each ⓑ Qp Qh ♿ Y
Inexpensive and routinely purchased DME

* **K0052** Swing-away, detachable footrests, replacement only, each ⓑ Qp Qh ♿ Y
Inexpensive and routinely purchased DME

* **K0053** Elevating footrests, articulating (telescoping), each ⓑ Qp Qh ♿ Y
Inexpensive and routinely purchased DME

* **K0056** Seat height less than 17" or equal to or greater than 21" for a high strength, lightweight, or ultralightweight wheelchair ⓑ Qp Qh ♿ Y
Inexpensive and routinely purchased DME

* **K0065** Spoke protectors, each ⓑ Qp Qh ♿ Y
Inexpensive and routinely purchased DME

* **K0069** Rear wheel assembly, complete, with solid tire, spokes or molded, replacement only, each ⓑ Qp Qh ♿ Y
Inexpensive and routinely purchased DME

* **K0070** Rear wheel assembly, complete, with pneumatic tire, spokes or molded, replacement only, each ⓑ Qp Qh ♿ Y
Inexpensive and routinely purchased DME

* **K0071** Front caster assembly, complete, with pneumatic tire, replacement only, each ⓑ Qp Qh ♿ Y
Caster assembly includes a caster fork (E2396), wheel rim, and tire.
Inexpensive and routinely purchased DME

* **K0072** Front caster assembly, complete, with semi-pneumatic tire, replacement only, each ⓑ Qp Qh ♿ Y
Inexpensive and routinely purchased DME

* **K0073** Caster pin lock, each ⓑ Qp Qh ♿ Y
Inexpensive and routinely purchased DME

* **K0077** Front caster assembly, complete, with solid tire, replacement only, each ⓑ Qp Qh ♿ Y

* **K0098** Drive belt for power wheelchair, replacement only ⓑ ♿ Y
Inexpensive and routinely purchased DME

* **K0105** IV hanger, each ⓑ Qp Qh ♿ Y
Inexpensive and routinely purchased DME

* **K0108** Wheelchair component or accessory, not otherwise specified ⓑ Y

⊛ **K0195** Elevating leg rests, pair (for use with capped rental wheelchair base) ⓑ Qp Qh ♿ Y
Medically necessary replacement items are covered if rollabout chair or transport chair covered
IOM: 100-03, 4, 280.1

Infusion Pump, Supplies, and Batteries

⊛ **K0455** Infusion pump used for uninterrupted parenteral administration of medication (e.g., epoprostenol or treprostinol) ⓑ Qp Qh ♿ Y
An EIP may also be referred to as an external insulin pump, ambulatory pump, or mini-infuser. CMN/DIF required. Frequent and substantial service DME.
IOM: 100-03, 1, 50.3

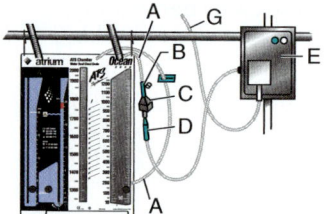

Figure 18 Infusion pump.

▶ New   ⤳ Revised   ✓ Reinstated   ~~deleted~~ Deleted   ⊘ Not covered or valid by Medicare
⊛ Special coverage instructions   * Carrier discretion   ⓑ Bill Part B MAC   ⓑ Bill DME MAC

TEMPORARY CODES ASSIGNED TO DME REGIONAL CARRIERS

○ **K0462** Temporary replacement for patient owned equipment being repaired, any type ⒷQpQh Y

Only report for maintenance and service for an item for which initial claim was paid. The term power mobility device (PMD) includes power operated vehicles (POVs) and power wheelchairs (PWCs). Not otherwise classified.

IOM: 100-04, 20, 40.1

○ **K0552** Supplies for external non-insulin drug infusion pump, syringe type cartridge, sterile, each ⒷQh& Y

Supplies

IOM: 100-03, 1, 50.3

✱ **K0601** Replacement battery for external infusion pump owned by patient, silver oxide, 1.5 volt, each ⒷQh& Y

Inexpensive and routinely purchased DME

✱ **K0602** Replacement battery for external infusion pump owned by patient, silver oxide, 3 volt, each ⒷQpQh& Y

Inexpensive and routinely purchased DME

✱ **K0603** Replacement battery for external infusion pump owned by patient, alkaline, 1.5 volt, each ⒷQh& Y

Inexpensive and routinely purchased DME

✱ **K0604** Replacement battery for external infusion pump owned by patient, lithium, 3.6 volt, each ⒷQh& Y

Inexpensive and routinely purchased DME

✱ **K0605** Replacement battery for external infusion pump owned by patient, lithium, 4.5 volt, each ⒷQpQh& Y

Inexpensive and routinely purchased DME

Defibrillator and Accessories

✱ **K0606** Automatic external defibrillator, with integrated electrocardiogram analysis, garment type ⒷQpQh& Y

Capped rental

✱ **K0607** Replacement battery for automated external defibrillator, garment type only, each ⒷQpQh& Y

Inexpensive and routinely purchased DME

✱ **K0608** Replacement garment for use with automated external defibrillator, each ⒷQpQh& Y

Inexpensive and routinely purchased DME

✱ **K0609** Replacement electrodes for use with automated external defibrillator, garment type only, each ⒷQpQh& Y

Supplies

Miscellaneous

✱ **K0669** Wheelchair accessory, wheelchair seat or back cushion, does not meet specific code criteria or no written coding verification from DME PDAC Ⓑ Y

Inexpensive and routinely purchased DME

✱ **K0672** Addition to lower extremity orthosis, removable soft interface, all components, replacement only, each ⒷQp& A

Prosthetics/Orthotics

✱ **K0730** Controlled dose inhalation drug delivery system ⒷQpQh& Y

Inexpensive and routinely purchased DME

✱ **K0733** Power wheelchair accessory, 12 to 24 amp hour sealed lead acid battery, each (e.g., gel cell, absorbed glassmat) ⒷQpQh& Y

Inexpensive and routinely purchased DME

✱ **K0738** Portable gaseous oxygen system, rental; home compressor used to fill portable oxygen cylinders; includes portable containers, regulator, flowmeter, humidifier, cannula or mask, and tubing ⒷQpQh& Y

Oxygen and oxygen equipment

✱ **K0739** Repair or nonroutine service for durable medical equipment other than oxygen equipment requiring the skill of a technician, labor component, per 15 minutes ◉Ⓑ Y

⊘ **K0740** Repair or nonroutine service for oxygen equipment requiring the skill of a technician, labor component, per 15 minutes ⒷQpQh E1

✱ **K0743** Suction pump, home model, portable, for use on wounds ⒷQpQh Y

✱ **K0744** Absorptive wound dressing for use with suction pump, home model, portable, pad size 16 square inches or less ⒷQp A

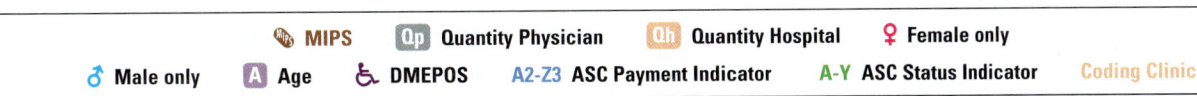

♂ Male only · Ⓐ Age · & DMEPOS · A2-Z3 ASC Payment Indicator · A-Y ASC Status Indicator · Coding Clinic

* **K0745** Absorptive wound dressing for use with suction pump, home model, portable, pad size more than 16 square inches but less than or equal to 48 square inches Ⓑ Qp A

* **K0746** Absorptive wound dressing for use with suction pump, home model, portable, pad size greater than 48 square inches Ⓑ Qp A

Power Mobility Devices

* **K0800** Power operated vehicle, group 1 standard, patient weight capacity up to and including 300 pounds Ⓑ Qp Qh ♿ Y

    Power mobility device (PMD) includes power operated vehicles (POVs) and power wheelchairs (PWCs). Inexpensive and routinely purchased DME

* **K0801** Power operated vehicle, group 1 heavy duty, patient weight capacity 301 to 450 pounds Ⓑ Qp Qh ♿ Y

    Inexpensive and routinely purchased DME

* **K0802** Power operated vehicle, group 1 very heavy duty, patient weight capacity 451 to 600 pounds Ⓑ Qp Qh ♿ Y

    Inexpensive and routinely purchased DME

* **K0806** Power operated vehicle, group 2 standard, patient weight capacity up to and including 300 pounds Ⓑ Qp Qh ♿ Y

    Inexpensive and routinely purchased DME

* **K0807** Power operated vehicle, group 2 heavy duty, patient weight capacity 301 to 450 pounds Ⓑ Qp Qh ♿ Y

    Inexpensive and routinely purchased DME

* **K0808** Power operated vehicle, group 2 very heavy duty, patient weight capacity 451 to 600 pounds Ⓑ Qp Qh ♿ Y

    Inexpensive and routinely purchased DME

* **K0812** Power operated vehicle, not otherwise classified Ⓑ Qp Qh Y

    Not otherwise classified.

* **K0813** Power wheelchair, group 1 standard, portable, sling/solid seat and back, patient weight capacity up to and including 300 pounds Ⓑ Qp Qh ♿ Y

    Capped rental

* **K0814** Power wheelchair, group 1 standard, portable, captains chair, patient weight capacity up to and including 300 pounds Ⓑ Qp Qh ♿ Y

    Capped rental

* **K0815** Power wheelchair, group 1 standard, sling/solid seat and back, patient weight capacity up to and including 300 pounds Ⓑ Qp Qh ♿ Y

    Capped rental

* **K0816** Power wheelchair, group 1 standard, captains chair, patient weight capacity up to and including 300 pounds Ⓑ Qp Qh ♿ Y

    Capped rental

* **K0820** Power wheelchair, group 2 standard, portable, sling/solid seat/back, patient weight capacity up to and including 300 pounds Ⓑ Qp Qh ♿ Y

    Capped rental

* **K0821** Power wheelchair, group 2 standard, portable, captains chair, patient weight capacity up to and including 300 pounds Ⓑ Qp Qh ♿ Y

    Capped rental

* **K0822** Power wheelchair, group 2 standard, sling/solid seat/back, patient weight capacity up to and including 300 pounds Ⓑ Qp Qh ♿ Y

    Capped rental

* **K0823** Power wheelchair, group 2 standard, captains chair, patient weight capacity up to and including 300 pounds Ⓑ Qp Qh ♿ Y

    Capped rental

* **K0824** Power wheelchair, group 2 heavy duty, sling/solid seat/back, patient weight capacity 301 to 450 pounds Ⓑ Qp Qh ♿ Y

    Capped rental

* **K0825** Power wheelchair, group 2 heavy duty, captains chair, patient weight capacity 301 to 450 pounds Ⓑ Qp Qh ♿ Y

    Capped rental

* **K0826** Power wheelchair, group 2 very heavy duty, sling/solid seat/back, patient weight capacity 451 to 600 pounds Ⓑ Qp Qh ♿ Y

    Capped rental

* **K0827** Power wheelchair, group 2 very heavy duty, captains chair, patient weight capacity 451 to 600 pounds Ⓑ Qp Qh ♿ Y

    Capped rental

▶ New   ⤺ Revised   ✔ Reinstated   ~~deleted~~ Deleted   ⊘ Not covered or valid by Medicare
● Special coverage instructions   ✱ Carrier discretion   Ⓑ Bill Part B MAC   Ⓓ Bill DME MAC

TEMPORARY CODES ASSIGNED TO DME REGIONAL CARRIERS

* **K0828** Power wheelchair, group 2 extra heavy duty, sling/solid seat/back, patient weight capacity 601 pounds or more ⓑ Qp Qh ♿ Y
Capped rental

* **K0829** Power wheelchair, group 2 extra heavy duty, captains chair, patient weight 601 pounds or more ⓑ Qp Qh ♿ Y
Capped rental

* **K0830** Power wheelchair, group 2 standard, seat elevator, sling/solid seat/back, patient weight capacity up to and including 300 pounds ⓑ Qp Qh Y
Capped rental

* **K0831** Power wheelchair, group 2 standard, seat elevator, captains chair, patient weight capacity up to and including 300 pounds ⓑ Qp Qh Y

* **K0835** Power wheelchair, group 2 standard, single power option, sling/solid seat/back, patient weight capacity up to and including 300 pounds ⓑ Qp Qh ♿ Y
Capped rental

* **K0836** Power wheelchair, group 2 standard, single power option, captains chair, patient weight capacity up to and including 300 pounds ⓑ Qp Qh ♿ Y
Capped rental

* **K0837** Power wheelchair, group 2 heavy duty, single power option, sling/solid seat/back, patient weight capacity 301 to 450 pounds ⓑ Qp Qh ♿ Y
Capped rental

* **K0838** Power wheelchair, group 2 heavy duty, single power option, captains chair, patient weight capacity 301 to 450 pounds ⓑ Qp Qh ♿ Y
Capped rental

* **K0839** Power wheelchair, group 2 very heavy duty, single power option, sling/solid seat/back, patient weight capacity 451 to 600 pounds ⓑ Qp Qh ♿ Y
Capped rental

* **K0840** Power wheelchair, group 2 extra heavy duty, single power option, sling/solid seat/back, patient weight capacity 601 pounds or more ⓑ Qp Qh ♿ Y
Capped rental

* **K0841** Power wheelchair, group 2 standard, multiple power option, sling/solid seat/back, patient weight capacity up to and including 300 pounds ⓑ Qp Qh ♿ Y
Capped rental

* **K0842** Power wheelchair, group 2 standard, multiple power option, captains chair, patient weight capacity up to and including 300 pounds ⓑ Qp Qh ♿ Y
Capped rental

* **K0843** Power wheelchair, group 2 heavy duty, multiple power option, sling/solid seat/back, patient weight capacity 301 to 450 pounds ⓑ Qp Qh ♿ Y
Capped rental

* **K0848** Power wheelchair, group 3 standard, sling/solid seat/back, patient weight capacity up to and including 300 pounds ⓑ Qp Qh ♿ Y
Capped rental

* **K0849** Power wheelchair, group 3 standard, captains chair, patient weight capacity up to and including 300 pounds ⓑ Qp Qh ♿ Y
Capped rental

* **K0850** Power wheelchair, group 3 heavy duty, sling/solid seat/back, patient weight capacity 301 to 450 pounds ⓑ Qp Qh ♿ Y
Capped rental

* **K0851** Power wheelchair, group 3 heavy duty, captains chair, patient weight capacity 301 to 450 pounds ⓑ Qp Qh ♿ Y
Capped rental

* **K0852** Power wheelchair, group 3 very heavy duty, sling/solid seat/back, patient weight capacity 451 to 600 pounds ⓑ Qp Qh ♿ Y
Capped rental

* **K0853** Power wheelchair, group 3 very heavy duty, captains chair, patient weight capacity 451 to 600 pounds ⓑ Qp Qh ♿ Y
Capped rental

* **K0854** Power wheelchair, group 3 extra heavy duty, sling/solid seat/back, patient weight capacity 601 pounds or more ⓑ Qp Qh ♿ Y
Capped rental

* **K0855** Power wheelchair, group 3 extra heavy duty, captains chair, patient weight capacity 601 pounds or more ⓑ Qp Qh ♿ Y
Capped rental

* **K0856** Power wheelchair, group 3 standard, single power option, sling/solid seat/back, patient weight capacity up to and including 300 pounds ⓑ Qp Qh ♿ Y
Capped rental

* **K0857** Power wheelchair, group 3 standard, single power option, captains chair, patient weight capacity up to and including 300 pounds ⓑ Qp Qh ♿ Y
Capped rental

♂ Male only   A Age   ♿ DMEPOS   A2-Z3 ASC Payment Indicator   A-Y ASC Status Indicator   MIPS   Qp Quantity Physician   Qh Quantity Hospital   ♀ Female only   Coding Clinic

* **K0858** Power wheelchair, group 3 heavy duty, single power option, sling/solid seat/back, patient weight 301 to 450 pounds ⓑ Qp Qh ♿ Y
Capped rental

* **K0859** Power wheelchair, group 3 heavy duty, single power option, captains chair, patient weight capacity 301 to 450 pounds ⓑ Qp Qh ♿ Y
Capped rental

* **K0860** Power wheelchair, group 3 very heavy duty, single power option, sling/solid seat/back, patient weight capacity 451 to 600 pounds ⓑ Qp Qh ♿ Y
Capped rental

* **K0861** Power wheelchair, group 3 standard, multiple power option, sling/solid seat/back, patient weight capacity up to and including 300 pounds ⓑ Qp Qh ♿ Y
Capped rental

* **K0862** Power wheelchair, group 3 heavy duty, multiple power option, sling/solid seat/back, patient weight capacity 301 to 450 pounds ⓑ Qp Qh ♿ Y
Capped rental

* **K0863** Power wheelchair, group 3 very heavy duty, multiple power option, sling/solid seat/back, patient weight capacity 451 to 600 pounds ⓑ Qp Qh ♿ Y
Capped rental

* **K0864** Power wheelchair, group 3 extra heavy duty, multiple power option, sling/solid seat/back, patient weight capacity 601 pounds or more ⓑ Qp Qh ♿ Y
Capped rental

* **K0868** Power wheelchair, group 4 standard, sling/solid seat/back, patient weight capacity up to and including 300 pounds Qp Qh Y
Capped rental

* **K0869** Power wheelchair, group 4 standard, captains chair, patient weight capacity up to and including 300 pounds ⓑ Qp Qh Y
Capped rental

* **K0870** Power wheelchair, group 4 heavy duty, sling/solid seat/back, patient weight capacity 301 to 450 pounds ⓑ Qp Qh Y
Capped rental

* **K0871** Power wheelchair, group 4 very heavy duty, sling/solid seat/back, patient weight capacity 451 to 600 pounds ⓑ Qp Qh Y
Capped rental

* **K0877** Power wheelchair, group 4 standard, single power option, sling/solid seat/back, patient weight capacity up to and including 300 pounds ⓑ Qp Qh Y
Capped rental

* **K0878** Power wheelchair, group 4 standard, single power option, captains chair, patient weight capacity up to and including 300 pounds ⓑ Qp Qh Y
Capped rental

* **K0879** Power wheelchair, group 4 heavy duty, single power option, sling/solid seat/back, patient weight capacity 301 to 450 pounds ⓑ Qp Qh Y
Capped rental

* **K0880** Power wheelchair, group 4 very heavy duty, single power option, sling/solid seat/back, patient weight 451 to 600 pounds ⓑ Qp Qh Y
Capped rental

* **K0884** Power wheelchair, group 4 standard, multiple power option, sling/solid seat/back, patient weight capacity up to and including 300 pounds ⓑ Qp Qh Y
Capped rental

* **K0885** Power wheelchair, group 4 standard, multiple power option, captains chair, patient weight capacity up to and including 300 pounds ⓑ Qp Qh Y
Capped rental

* **K0886** Power wheelchair, group 4 heavy duty, multiple power option, sling/solid seat/back, patient weight capacity 301 to 450 pounds ⓑ Qp Qh Y
Capped rental

* **K0890** Power wheelchair, group 5 pediatric, single power option, sling/solid seat/back, patient weight capacity up to and including 125 pounds ⓑ Qp Qh A Y
Capped rental

* **K0891** Power wheelchair, group 5 pediatric, multiple power option, sling/solid seat/back, patient weight capacity up to and including 125 pounds ⓑ Qp Qh A Y
Capped rental

* **K0898** Power wheelchair, not otherwise classified ⓑ Qp Qh Y

* **K0899** Power mobility device, not coded by DME PDAC or does not meet criteria ⓑ Y

▶ New ⟳ Revised ✓ Reinstated ~~deleted~~ Deleted ⊘ Not covered or valid by Medicare
◉ Special coverage instructions ✱ Carrier discretion ⓑ Bill Part B MAC ⓑ Bill DME MAC

TEMPORARY CODES ASSIGNED TO DME REGIONAL CARRIERS

Customized DME: Other than Wheelchair

◎ **K0900** Customized durable medical equipment, other than wheelchair ⓑ Qp Qh   Y

Devices

✱ **K1004** Low frequency ultrasonic diathermy treatment device for home use ⓑ   E1

✱ **K1007** Bilateral hip, knee, ankle, foot device, powered, includes pelvic component, single or double upright(s), knee joints any type, with or without ankle joints any type, includes all components and accessories, motors, microprocessors, sensors ⓑ   Y

✱ **K1027** Oral device/appliance used to reduce upper airway collapsibility, without fixed mechanical hinge, custom fabricated, includes fitting and adjustment ⓑ   Y

Self-administered test

K1030 External recharging system for battery (internal) for use with implanted cardiac contractility modulation generator, replacement only   Y

K1034 Provision of covid-19 test, nonprescription self-administered and self-collected use, FDA approved, authorized or cleared, one test count   E1

K1035 Molecular diagnostic test reader, nonprescription self-administered and self-collected use, FDA approved, authorized or cleared ⓑ   E1

K1036 Supplies and accessories (e.g., transducer) for low frequency ultrasonic diathermy treatment device, per month ⓑ   E1

K1037 Docking station for use with oral device/appliance used to reduce upper airway collapsibility ⓑ   E1

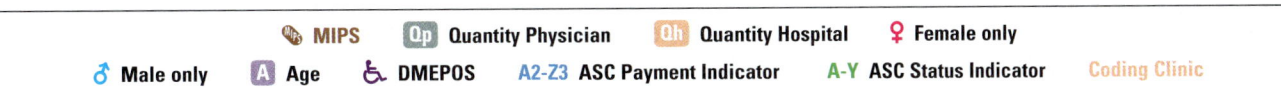

♦ MIPS   Qp Quantity Physician   Qh Quantity Hospital   ♀ Female only
♂ Male only   Ⓐ Age   ♿ DMEPOS   A2-Z3 ASC Payment Indicator   A-Y ASC Status Indicator   Coding Clinic

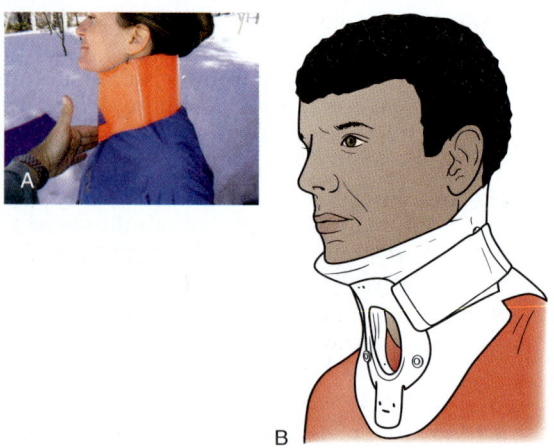

Figure 19 (A) Flexible cervical collar. (B) Adjustable cervical collar.

ORTHOTICS & DEVICES (L0112-L4631)

Note: DMEPOS fee schedule https://www.cms.gov/Medicare/Medicare-Fee-for-Service-Payment/DMEPOSFeeSched/DMEPOS-Fee-Schedule.html

Cervical Orthotics

* L0112 Cranial cervical orthosis, congenital torticollis type, with or without soft interface material, adjustable range of motion joint, custom fabricated A

* L0113 Cranial cervical orthosis, torticollis type, with or without joint, with or without soft interface material, prefabricated, includes fitting and adjustment A

* L0120 Cervical, flexible, non-adjustable, prefabricated, off-the-shelf (foam collar) A

   Cervical orthoses including soft and rigid devices may be used as nonoperative management for cervical trauma

* L0130 Cervical, flexible, thermoplastic collar, molded to patient A

* L0140 Cervical, semi-rigid, adjustable (plastic collar) A

* L0150 Cervical, semi-rigid, adjustable molded chin cup (plastic collar with mandibular/occipital piece) A

* L0160 Cervical, semi-rigid, wire frame occipital/mandibular support, prefabricated, off-the-shelf A

* L0170 Cervical, collar, molded to patient model A

* L0172 Cervical, collar, semi-rigid thermoplastic foam, two-piece, prefabricated, off-the-shelf A

* L0174 Cervical, collar, semi-rigid, thermoplastic foam, two piece with thoracic extension, prefabricated, off-the-shelf A

Multiple Post Collar: Cervical

* L0180 Cervical, multiple post collar, occipital/mandibular supports, adjustable A

* L0190 Cervical, multiple post collar, occipital/mandibular supports, adjustable cervical bars (SOMI, Guilford, Taylor types) A

* L0200 Cervical, multiple post collar, occipital/mandibular supports, adjustable cervical bars, and thoracic extension A

Thoracic Rib Belt

* L0220 Thoracic, rib belt, custom fabricated A

Thoracic-Lumbar-Sacral Orthotics

* L0450 TLSO, flexible, provides trunk support, upper thoracic region, produces intracavitary pressure to reduce load on the intervertebral disks with rigid stays or panel(s), includes shoulder straps and closures, prefabricated, off-the-shelf A

   Used to immobilize specified area of spine, and is generally worn under clothing

* L0452 TLSO, flexible, provides trunk support, upper thoracic region, produces intracavitary pressure to reduce load on the intervertebral disks with rigid stays or panel(s), includes shoulder straps and closures, custom fabricated A

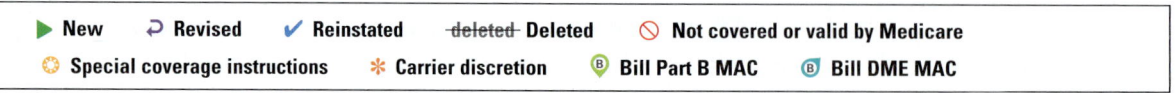

ORTHOTICS & DEVICES

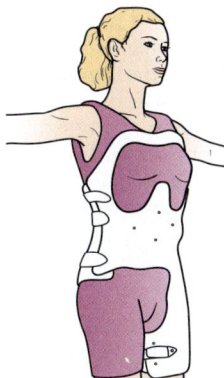

Figure 20 Thoracic-lumbar-sacral-orthosis (TLSO).

* **L0454** TLSO flexible, provides trunk support, extends from sacrococcygeal junction to above T-9 vertebra, restricts gross trunk motion in the sagittal plane, produces intracavitary pressure to reduce load on the intervertebral disks with rigid stays or panel(s), includes shoulder straps and closures, prefabricated item that has been trimmed, bent, molded, assembled, or otherwise customized to fit a specific patient by an individual with expertise ⑧ Qp Qh ♿ A

   Used to immobilize specified areas of spine; and is generally designed to be worn under clothing; not specifically designed for patients in wheelchairs

* **L0455** TLSO, flexible, provides trunk support, extends from sacrococcygeal junction to above T-9 vertebra, restricts gross trunk motion in the sagittal plane, produces intracavitary pressure to reduce load on the intervertebral disks with rigid stays or panel(s), includes shoulder straps and closures, prefabricated, off-the-shelf ⑧ Qp Qh ♿ A

* **L0456** TLSO, flexible, provides trunk support, thoracic region, rigid posterior panel and soft anterior apron, extends from the sacrococcygeal junction and terminates just inferior to the scapular spine, restricts gross trunk motion in the sagittal plane, produces intracavitary pressure to reduce load on the intervertebral disks, includes straps and closures, prefabricated item that has been trimmed, bent, molded, assembled, or otherwise customized to fit a specific patient by an individual with expertise ⑧ Qp Qh ♿ A

* **L0457** TLSO, flexible, provides trunk support, thoracic region, rigid posterior panel and soft anterior apron, extends from the sacrococcygeal junction and terminates just inferior to the scapular spine, restricts gross trunk motion in the sagittal plane, produces intracavitary pressure to reduce load on the intervertebral disks, includes straps and closures, prefabricated, off-the-shelf ⑧ Qp Qh ♿ A

* **L0458** TLSO, triplanar control, modular segmented spinal system, two rigid plastic shells, posterior extends from the sacrococcygeal junction and terminates just inferior to the scapular spine, anterior extends from the symphysis pubis to the xiphoid, soft liner, restricts gross trunk motion in the sagittal, coronal, and transverse planes, lateral strength is provided by overlapping plastic and stabilizing closures, includes straps and closures, prefabricated, includes fitting and adjustment ⑧ Qp Qh ♿ A

   To meet Medicare's definition of body jacket, orthosis has to have rigid plastic shell that circles trunk with overlapping edges and stabilizing closures, and entire circumference of shell must be made of same rigid material.

MIPS Qp Quantity Physician Qh Quantity Hospital ♀ Female only
♂ Male only A Age ♿ DMEPOS A2-Z3 ASC Payment Indicator A-Y ASC Status Indicator Coding Clinic

* **L0460** TLSO, triplanar control, modular segmented spinal system, two rigid plastic shells, posterior extends from the sacrococcygeal junction and terminates just inferior to the scapular spine, anterior extends from the symphysis pubis to the sternal notch, soft liner, restricts gross trunk motion in the sagittal, coronal, and transverse planes, lateral strength is provided by overlapping plastic and stabilizing closures, includes straps and closures, prefabricated item that has been trimmed, bent, molded, assembled, or otherwise customized to fit a specific patient by an individual with expertise ⓑ Qp Qh ♿ A

* **L0462** TLSO, triplanar control, modular segmented spinal system, three rigid plastic shells, posterior extends from the sacrococcygeal junction and terminates just inferior to the scapular spine, anterior extends from the symphysis pubis to the sternal notch, soft liner, restricts gross trunk motion in the sagittal, coronal, and transverse planes, lateral strength is provided by overlapping plastic and stabilizing closures, includes straps and closures, prefabricated, includes fitting and adjustment ⓑ Qp Qh ♿ A

* **L0464** TLSO, triplanar control, modular segmented spinal system, four rigid plastic shells, posterior extends from sacrococcygeal junction and terminates just inferior to scapular spine, anterior extends from symphysis pubis to the sternal notch, soft liner, restricts gross trunk motion in sagittal, coronal, and transverse planes, lateral strength is provided by overlapping plastic and stabilizing closures, includes straps and closures, prefabricated, includes fitting and adjustment ⓑ Qp Qh ♿ A

* **L0466** TLSO, sagittal control, rigid posterior frame and flexible soft anterior apron with straps, closures and padding, restricts gross trunk motion in sagittal plane, produces intracavitary pressure to reduce load on intervertebral disks, prefabricated item that has been trimmed, bent, molded, assembled, or otherwise customized to fit a specific patient by an individual with expertise ⓑ Qp Qh ♿ A

* **L0467** TLSO, sagittal control, rigid posterior frame and flexible soft anterior apron with straps, closures and padding, restricts gross trunk motion in sagittal plane, produces intracavitary pressure to reduce load on intervertebral disks, prefabricated, off-the-shelf ⓑ Qp Qh ♿ A

* **L0468** TLSO, sagittal-coronal control, rigid posterior frame and flexible soft anterior apron with straps, closures and padding, extends from sacrococcygeal junction over scapulae, lateral strength provided by pelvic, thoracic, and lateral frame pieces, restricts gross trunk motion in sagittal, and coronal planes, produces intracavitary pressure to reduce load on intervertebral disks, prefabricated item that has been trimmed, bent, molded, assembled, or otherwise customized to fit a specific patient by an individual with expertise ⓑ Qp Qh ♿ A

* **L0469** TLSO, sagittal-coronal control, rigid posterior frame and flexible soft anterior apron with straps, closures and padding, extends from sacrococcygeal junction over scapulae, lateral strength provided by pelvic, thoracic, and lateral frame pieces, restricts gross trunk motion in sagittal and coronal planes, produces intracavitary pressure to reduce load on intervertebral disks, prefabricated, off-the-shelf ⓑ Qp Qh ♿ A

ORTHOTICS & DEVICES

* **L0470** TLSO, triplanar control, rigid posterior frame and flexible soft anterior apron with straps, closures and padding, extends from sacrococcygeal junction to scapula, lateral strength provided by pelvic, thoracic, and lateral frame pieces, rotational strength provided by subclavicular extensions, restricts gross trunk motion in sagittal, coronal, and transverse planes, provides intracavitary pressure to reduce load on the intervertebral disks, includes fitting and shaping the frame, prefabricated, includes fitting and adjustment ⓑ Qp Qh ♿   A

* **L0472** TLSO, triplanar control, hyperextension, rigid anterior and lateral frame extends from symphysis pubis to sternal notch with two anterior components (one pubic and one sternal), posterior and lateral pads with straps and closures, limits spinal flexion, restricts gross trunk motion in sagittal, coronal, and transverse planes, includes fitting and shaping the frame, prefabricated, includes fitting and adjustment ⓑ Qp Qh ♿   A

* **L0480** TLSO, triplanar control, one piece rigid plastic shell without interface liner, with multiple straps and closures, posterior extends from sacrococcygeal junction and terminates just inferior to scapular spine, anterior extends from symphysis pubis to sternal notch, anterior or posterior opening, restricts gross trunk motion in sagittal, coronal, and transverse planes, includes a carved plaster or CAD-CAM model, custom fabricated ⓑ Qp Qh ♿   A

* **L0482** TLSO, triplanar control, one piece rigid plastic shell with interface liner, multiple straps and closures, posterior extends from sacrococcygeal junction and terminates just inferior to scapular spine, anterior extends from symphysis pubis to sternal notch, anterior or posterior opening, restricts gross trunk motion in sagittal, coronal, and transverse planes, includes a carved plaster or CAD-CAM model, custom fabricated ⓑ Qp Qh ♿   A

* **L0484** TLSO, triplanar control, two piece rigid plastic shell without interface liner, with multiple straps and closures, posterior extends from sacrococcygeal junction and terminates just inferior to scapular spine, anterior extends from symphysis pubis to sternal notch, lateral strength is enhanced by overlapping plastic, restricts gross trunk motion in the sagittal, coronal, and transverse planes, includes a carved plaster or CAD-CAM model, custom fabricated ⓑ Qp Qh ♿   A

* **L0486** TLSO, triplanar control, two piece rigid plastic shell with interface liner, multiple straps and closures, posterior extends from sacrococcygeal junction and terminates just inferior to scapular spine, anterior extends from symphysis pubis to sternal notch, lateral strength is enhanced by overlapping plastic, restricts gross trunk motion in the sagittal, coronal, and transverse planes, includes a carved plaster or CAD-CAM model, custom fabricated ⓑ Qp Qh ♿   A

* **L0488** TLSO, triplanar control, one piece rigid plastic shell with interface liner, multiple straps and closures, posterior extends from sacrococcygeal junction and terminates just inferior to scapular spine, anterior extends from symphysis pubis to sternal notch, anterior or posterior opening, restricts gross trunk motion in sagittal, coronal, and transverse planes, prefabricated, includes fitting and adjustment ⓑ Qp Qh ♿   A

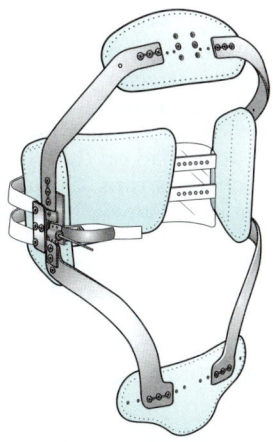

Figure 21 Thoracic-lumbar-sacral orthosis (TLSO) Jewett flexion control.

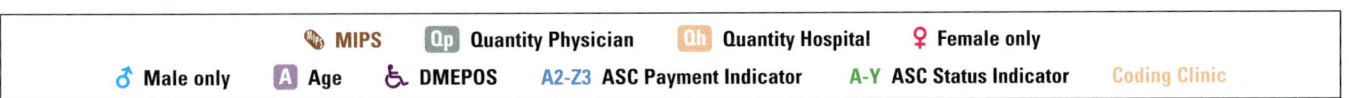

* **L0490** TLSO, sagittal-coronal control, one piece rigid plastic shell, with overlapping reinforced anterior, with multiple straps and closures, posterior extends from sacrococcygeal junction and terminates at or before the T-9 vertebra, anterior extends from symphysis pubis to xiphoid, anterior opening, restricts gross trunk motion in sagittal and coronal planes, prefabricated, includes fitting and adjustment Ⓑ Qp Qh ♿ A

* **L0491** TLSO, sagittal-coronal control, modular segmented spinal system, two rigid plastic shells, posterior extends from the sacrococcygeal junction and terminates just inferior to the scapular spine, anterior extends from the symphysis pubis to the xiphoid, soft liner, restricts gross trunk motion in the sagittal and coronal planes, lateral strength is provided by overlapping plastic and stabilizing closures, includes straps and closures, prefabricated, includes fitting and adjustment Ⓑ Qp Qh ♿ A

* **L0492** TLSO, sagittal-coronal control, modular segmented spinal system, three rigid plastic shells, posterior extends from the sacrococcygeal junction and terminates just inferior to the scapular spine, anterior extends from the symphysis pubis to the xiphoid, soft liner, restricts gross trunk motion in the sagittal and coronal planes, lateral strength is provided by overlapping plastic and stabilizing closures, includes straps and closures, prefabricated, includes fitting and adjustment Ⓑ Qp Qh ♿ A

Sacroilliac Orthotics

* **L0621** Sacroiliac orthosis, flexible, provides pelvic-sacral support, reduces motion about the sacroiliac joint, includes straps, closures, may include pendulous abdomen design, prefabricated, off-the-shelf Ⓑ Qp Qh ♿ A

* **L0622** Sacroiliac orthosis, flexible, provides pelvic-sacral support, reduces motion about the sacroiliac joint, includes straps, closures, may include pendulous abdomen design, custom fabricated Ⓑ Qp Qh ♿ A

Type of custom-fabricated device for which impression of specific body part is made (e.g., by means of plaster cast, or CAD-CAM [computer-aided design] technology); impression then used to make specific patient model

* **L0623** Sacroiliac orthosis, provides pelvic-sacral support, with rigid or semi-rigid panels over the sacrum and abdomen, reduces motion about the sacroiliac joint, includes straps, closures, may include pendulous abdomen design, prefabricated, off-the-shelf Ⓑ Qp Qh ♿ A

* **L0624** Sacroiliac orthosis, provides pelvic-sacral support, with rigid or semi-rigid panels placed over the sacrum and abdomen, reduces motion about the sacroiliac joint, includes straps, closures, may include pendulous abdomen design, custom fabricated Ⓑ Qp Qh ♿ A

Custom fitted

Lumbar Orthotics

* **L0625** Lumbar orthosis, flexible, provides lumbar support, posterior extends from L-1 to below L-5 vertebra, produces intracavitary pressure to reduce load on the intervertebral discs, includes straps, closures, may include pendulous abdomen design, shoulder straps, stays, prefabricated, off-the-shelf Ⓑ Qp Qh ♿ A

* **L0626** Lumbar orthosis, sagittal control, with rigid posterior panel(s), posterior extends from L-1 to below L-5 vertebra, produces intracavitary pressure to reduce load on the intervertebral discs, includes straps, closures, may include padding, stays, shoulder straps, pendulous abdomen design, prefabricated item that has been trimmed, bent, molded, assembled, or otherwise customized to fit a specific patient by an individual with expertise Ⓑ Qp Qh ♿ A

▶ New   ⟲ Revised   ✓ Reinstated   ~~deleted~~ Deleted   ⊘ Not covered or valid by Medicare   ⓢ Special coverage instructions   ✱ Carrier discretion   Ⓑ Bill Part B MAC   Ⓑ Bill DME MAC

ORTHOTICS & DEVICES

* **L0627** Lumbar orthosis, sagittal control, with rigid anterior and posterior panels, posterior extends from L-1 to below L-5 vertebra, produces intracavitary pressure to reduce load on the intervertebral discs, includes straps, closures, may include padding, shoulder straps, pendulous abdomen design, prefabricated item that has been trimmed, bent, molded, assembled, or otherwise customized to fit a specific patient by an individual with expertise ⑧ Qp Qh ♿ A

Figure 22 Lumbar-sacral orthosis.

Lumbar-Sacral Orthotics

* **L0628** Lumbar-sacral orthosis, flexible, provides lumbo-sacral support, posterior extends from sacrococcygeal junction to T-9 vertebra, produces intracavitary pressure to reduce load on the intervertebral discs, includes straps, closures, may include stays, shoulder straps, pendulous abdomen design, prefabricated, off-the-shelf ⑧ Qp Qh ♿ A

* **L0629** Lumbar-sacral orthosis, flexible, provides lumbo-sacral support, posterior extends from sacrococcygeal junction to T-9 vertebra, produces intracavitary pressure to reduce load on the intervertebral discs, includes straps, closures, may include stays, shoulder straps, pendulous abdomen design, custom fabricated ⑧ Qp Qh ♿ A

   Custom fitted

* **L0630** Lumbar-sacral orthosis, sagittal control, with rigid posterior panel(s), posterior extends from sacrococcygeal junction to T-9 vertebra, produces intracavitary pressure to reduce load on the intervertebral discs, includes straps, closures, may include padding, stays, shoulder straps, pendulous abdomen design, prefabricated item that has been trimmed, bent, molded, assembled, or otherwise customized to fit a specific patient by an individual with expertise ⑧ Qp Qh ♿ A

* **L0631** Lumbar-sacral orthosis, sagittal control, with rigid anterior and posterior panels, posterior extends from sacrococcygeal junction to T-9 vertebra, produces intracavitary pressure to reduce load on the intervertebral discs, includes straps, closures, may include padding, shoulder straps, pendulous abdomen design, prefabricated item that has been trimmed, bent, molded, assembled, or otherwise customized to fit a specific patient by an individual with expertise ⑧ Qp Qh ♿ A

* **L0632** Lumbar-sacral orthosis, sagittal control, with rigid anterior and posterior panels, posterior extends from sacrococcygeal junction to T-9 vertebra, produces intracavitary pressure to reduce load on the intervertebral discs, includes straps, closures, may include padding, shoulder straps, pendulous abdomen design, custom fabricated ⑧ Qp Qh ♿ A

   Custom fitted

* **L0633** Lumbar-sacral orthosis, sagittal-coronal control, with rigid posterior frame/panel(s), posterior extends from sacrococcygeal junction to T-9 vertebra, lateral strength provided by rigid lateral frame/panels, produces intracavitary pressure to reduce load on intervertebral discs, includes straps, closures, may include padding, stays, shoulder straps, pendulous abdomen design, prefabricated item that has been trimmed, bent, molded, assembled, or otherwise customized to fit a specific patient by an individual with expertise ⑧ Qp Qh ♿ A

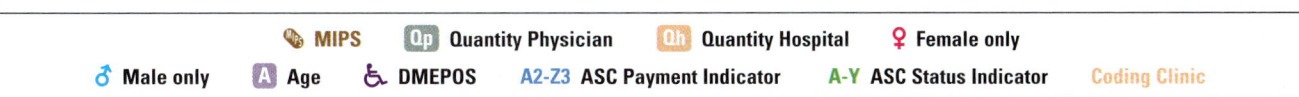

* **L0634** Lumbar-sacral orthosis, sagittal-coronal control, with rigid posterior frame/panel(s), posterior extends from sacrococcygeal junction to T-9 vertebra, lateral strength provided by rigid lateral frame/panel(s), produces intracavitary pressure to reduce load on intervertebral discs, includes straps, closures, may include padding, stays, shoulder straps, pendulous abdomen design, custom fabricated ⒷQpQh♿ A
Custom fitted

* **L0635** Lumbar-sacral orthosis, sagittal-coronal control, lumbar flexion, rigid posterior frame/panel(s), lateral articulating design to flex the lumbar spine, posterior extends from sacrococcygeal junction to T-9 vertebra, lateral strength provided by rigid lateral frame/panel(s), produces intracavitary pressure to reduce load on intervertebral discs, includes straps, closures, may include padding, anterior panel, pendulous abdomen design, prefabricated, includes fitting and adjustment ⒷQpQh♿ A

* **L0636** Lumbar sacral orthosis, sagittal-coronal control, lumbar flexion, rigid posterior frame/panels, lateral articulating design to flex the lumbar spine, posterior extends from sacrococcygeal junction to T-9 vertebra, lateral strength provided by rigid lateral frame/panels, produces intracavitary pressure to reduce load on intervertebral discs, includes straps, closures, may include padding, anterior panel, pendulous abdomen design, custom fabricated ⒷQpQh♿ A
Custom fitted

* **L0637** Lumbar-sacral orthosis, sagittal-coronal control, with rigid anterior and posterior frame/panels, posterior extends from sacrococcygeal junction to T-9 vertebra, lateral strength provided by rigid lateral frame/panels, produces intracavitary pressure to reduce load on intervertebral discs, includes straps, closures, may include padding, shoulder straps, pendulous abdomen design, prefabricated item that has been trimmed, bent, molded, assembled, or otherwise customized to fit a specific patient by an individual with expertise ⒷQpQh♿ A

* **L0638** Lumbar-sacral orthosis, sagittal-coronal control, with rigid anterior and posterior frame/panels, posterior extends from sacrococcygeal junction to T-9 vertebra, lateral strength provided by rigid lateral frame/panels, produces intracavitary pressure to reduce load on intervertebral discs, includes straps, closures, may include padding, shoulder straps, pendulous abdomen design, custom fabricated ⒷQpQh♿ A

* **L0639** Lumbar-sacral orthosis, sagittal-coronal control, rigid shell(s)/panel(s), posterior extends from sacrococcygeal junction to T-9 vertebra, anterior extends from symphysis pubis to xyphoid, produces intracavitary pressure to reduce load on the intervertebral discs, overall strength is provided by overlapping rigid material and stabilizing closures, includes straps, closures, may include soft interface, pendulous abdomen design, prefabricated item that has been trimmed, bent, molded, assembled, or otherwise customized to fit a specific patient by an individual with expertise ⒷQpQh♿ A
Characterized by rigid plastic shell that encircles trunk with overlapping edges and stabilizing closures and provides high degree of immobility

* **L0640** Lumbar-sacral orthosis, sagittal-coronal control, rigid shell(s)/panel(s), posterior extends from sacrococcygeal junction to T-9 vertebra, anterior extends from symphysis pubis to xyphoid, produces intracavitary pressure to reduce load on the intervertebral discs, overall strength is provided by overlapping rigid material and stabilizing closures, includes straps, closures, may include soft interface, pendulous abdomen design, custom fabricated ⒷQpQh♿ A
Custom fitted

Lumbar Orthotics

* **L0641** Lumbar orthosis, sagittal control, with rigid posterior panel(s), posterior extends from L-1 to below L-5 vertebra, produces intracavitary pressure to reduce load on the intervertebral discs, includes straps, closures, may include padding, stays, shoulder straps, pendulous abdomen design, prefabricated, off-the-shelf ⒷQpQh♿ A

▶ New　⇄ Revised　✓ Reinstated　~~deleted~~ Deleted　⊘ Not covered or valid by Medicare
✪ Special coverage instructions　✱ Carrier discretion　Ⓑ Bill Part B MAC　Ⓑ Bill DME MAC

ORTHOTICS & DEVICES

* **L0642** Lumbar orthosis, sagittal control, with rigid anterior and posterior panels, posterior extends from L-1 to below L-5 vertebra, produces intracavitary pressure to reduce load on the intervertebral discs, includes straps, closures, may include padding, shoulder straps, pendulous abdomen design, prefabricated, off-the-shelf ⓑ Qp Qh ♿ A

Lumbar-Sacral Orthotics

* **L0643** Lumbar-sacral orthosis, sagittal control, with rigid posterior panel(s), posterior extends from sacrococcygeal junction to T-9 vertebra, produces intracavitary pressure to reduce load on the intervertebral discs, includes straps, closures, may include padding, stays, shoulder straps, pendulous abdomen design, prefabricated, off-the-shelf ⓑ Qp Qh ♿ A

* **L0648** Lumbar-sacral orthosis, sagittal control, with rigid anterior and posterior panels, posterior extends from sacrococcygeal junction to T-9 vertebra, produces intracavitary pressure to reduce load on the intervertebral discs, includes straps, closures, may include padding, shoulder straps, pendulous abdomen design, prefabricated, off-the-shelf ⓑ Qp Qh ♿ A

* **L0649** Lumbar-sacral orthosis, sagittal-coronal control, with rigid posterior frame/panel(s), posterior extends from sacrococcygeal junction to T-9 vertebra, lateral strength provided by rigid lateral frame/panels, produces intracavitary pressure to reduce load on intervertebral discs, includes straps, closures, may include padding, stays, shoulder straps, pendulous abdomen design, prefabricated, off-the-shelf ⓑ Qp Qh ♿ A

* **L0650** Lumbar-sacral orthosis, sagittal-coronal control, with rigid anterior and posterior frame/panel(s), posterior extends from sacrococcygeal junction to T-9 vertebra, lateral strength provided by rigid lateral frame/panel(s), produces intracavitary pressure to reduce load on intervertebral discs, includes straps, closures, may include padding, shoulder straps, pendulous abdomen design, prefabricated, off-the-shelf ⓑ Qp Qh ♿ A

* **L0651** Lumbar-sacral orthosis, sagittal-coronal control, rigid shell(s)/panel(s), posterior extends from sacrococcygeal junction to T-9 vertebra, anterior extends from symphysis pubis to xyphoid, produces intracavitary pressure to reduce load on the intervertebral discs, overall strength is provided by overlapping rigid material and stabilizing closures, includes straps, closures, may include soft interface, pendulous abdomen design, prefabricated, off-the-shelf ⓑ Qp Qh ♿ A

Cervical-Thoracic-Lumbar-Sacral

* **L0700** Cervical-thoracic-lumbar-sacral-orthoses (CTLSO), anterior-posterior-lateral control, molded to patient model (Minerva type) ⓑ Qp Qh ♿ A

* **L0710** CTLSO, anterior-posterior-lateral-control, molded to patient model, with interface material (Minerva type) ⓑ Qp Qh ♿ A

▶ * **L0720** Cervical-thoracic-lumbar-sacral-orthoses (CTLSO), anterior-posterior-lateral control, prefabricated item that has been trimmed, bent, molded, assembled, or otherwise customized to fit a specific patient by an individual with expertise ⓑ Qp Qh ♿ A

HALO Procedure

* **L0810** HALO procedure, cervical halo incorporated into jacket vest ⓑ Qp Qh ♿ A

* **L0820** HALO procedure, cervical halo incorporated into plaster body jacket ⓑ Qp Qh ♿ A

* **L0830** HALO procedure, cervical halo incorporated into Milwaukee type orthosis ⓑ Qp Qh ♿ A

* **L0859** Addition to HALO procedure, magnetic resonance image compatible systems, rings and pins, any material ⓑ Qp Qh ♿ A

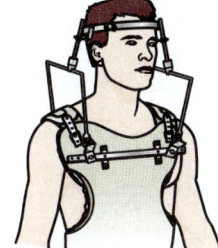

Figure 23 Halo device.

🏷 MIPS　Qp Quantity Physician　Qh Quantity Hospital　♀ Female only
♂ Male only　Ⓐ Age　♿ DMEPOS　A2-Z3 ASC Payment Indicator　A-Y ASC Status Indicator　Coding Clinic

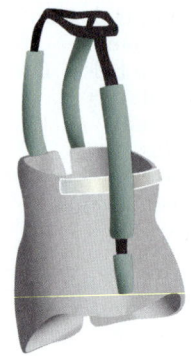

Figure 24   Milwaukee CTLSO.

* **L0861**   Addition to HALO procedure, replacement liner/interface material Ⓑ Qp Qh ♿   A

Additions to Spinal Orthotics

NOTE: TLSO - Thoraci-lumbar-sacral orthoses/Spinal orthoses may be prefabricated, prefitted, or custom fabricated. Conservative treatment for back pain may include the use of spinal orthoses.

* **L0970**   TLSO, corset front Ⓑ Qp Qh ♿   A
* **L0972**   LSO, corset front Ⓑ Qp Qh ♿   A
* **L0974**   TLSO, full corset Ⓑ Qp Qh ♿   A
* **L0976**   LSO, full corset Ⓑ Qp Qh ♿   A
* **L0978**   Axillary crutch extension Ⓑ Qp Qh ♿   A
* **L0980**   Peroneal straps, prefabricated, off-the-shelf, pair Ⓑ Qp Qh ♿   A
* **L0982**   Stocking supporter grips, prefabricated, off-the-shelf, set of four (4) Ⓑ Qp Qh ♿   A
    Convenience item
* **L0984**   Protective body sock, prefabricated, off-the-shelf, each Ⓑ Qp Qh ♿   A
    Garment made of cloth or similar material that is worn under spinal orthosis and is not primarily medical in nature
* **L0999**   Addition to spinal orthosis, not otherwise specified Ⓑ   A

Orthotic Devices: Scoliosis Procedures

NOTE: Orthotic care of scoliosis differs from other orthotic care in that the treatment is more dynamic in nature and uses ongoing continual modification of the orthosis to the patient's changing condition. This coding structure uses the proper names, or eponyms, of the procedures because they have historic and universal acceptance in the profession. It should be recognized that variations to the basic procedures described by the founders/developers are accepted in various medical and orthotic practices throughout the country. All procedures include a model of patient when indicated.

* **L1000**   Cervical-thoracic-lumbar-sacral orthosis (CTLSO) (Milwaukee), inclusive of furnishing initial orthosis, including model Ⓑ Qp Qh ♿   A
* **L1001**   Cervical thoracic lumbar sacral orthosis, immobilizer, infant size, prefabricated, includes fitting and adjustment Ⓑ Qp Qh ♿   A
* **L1005**   Tension based scoliosis orthosis and accessory pads, includes fitting and adjustment Ⓑ Qp Qh ♿   A
* **L1006**   Scoliosis orthosis, sagittal-coronal control provided by a rigid lateral frame, extends from axilla to trochanter, includes all accessory pads, straps and interface, prefabricated item that has been trimmed, bent, molded, assembled, or otherwise customized to fit a specific patient by an individual with expertise Ⓑ Qp Qh ♿   A
▶ * **L1007**   Scoliosis orthosis, sagittal-coronal control provided by a rigid lateral frame, extends from axilla, to trochanter, includes all accessory pads, straps, and interface, custom fabricated Ⓑ Qp Qh ♿   A
* **L1010**   Addition to cervical-thoracic-lumbar-sacral orthosis (CTLSO) or scoliosis orthosis, axilla sling Ⓑ Qp Qh ♿   A
* **L1020**   Addition to CTLSO or scoliosis orthosis, kyphosis pad Ⓑ Qp Qh ♿   A
* **L1025**   Addition to CTLSO or scoliosis orthosis, kyphosis pad, floating Ⓑ Qp Qh ♿   A
* **L1030**   Addition to CTLSO or scoliosis orthosis, lumbar bolster pad Ⓑ Qp Qh ♿   A
* **L1040**   Addition to CTLSO or scoliosis orthosis, lumbar or lumbar rib pad Ⓑ Qp Qh ♿   A
* **L1050**   Addition to CTLSO or scoliosis orthosis, sternal pad Ⓑ Qp Qh ♿   A
* **L1060**   Addition to CTLSO or scoliosis orthosis, thoracic pad Ⓑ Qp Qh ♿   A
* **L1070**   Addition to CTLSO or scoliosis orthosis, trapezius sling Ⓑ Qp Qh ♿   A

▶ New   ⟲ Revised   ✓ Reinstated   deleted Deleted   ⊘ Not covered or valid by Medicare
⊛ Special coverage instructions   * Carrier discretion   Ⓑ Bill Part B MAC   Ⓑ Bill DME MAC

ORTHOTICS & DEVICES

* **L1080** Addition to CTLSO or scoliosis orthosis, outrigger A
* **L1085** Addition to CTLSO or scoliosis orthosis, outrigger, bilateral with vertical extensions A
* **L1090** Addition to CTLSO or scoliosis orthosis, lumbar sling A
* **L1100** Addition to CTLSO or scoliosis orthosis, ring flange, plastic or leather A
* **L1110** Addition to CTLSO or scoliosis orthosis, ring flange, plastic or leather, molded to patient model A
* **L1120** Addition to CTLSO, scoliosis orthosis, cover for upright, each A

Thoracic-Lumbar-Sacral (Low Profile)

* **L1200** Thoracic-lumbar-sacral-orthosis (TLSO), inclusive of furnishing initial orthosis only A
* **L1210** Addition to TLSO, (low profile), lateral thoracic extension A
* **L1220** Addition to TLSO, (low profile), anterior thoracic extension A
* **L1230** Addition to TLSO, (low profile), Milwaukee type superstructure A
* **L1240** Addition to TLSO, (low profile), lumbar derotation pad A
* **L1250** Addition to TLSO, (low profile), anterior ASIS pad A
* **L1260** Addition to TLSO, (low profile), anterior thoracic derotation pad A
* **L1270** Addition to TLSO, (low profile), abdominal pad A
* **L1280** Addition to TLSO, (low profile), rib gusset (elastic), each A
* **L1290** Addition to TLSO, (low profile), lateral trochanteric pad A

Other Scoliosis Procedures

* **L1300** Other scoliosis procedure, body jacket molded to patient model A
* **L1310** Other scoliosis procedure, postoperative body jacket A
* **L1320** Thoracic, pectus carinatum orthosis, sternal compression, rigid circumferential frame with anterior and posterior rigid pads, custom fabricated A
* **L1499** Spinal orthosis, not otherwise specified A

Orthotic Devices: Lower Limb (L1600-L3649)

NOTE: the procedures in L1600-L2999 are considered as base or basic procedures and may be modified by listing procedure from the Additions Sections and adding them to the base procedure.

Hip: Flexible

* **L1600** Hip orthosis, abduction control of hip joints, flexible, frejka type with cover, prefabricated item that has been trimmed, bent, molded, assembled, or otherwise customized to fit a specific patient by an individual with expertise A
* **L1610** Hip orthosis, abduction control of hip joints, flexible, (frejka cover only), prefabricated item that has been trimmed, bent, molded, assembled, or otherwise customized to fit a specific patient by an individual with expertise A
* **L1620** Hip orthosis, abduction control of hip joints, flexible, (Pavlik harness), prefabricated item that has been trimmed, bent, molded, assembled, or otherwise customized to fit a specific patient by an individual with expertise A
* **L1630** Hip orthosis, abduction control of hip joints, semi-flexible (Von Rosen type), custom-fabricated A
* **L1640** Hip orthosis, abduction control of hip joints, static, pelvic band or spreader bar, thigh cuffs, custom-fabricated A

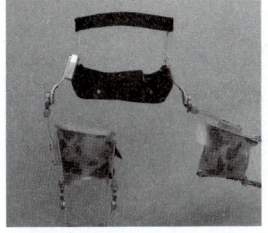

Figure 25 Thoracic-hip-knee-ankle orthosis (THKAO).

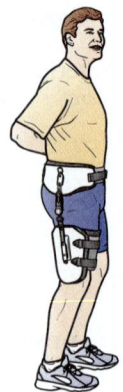

Figure 26 Hip orthosis.

* L1650 Hip orthosis, abduction control of hip joints, static, adjustable, (Ilfled type), prefabricated, includes fitting and adjustment ⓑ Qp Qh ♿ A

* L1652 Hip orthosis, bilateral thigh cuffs with adjustable abductor spreader bar, adult size, prefabricated, includes fitting and adjustment, prefabricated item that has been trimmed, bent, molded, assembled, or otherwise customized to fit a specific patient by an individual with expertise ⓑ Qp Qh A ♿ A

L1653 Hip orthosis, bilateral thigh cuffs with adjustable abductor spreader bar, adult size, prefabricated, off the shelf ⓑ Qp Qh A ♿ A

* L1660 Hip orthosis, abduction control of hip joints, static, plastic, prefabricated, includes fitting and adjustment ⓑ Qp Qh ♿ A

* L1680 Hip orthosis, abduction control of hip joints, dynamic, pelvic control, adjustable hip motion control, thigh cuffs (Rancho hip action type), custom fabrication ⓑ Qp Qh ♿ A

* L1681 Hip orthosis, bilateral hip joints and thigh cuffs, adjustable flexion, extension, abduction control of hip joint, postoperative hip abduction type, prefabricated item that has been trimmed, bent, molded, assembled, or otherwise customized to fit a specific patient by an individual with expertise ⓑ Qp Qh ♿ A

* L1685 Hip orthosis, abduction control of hip joint, postoperative hip abduction type, custom fabricated ⓑ Qp Qh ♿ A

* L1686 Hip orthosis, abduction control of hip joint, postoperative hip abduction type, prefabricated, includes fitting and adjustment ⓑ Qp Qh ♿ A

* L1690 Combination, bilateral, lumbo-sacral, hip, femur orthosis providing adduction and internal rotation control, prefabricated, includes fitting and adjustment ⓑ Qp Qh ♿ A

Legg Perthes

* L1700 Legg-Perthes orthosis (Toronto type), custom-fabricated ⓑ Qp Qh ♿ A

* L1710 Legg-Perthes orthosis (Newington type), custom-fabricated ⓑ Qp Qh ♿ A

* L1720 Legg-Perthes orthosis, trilateral (Tachdjian type), custom-fabricated ⓑ Qp Qh ♿ A

* L1730 Legg-Perthes orthosis (Scottish Rite type), custom-fabricated ⓑ Qp Qh ♿ A

* L1755 Legg-Perthes orthosis (Patten bottom type), custom-fabricated ⓑ Qp Qh ♿ A

Knee (KO)

* L1810 Knee orthosis, elastic with joints, prefabricated item that has been trimmed, bent, molded, assembled, or otherwise customized to fit a specific patient by an individual with expertise ⓑ Qp Qh ♿ A

* L1812 Knee orthosis, elastic with joints, prefabricated, off-the-shelf ⓑ Qp Qh ♿ A

* L1820 Knee orthosis, elastic with condylar pads and joints, with or without patellar control, prefabricated item that has been trimmed, bent, molded, assembled, or otherwise customized to fit a specific patient by an individual with expertise ⓑ Qp Qh ♿ A

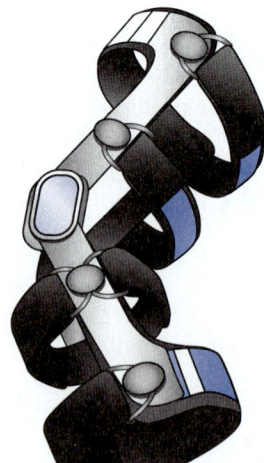

Figure 27 Knee orthosis.

ORTHOTICS & DEVICES

L1821 Knee orthosis, elastic with condylar pads and joints, with or without patellar control, prefabricated, off the shelf ⓑ Qp Qh ♿ A

* **L1830** Knee orthosis, immobilizer, canvas longitudinal, prefabricated, off-the-shelf ⓑ Qp Qh ♿ A

* **L1831** Knee orthosis, locking knee joint(s), positional orthosis, prefabricated, includes fitting and adjustment ⓑ Qp Qh ♿ A

* **L1832** Knee orthosis, adjustable knee joints (unicentric or polycentric), positional orthosis, rigid support, prefabricated item that has been trimmed, bent, molded, assembled, or otherwise customized to fit a specific patient by an individual with expertise ⓑ Qp Qh ♿ A

* **L1833** Knee orthosis, adjustable knee joints (unicentric or polycentric), positional orthosis, rigid support, prefabricated, off-the-shelf ⓑ Qp Qh ♿ A

* **L1834** Knee orthosis, without knee joint, rigid, custom-fabricated ⓑ Qp Qh ♿ A

* **L1836** Knee orthosis, rigid, without joint(s), includes soft interface material, prefabricated, off-the-shelf ⓑ Qp Qh ♿ A

* **L1840** Knee orthosis, derotation, medial-lateral, anterior cruciate ligament, custom fabricated ⓑ Qp Qh ♿ A

* **L1843** Knee orthosis, single upright, thigh and calf, with adjustable flexion and extension joint (unicentric or polycentric), medial-lateral and rotation control, with or without varus/valgus adjustment, prefabricated item that has been trimmed, bent, molded, assembled, or otherwise customized to fit a specific patient by an individual with expertise ⓑ Qp Qh ♿ A

* **L1844** Knee orthosis, single upright, thigh and calf, with adjustable flexion and extension joint (unicentric or polycentric), medial-lateral and rotation control, with or without varus/ valgus adjustment, custom fabricated ⓑ Qp Qh ♿ A

* **L1845** Knee orthosis, double upright, thigh and calf, with adjustable flexion and extension joint (unicentric or polycentric), medial-lateral and rotation control, with or without varus/valgus adjustment, prefabricated item that has been trimmed, bent, molded, assembled, or otherwise customized to fit a specific patient by an individual with expertise ⓑ Qp Qh ♿ A

* **L1846** Knee orthosis, double upright, thigh and calf, with adjustable flexion and extension joint (unicentric or polycentric), medial-lateral and rotation control, with or without varus/ valgus adjustment, custom fabricated ⓑ Qp Qh ♿ A

* **L1847** Knee orthosis, double upright with adjustable joint, with inflatable air support chamber(s), prefabricated item that has been trimmed, bent, molded, assembled, or otherwise customized to fit a specific patient by an individual with expertise ⓑ Qp Qh ♿ A

* **L1848** Knee orthosis, double upright with adjustable joint, with inflatable air support chamber(s), prefabricated, off-the-shelf ⓑ Qp Qh ♿ A

* **L1850** Knee orthosis, Swedish type, prefabricated, off-the-shelf ⓑ Qp Qh ♿ A

* **L1851** Knee orthosis (KO), single upright, thigh and calf, with adjustable flexion and extension joint (unicentric or polycentric), medial-lateral and rotation control, with or without varus/valgus adjustment, prefabricated, off-the-shelf ⓑ Qp Qh ♿ A

* **L1852** Knee orthosis (KO), double upright, thigh and calf, with adjustable flexion and extension joint (unicentric or polycentric), medial-lateral and rotation control, with or without varus/valgus adjustment, prefabricated, off-the-shelf ⓑ Qp Qh ♿ A

* **L1860** Knee orthosis, modification of supracondylar prosthetic socket, custom fabricated (SK) ⓑ Qp Qh ♿ A

Ankle-Foot (AFO)

* **L1900** Ankle foot orthosis (AFO), spring wire, dorsiflexion assist calf band, custom-fabricated ⓑ Qp Qh ♿ A

* **L1902** Ankle orthosis, ankle gauntlet or similiar, with or without joints, prefabricated, off-the-shelf ⓑ Qp Qh ♿ A

* **L1904** Ankle orthosis, ankle gauntlet or similiar, with or without joints, custom fabricated ⓑ Qp Qh ♿ A

* **L1906** Ankle foot orthosis, multiligamentus ankle support, prefabricated, off-the-shelf ⓑ Qp Qh ♿ A

* **L1907** Ankle orthosis, supramalleolar with straps, with or without interface/pads, custom fabricated ⓑ Qp Qh ♿ A

🔍 MIPS	Qp Quantity Physician	Qh Quantity Hospital	♀ Female only
♂ Male only	Ⓐ Age	♿ DMEPOS	A2-Z3 ASC Payment Indicator	A-Y ASC Status Indicator	Coding Clinic

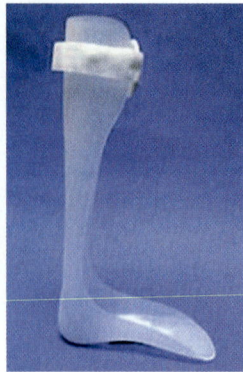

Figure 28 Ankle-foot orthosis (AFO).

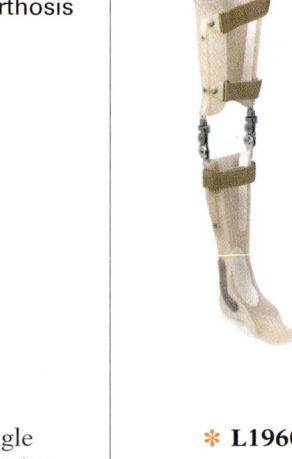

Figure 29 Knee-ankle-foot orthosis (KAFO).

* **L1910** Ankle foot orthosis, posterior, single bar, clasp attachment to shoe counter, prefabricated, includes fitting and adjustment Ⓑ Qp Qh   A

* **L1920** Ankle foot orthosis, single upright with static or adjustable stop (Phelps or Perlstein type), custom fabricated Ⓑ Qp Qh   A

* **L1930** Ankle foot orthosis, plastic or other material, prefabricated, includes fitting and adjustment Ⓑ Qp Qh   A

↻ * **L1932** Ankle foot orthosis, rigid anterior tibial section, total carbon fiber or equal material, prefabricated, item that has been trimmed, bent, molded, assembled, or otherwise customized to fit a specific patient by an individual with expertise Ⓑ Qp Qh   A

▶ * **L1933** Ankle foot orthosis, rigid anterior tibial section, total carbon fiber or equal material, prefabricated, off-the-shelf Ⓑ Qp Qh   A

* **L1940** Ankle foot orthosis, plastic or other material, custom fabricated Ⓑ Qp Qh   A

* **L1945** Ankle foot orthosis, plastic, rigid anterior tibial section (floor reaction), custom fabricated Ⓑ Qp Qh   A

* **L1950** Ankle foot orthosis, spiral (Institute of Rehabilitation Medicine type), plastic, custom fabricated Ⓑ Qp Qh   A

↻ * **L1951** Ankle foot orthosis, spiral (Institute of Rehabilitative Medicine type), plastic or other material, prefabricated, item that has been trimmed, bent, molded, assembled, or otherwise customized to fit a specific patient by an individual with expertise Ⓑ Qp Qh   A

▶ * **L1952** Ankle foot orthosis, spiral, (institute of rehabilitative medicine type), plastic or other material, prefabricated, off-the-shelf Ⓑ Qp Qh   A

* **L1960** Ankle foot orthosis, posterior solid ankle, plastic, custom fabricated Ⓑ Qp Qh   A

* **L1970** Ankle foot orthosis, plastic, with ankle joint, custom fabricated Ⓑ Qp Qh   A

↻ * **L1971** Ankle foot orthosis, plastic or other material with ankle joint, with or without dorsiflexion assist, prefabricated, includes fitting and adjustment Ⓑ Qp Qh   A

* **L1980** Ankle foot orthosis, single upright free plantar dorsiflexion, solid stirrup, calf band/cuff (single bar 'BK' orthosis), custom fabricated Ⓑ Qp Qh   A

* **L1990** Ankle foot orthosis, double upright free plantar dorsiflexion, solid stirrup, calf band/cuff (double bar 'BK' orthosis), custom fabricated Ⓑ Qp Qh   A

Hip-Knee-Ankle-Foot (or Any Combination)

NOTE: L2000, L2020, and L2036 are base procedures to be used with any knee joint. L2010 and L2030 are to be used only with no knee joint.

* **L2000** Knee ankle foot orthosis, single upright, free knee, free ankle, solid stirrup, thigh and calf bands/cuffs (single bar 'AK' orthosis), custom-fabricated Ⓑ Qp Qh   A

* **L2005** Knee ankle foot orthosis, any material, single or double upright, stance control, automatic lock and swing phase release, any type activation; includes ankle joint, any type, custom fabricated Ⓑ Qp Qh   A

* **L2006** Knee ankle foot device, any material, single or double upright, swing and/or stance phase microprocessor control with adjustability, includes all components (e.g., sensors, batteries, charger), any type activation, with or without ankle joint(s), custom fabricated Ⓑ Qp Qh   A

▶ New ↻ Revised ✓ Reinstated ~~deleted~~ Deleted ⊘ Not covered or valid by Medicare
☉ Special coverage instructions * Carrier discretion Ⓑ Bill Part B MAC Ⓑ Bill DME MAC

ORTHOTICS & DEVICES

* **L2010** Knee ankle foot orthosis, single upright, free ankle, solid stirrup, thigh and calf bands/cuffs (single bar 'AK' orthosis), without knee joint, custom-fabricated ⓑ Qp Qh ♿ A

* **L2020** Knee ankle foot orthosis, double upright, free knee, free ankle, solid stirrup, thigh and calf bands/cuffs (double bar 'AK' orthosis), custom fabricated ⓑ Qp Qh ♿ A

* **L2030** Knee ankle foot orthosis, double upright, free ankle, solid stirrup, thigh and calf bands/cuffs (double bar 'AK' orthosis), without knee joint, custom fabricated ⓑ Qp Qh ♿ A

* **L2034** Knee ankle foot orthosis, full plastic, single upright, with or without free motion knee, medial lateral rotation control, with or without free motion ankle, custom fabricated ⓑ Qp Qh ♿ A

* **L2035** Knee ankle foot orthosis, full plastic, static (pediatric size), without free motion ankle, prefabricated, includes fitting and adjustment ⓑ Qp Qh A ♿ A

* **L2036** Knee ankle foot orthosis, full plastic, double upright, with or without free motion knee, with or without free motion ankle, custom fabricated ⓑ Qp Qh ♿ A

* **L2037** Knee ankle foot orthosis, full plastic, single upright, with or without free motion knee, with or without free motion ankle, custom fabricated ⓑ Qp Qh ♿ A

* **L2038** Knee ankle foot orthosis, full plastic, with or without free motion knee, multi-axis ankle, custom fabricated ⓑ Qp Qh ♿ A

Torsion Control: Hip-Knee-Ankle-Foot (TLSO)

* **L2040** Hip knee ankle foot orthosis, torsion control, bilateral rotation straps, pelvic band/belt, custom fabricated ⓑ Qp Qh ♿ A

* **L2050** Hip knee ankle foot orthosis, torsion control, bilateral torsion cables, hip joint, pelvic band/belt, custom fabricated ⓑ Qp Qh ♿ A

* **L2060** Hip knee ankle foot orthosis, torsion control, bilateral torsion cables, ball bearing hip joint, pelvic band/belt, custom fabricated ⓑ Qp Qh ♿ A

* **L2070** Hip knee ankle foot orthosis, torsion control, unilateral rotation straps, pelvic band/belt, custom fabricated ⓑ Qp Qh ♿ A

* **L2080** Hip knee ankle foot orthosis, torsion control, unilateral torsion cable, hip joint, pelvic band/belt, custom fabricated ⓑ Qp Qh ♿ A

* **L2090** Hip knee ankle foot orthosis, torsion control, unilateral torsion cable, ball bearing hip joint, pelvic band/belt, custom fabricated ⓑ Qp Qh ♿ A

Fracture Orthotics: Ankle-Foot and Knee-Ankle-Foot

* **L2106** Ankle foot orthosis, fracture orthosis, tibial fracture cast orthosis, thermoplastic type casting material, custom fabricated ⓑ Qp Qh ♿ A

* **L2108** Ankle foot orthosis, fracture orthosis, tibial fracture cast orthosis, custom fabricated ⓑ Qp Qh ♿ A

* **L2112** Ankle foot orthosis, fracture orthosis, tibial fracture orthosis, soft, prefabricated, includes fitting and adjustment ⓑ Qp Qh ♿ A

* **L2114** Ankle foot orthosis, fracture orthosis, tibial fracture orthosis, semi-rigid, prefabricated, includes fitting and adjustment ⓑ Qp Qh ♿ A

* **L2116** Ankle foot orthosis, fracture orthosis, tibial fracture orthosis, rigid, prefabricated, includes fitting and adjustment ⓑ Qp Qh ♿ A

* **L2126** Knee ankle foot orthosis, fracture orthosis, femoral fracture cast orthosis, thermoplastic type casting material, custom fabricated ⓑ Qp Qh ♿ A

* **L2128** Knee ankle foot orthosis, fracture orthosis, femoral fracture cast orthosis, custom fabricated ⓑ Qp Qh ♿ A

* **L2132** Knee ankle foot orthosis, femoral fracture cast orthosis, soft, prefabricated, includes fitting and adjustment ⓑ Qp Qh ♿ A

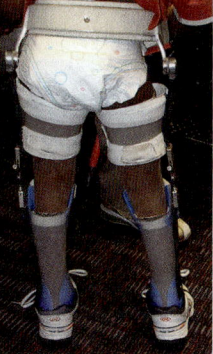

Figure 30 Hip-knee-ankle-foot orthosis (HKAFO).

🔖 MIPS   Qp Quantity Physician   Qh Quantity Hospital   ♀ Female only
♂ Male only   A Age   ♿ DMEPOS   A2-Z3 ASC Payment Indicator   A-Y ASC Status Indicator   Coding Clinic

2026 HCPCS LEVEL II NATIONAL CODES

* **L2134** Knee ankle foot orthosis, femoral fracture cast orthosis, semi-rigid, prefabricated, includes fitting and adjustment Ⓑ Qp Qh & A

* **L2136** Knee ankle foot orthosis, fracture orthosis, femoral fracture cast orthosis, rigid, prefabricated, includes fitting and adjustment Ⓑ Qp Qh & A

Additions to Fracture Orthotics

* **L2180** Addition to lower extremity fracture orthosis, plastic shoe insert with ankle joints Ⓑ Qp Qh & A

* **L2182** Addition to lower extremity fracture orthosis, drop lock knee joint Ⓑ Qp Qh & A

* **L2184** Addition to lower extremity fracture orthosis, limited motion knee joint Ⓑ Qp Qh & A

* **L2186** Addition to lower extremity fracture orthosis, adjustable motion knee joint, Lerman type Ⓑ Qp Qh & A

* **L2188** Addition to lower extremity fracture orthosis, quadrilateral brim Ⓑ Qp Qh & A

* **L2190** Addition to lower extremity fracture orthosis, waist belt Ⓑ Qp Qh & A

* **L2192** Addition to lower extremity fracture orthosis, hip joint, pelvic band, thigh flange, and pelvic belt Ⓑ Qp Qh & A

Additions to Lower Extremity Orthotics

* **L2200** Addition to lower extremity, limited ankle motion, each joint Ⓑ Qp Qh & A

* **L2210** Addition to lower extremity, dorsiflexion assist (plantar flexion resist), each joint Ⓑ Qp Qh & A

* **L2220** Addition to lower extremity, dorsiflexion and plantar flexion assist/resist, each joint Ⓑ Qp Qh & A

* **L2230** Addition to lower extremity, split flat caliper stirrups and plate attachment Ⓑ Qp Qh & A

* **L2232** Addition to lower extremity orthosis, rocker bottom for total contact ankle foot orthosis, for custom fabricated orthosis only Ⓑ Qp Qh & A

* **L2240** Addition to lower extremity, round caliper and plate attachment Ⓑ Qp Qh & A

* **L2250** Addition to lower extremity, foot plate, molded to patient model, stirrup attachment Ⓑ Qp Qh & A

* **L2260** Addition to lower extremity, reinforced solid stirrup (Scott-Craig type) Ⓑ Qp Qh & A

* **L2265** Addition to lower extremity, long tongue stirrup Ⓑ Qp Qh & A

* **L2270** Addition to lower extremity, varus/valgus correction ('T') strap, padded/lined or malleolus pad Ⓑ Qp Qh & A

* **L2275** Addition to lower extremity, varus/valgus correction, plastic modification, padded/lined Ⓑ Qp Qh & A

* **L2280** Addition to lower extremity, molded inner boot Ⓑ Qp Qh & A

* **L2300** Addition to lower extremity, abduction bar (bilateral hip involvement), jointed, adjustable Ⓑ Qp Qh & A

* **L2310** Addition to lower extremity, abduction bar-straight Ⓑ Qp Qh & A

* **L2320** Addition to lower extremity, non-molded lacer, for custom fabricated orthosis only Ⓑ Qp Qh & A

* **L2330** Addition to lower extremity, lacer molded to patient model, for custom fabricated orthosis only Ⓑ Qp Qh & A

Used whether closure is lacer or Velcro

* **L2335** Addition to lower extremity, anterior swing band Ⓑ Qp Qh & A

* **L2340** Addition to lower extremity, pre-tibial shell, molded to patient model Ⓑ Qp Qh & A

* **L2350** Addition to lower extremity, prosthetic type (BK) socket, molded to patient model, (used for 'PTB' and 'AFO' orthoses) Ⓑ Qp Qh & A

* **L2360** Addition to lower extremity, extended steel shank Ⓑ Qp Qh & A

* **L2370** Addition to lower extremity, Patten bottom Ⓑ Qp Qh & A

* **L2375** Addition to lower extremity, torsion control, ankle joint and half solid stirrup Ⓑ Qp Qh & A

* **L2380** Addition to lower extremity, torsion control, straight knee joint, each joint Ⓑ Qp Qh & A

* **L2385** Addition to lower extremity, straight knee joint, heavy duty, each joint Ⓑ Qp & A

* **L2387** Addition to lower extremity, polycentric knee joint, for custom fabricated knee ankle foot orthosis, each joint Ⓑ Qp & A

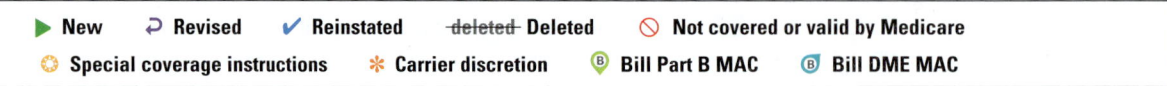

▶ New ↪ Revised ✓ Reinstated ~~deleted~~ Deleted ⊘ Not covered or valid by Medicare
◎ Special coverage instructions ∗ Carrier discretion Ⓑ Bill Part B MAC Ⓑ Bill DME MAC

ORTHOTICS & DEVICES

* **L2390** Addition to lower extremity, offset knee joint, each joint ⒷQp ♿ A
* **L2395** Addition to lower extremity, offset knee joint, heavy duty, each joint ⒷQp ♿ A
* **L2397** Addition to lower extremity orthosis, suspension sleeve ⒷQp ♿ A

Additions to Straight Knee or Offset Knee Joints

* **L2405** Addition to knee joint, drop lock, each ⒷQp ♿ A
* **L2415** Addition to knee lock with integrated release mechanism (bail, cable, or equal), any material, each joint ⒷQp ♿ A
* **L2425** Addition to knee joint, disc or dial lock for adjustable knee flexion, each joint ⒷQp ♿ A
* **L2430** Addition to knee joint, ratchet lock for active and progressive knee extension, each joint ⒷQp ♿ A
* **L2492** Addition to knee joint, lift loop for drop lock ring ⒷQp ♿ A

Additions to Thigh/Weight Bearing Gluteal/Ischial Weight Bearing

* **L2500** Addition to lower extremity, thigh/weight bearing, gluteal/ischial weight bearing, ring ⒷQp Qh A
* **L2510** Addition to lower extremity, thigh/weight bearing, quadri-lateral brim, molded to patient model ⒷQp Qh ♿ A
* **L2520** Addition to lower extremity, thigh/weight bearing, quadri-lateral brim, custom fitted ⒷQp Qh ♿ A
* **L2525** Addition to lower extremity, thigh/weight bearing, ischial containment/narrow M-L brim molded to patient model ⒷQp Qh ♿ A
* **L2526** Addition to lower extremity, thigh/weight bearing, ischial containment/narrow M-L brim, custom fitted ⒷQp Qh ♿ A
* **L2530** Addition to lower extremity, thigh-weight bearing, lacer, non-molded ⒷQp Qh ♿ A
* **L2540** Addition to lower extremity, thigh/weight bearing, lacer, molded to patient model ⒷQp Qh ♿ A
* **L2550** Addition to lower extremity, thigh/weight bearing, high roll cuff ⒷQp Qh A

Additions to Pelvic and Thoracic Control

* **L2570** Addition to lower extremity, pelvic control, hip joint, Clevis type two position joint, each ⒷQp Qh ♿ A
* **L2580** Addition to lower extremity, pelvic control, pelvic sling ⒷQp Qh A
* **L2600** Addition to lower extremity, pelvic control, hip joint, Clevis type, or thrust bearing, free, each ⒷQp Qh ♿ A
* **L2610** Addition to lower extremity, pelvic control, hip joint, Clevis or thrust bearing, lock, each ⒷQp Qh ♿ A
* **L2620** Addition to lower extremity, pelvic control, hip joint, heavy duty, each ⒷQp Qh A
* **L2622** Addition to lower extremity, pelvic control, hip joint, adjustable flexion, each ⒷQp Qh A
* **L2624** Addition to lower extremity, pelvic control, hip joint, adjustable flexion, extension, abduction control, each ⒷQp Qh A
* **L2627** Addition to lower extremity, pelvic control, plastic, molded to patient model, reciprocating hip joint and cables ⒷQp Qh ♿ A
* **L2628** Addition to lower extremity, pelvic control, metal frame, reciprocating hip joint and cables ⒷQp Qh ♿ A
* **L2630** Addition to lower extremity, pelvic control, band and belt, unilateral ⒷQp Qh ♿ A
* **L2640** Addition to lower extremity, pelvic control, band and belt, bilateral ⒷQp Qh ♿ A
* **L2650** Addition to lower extremity, pelvic and thoracic control, gluteal pad, each ⒷQp Qh ♿ A
* **L2660** Addition to lower extremity, thoracic control, thoracic band ⒷQp Qh A
* **L2670** Addition to lower extremity, thoracic control, paraspinal uprights ⒷQp Qh ♿ A
* **L2680** Addition to lower extremity, thoracic control, lateral support uprights ⒷQp Qh ♿ A

General Additions

* **L2750** Addition to lower extremity orthosis, plating chrome or nickel, per bar ⒷQp ♿ A
* **L2755** Addition to lower extremity orthosis, high strength, lightweight material, all hybrid lamination/prepreg composite, per segment, for custom fabricated orthosis only ⒷQp ♿ A

MIPS | Qp Quantity Physician | Qh Quantity Hospital | ♀ Female only
♂ Male only | Ⓐ Age | ♿ DMEPOS | A2-Z3 ASC Payment Indicator | A-Y ASC Status Indicator | Coding Clinic

* L2760	Addition to lower extremity orthosis, extension, per extension, per bar (for lineal adjustment for growth)	A
* L2768	Orthotic side bar disconnect device, per bar	A
* L2780	Addition to lower extremity orthosis, non-corrosive finish, per bar	A
* L2785	Addition to lower extremity orthosis, drop lock retainer, each	A
* L2795	Addition to lower extremity orthosis, knee control, full kneecap	A
* L2800	Addition to lower extremity orthosis, knee control, knee cap, medial or lateral pull, for use with custom fabricated orthosis only	A
* L2810	Addition to lower extremity orthosis, knee control, condylar pad	A
* L2820	Addition to lower extremity orthosis, soft interface for molded plastic, below knee section	A

Only report if soft interface provided, either leather or other material

* L2830	Addition to lower extremity orthosis, soft interface for molded plastic, above knee section	A
* L2840	Addition to lower extremity orthosis, tibial length sock, fracture or equal, each	A
* L2850	Addition to lower extremity orthosis, femoral length sock, fracture or equal, each	A
⊘ L2861	Addition to lower extremity joint, knee or ankle, concentric adjustable torsion style mechanism for custom fabricated orthotics only, each	E1
* L2999	Lower extremity orthoses, not otherwise specified	A

Foot (Orthopedic Shoes) (L3000-L3649)

Inserts

✳ L3000	Foot, insert, removable, molded to patient model, 'UCB' type, Berkeley shell, each	A

If both feet casted and supplied with an orthosis, bill L3000-LT and L3000-RT

IOM: 100-02, 15, 290

| ✳ L3001 | Foot, insert, removable, molded to patient model, Spenco, each | A |

IOM: 100-02, 15, 290

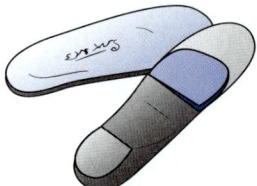

Figure 31 Foot inserts.

| ✳ L3002 | Foot, insert, removable, molded to patient model, Plastazote or equal, each | A |

IOM: 100-02, 15, 290

| ✳ L3003 | Foot, insert, removable, molded to patient model, silicone gel, each | A |

IOM: 100-02, 15, 290

| ✳ L3010 | Foot, insert, removable, molded to patient model, longitudinal arch support, each | A |

IOM: 100-02, 15, 290

| ✳ L3020 | Foot, insert, removable, molded to patient model, longitudinal/metatarsal support, each | A |

IOM: 100-02, 15, 290

| ✳ L3030 | Foot, insert, removable, formed to patient foot, each | A |

IOM: 100-02, 15, 290

| * L3031 | Foot, insert/plate, removable, addition to lower extremity orthosis, high strength, lightweight material, all hybrid lamination/prepreg composite, each | A |

Arch Support, Removable, Premolded

| ✳ L3040 | Foot, arch support, removable, premolded, longitudinal, each | A |

IOM: 100-02, 15, 290

| ✳ L3050 | Foot, arch support, removable, premolded, metatarsal, each | A |

IOM: 100-02, 15, 290

| ✳ L3060 | Foot, arch support, removable, premolded, longitudinal/metatarsal, each | A |

IOM: 100-02, 15, 290

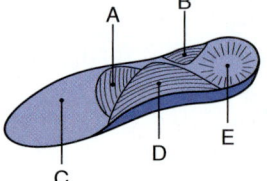

Figure 32 Arch support.

ORTHOTICS & DEVICES

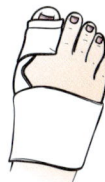

Figure 33 Hallux valgus splint.

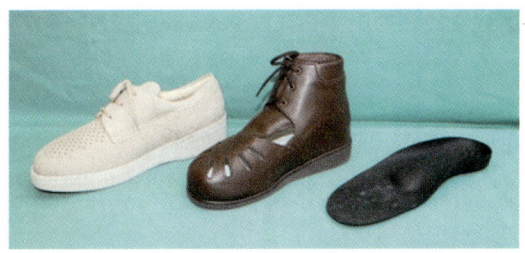

Figure 34 Molded custom shoe.

Arch Support, Non-removable, Attached to Shoe

- ⊛ **L3070** Foot, arch support, non-removable attached to shoe, longitudinal, each ⓑ Qp Qh ♿   A
  IOM: 100-02, 15, 290

- ⊛ **L3080** Foot, arch support, non-removable attached to shoe, metatarsal, each ⓑ Qp Qh ♿   A
  IOM: 100-02, 15, 290

- ⊛ **L3090** Foot, arch support, non-removable attached to shoe, longitudinal/metatarsal, each ⓑ Qp Qh ♿   A
  IOM: 100-02, 15, 290

- ⊛ **L3100** Hallus-valgus night dynamic splint, prefabricated, off-the-shelf ⓑ Qp Qh ♿   A
  IOM: 100-02, 15, 290

Abduction and Rotation Bars

- ⊛ **L3140** Foot, abduction rotation bar, including shoes ⓑ Qp Qh ♿   A
  IOM: 100-02, 15, 290

- ⊛ **L3150** Foot, abduction rotation bar, without shoes ⓑ Qp Qh ♿   A
  IOM: 100-02, 15, 290

- ✱ **L3160** Foot, adjustable shoe-styled positioning device ⓑ Qp Qh   A

- **L3161** Foot, adductus positioning device, adjustable ⓑ Qp Qh   A

- ⊛ **L3170** Foot, plastic, silicone or equal, heel stabilizer, prefabricated, off-the-shelf, each ⓑ Qp Qh ♿   A
  IOM: 100-02, 15, 290

Orthopedic Footwear

- ⊛ **L3201** Orthopedic shoe, oxford with supinator or pronator, infant ⓑ A   A
  IOM: 100-02, 15, 290

- ⊛ **L3202** Orthopedic shoe, oxford with supinator or pronator, child ⓑ A   A
  IOM: 100-02, 15, 290

- ⊛ **L3203** Orthopedic shoe, oxford with supinator or pronator, junior ⓑ A   A
  IOM: 100-02, 15, 290

- ⊛ **L3204** Orthopedic shoe, hightop with supinator or pronator, infant ⓑ A   A
  IOM: 100-02, 15, 290

- ⊛ **L3206** Orthopedic shoe, hightop with supinator or pronator, child ⓑ A   A
  IOM: 100-02, 15, 290

- ⊛ **L3207** Orthopedic shoe, hightop with supinator or pronator, junior ⓑ A   A
  IOM: 100-02, 15, 290

- ⊛ **L3208** Surgical boot, infant, each ⓑ A   A
  IOM: 100-02, 15, 100

- ⊛ **L3209** Surgical boot, each, child ⓑ A   A
  IOM: 100-02, 15, 100

- ⊛ **L3211** Surgical boot, each, junior ⓑ A   A
  IOM: 100-02, 15, 100

- ⊛ **L3212** Benesch boot, pair, infant ⓑ A   A
  IOM: 100-02, 15, 100

- ⊛ **L3213** Benesch boot, pair, child ⓑ A   A
  IOM: 100-02, 15, 100

- ⊛ **L3214** Benesch boot, pair, junior ⓑ A   A
  IOM: 100-02, 15, 100

- ⊘ **L3215** Orthopedic footwear, ladies' shoe, oxford, each ⓑ Qp Qh ♀   E1
  Medicare Statute 1862a8

- ⊘ **L3216** Orthopedic footwear, ladies' shoe, depth inlay, each ⓑ Qp Qh ♀   E1
  Medicare Statute 1862a8

- ⊘ **L3217** Orthopedic footwear, ladies' shoe, hightop, depth inlay, each ⓑ Qp Qh ♀   E1
  Medicare Statute 1862a8

- ⊘ **L3219** Orthopedic footwear, men's shoe, oxford, each ⓑ Qp Qh ♂   E1
  Medicare Statute 1862a8

- ⊘ **L3221** Orthopedic footwear, men's shoe, depth inlay, each ⓑ Qp Qh ♂   E1
  Medicare Statute 1862a8

 MIPS   **Qp** Quantity Physician   **Qh** Quantity Hospital   ♀ Female only
♂ Male only   **A** Age   ♿ DMEPOS   **A2-Z3** ASC Payment Indicator   **A-Y** ASC Status Indicator   Coding Clinic

| ⊘ **L3222** | Orthopedic footwear, men's shoe, hightop, depth inlay, each ⓑ Qp Qh ♂ E1 |

Medicare Statute 1862a8

| ✺ **L3224** | Orthopedic footwear, ladies' shoe, oxford, used as an integral part of a brace (orthosis) ⓑ Qp Qh ♀ ♿ A |

IOM: 100-02, 15, 290

| ✺ **L3225** | Orthopedic footwear, men's shoe, oxford, used as an integral part of a brace (orthosis) ⓑ Qp Qh ♂ ♿ A |

IOM: 100-02, 15, 290

| ✺ **L3230** | Orthopedic footwear, custom shoe, depth inlay, each Qp Qh A |

IOM: 100-02, 15, 290

| ✺ **L3250** | Orthopedic footwear, custom molded shoe, removable inner mold, prosthetic shoe, each ⓑ Qp Qh A |

IOM: 100-02, 15, 290

| ✺ **L3251** | Foot, shoe molded to patient model, silicone shoe, each ⓑ Qp Qh A |

IOM: 100-02, 15, 290

| ✺ **L3252** | Foot, shoe molded to patient model, Plastazote (or similar), custom fabricated, each ⓑ Qp Qh A |

IOM: 100-02, 15, 290

| ✺ **L3253** | Foot, molded shoe Plastazote (or similar), custom fitted, each ⓑ Qp Qh A |

IOM: 100-02, 15, 290

| ✺ **L3254** | Non-standard size or width ⓑ A |

IOM: 100-02, 15, 290

| ✺ **L3255** | Non-standard size or length ⓑ A |

IOM: 100-02, 15, 290

| ✺ **L3257** | Orthopedic footwear, additional charge for split size ⓑ A |

IOM: 100-02, 15, 290

| ✺ **L3260** | Surgical boot/shoe, each ⓑ E1 |

IOM: 100-02, 15, 100

| ✱ **L3265** | Plastazote sandal, each ⓑ A |

Shoe Lifts

| ✺ **L3300** | Lift, elevation, heel, tapered to metatarsals, per inch ⓑ Qp ♿ A |

IOM: 100-02, 15, 290

| ✺ **L3310** | Lift, elevation, heel and sole, Neoprene, per inch ⓑ Qp ♿ A |

IOM: 100-02, 15, 290

| ✺ **L3320** | Lift, elevation, heel and sole, cork, per inch ⓑ Qp A |

IOM: 100-02, 15, 290

| ✺ **L3330** | Lift, elevation, metal extension (skate) ⓑ Qp Qh ♿ A |

IOM: 100-02, 15, 290

| ✺ **L3332** | Lift, elevation, inside shoe, tapered, up to one-half inch ⓑ Qp Qh ♿ A |

IOM: 100-02, 15, 290

| ✺ **L3334** | Lift, elevation, heel, per inch ⓑ Qp ♿ A |

IOM: 100-02, 15, 290

Shoe Wedges

| ✺ **L3340** | Heel wedge, SACH ⓑ Qp Qh ♿ A |

IOM: 100-02, 15, 290

| ✺ **L3350** | Heel wedge Qp Qh ♿ A |

IOM: 100-02, 15, 290

| ✺ **L3360** | Sole wedge, outside sole ⓑ Qp Qh ♿ A |

IOM: 100-02, 15, 290

| ✺ **L3370** | Sole wedge, between sole Qp Qh A |

IOM: 100-02, 15, 290

| ✺ **L3380** | Clubfoot wedge ⓑ Qp Qh ♿ A |

IOM: 100-02, 15, 290

| ✺ **L3390** | Outflare wedge ⓑ Qp Qh ♿ A |

IOM: 100-02, 15, 290

| ✺ **L3400** | Metatarsal bar wedge, rocker ⓑ Qp Qh ♿ A |

IOM: 100-02, 15, 290

| ✺ **L3410** | Metatarsal bar wedge, between sole ⓑ Qp Qh ♿ A |

IOM: 100-02, 15, 290

| ✺ **L3420** | Full sole and heel wedge, between sole ⓑ Qp Qh ♿ A |

IOM: 100-02, 15, 290

Shoe Heels

| ✺ **L3430** | Heel, counter, plastic reinforced ⓑ Qp Qh ♿ A |

IOM: 100-02, 15, 290

| ✺ **L3440** | Heel, counter, leather reinforced ⓑ Qp Qh ♿ A |

IOM: 100-02, 15, 290

| ✺ **L3450** | Heel, SACH cushion type ⓑ Qp Qh ♿ A |

IOM: 100-02, 15, 290

| ✺ **L3455** | Heel, new leather, standard ⓑ Qp Qh ♿ A |

IOM: 100-02, 15, 290

| ✺ **L3460** | Heel, new rubber, standard ⓑ Qp Qh ♿ A |

IOM: 100-02, 15, 290

▶ New ⤺ Revised ✓ Reinstated ~~deleted~~ Deleted ⊘ Not covered or valid by Medicare
✺ Special coverage instructions ✱ Carrier discretion ⓑ Bill Part B MAC ⓑ Bill DME MAC

ORTHOTICS & DEVICES

- ✹ **L3465** Heel, Thomas with wedge Ⓑ Qp Qh ♿ A
  IOM: 100-02, 15, 290
- ✹ **L3470** Heel, Thomas extended to ball Ⓑ Qp Qh ♿ A
  IOM: 100-02, 15, 290
- ✹ **L3480** Heel, pad and depression for spur Ⓑ Qp Qh ♿ A
  IOM: 100-02, 15, 290
- ✹ **L3485** Heel, pad, removable for spur Ⓑ Qp Qh A
  IOM: 100-02, 15, 290

Orthopedic Shoe Additions: Other

- ✹ **L3500** Orthopedic shoe addition, insole, leather Ⓑ Qp Qh ♿ A
  IOM: 100-02, 15, 290
- ✹ **L3510** Orthopedic shoe addition, insole, rubber Ⓑ Qp Qh ♿ A
  IOM: 100-02, 15, 290
- ✹ **L3520** Orthopedic shoe addition, insole, felt covered with leather Ⓑ Qp Qh ♿ A
  IOM: 100-02, 15, 290
- ✹ **L3530** Orthopedic shoe addition, sole, half Ⓑ Qp Qh ♿ A
  IOM: 100-02, 15, 290
- ✹ **L3540** Orthopedic shoe addition, sole, full Ⓑ Qp Qh ♿ A
  IOM: 100-02, 15, 290
- ✹ **L3550** Orthopedic shoe addition, toe tap standard Ⓑ Qp Qh ♿ A
  IOM: 100-02, 15, 290
- ✹ **L3560** Orthopedic shoe addition, toe tap, horseshoe Ⓑ Qp Qh ♿ A
  IOM: 100-02, 15, 290
- ✹ **L3570** Orthopedic shoe addition, special extension to instep (leather with eyelets) Ⓑ Qp Qh ♿ A
  IOM: 100-02, 15, 290
- ✹ **L3580** Orthopedic shoe addition, convert instep to Velcro closure Ⓑ Qp Qh ♿ A
  IOM: 100-02, 15, 290
- ✹ **L3590** Orthopedic shoe addition, convert firm shoe counter to soft counter Ⓑ Qp Qh ♿ A
  IOM: 100-02, 15, 290
- ✹ **L3595** Orthopedic shoe addition, March bar Ⓑ Qp Qh ♿ A
  IOM: 100-02, 15, 290

Transfer or Replacement

- ✹ **L3600** Transfer of an orthosis from one shoe to another, caliper plate, existing Ⓑ Qp Qh ♿ A
  IOM: 100-02, 15, 290
- ✹ **L3610** Transfer of an orthosis from one shoe to another, caliper plate, new Ⓑ Qp Qh ♿ A
  IOM: 100-02, 15, 290
- ✹ **L3620** Transfer of an orthosis from one shoe to another, solid stirrup, existing Ⓑ Qp Qh ♿ A
  IOM: 100-02, 15, 290
- ✹ **L3630** Transfer of an orthosis from one shoe to another, solid stirrup, new Ⓑ Qp Qh ♿ A
  IOM: 100-02, 15, 290
- ✹ **L3640** Transfer of an orthosis from one shoe to another, Dennis Browne splint (Riveton), both shoes Ⓑ Qp Qh ♿ A
  IOM: 100-02, 15, 290
- ✹ **L3649** Orthopedic shoe, modification, addition or transfer, not otherwise specified Ⓑ A
  IOM: 100-02, 15, 290

Orthotic Devices: Upper Limb

NOTE: The procedures in this section are considered as base or basic procedures and may be modified by listing procedures from the Additions section and adding them to the base procedure.

Shoulder

- ✶ **L3650** Shoulder orthosis, figure of eight design abduction restrainer, prefabricated, off-the-shelf Ⓑ Qp Qh ♿ A
- ✶ **L3660** Shoulder orthosis, figure of eight design abduction restrainer, canvas and webbing, prefabricated, off-the-shelf Ⓑ Qp Qh ♿ A
- ✶ **L3670** Shoulder orthosis, acromio/clavicular (canvas and webbing type), prefabricated, off-the-shelf Ⓑ Qp Qh ♿ A
- ✶ **L3671** Shoulder orthosis, shoulder joint design, without joints, may include soft interface, straps, custom fabricated, includes fitting and adjustment Ⓑ Qp Qh ♿ A

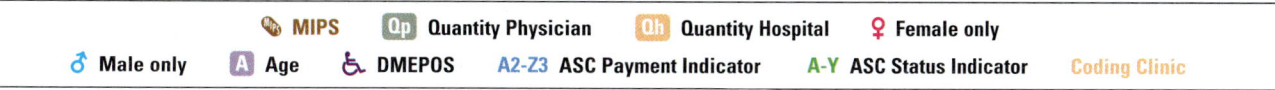

| 🏵 MIPS | Qp Quantity Physician | Qh Quantity Hospital | ♀ Female only |
| ♂ Male only | Ⓐ Age | ♿ DMEPOS | A2-Z3 ASC Payment Indicator | A-Y ASC Status Indicator | Coding Clinic |

✱ L3674	Shoulder orthosis, abduction positioning (airplane design), thoracic component and support bar, with or without nontorsion joint/turnbuckle, may include soft interface, straps, custom fabricated, includes fitting and adjustment		A
✱ L3675	Shoulder orthosis, vest type abduction restrainer, canvas webbing type or equal, prefabricated, off-the-shelf		A
⊘ L3677	Shoulder orthosis, shoulder joint design, without joints, may include soft interface, straps, prefabricated item that has been trimmed, bent, molded, assembled, or otherwise customized to fit a specific patient by an individual with expertise		A
✱ L3678	Shoulder orthosis, shoulder joint design, without joints, may include soft interface, straps, prefabricated, off-the-shelf		A

Elbow

✱ L3702	Elbow orthosis, without joints, may include soft interface, straps, custom fabricated, includes fitting and adjustment		A
✱ L3710	Elbow orthosis, elastic with metal joints, prefabricated, off-the-shelf		A
✱ L3720	Elbow orthosis, double upright with forearm/arm cuffs, free motion, custom fabricated		A
✱ L3730	Elbow orthosis, double upright with forearm/arm cuffs, extension/flexion assist, custom fabricated		A
✱ L3740	Elbow orthosis, double upright with forearm/arm cuffs, adjustable position lock with active control, custom fabricated		A
✱ L3760	Elbow orthosis (EO), with adjustable position locking joint(s), prefabricated, item that has been trimmed, bent, molded, assembled, or otherwise customized to fit a specific patient by an individual with expertise		A
✱ L3761	Elbow orthosis (EO), with adjustable position locking joint(s), prefabricated, off-the-shelf		A
✱ L3762	Elbow orthosis, rigid, without joints, includes soft interface material, prefabricated, off-the-shelf		A
✱ L3763	Elbow wrist hand orthosis, rigid, without joints, may include soft interface, straps, custom fabricated, includes fitting and adjustment		A
✱ L3764	Elbow wrist hand orthosis, includes one or more nontorsion joints, elastic bands, turnbuckles, may include soft interface, straps, custom fabricated, includes fitting and adjustment		A
✱ L3765	Elbow wrist hand finger orthosis, rigid, without joints, may include soft interface, straps, custom fabricated, includes fitting and adjustment		A
✱ L3766	Elbow wrist hand finger orthosis, includes one or more nontorsion joints, elastic bands, turnbuckles, may include soft interface, straps, custom fabricated, includes fitting and adjustment		A

Wrist-Hand-Finger Orthosis (WHFO)

✱ L3806	Wrist hand finger orthosis, includes one or more nontorsion joint(s), turnbuckles, elastic bands/springs, may include soft interface material, straps, custom fabricated, includes fitting and adjustment		A
✱ L3807	Wrist hand finger orthosis, without joint(s), prefabricated item that has been trimmed, bent, molded, assembled, or otherwise customized to fit a specific patient by an individual with expertise		A
✱ L3808	Wrist hand finger orthosis, rigid without joints, may include soft interface material; straps, custom fabricated, includes fitting and adjustment		A
✱ L3809	Wrist hand finger orthosis, without joint(s), prefabricated, off-the-shelf, any type		A
⊘ L3891	Addition to upper extremity joint, wrist or elbow, concentric adjustable torsion style mechanism for custom fabricated orthotics only, each		E1

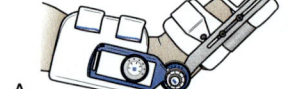
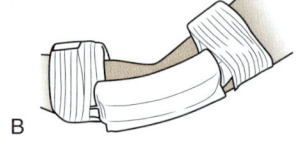

Figure 35 Elbow orthoses.

▶ New   ↻ Revised   ✓ Reinstated   ~~deleted~~ Deleted   ⊘ Not covered or valid by Medicare
⊙ Special coverage instructions   ✱ Carrier discretion   ⑧ Bill Part B MAC   ⑨ Bill DME MAC

ORTHOTICS & DEVICES

* **L3900** Wrist hand finger orthosis, dynamic flexor hinge, reciprocal wrist extension/flexion, finger flexion/extension, wrist or finger driven, custom fabricated ⓑ Qp Qh ♿ A

* **L3901** Wrist hand finger orthosis, dynamic flexor hinge, reciprocal wrist extension/flexion, finger flexion/extension, cable driven, custom fabricated ⓑ Qp Qh ♿ A

* **L3904** Wrist hand finger orthosis, external powered, electric, custom fabricated ⓑ Qp Qh ♿ A

Other Upper Extremity Orthotics

* **L3905** Wrist hand orthosis, includes one or more nontorsion joints, elastic bands, turnbuckles, may include soft interface, straps, custom fabricated, includes fitting and adjustment ⓑ Qp Qh ♿ A

* **L3906** Wrist hand orthosis, without joints, may include soft interface, straps, custom fabricated, includes fitting and adjustment ⓑ Qp Qh ♿ A

* **L3908** Wrist hand orthosis, wrist extension control cock-up, non-molded, prefabricated, off-the-shelf ⓑ Qp Qh ♿ A

* **L3912** Hand finger orthosis (HFO), flexion glove with elastic finger control, prefabricated, off-the-shelf ⓑ Qp Qh ♿ A

* **L3913** Hand finger orthosis, without joints, may include soft interface, straps, custom fabricated, includes fitting and adjustment ⓑ Qp Qh ♿ A

* **L3915** Wrist hand orthosis, includes one or more nontorsion joint(s), elastic bands, turnbuckles, may include soft interface, straps, prefabricated item that has been trimmed, bent, molded, assembled, or otherwise customized to fit a specific patient by an individual with expertise ⓑ Qp Qh ♿ A

* **L3916** Wrist hand orthosis, includes one or more nontorsion joint(s), elastic bands, turnbuckles, may include soft interface, straps, prefabricated, off-the-shelf ⓑ Qp Qh ♿ A

* **L3917** Hand orthosis, metacarpal fracture orthosis, prefabricated item that has been trimmed, bent, molded, assembled, or otherwise customized to fit a specific patient by an individual with expertise ⓑ Qp Qh ♿ A

* **L3918** Hand orthosis, metacarpal fracture orthosis, prefabricated, off-the-shelf ⓑ Qp Qh ♿ A

* **L3919** Hand orthosis, without joints, may include soft interface, straps, custom fabricated, includes fitting and adjustment ⓑ Qp Qh ♿ A

* **L3921** Hand finger orthosis, includes one or more nontorsion joints, elastic bands, turnbuckles, may include soft interface, straps, custom fabricated, includes fitting and adjustment ⓑ Qp Qh ♿ A

* **L3923** Hand finger orthosis, without joints, may include soft interface, straps, prefabricated item that has been trimmed, bent, molded, assembled, or otherwise customized to fit a specific patient by an individual with expertise ⓑ Qp Qh ♿ A

* **L3924** Hand finger orthosis, without joints, may include soft interface, straps, prefabricated, off-the-shelf ⓑ Qp Qh ♿ A

* **L3925** Finger orthosis, proximal interphalangeal (PIP)/distal interphalangeal (DIP), non torsion joint/spring, extension/flexion, may include soft interface material, prefabricated, off-the-shelf ⓑ Qp Qh ♿ A

* **L3927** Finger orthosis, proximal interphalangeal (PIP)/distal interphalangeal (DIP), without joint/spring, extension/flexion (e.g., static or ring type), may include soft interface material, prefabricated, off-the-shelf ⓑ Qp Qh ♿ A

* **L3929** Hand finger orthosis, includes one or more nontorsion joint(s), turnbuckles, elastic bands/springs, may include soft interface material, straps, prefabricated item that has been trimmed, bent, molded, assembled, or otherwise customized to fit a specific patient by an individual with expertise ⓑ Qp Qh ♿ A

* **L3930** Hand finger orthosis, includes one or more nontorsion joint(s), turnbuckles, elastic bands/springs, may include soft interface material, straps, prefabricated, off-the-shelf ⓑ Qp Qh ♿ A

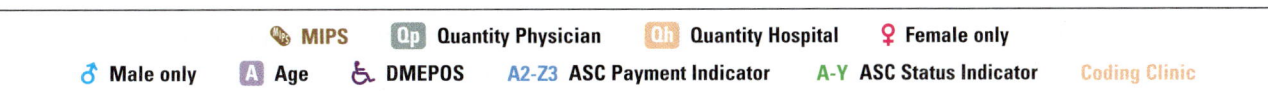

MIPS   Qp Quantity Physician   Qh Quantity Hospital   ♀ Female only   ♂ Male only   A Age   ♿ DMEPOS   A2-Z3 ASC Payment Indicator   A-Y ASC Status Indicator   Coding Clinic

* **L3931** Wrist hand finger orthosis, includes one or more nontorsion joint(s), turnbuckles, elastic bands/springs, may include soft interface material, straps, prefabricated, includes fitting and adjustment A

* **L3933** Finger orthosis, without joints, may include soft interface, custom fabricated, includes fitting and adjustment A

* **L3935** Finger orthosis, nontorsion joint, may include soft interface, custom fabricated, includes fitting and adjustment A

* **L3956** Addition of joint to upper extremity orthosis, any material, per joint A

Shoulder-Elbow-Wrist-Hand Orthotics (SEWHO) (L3960-L3973)

* **L3960** Shoulder elbow wrist hand orthosis, abduction positioning, airplane design, prefabricated, includes fitting and adjustment A

* **L3961** Shoulder elbow wrist hand orthosis, shoulder cap design, without joints, may include soft interface, straps, custom fabricated, includes fitting and adjustment A

* **L3962** Shoulder elbow wrist hand orthosis, abduction positioning, Erb's palsy design, prefabricated, includes fitting and adjustment A

* **L3967** Shoulder elbow wrist hand orthosis, abduction positioning (airplane design), thoracic component and support bar, without joints, may include soft interface, straps, custom fabricated, includes fitting and adjustment A

* **L3971** Shoulder elbow wrist hand orthosis, shoulder cap design, includes one or more nontorsion joints, elastic bands, turnbuckles, may include soft interface, straps, custom fabricated, includes fitting and adjustment A

* **L3973** Shoulder elbow wrist hand orthosis, abduction positioning (airplane design), thoracic component and support bar, includes one or more nontorsion joints, elastic bands, turnbuckles, may include soft interface, straps, custom fabricated, includes fitting and adjustment A

Shoulder-Elbow-Wrist-Hand-Finger Orthotics

* **L3975** Shoulder elbow wrist hand finger orthosis, shoulder cap design, without joints, may include soft interface, straps, custom fabricated, includes fitting and adjustment A

* **L3976** Shoulder elbow wrist hand finger orthosis, abduction positioning (airplane design), thoracic component and support bar, without joints, may include soft interface, straps, custom fabricated, includes fitting and adjustment A

* **L3977** Shoulder elbow wrist hand finger orthosis, shoulder cap design, includes one or more nontorsion joints, elastic bands, turnbuckles, may include soft interface, straps, custom fabricated, includes fitting and adjustment A

* **L3978** Shoulder elbow wrist hand finger orthosis, abduction positioning (airplane design), thoracic component and support bar, includes one or more nontorsion joints, elastic bands, turnbuckles, may include soft interface, straps, custom fabricated, includes fitting and adjustment A

Fracture Orthorics

* **L3980** Upper extremity fracture orthosis, humeral, prefabricated, includes fitting and adjustment A

* **L3981** Upper extremity fracture orthosis, humeral, prefabricated, includes shoulder cap design, with or without joints, forearm section, may include soft interface, straps, includes fitting and adjustments A

* **L3982** Upper extremity fracture orthosis, radius/ulnar, prefabricated, includes fitting and adjustment A

* **L3984** Upper extremity fracture orthosis, wrist, prefabricated, includes fitting and adjustment A

* **L3995** Addition to upper extremity orthosis, sock, fracture or equal, each A

* **L3999** Upper limb orthosis, not otherwise specified A

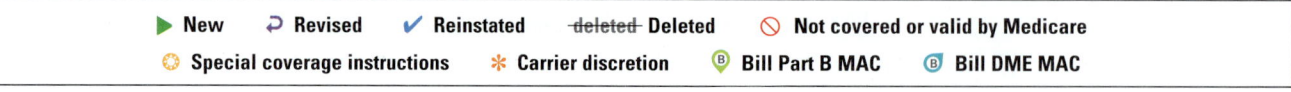
▶ New ↻ Revised ✓ Reinstated ~~deleted~~ Deleted ⊘ Not covered or valid by Medicare
⊛ Special coverage instructions ✱ Carrier discretion Ⓑ Bill Part B MAC Ⓑ Bill DME MAC

ORTHOTICS & DEVICES

Repairs

* **L4000** Replace girdle for spinal orthosis (CTLSO or SO) Ⓑ Qp Qh ♿ A
* **L4002** Replacement strap, any orthosis, includes all components, any length, any type Ⓑ Qp ♿ A
* **L4010** Replace trilateral socket brim Ⓑ Qp Qh ♿ A
* **L4020** Replace quadrilateral socket brim, molded to patient model Ⓑ Qp Qh ♿ A
* **L4030** Replace quadrilateral socket brim, custom fitted Ⓑ Qp Qh ♿ A
* **L4040** Replace molded thigh lacer, for custom fabricated orthosis only Ⓑ Qp Qh ♿ A
* **L4045** Replace non-molded thigh lacer, for custom fabricated orthosis only Ⓑ Qp Qh ♿ A
* **L4050** Replace molded calf lacer, for custom fabricated orthosis only Ⓑ Qp Qh ♿ A
* **L4055** Replace non-molded calf lacer, for custom fabricated orthosis only Ⓑ Qp Qh ♿ A
* **L4060** Replace high roll cuff Ⓑ Qp Qh ♿ A
* **L4070** Replace proximal and distal upright for KAFO Ⓑ Qp Qh ♿ A
* **L4080** Replace metal bands KAFO, proximal thigh Ⓑ Qp Qh ♿ A
* **L4090** Replace metal bands KAFO-AFO, calf or distal thigh Ⓑ Qp ♿ A
* **L4100** Replace leather cuff KAFO, proximal thigh Ⓑ Qp Qh ♿ A
* **L4110** Replace leather cuff KAFO-AFO, calf or distal thigh Ⓑ Qp ♿ A
* **L4130** Replace pretibial shell Ⓑ Qp Qh ♿ A
* **L4205** Repair of orthotic device, labor component, per 15 minutes Ⓑ Qp A

    IOM: 100-02, 15, 110.2

* **L4210** Repair of orthotic device, repair or replace minor parts Ⓑ Qp Qh A

    IOM: 100-02, 15, 110.2; 100-02, 15, 120

Ancillary Orthotic Services

* **L4350** Ankle control orthosis, stirrup style, rigid, includes any type interface (e.g., pneumatic, gel), prefabricated, off-the-shelf Ⓑ Qp Qh ♿ A

* **L4360** Walking boot, pneumatic and/or vacuum, with or without joints, with or without interface material, prefabricated item that has been trimmed, bent, molded, assembled, or otherwise customized to fit a specific patient by an individual with expertise Ⓑ Qp Qh ♿ A

    Noncovered when walking boots used primarily to relieve pressure, especially on sole of foot, or are used for patients with foot ulcers

* **L4361** Walking boot, pneumatic and/or vacuum, with or without joints, with or without interface material, prefabricated, off-the-shelf Ⓑ Qp Qh ♿ A
* **L4370** Pneumatic full leg splint, prefabricated, off-the-shelf Ⓑ Qp Qh ♿ A
* **L4386** Walking boot, non-pneumatic, with or without joints, with or without interface material, prefabricated item that has been trimmed, bent, molded, assembled, or otherwise customized to fit a specific patient by an individual with expertise Ⓑ Qp Qh ♿ A
* **L4387** Walking boot, non-pneumatic, with or without joints, with or without interface material, prefabricated, off-the-shelf Ⓑ Qp Qh ♿ A
* **L4392** Replacement, soft interface material, static AFO Ⓑ Qp Qh ♿ A
* **L4394** Replace soft interface material, foot drop splint Ⓑ Qp Qh ♿ A
* **L4396** Static or dynamic ankle foot orthosis, including soft interface material, adjustable for fit, for positioning, may be used for minimal ambulation, prefabricated item that has been trimmed, bent, molded, assembled, or otherwise customized to fit a specific patient by an individual with expertise Ⓑ Qp Qh ♿ A
* **L4397** Static or dynamic ankle foot orthosis, including soft interface material, adjustable for fit, for positioning, may be used for minimal ambulation, prefabricated, off-the-shelf Ⓑ Qp Qh ♿ A
* **L4398** Foot drop splint, recumbent positioning device, prefabricated, off-the-shelf Ⓑ Qp Qh ♿ A
* **L4631** Ankle foot orthosis, walking boot type, varus/valgus correction, rocker bottom, anterior tibial shell, soft interface, custom arch support, plastic or other material, includes straps and closures, custom fabricated Ⓑ Qp Qh ♿ A

| 🪙 MIPS | Qp Quantity Physician | Qh Quantity Hospital | ♀ Female only |
| ♂ Male only | Ⓐ Age | ♿ DMEPOS | A2-Z3 ASC Payment Indicator | A-Y ASC Status Indicator | Coding Clinic |

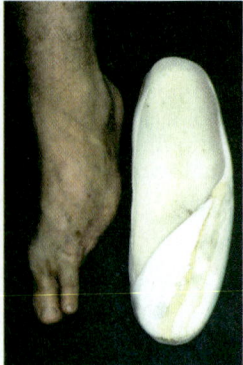

Figure 36 Partial foot.

PROSTHETICS (L5000-L9999)

Lower Limb (L5000-L5999)

NOTE: The procedures in this section are considered as base or basic procedures and may be modified by listing items/procedures or special materials from the Additions section and adding them to the base procedure.

Partial Foot

- ✺ **L5000** Partial foot, shoe insert with longitudinal arch, toe filler ⑧ Qp Qh ♿ A
  IOM: 100-02, 15, 290
- ✺ **L5010** Partial foot, molded socket, ankle height, with toe filler ⑧ Qp Qh ♿ A
  IOM: 100-02, 15, 290
- ✺ **L5020** Partial foot, molded socket, tibial tubercle height, with toe filler ⑧ Qp Qh ♿ A
  IOM: 100-02, 15, 290

Ankle

- ✱ **L5050** Ankle, Symes, molded socket, SACH foot ⑧ Qp Qh ♿ A
- ✱ **L5060** Ankle, Symes, metal frame, molded leather socket, articulated ankle/foot ⑧ Qp Qh ♿ A

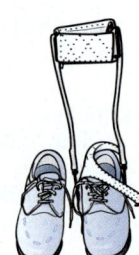

Figure 37 Ankle Symes.

Below Knee

- ✱ **L5100** Below knee, molded socket, shin, SACH foot ⑧ Qp Qh ♿ A
- ✱ **L5105** Below knee, plastic socket, joints and thigh lacer, SACH foot ⑧ Qp Qh ♿ A

Knee Disarticulation

- ✱ **L5150** Knee disarticulation (or through knee), molded socket, external knee joints, shin, SACH foot ⑧ Qp Qh ♿ A
- ✱ **L5160** Knee disarticulation (or through knee), molded socket, bent knee configuration, external knee joints, shin, SACH foot ⑧ Qp Qh ♿ A

Above Knee

- ✱ **L5200** Above knee, molded socket, single axis constant friction knee, shin, SACH foot ⑧ Qp Qh ♿ A
- ✱ **L5210** Above knee, short prosthesis, no knee joint ('stubbies'), with foot blocks, no ankle joints, each ⑧ Qp Qh ♿ A
- ✱ **L5220** Above knee, short prosthesis, no knee joint ('stubbies'), with articulated ankle/foot, dynamically aligned, each ⑧ Qp Qh ♿ A
- ✱ **L5230** Above knee, for proximal femoral focal deficiency, constant friction knee, shin, SACH foot ⑧ Qp Qh ♿ A

Hip Disarticulation

- ✱ **L5250** Hip disarticulation, Canadian type; molded socket, hip joint, single axis constant friction knee, shin, SACH foot ⑧ Qp Qh ♿ A
- ✱ **L5270** Hip disarticulation, tilt table type; molded socket, locking hip joint, single axis constant friction knee, shin, SACH foot ⑧ Qp Qh ♿ A

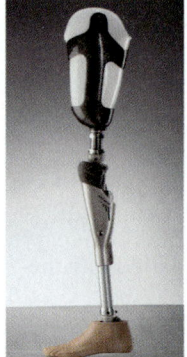

Figure 38 Above knee.

▶ New ⟲ Revised ✔ Reinstated ~~deleted~~ Deleted ⊘ Not covered or valid by Medicare
✺ Special coverage instructions ✱ Carrier discretion ⑨ Bill Part B MAC ⑧ Bill DME MAC

PROSTHETICS

Hemipelvectomy

* **L5280** Hemipelvectomy, Canadian type; molded socket, hip joint, single axis constant friction knee, shin, SACH foot ⓑ Qp Qh ♿ A

Endoskeletal

* **L5301** Below knee, molded socket, shin, SACH foot, endoskeletal system ⓑ Qp Qh ♿ A
* **L5312** Knee disarticulation (or through knee), molded socket, single axis knee, pylon, sach foot, endoskeletal system ⓑ Qp Qh ♿ A
* **L5321** Above knee, molded socket, open end, SACH foot, endoskeletal system, single axis knee ⓑ Qp Qh ♿ A
* **L5331** Hip disarticulation, Canadian type, molded socket, endoskeletal system, hip joint, single axis knee, SACH foot ⓑ Qp Qh ♿ A
* **L5341** Hemipelvectomy, Canadian type, molded socket, endoskeletal system, hip joint, single axis knee, SACH foot ⓑ Qp Qh ♿ A

Immediate Postsurgical or Early Fitting Procedures

* **L5400** Immediate post surgical or early fitting, application of initial rigid dressing, including fitting, alignment, suspension, and one cast change, below knee ⓑ Qp Qh ♿ A
* **L5410** Immediate post surgical or early fitting, application of initial rigid dressing, including fitting, alignment and suspension, below knee, each additional cast change and realignment ⓑ Qp Qh ♿ A
* **L5420** Immediate post surgical or early fitting, application of initial rigid dressing, including fitting, alignment and suspension and one cast change 'AK' or knee disarticulation ⓑ Qp Qh ♿ A
* **L5430** Immediate postsurgical or early fitting, application of initial rigid dressing, including fitting, alignment, and suspension, 'AK' or knee disarticulation, each additional cast change and realignment ⓑ Qp Qh ♿ A
* **L5450** Immediate post surgical or early fitting, application of non-weight bearing rigid dressing, below knee ⓑ Qp Qh ♿ A
* **L5460** Immediate post surgical or early fitting, application of non-weight bearing rigid dressing, above knee ⓑ Qp Qh ♿ A

Initial Prosthesis

* **L5500** Initial, below knee 'PTB' type socket, non-alignable system, pylon, no cover, SACH foot, plaster socket, direct formed ⓑ Qp Qh ♿ A
* **L5505** Initial, above knee-knee disarticulation, ischial level socket, non-alignable system, pylon, no cover, SACH foot, plaster socket, direct formed ⓑ Qp Qh ♿ A

Preparatory Prosthesis

* **L5510** Preparatory, below knee 'PTB' type socket, non-alignable system, pylon, no cover, SACH foot, plaster socket, molded to model ⓑ Qp Qh ♿ A
* **L5520** Preparatory, below knee 'PTB' type socket, non-alignable system, pylon, no cover, SACH foot, thermoplastic or equal, direct formed ⓑ Qp Qh ♿ A
* **L5530** Preparatory, below knee 'PTB' type socket, non-alignable system, pylon, no cover, SACH foot, thermoplastic or equal, molded to model ⓑ Qp Qh ♿ A
* **L5535** Preparatory, below knee 'PTB' type socket, non-alignable system, no cover, SACH foot, prefabricated, adjustable open end socket ⓑ Qp Qh ♿ A
* **L5540** Preparatory, below knee 'PTB' type socket, non-alignable system, pylon, no cover, SACH foot, laminated socket, molded to model ⓑ Qp Qh ♿ A
* **L5560** Preparatory, above knee - knee disarticulation, ischial level socket, non-alignable system, pylon, no cover, SACH foot, plaster socket, molded to model ⓑ Qp Qh ♿ A
* **L5570** Preparatory, above knee - knee disarticulation, ischial level socket, non-alignable system, pylon, no cover, SACH foot, thermoplastic or equal, direct formed ⓑ Qp Qh ♿ A
* **L5580** Preparatory, above knee - knee disarticulation, ischial level socket, non-alignable system, pylon, no cover, SACH foot, thermoplastic or equal, molded to model ⓑ Qp Qh ♿ A
* **L5585** Preparatory, above knee - knee disarticulation, ischial level socket, non-alignable system, pylon, no cover, SACH foot, prefabricated adjustable open end socket ⓑ Qp Qh ♿ A
* **L5590** Preparatory, above knee - knee disarticulation, ischial level socket, non-alignable system, pylon, no cover, SACH foot, laminated socket, molded to model ⓑ Qp Qh ♿ A

| 🏅 MIPS | Qp Quantity Physician | Qh Quantity Hospital | ♀ Female only |
| ♂ Male only | A Age | ♿ DMEPOS | A2-Z3 ASC Payment Indicator | A-Y ASC Status Indicator | Coding Clinic |

| * L5595 | Preparatory, hip disarticulation-hemipelvectomy, pylon, no cover, SACH foot, thermoplastic or equal, molded to patient model Ⓑ Qp Qh ♿ A

* L5600 Preparatory, hip disarticulation-hemipelvectomy, pylon, no cover, SACH foot, laminated socket, molded to patient model Ⓑ Qp Qh ♿ A

Additions to Lower Extremity

* L5610 Addition to lower extremity, endoskeletal system, above knee, hydracadence system Ⓑ Qp Qh ♿ A

* L5611 Addition to lower extremity, endoskeletal system, above knee-knee disarticulation, 4 bar linkage, with friction swing phase control Ⓑ Qp Qh ♿ A

* L5613 Addition to lower extremity, endoskeletal system, above knee-knee disarticulation, 4 bar linkage, with hydraulic swing phase control Ⓑ Qp Qh ♿ A

* L5614 Addition to lower extremity, exoskeletal system, above knee-knee disarticulation, 4 bar linkage, with pneumatic swing phase control Ⓑ Qp Qh ♿ A

* L5615 Addition, endoskeletal knee-shin system, 4 bar linkage or multiaxial, fluid swing and stance phase control Ⓑ Qp Qh ♿ A

* L5616 Addition to lower extremity, endoskeletal system, above knee, universal multiplex system, friction swing phase control Ⓑ Qp Qh ♿ A

* L5617 Addition to lower extremity, quick change self-aligning unit, above knee or below knee, each Ⓑ Qp Qh ♿ A

Additions to Test Sockets

* L5618 Addition to lower extremity, test socket, Symes Ⓑ Qp ♿ A

* L5620 Addition to lower extremity, test socket, below knee Ⓑ Qp ♿ A

* L5622 Addition to lower extremity, test socket, knee disarticulation Ⓑ Qp ♿ A

* L5624 Addition to lower extremity, test socket, above knee Ⓑ Qp ♿ A

* L5626 Addition to lower extremity, test socket, hip disarticulation Ⓑ Qp ♿ A

* L5628 Addition to lower extremity, test socket, hemipelvectomy Ⓑ Qp Qh ♿ A

Additions to Socket Variations

* L5629 Addition to lower extremity, below knee, acrylic socket Ⓑ Qp Qh ♿ A

* L5630 Addition to lower extremity, Symes type, expandable wall socket Ⓑ Qp Qh ♿ A

* L5631 Addition to lower extremity, above knee or knee disarticulation, acrylic socket Ⓑ Qp Qh ♿ A

* L5632 Addition to lower extremity, Symes type, 'PTB' brim design socket Ⓑ Qp Qh ♿ A

* L5634 Addition to lower extremity, Symes type, posterior opening (Canadian) socket Ⓑ Qp Qh ♿ A

* L5636 Addition to lower extremity, Symes type, medial opening socket Ⓑ Qp Qh ♿ A

* L5637 Addition to lower extremity, below knee, total contact Ⓑ Qp Qh ♿ A

* L5638 Addition to lower extremity, below knee, leather socket Ⓑ Qp Qh ♿ A

* L5639 Addition to lower extremity, below knee, wood socket Ⓑ Qp Qh ♿ A

* L5640 Addition to lower extremity, knee disarticulation, leather socket Ⓑ Qp Qh ♿ A

* L5642 Addition to lower extremity, above knee, leather socket Ⓑ Qp Qh ♿ A

* L5643 Addition to lower extremity, hip disarticulation, flexible inner socket, external frame Ⓑ Qp Qh ♿ A

* L5644 Addition to lower extremity, above knee, wood socket Ⓑ Qp Qh ♿ A

* L5645 Addition to lower extremity, below knee, flexible inner socket, external frame Ⓑ Qp Qh ♿ A

* L5646 Addition to lower extremity, below knee, air, fluid, gel or equal, cushion socket Ⓑ Qp Qh ♿ A

* L5647 Addition to lower extremity, below knee, suction socket Ⓑ Qp Qh ♿ A

* L5648 Addition to lower extremity, above knee, air, fluid, gel or equal, cushion socket Ⓑ Qp Qh ♿ A

* L5649 Addition to lower extremity, ischial containment/narrow M-L socket Ⓑ Qp Qh ♿ A

* L5650 Additions to lower extremity, total contact, above knee or knee disarticulation socket Ⓑ Qp Qh ♿ A

* L5651 Addition to lower extremity, above knee, flexible inner socket, external frame Ⓑ Qp Qh ♿ A

▶ New   ⇄ Revised   ✓ Reinstated   ~~deleted~~ Deleted   ⊘ Not covered or valid by Medicare
◉ Special coverage instructions   * Carrier discretion   Ⓑ Bill Part B MAC   Ⓑ Bill DME MAC

PROSTHETICS

* **L5652** Addition to lower extremity, suction suspension, above knee or knee disarticulation socket Qp Qh ♿ A
* **L5653** Addition to lower extremity, knee disarticulation, expandable wall socket Qp Qh ♿ A

Additions to Socket Insert and Suspension

* **L5654** Addition to lower extremity, socket insert, Symes, (Kemblo, Pelite, Aliplast, Plastazote or equal) Qp Qh ♿ A
* **L5655** Addition to lower extremity, socket insert, below knee (Kemblo, Pelite, Aliplast, Plastazote or equal) Qp Qh ♿ A
* **L5656** Addition to lower extremity, socket insert, knee disarticulation (Kemblo, Pelite, Aliplast, Plastazote or equal) Qp Qh ♿ A
* **L5657** Addition to lower extremity prosthesis, manual/automated adjustable air, fluid, gel or equal socket insert for limb volume management, any materials Qp Qh ♿ A
* **L5658** Addition to lower extremity, socket insert, above knee (Kemblo, Pelite, Aliplast, Plastazote or equal) Qp Qh ♿ A
* **L5661** Addition to lower extremity, socket insert, multi-durometer Symes Qp Qh ♿ A
* **L5665** Addition to lower extremity, socket insert, multi-durometer, below knee Qp Qh ♿ A
* **L5666** Addition to lower extremity, below knee, cuff suspension Qp Qh ♿ A
* **L5668** Addition to lower extremity, below knee, molded distal cushion Qp Qh ♿ A
* **L5670** Addition to lower extremity, below knee, molded supracondylar suspension ('PTS' or similar) Qp Qh ♿ A
* **L5671** Addition to lower extremity, below knee/above knee suspension locking mechanism (shuttle, lanyard or equal), excludes socket insert Qp Qh ♿ A
* **L5672** Addition to lower extremity, below knee, removable medial brim suspension Qp Qh ♿ A
* **L5673** Addition to lower extremity, below knee/above knee, custom fabricated from existing mold or prefabricated, socket insert, silicone gel, elastomeric, or equal, with or without perforations, with or without breathable material, for use with locking mechanism Qp ♿ A
* **L5676** Additions to lower extremity, below knee, knee joints, single axis, pair Qp Qh ♿ A
* **L5677** Additions to lower extremity, below knee, knee joints, polycentric, pair Qp Qh ♿ A
* **L5678** Additions to lower extremity, below knee, joint covers, pair Qp Qh ♿ A
* **L5679** Addition to lower extremity, below knee/above knee, custom fabricated from existing mold or prefabricated, socket insert, silicone gel, elastomeric, or equal, with or without perforations, with or without breathable material, not for use with locking mechanism Qp ♿ A
* **L5680** Addition to lower extremity, below knee, thigh lacer, non-molded Qp Qh ♿ A
* **L5681** Addition to lower extremity, below knee/above knee, custom fabricated socket insert for congenital or atypical traumatic amputee, silicone gel, elastomeric or equal, for use with or without locking mechanism, initial only (for other than initial, use code L5673 or L5679) Qp Qh ♿ A
* **L5682** Addition to lower extremity, below knee, thigh lacer, gluteal/ischial, molded Qp Qh ♿ A
* **L5683** Addition to lower extremity, below knee/above knee, custom fabricated socket insert for other than congenital or atypical traumatic amputee, silicone gel, elastomeric, or equal, for use with or without locking mechanism, initial only (for other than initial, use code L5673 or L5679) Qp Qh ♿ A
* **L5684** Addition to lower extremity, below knee, fork strap Qp Qh ♿ A
* **L5685** Addition to lower extremity prosthesis, below knee, suspension/sealing sleeve, with or without valve, any material, each Qp ♿ A
* **L5686** Addition to lower extremity, below knee, back check (extension control) Qp Qh ♿ A
* **L5688** Addition to lower extremity, below knee, waist belt, webbing Qp Qh ♿ A
* **L5690** Addition to lower extremity, below knee, waist belt, padded and lined Qp Qh ♿ A
* **L5692** Addition to lower extremity, above knee, pelvic control belt, light Qp Qh ♿ A

MIPS Qp Quantity Physician Qh Quantity Hospital ♀ Female only
♂ Male only A Age ♿ DMEPOS A2-Z3 ASC Payment Indicator A-Y ASC Status Indicator Coding Clinic

* L5694 Addition to lower extremity, above knee, pelvic control belt, padded and lined Ⓑ Qp Qh ♿ A
* L5695 Addition to lower extremity, above knee, pelvic control, sleeve suspension, neoprene or equal, each Ⓑ Qp Qh ♿ A
* L5696 Addition to lower extremity, above knee or knee disarticulation, pelvic joint Ⓑ Qp Qh ♿ A
* L5697 Addition to lower extremity, above knee or knee disarticulation, pelvic band Ⓑ Qp Qh ♿ A
* L5698 Addition to lower extremity, above knee or knee disarticulation, Silesian bandage Ⓑ Qp Qh ♿ A
* L5699 All lower extremity prostheses, shoulder harness Ⓑ Qp Qh ♿ A

Replacement Sockets

* L5700 Replacement, socket, below knee, molded to patient model Ⓑ Qp Qh ♿ A
* L5701 Replacement, socket, above knee/knee disarticulation, including attachment plate, molded to patient model Ⓑ Qp Qh ♿ A
* L5702 Replacement, socket, hip disarticulation, including hip joint, molded to patient model Ⓑ Qp Qh ♿ A
* L5703 Ankle, Symes, molded to patient model, socket without solid ankle cushion heel (SACH) foot, replacement only Ⓑ Qp Qh ♿ A

Protective Covers

* L5704 Custom shaped protective cover, below knee Ⓑ Qp Qh ♿ A
* L5705 Custom shaped protective cover, above knee Ⓑ Qp Qh ♿ A
* L5706 Custom shaped protective cover, knee disarticulation Ⓑ Qp Qh ♿ A
* L5707 Custom shaped protective cover, hip disarticulation Ⓑ Qp Qh ♿ A

Additions to Exoskeletal–Knee-Shin System

* L5710 Addition, exoskeletal knee-shin system, single axis, manual lock Ⓑ Qp Qh ♿ A
* L5711 Additions exoskeletal knee-shin system, single axis, manual lock, ultra-light material Ⓑ Qp Qh ♿ A
* L5712 Addition, exoskeletal knee-shin system, single axis, friction swing and stance phase control (safety knee) Ⓑ Qp Qh ♿ A
* L5714 Addition, exoskeletal knee-shin system, single axis, variable friction swing phase control Ⓑ Qp Qh ♿ A
* L5716 Addition, exoskeletal knee-shin system, polycentric, mechanical stance phase lock Ⓑ Qp Qh ♿ A
* L5718 Addition, exoskeletal knee-shin system, polycentric, friction swing and stance phase control Ⓑ Qp Qh ♿ A
* L5722 Addition, exoskeletal knee-shin system, single axis, pneumatic swing, friction stance phase control Ⓑ Qp Qh ♿ A
* L5724 Addition, exoskeletal knee-shin system, single axis, fluid swing phase control Ⓑ Qp Qh ♿ A
* L5726 Addition, exoskeletal knee-shin system, single axis, external joints, fluid swing phase control Ⓑ Qp Qh ♿ A
* L5728 Addition, exoskeletal knee-shin system, single axis, fluid swing and stance phase control Ⓑ Qp Qh ♿ A
* L5780 Addition, exoskeletal knee-shin system, single axis, pneumatic/hydra pneumatic swing phase control Ⓑ Qp Qh ♿ A

Vacuum Pumps

* L5781 Addition to lower limb prosthesis, vacuum pump, residual limb volume management and moisture evacuation system Ⓑ Qp Qh ♿ A
* L5782 Addition to lower limb prosthesis, vacuum pump, residual limb volume management and moisture evacuation system, heavy duty Ⓑ Qp Qh ♿ A
⤺ * L5783 Addition to lower extremity, user adjustable, mechanical, residual limb volume management system (with or without lamination kit) A

Component Modification

* L5785 Addition, exoskeletal system, below knee, ultra-light material (titanium, carbon fiber, or equal) Ⓑ Qp Qh ♿ A
* L5790 Addition, exoskeletal system, above knee, ultra-light material (titanium, carbon fiber, or equal) Ⓑ Qp Qh ♿ A
* L5795 Addition, exoskeletal system, hip disarticulation, ultra-light material (titanium, carbon fiber, or equal) Ⓑ Qp Qh ♿ A

Endoskeletal

* L5810 Addition, endoskeletal knee-shin system, single axis, manual lock Ⓑ Qp Qh ♿ A

▶ New   ⤺ Revised   ✔ Reinstated   ~~deleted~~ Deleted   ⊘ Not covered or valid by Medicare
◉ Special coverage instructions   * Carrier discretion   Ⓑ Bill Part B MAC   Ⓑ Bill DME MAC

PROSTHETICS

* **L5811** Addition, endoskeletal knee-shin system, single axis, manual lock, ultralight material ⓑ Qp Qh ♿ A

* **L5812** Addition, endoskeletal knee-shin system, single axis, friction swing and stance phase control (safety knee) ⓑ Qp Qh ♿ A

* **L5814** Addition, endoskeletal knee-shin system, polycentric, hydraulic swing phase control, mechanical stance phase lock ⓑ Qp Qh ♿ A

* **L5816** Addition, endoskeletal knee-shin system, polycentric, mechanical stance phase lock ⓑ Qp Qh ♿ A

* **L5818** Addition, endoskeletal knee-shin system, polycentric, friction swing, and stance phase control ⓑ Qp Qh ♿ A

* **L5822** Addition, endoskeletal knee-shin system, single axis, pneumatic swing, friction stance phase control ⓑ Qp Qh ♿ A

* **L5824** Addition, endoskeletal knee-shin system, single axis, fluid swing phase control ⓑ Qp Qh ♿ A

* **L5826** Addition, endoskeletal knee-shin system, single axis, hydraulic swing phase control, with miniature high activity frame ⓑ Qp Qh ♿ A

▶ * **L5827** Endoskeletal knee-shin system, single axis, electromechanical swing and stance phase control, with or without shock absorption and stance extension damping ⓑ Qp Qh ♿ A

* **L5828** Addition, endoskeletal knee-shin system, single axis, fluid swing and stance phase control ⓑ Qp Qh ♿ A

* **L5830** Addition, endoskeletal knee-shin system, single axis, pneumatic/swing phase control ⓑ Qp Qh ♿ A

* **L5840** Addition, endoskeletal knee/shin system, 4-bar linkage or multiaxial, pneumatic swing phase control ⓑ Qp Qh ♿ A

L5841 Addition, endoskeletal knee-shin system, polycentric, pneumatic swing, and stance phase control ⓑ Qp Qh ♿ A

* **L5845** Addition, endoskeletal, knee-shin system, stance flexion feature, adjustable ⓑ Qp Qh ♿ A

* **L5848** Addition to endoskeletal, knee-shin system, fluid stance extension, dampening feature, with or without adjustability ⓑ Qp Qh ♿ A

* **L5850** Addition, endoskeletal system, above knee or hip disarticulation, knee extension assist ⓑ Qp Qh ♿ A

* **L5855** Addition, endoskeletal system, hip disarticulation, mechanical hip extension assist ⓑ Qp Qh ♿ A

* **L5856** Addition to lower extremity prosthesis, endoskeletal knee-shin system, microprocessor control feature, swing and stance phase; includes electronic sensor(s), any type ⓑ Qp Qh ♿ A

* **L5857** Addition to lower extremity prosthesis, endoskeletal knee-shin system, microprocessor control feature, swing phase only; includes electronic sensor(s), any type ⓑ Qp Qh ♿ A

* **L5858** Addition to lower extremity prosthesis, endoskeletal knee shin system, microprocessor control feature, stance phase only, includes electronic sensor(s), any type ⓑ Qp Qh ♿ A

* **L5859** Addition to lower extremity prosthesis, endoskeletal knee-shin system, powered and programmable flexion/extension assist control, includes any type motor(s) ⓑ Qp Qh ♿ A

* **L5910** Addition, endoskeletal system, below knee, alignable system ⓑ Qp Qh ♿ A

* **L5920** Addition, endoskeletal system, above knee or hip disarticulation, alignable system ⓑ Qp Qh ♿ A

* **L5925** Addition, endoskeletal system, above knee, knee disarticulation or hip disarticulation, manual lock ⓑ Qp Qh ♿ A

* **L5926** Addition to lower extremity prosthesis, endoskeletal, knee disarticulation, above knee, hip disarticulation, positional rotation unit, any type ⓑ Qp Qh ♿ A

* **L5930** Addition, endoskeletal system, high activity knee control frame ⓑ Qp Qh ♿ A

* **L5940** Addition, endoskeletal system, below knee, ultra-light material (titanium, carbon fiber or equal) ⓑ Qp Qh ♿ A

* **L5950** Addition, endoskeletal system, above knee, ultra-light material (titanium, carbon fiber or equal) ⓑ Qp Qh ♿ A

* **L5960** Addition, endoskeletal system, hip disarticulation, ultra-light material (titanium, carbon fiber, or equal) ⓑ Qp Qh ♿ A

* **L5961** Addition, endoskeletal system, polycentric hip joint, pneumatic or hydraulic control, rotation control, with or without flexion, and/or extension control ⓑ Qp Qh ♿ A

* **L5962** Addition, endoskeletal system, below knee, flexible protective outer surface covering system ⓑ Qp Qh ♿ A

MIPS | Qp Quantity Physician | Qh Quantity Hospital | ♀ Female only
♂ Male only | A Age | ♿ DMEPOS | A2-Z3 ASC Payment Indicator | A-Y ASC Status Indicator | Coding Clinic

* **L5964**	Addition, endoskeletal system, above knee, flexible protective outer surface covering system ⒷQpQh♿	A
* **L5966**	Addition, endoskeletal system, hip disarticulation, flexible protective outer surface covering system ⒷQpQh♿	A

Additions to Ankle and/or Foot

* **L5968**	Addition to lower limb prosthesis, multiaxial ankle with swing phase active dorsiflexion feature ⒷQpQh♿	A
* **L5969**	Addition, endoskeletal ankle-foot or ankle system, power assist, includes any type motor(s) ⒷQpQh	A
* **L5970**	All lower extremity prostheses, foot, external keel, SACH foot ⒷQpQh♿	A
* **L5971**	All lower extremity prosthesis, solid ankle cushion keel (SACH) foot, replacement only ⒷQpQh♿	A
* **L5972**	All lower extremity prostheses (foot, flexible keel) ⒷQpQh♿	A
* **L5973**	Endoskeletal ankle foot system, microprocessor controlled feature, dorsiflexion and/or plantar flexion control, includes power source ⒷQh♿	A
* **L5974**	All lower extremity prostheses, foot, single axis ankle/foot ⒷQpQh♿	A
* **L5975**	All lower extremity prostheses, combination single axis ankle and flexible keel foot ⒷQpQh♿	A
* **L5976**	All lower extremity prostheses, energy storing foot (Seattle Carbon Copy II or equal) ⒷQpQh♿	A
* **L5978**	All lower extremity prostheses, foot, multiaxial ankle/foot ⒷQpQh♿	A
* **L5979**	All lower extremity prostheses, multiaxial ankle, dynamic response foot, one piece system ⒷQpQh♿	A
* **L5980**	All lower extremity prostheses, flex foot system ⒷQpQh♿	A
* **L5981**	All lower extremity prostheses, flexwalk system or equal ⒷQpQh♿	A
* **L5982**	All exoskeletal lower extremity prostheses, axial rotation unit ⒷQpQh♿	A
* **L5984**	All endoskeletal lower extremity prostheses, axial rotation unit, with or without adjustability ⒷQpQh♿	A
* **L5985**	All endoskeletal lower extremity prostheses, dynamic prosthetic pylon ⒷQpQh♿	A
* **L5986**	All lower extremity prostheses, multiaxial rotation unit ('MCP' or equal) ⒷQpQh♿	A
* **L5987**	All lower extremity prostheses, shank foot system with vertical loading pylon ⒷQpQh♿	A
* **L5988**	Addition to lower limb prosthesis, vertical shock reducing pylon feature ⒷQpQh♿	A
* **L5990**	Addition to lower extremity prosthesis, user adjustable heel height ⒷQpQh♿	A
* **L5991**	Addition to lower extremity prostheses, osseointegrated external prosthetic connector ⒷQpQh♿	A
* **L5999**	Lower extremity prosthesis, not otherwise specified Ⓑ	A

Upper Limb (L6000-L7600)

NOTE: The procedures in L6000-L6599 are considered as base or basic procedures and may be modified by listing procedures from the additions sections. The base procedures include only standard friction wrist and control cable system unless otherwise specified.

Partial Hand

* **L6000**	Partial hand, thumb remaining ⒷQpQh♿	A
* **L6010**	Partial hand, little and/or ring finger remaining ⒷQpQh♿	A
* **L6020**	Partial hand, no finger remaining ⒷQpQh♿	A
* **L6026**	Transcarpal/metacarpal or partial hand disarticulation prosthesis, external power, self-suspended, inner socket with removable forearm section, electrodes and cables, two batteries, charger, myoelectric control of terminal device, excludes terminal device(s) ⒷQpQh♿	A

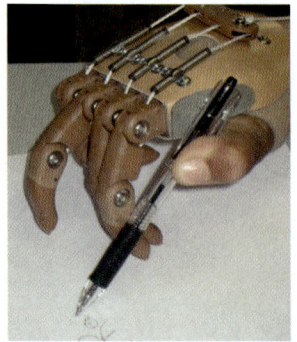

Figure 39 Partial hand.

▶ New ⤳ Revised ✓ Reinstated ~~deleted~~ Deleted ⊘ Not covered or valid by Medicare
✸ Special coverage instructions * Carrier discretion Ⓑ Bill Part B MAC Ⓑ Bill DME MAC

PROSTHETICS

▶ * **L6028** Partial hand, finger, and thumb prosthesis without prosthetic digit(s)/thumb, amputation at metacarpal level, including flexible or non-flexible interface, molded to patient model, including palm, for use without external power and/or passive prosthetic digit/thumb, not including inserts described by L6692 Ⓑ Qp Qh ♿ E1

▶ * **L6029** Upper extremity addition, test socket/interface, partial hand including fingers Ⓑ Qp Qh ♿ A

▶ * **L6030** Upper extremity addition, external frame, partial hand including fingers Ⓑ Qp Qh ♿ A

▶ * **L6031** Replacement socket/interface, partial hand including fingers, molded to patient model, for use with or without external power Ⓑ Qp Qh ♿ A

▶ * **L6032** Addition to upper extremity prosthesis, partial hand including fingers, ultralight material (titanium, carbon fiber or equal) Ⓑ Qp Qh ♿ A

▶ * **L6033** Addition to upper extremity prosthesis, partial hand including fingers, acrylic material Ⓑ Qp Qh ♿ A

▶ * **L6034** Partial hand, finger, and thumb prosthesis without prosthetic digit(s)/thumb, amputation at distal to metacarpal joint, including flexible or non-flexible interface, molded to patient model, for use without external power and/or passive prosthetic digit/thumb, not including inserts described by L6692 Ⓑ Qp Qh ♿ A

▶ * **L6035** Single prosthetic digit, mechanical, can include metacarpophalangeal (MCP), proximal interphalangeal (PIP), and/or distal interphalangeal (DIP) joint(s), with or without locking mechanism, can include flexion or extension assist, any material, attachment, initial issue or replacement Ⓑ Qp Qh ♿ A

▶ * **L6036** Prosthetic thumb, mechanical, can include metacarpophalangeal (MCP), interphalangeal (IP) joint(s), with or without locking mechanism, can include flexion or extension assist, any material, attachment, initial issue or replacement Ⓑ Qp Qh ♿ A

▶ * **L6037** Immediate post-surgical or early fitting, application of initial rigid dressing, including fitting alignment and suspension of components, and one cast change, partial hand including fingers Ⓑ Qp Qh ♿ A

▶ * **L6038** Addition to single prosthetic digit or thumb, mechanical, attachment, multiaxial and/or internal/external rotation/abduction/adduction mechanism, with or without locking feature, any material Ⓑ Qp Qh ♿ A

▶ * **L6039** Passive prosthetic digit or thumb prosthesis not including hand restoration partial hand, full or partial, custom made, any material, initial or replacement, per single passive prosthetic digit or thumb Ⓑ Qp Qh ♿ A

Wrist Disarticulation

* **L6050** Wrist disarticulation, molded socket, flexible elbow hinges, triceps pad Ⓑ Qp Qh ♿ A

* **L6055** Wrist disarticulation, molded socket with expandable interface, flexible elbow hinges, triceps pad Ⓑ Qp Qh ♿ A

Below Elbow

* **L6100** Below elbow, molded socket, flexible elbow hinge, triceps pad Ⓑ Qp Qh ♿ A

* **L6110** Below elbow, molded socket, (Muenster or Northwestern suspension types) Ⓑ Qp Qh ♿ A

* **L6120** Below elbow, molded double wall split socket, step-up hinges, half cuff Ⓑ Qp Qh ♿ A

* **L6130** Below elbow, molded double wall split socket, stump activated locking hinge, half cuff Ⓑ Qp Qh ♿ A

Elbow Disarticulation

* **L6200** Elbow disarticulation, molded socket, outside locking hinge, forearm Ⓑ Qp Qh ♿ A

* **L6205** Elbow disarticulation, molded socket with expandable interface, outside locking hinges, forearm Ⓑ Qp Qh ♿ A

Above Elbow

* **L6250** Above elbow, molded double wall socket, internal locking elbow, forearm Ⓑ Qp Qh ♿ A

Shoulder Disarticulation

* **L6300** Shoulder disarticulation, molded socket, shoulder bulkhead, humeral section, internal locking elbow, forearm Ⓑ Qp Qh ♿ A

| MIPS | Qp Quantity Physician | Qh Quantity Hospital | ♀ Female only |
| ♂ Male only | A Age | ♿ DMEPOS | A2-Z3 ASC Payment Indicator | A-Y ASC Status Indicator | Coding Clinic |

* **L6310** Shoulder disarticulation, passive restoration (complete prosthesis) Ⓑ Qp Qh ♿ A
* **L6320** Shoulder disarticulation, passive restoration (shoulder cap only) Ⓑ Qp Qh ♿ A

Interscapular Thoracic

* **L6350** Interscapular thoracic, molded socket, shoulder bulkhead, humeral section, internal locking elbow, forearm Ⓑ Qp Qh ♿ A
* **L6360** Interscapular thoracic, passive restoration (complete prosthesis) Ⓑ Qp Qh ♿ A
* **L6370** Interscapular thoracic, passive restoration (shoulder cap only) Ⓑ Qp Qh ♿ A

Immediate and Early Postsurgical Procedures

* **L6380** Immediate post surgical or early fitting, application of initial rigid dressing, including fitting alignment and suspension of components, and one cast change, wrist disarticulation or below elbow Qp Qh ♿ A
* **L6382** Immediate post surgical or early fitting, application of initial rigid dressing including fitting alignment and suspension of components, and one cast change, elbow disarticulation or above elbow Qp Qh ♿ A
* **L6384** Immediate post surgical or early fitting, application of initial rigid dressing including fitting alignment and suspension of components, and one cast change, shoulder disarticulation or interscapular thoracic Ⓑ Qp Qh ♿ A
* **L6386** Immediate post surgical or early fitting, each additional cast change and realignment Ⓑ Qp Qh ♿ A
* **L6388** Immediate post surgical or early fitting, application of rigid dressing only Ⓑ Qp Qh ♿ A

Molded Socket

* **L6400** Below elbow, molded socket, endoskeletal system, including soft prosthetic tissue shaping Ⓑ Qp Qh ♿ A
* **L6450** Elbow disarticulation, molded socket, endoskeletal system, including soft prosthetic tissue shaping Ⓑ Qp Qh ♿ A
* **L6500** Above elbow, molded socket, endoskeletal system, including soft prosthetic tissue shaping Ⓑ Qp Qh ♿ A
* **L6550** Shoulder disarticulation, molded socket, endoskeletal system, including soft prosthetic tissue shaping Ⓑ Qp Qh ♿ A
* **L6570** Interscapular thoracic, molded socket, endoskeletal system, including soft prosthetic tissue shaping Ⓑ Qp Qh ♿ A

Preparatory Prosthetic

* **L6580** Preparatory, wrist disarticulation or below elbow, single wall plastic socket, friction wrist, flexible elbow hinges, figure of eight harness, humeral cuff, Bowden cable control, USMC or equal pylon, no cover, molded to patient model Ⓑ Qp Qh ♿ A
* **L6582** Preparatory, wrist disarticulation or below elbow, single wall socket, friction wrist, flexible elbow hinges, figure of eight harness, humeral cuff, Bowden cable control, USMC or equal pylon, no cover, direct formed Ⓑ Qp Qh ♿ A
* **L6584** Preparatory, elbow disarticulation or above elbow, single wall plastic socket, friction wrist, locking elbow, figure of eight harness, fair lead cable control, USMC or equal pylon, no cover, molded to patient model Ⓑ Qp Qh ♿ A
* **L6586** Preparatory, elbow disarticulation or above elbow, single wall socket, friction wrist, locking elbow, figure of eight harness, fair lead cable control, USMC or equal pylon, no cover, direct formed Ⓑ Qp Qh ♿ A
* **L6588** Preparatory, shoulder disarticulation or interscapular thoracic, single wall plastic socket, shoulder joint, locking elbow, friction wrist, chest strap, fair lead cable control, USMC or equal pylon, no cover, molded to patient model Ⓑ Qp Qh ♿ A
* **L6590** Preparatory, shoulder disarticulation or interscapular thoracic, single wall socket, shoulder joint, locking elbow, friction wrist, chest strap, fair lead cable control, USMC or equal pylon, no cover, direct formed Ⓑ Qp Qh ♿ A

▶ New　⤺ Revised　✓ Reinstated　~~deleted~~ Deleted　⊘ Not covered or valid by Medicare
⊛ Special coverage instructions　* Carrier discretion　Ⓑ Bill Part B MAC　Ⓑ Bill DME MAC

PROSTHETICS

Additions to Upper Limb

NOTE: The following procedures/modifications/components may be added to other base procedures. The items in this section should reflect the additional complexity of each modification procedure, in addition to base procedure, at the time of the original order.

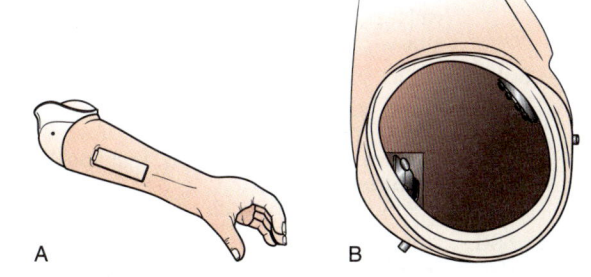

Figure 40   Upper extremity addition.

* **L6600** Upper extremity additions, polycentric hinge, pair ⒷQp Qh ♿ A
* **L6605** Upper extremity additions, single pivot hinge, pair ⒷQp Qh ♿ A
* **L6610** Upper extremity additions, flexible metal hinge, pair ⒷQp Qh ♿ A
* **L6611** Addition to upper extremity prosthesis, external powered, additional switch, any type ⒷQp Qh ♿ A
* **L6615** Upper extremity addition, disconnect locking wrist unit ⒷQp Qh ♿ A
* **L6616** Upper extremity addition, additional disconnect insert for locking wrist unit, each ⒷQp Qh ♿ A
* **L6620** Upper extremity addition, flexion/extension wrist unit, with or without friction ⒷQp Qh ♿ A
* **L6621** Upper extremity prosthesis addition, flexion/extension wrist with or without friction, for use with external powered terminal device ⒷQp Qh ♿ A
* **L6623** Upper extremity addition, spring assisted rotational wrist unit with latch release ⒷQp Qh ♿ A
* **L6624** Upper extremity addition, flexion/extension and rotation wrist unit ⒷQp Qh ♿ A
* **L6625** Upper extremity addition, rotation wrist unit with cable lock ⒷQp Qh ♿ A
* **L6628** Upper extremity addition, quick disconnect hook adapter, Otto Bock or equal ⒷQp Qh ♿ A
* **L6629** Upper extremity addition, quick disconnect lamination collar with coupling piece, Otto Bock or equal ⒷQp Qh ♿ A
* **L6630** Upper extremity addition, stainless steel, any wrist ⒷQp Qh ♿ A
* **L6632** Upper extremity addition, latex suspension sleeve, each ⒷQp ♿ A
* **L6635** Upper extremity addition, lift assist for elbow ⒷQp Qh ♿ A
* **L6637** Upper extremity addition, nudge control elbow lock ⒷQp Qh ♿ A
* **L6638** Upper extremity addition to prosthesis, electric locking feature, only for use with manually powered elbow ⒷQp Qh ♿ A
* **L6640** Upper extremity additions, shoulder abduction joint, pair ⒷQp Qh ♿ A
* **L6641** Upper extremity addition, excursion amplifier, pulley type ⒷQp Qh ♿ A
* **L6642** Upper extremity addition, excursion amplifier, lever type ⒷQp Qh ♿ A
* **L6645** Upper extremity addition, shoulder flexion-abduction joint, each ⒷQp Qh ♿ A
* **L6646** Upper extremity addition, shoulder joint, multipositional locking, flexion, adjustable abduction friction control, for use with body powered or external powered system ⒷQp Qh ♿ A
* **L6647** Upper extremity addition, shoulder lock mechanism, body powered actuator ⒷQp Qh ♿ A
* **L6648** Upper extremity addition, shoulder lock mechanism, external powered actuator ⒷQp Qh ♿ A
* **L6650** Upper extremity addition, shoulder universal joint, each ⒷQp Qh ♿ A
* **L6655** Upper extremity addition, standard control cable, extra ⒷQp ♿ A
* **L6660** Upper extremity addition, heavy duty control cable ⒷQp ♿ A
* **L6665** Upper extremity addition, Teflon, or equal, cable lining ⒷQp ♿ A
* **L6670** Upper extremity addition, hook to hand, cable adapter ⒷQp Qh ♿ A
* **L6672** Upper extremity addition, harness, chest or shoulder, saddle type ⒷQp Qh ♿ A
* **L6675** Upper extremity addition, harness, (e.g., figure of eight type), single cable design ⒷQp Qh ♿ A
* **L6676** Upper extremity addition, harness, (e.g., figure of eight type), dual cable design ⒷQp Qh ♿ A
* **L6677** Upper extremity addition, harness, triple control, simultaneous operation of terminal device and elbow ⒷQp Qh ♿ A

| 🔹 MIPS | Qp Quantity Physician | Qh Quantity Hospital | ♀ Female only |
| ♂ Male only | Ⓐ Age | ♿ DMEPOS | A2-Z3 ASC Payment Indicator | A-Y ASC Status Indicator | Coding Clinic |

* L6680	Upper extremity addition, test socket, wrist disarticulation or below elbow A
* L6682	Upper extremity addition, test socket, elbow disarticulation or above elbow A
* L6684	Upper extremity addition, test socket, shoulder disarticulation or interscapular thoracic A
* L6686	Upper extremity addition, suction socket A
* L6687	Upper extremity addition, frame type socket, below elbow or wrist disarticulation A
* L6688	Upper extremity addition, frame type socket, above elbow or elbow disarticulation A
* L6689	Upper extremity addition, frame type socket, shoulder disarticulation A
* L6690	Upper extremity addition, frame type socket, interscapular-thoracic A
* L6691	Upper extremity addition, removable insert, each A
↻ * L6692	Upper extremity addition, silicone gel insert or equal, with or without locking mechanism, each A
* L6693	Upper extremity addition, locking elbow, forearm counterbalance A
* L6694	Addition to upper extremity prosthesis, below elbow/above elbow, custom fabricated from existing mold or prefabricated, socket insert, silicone gel, elastomeric or equal, for use with locking mechanism A
* L6695	Addition to upper extremity prosthesis, below elbow/above elbow, custom fabricated from existing mold or prefabricated, socket insert, silicone gel, elastomeric or equal, not for use with locking mechanism A
* L6696	Addition to upper extremity prosthesis, below elbow/above elbow, custom fabricated socket insert for congenital or atypical traumatic amputee, silicone gel, elastomeric or equal, for use with or without locking mechanism, initial only (for other than initial, use code L6694 or L6695) A
* L6697	Addition to upper extremity prosthesis, below elbow/above elbow, custom fabricated socket insert for other than congenital or atypical traumatic amputee, silicone gel, elastomeric or equal, for use with or without locking mechanism, initial only (for other than initial, use code L6694 or L6695) A
↻ * L6698	Addition to upper extremity prosthesis, lock mechanism, excludes socket insert A
▶ * L6700	Upper extremity addition, external powered feature, myoelectronic control module, additional EMG inputs, pattern-recognition decoding intent movement A

Terminal Devices

* L6703	Terminal device, passive hand/mitt, any material, any size A
* L6704	Terminal device, sport/recreational/work attachment, any material, any size A
* L6706	Terminal device, hook, mechanical, voluntary opening, any material, any size, lined or unlined A
* L6707	Terminal device, hook, mechanical, voluntary closing, any material, any size, lined or unlined A
* L6708	Terminal device, hand, mechanical, voluntary opening, any material, any size A
* L6709	Terminal device, hand, mechanical, voluntary closing, any material, any size A
* L6711	Terminal device, hook, mechanical, voluntary opening, any material, any size, lined or unlined, pediatric A
* L6712	Terminal device, hook, mechanical, voluntary closing, any material, any size, lined or unlined, pediatric A
* L6713	Terminal device, hand, mechanical, voluntary opening, any material, any size, pediatric A
* L6714	Terminal device, hand, mechanical, voluntary closing, any material, any size, pediatric A
* L6715	Terminal device, multiple articulating digit, includes motor(s), initial issue or replacement A
* L6721	Terminal device, hook or hand, heavy duty, mechanical, voluntary opening, any material, any size, lined or unlined A
* L6722	Terminal device, hook or hand, heavy duty, mechanical, voluntary closing, any material, any size, lined or unlined A
○ L6805	Addition to terminal device, modifier wrist unit A
	IOM: 100-02, 15, 120; 100-04, 3, 10.4

▶ New   ↻ Revised   ✓ Reinstated   ~~deleted~~ Deleted   ○ Not covered or valid by Medicare
◎ Special coverage instructions   * Carrier discretion   Ⓑ Bill Part B MAC   Ⓑ Bill DME MAC

PROSTHETICS

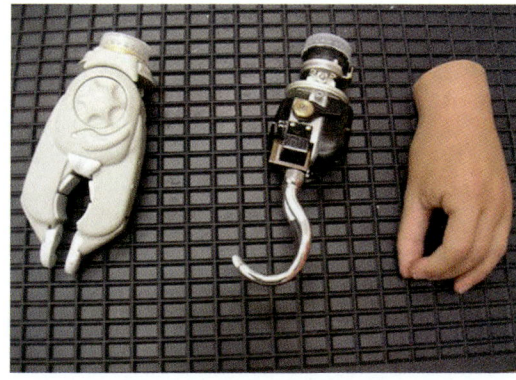

Figure 41 Terminal devices, hand and hook.

- **L6810** Addition to terminal device, precision pinch device ⓑ Qp Qh ♿ A

  IOM: 100-02, 15, 120; 100-04, 3, 10.4

- **L6880** Electric hand, switch or myoelectric controlled, independently articulating digits, any grasp pattern or combination of grasp patterns, includes motor(s) ⓑ Qp Qh ♿ A

- **L6881** Automatic grasp feature, addition to upper limb electric prosthetic terminal device ⓑ Qp Qh ♿ A

- **L6882** Microprocessor control feature, addition to upper limb prosthetic terminal device ⓑ Qp Qh ♿ A

  IOM: 100-02, 15, 120; 100-04, 3, 10.4

Replacement Sockets

- **L6883** Replacement socket, below elbow/wrist disarticulation, molded to patient model, for use with or without external power ⓑ Qp Qh ♿ A

- **L6884** Replacement socket, above elbow/elbow disarticulation, molded to patient model, for use with or without external power ⓑ Qp Qh ♿ A

- **L6885** Replacement socket, shoulder disarticulation/interscapular thoracic, molded to patient model, for use with or without external power ⓑ Qp Qh ♿ A

Hand Restoration

- **L6890** Addition to upper extremity prosthesis, glove for terminal device, any material, prefabricated, includes fitting and adjustment ⓑ Qp Qh ♿ A

- **L6895** Addition to upper extremity prosthesis, glove for terminal device, any material, custom fabricated ⓑ Qp Qh ♿ A

- **L6900** Hand restoration (casts, shading and measurements included), partial hand, with glove, thumb or one finger remaining ⓑ Qp Qh ♿ A

- **L6905** Hand restoration (casts, shading and measurements included), partial hand, with glove, multiple fingers remaining ⓑ Qp Qh ♿ A

- **L6910** Hand restoration (casts, shading and measurements included), partial hand, with glove, no fingers remaining ⓑ Qp Qh ♿ A

- **L6915** Hand restoration (shading, and measurements included), replacement glove for above ⓑ Qp Qh ♿ A

External Power

- **L6920** Wrist disarticulation, external power, self-suspended inner socket, removable forearm shell, Otto Bock or equal switch, cables, two batteries and one charger, switch control of terminal device ⓑ Qp Qh ♿ A

- **L6925** Wrist disarticulation, external power, self-suspended inner socket, removable forearm shell, Otto Bock or equal electrodes, cables, two batteries and one charger, myoelectronic control of terminal device ⓑ Qp Qh ♿ A

- **L6930** Below elbow, external power, self-suspended inner socket, removable forearm shell, Otto Bock or equal switch, cables, two batteries and one charger, switch control of terminal device ⓑ Qp Qh ♿ A

- **L6935** Below elbow, external power, self-suspended inner socket, removable forearm shell, Otto Bock or equal electrodes, cables, two batteries and one charger, myoelectronic control of terminal device ⓑ Qp Qh ♿ A

- **L6940** Elbow disarticulation, external power, molded inner socket, removable humeral shell, outside locking hinges, forearm, Otto Bock or equal switch, cables, two batteries and one charger, switch control of terminal device ⓑ Qp Qh ♿ A

- **L6945** Elbow disarticulation, external power, molded inner socket, removable humeral shell, outside locking hinges, forearm, Otto Bock or equal electrodes, cables, two batteries and one charger, myoelectronic control of terminal device ⓑ Qp Qh ♿ A

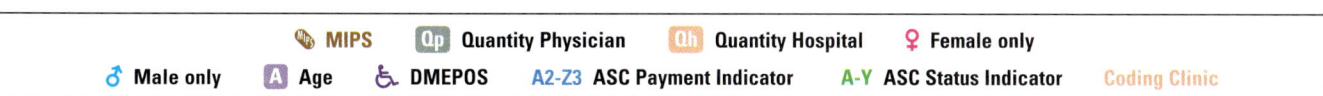

*	**L6950**	Above elbow, external power, molded inner socket, removable humeral shell, internal locking elbow, forearm, Otto Bock or equal switch, cables, two batteries and one charger, switch control of terminal device Ⓑ Qp Qh ♿	A
*	**L6955**	Above elbow, external power, molded inner socket, removable humeral shell, internal locking elbow, forearm, Otto Bock or equal electrodes, cables, two batteries and one charger, myoelectronic control of terminal device Ⓑ Qp Qh ♿	A
*	**L6960**	Shoulder disarticulation, external power, molded inner socket, removable shoulder shell, shoulder bulkhead, humeral section, mechanical elbow, forearm, Otto Bock or equal switch, cables, two batteries and one charger, switch control of terminal device Ⓑ Qp Qh ♿	A
*	**L6965**	Shoulder disarticulation, external power, molded inner socket, removable shoulder shell, shoulder bulkhead, humeral section, mechanical elbow, forearm, Otto Bock or equal electrodes, cables, two batteries and one charger, myoelectronic control of terminal device Ⓑ Qp Qh ♿	A
*	**L6970**	Interscapular-thoracic, external power, molded inner socket, removable shoulder shell, shoulder bulkhead, humeral section, mechanical elbow, forearm, Otto Bock or equal switch, cables, two batteries and one charger, switch control of terminal device Ⓑ Qp Qh ♿	A
*	**L6975**	Interscapular-thoracic, external power, molded inner socket, removable shoulder shell, shoulder bulkhead, humeral section, mechanical elbow, forearm, Otto Bock or equal electrodes, cables, two batteries and one charger, myoelectronic control of terminal device Ⓑ Qp Qh ♿	A

Additions to Electronic Hand or Hook

*	**L7007**	Electric hand, switch or myoelectric controlled, adult Ⓑ Qp Qh A ♿	A
*	**L7008**	Electric hand, switch or myoelectric controlled, pediatric Ⓑ Qp Qh A ♿	A
*	**L7009**	Electric hook, switch or myoelectric controlled, adult Ⓑ Qp Qh A ♿	A
*	**L7040**	Prehensile actuator, switch controlled Ⓑ Qp Qh ♿	A
*	**L7045**	Electric hook, switch or myoelectric controlled, pediatric Ⓑ Qp Qh A ♿	A

Additions to Electronic Elbow

*	**L7170**	Electronic elbow, Hosmer or equal, switch controlled Ⓑ Qp Qh	A
*	**L7180**	Electronic elbow, microprocessor sequential control of elbow and terminal device Ⓑ Qp Qh ♿	A
*	**L7181**	Electronic elbow, microprocessor simultaneous control of elbow and terminal device Ⓑ Qp Qh ♿	A
*	**L7185**	Electronic elbow, adolescent, Variety Village or equal, switch controlled Ⓑ Qp Qh ♿	A
*	**L7186**	Electronic elbow, child, Variety Village or equal, switch controlled Ⓑ Qp Qh A ♿	A
*	**L7190**	Electronic elbow, adolescent, Variety Village or equal, myoelectronically controlled Ⓑ Qp Qh ♿	A
*	**L7191**	Electronic elbow, child, Variety Village or equal, myoelectronically controlled Ⓑ Qp Qh A ♿	A

Wrist

*	**L7259**	Electronic wrist rotator, any type Ⓑ Qp Qh ♿	A

Battery Components

*	**L7360**	Six volt battery, each Ⓑ Qp ♿	A
*	**L7362**	Battery charger, six volt, each Ⓑ Qp Qh	A
*	**L7364**	Twelve volt battery, each Ⓑ Qp	A
*	**L7366**	Battery charger, twelve volt, each Ⓑ Qp Qh ♿	A
*	**L7367**	Lithium ion battery, rechargeable, replacement Ⓑ Qp ♿	A
*	**L7368**	Lithium ion battery charger, replacement only Ⓑ Qp Qh ♿	A

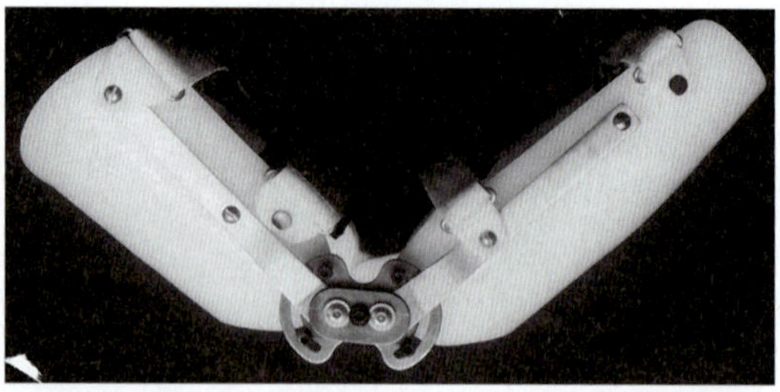

Figure 42 Electronic elbow.

▶ New   ⇌ Revised   ✓ Reinstated   ~~deleted~~ Deleted   ⊘ Not covered or valid by Medicare
⊛ Special coverage instructions   * Carrier discretion   Ⓑ Bill Part B MAC   Ⓑ Bill DME MAC

PROSTHETICS

Additions

* **L7400** Addition to upper extremity prosthesis, below elbow/wrist disarticulation, ultralight material (titanium, carbon fiber or equal) Ⓑ Qp Qh ⚕ A
* **L7401** Addition to upper extremity prosthesis, above elbow disarticulation, ultralight material (titanium, carbon fiber or equal) Ⓑ Qp Qh ⚕ A
* **L7402** Addition to upper extremity prosthesis, shoulder disarticulation/interscapular thoracic, ultralight material (titanium, carbon fiber or equal) Ⓑ Qp Qh ⚕ A
* **L7403** Addition to upper extremity prosthesis, below elbow/wrist disarticulation, acrylic material Ⓑ Qp Qh ⚕ A
* **L7404** Addition to upper extremity prosthesis, above elbow disarticulation, acrylic material Ⓑ Qp Qh ⚕ A
* **L7405** Addition to upper extremity prosthesis, shoulder disarticulation/interscapular thoracic, acrylic material Ⓑ Qp Qh ⚕ A
▶ * **L7406** Addition to upper extremity prosthesis, user adjustable, mechanical, residual limb volume management system (with or without lamination kit) Ⓑ Qp Qh ⚕ A

Other/Repair

* **L7499** Upper extremity prosthesis, not otherwise specified Ⓑ A
⊛ **L7510** Repair of prosthetic device, repair or replace minor parts ⓜ Ⓑ Qp Qh A

IOM: 100-02, 15, 110.2; 100-02, 15, 120; 100-04, 32, 100

* **L7520** Repair prosthetic device, labor component, per 15 minutes ⓜ Ⓑ A
⊘ **L7600** Prosthetic donning sleeve, any material, each Ⓑ E1

Medicare Statute 1862(1)(a)

General

Prosthetic Socket Insert

* **L7700** Gasket or seal, for use with prosthetic socket insert, any type, each Ⓑ ⚕ A

Penile Prosthetics

⊘ **L7900** Male vacuum erection system Ⓑ Qp Qh ♂ E1

Medicare Statute 1834a

⊘ **L7902** Tension ring, for vacuum erection device, any type, replacement only, each Ⓑ Qp Qh E1

Medicare Statute 1834a

Breast Prosthetics

⊛ **L8000** Breast prosthesis, mastectomy bra, without integrated breast prosthesis form, any size, any type Ⓑ Qp ♀ ⚕ A

IOM: 100-02, 15, 120

⊛ **L8001** Breast prosthesis, mastectomy bra, with integrated breast prosthesis form, unilateral, any size, any type Ⓑ Qp ♀ ⚕ A

IOM: 100-02, 15, 120

⊛ **L8002** Breast prosthesis, mastectomy bra, with integrated breast prosthesis form, bilateral, any size, any type Ⓑ Qp ♀ ⚕ A

IOM: 100-02, 15, 120

~~L8010 Breast prosthesis, mastectomy sleeve~~

⊛ **L8015** External breast prosthesis garment, with mastectomy form, post mastectomy Ⓑ Qp ♀ ⚕ A

IOM: 100-02, 15, 120

⊛ **L8020** Breast prosthesis, mastectomy form Ⓑ Qp ♀ ⚕ A

IOM: 100-02, 15, 120

⊛ **L8030** Breast prosthesis, silicone or equal, without integral adhesive Ⓑ Qp Qh ♀ ⚕ A

IOM: 100-02, 15, 120

⊛ **L8031** Breast prosthesis, silicone or equal, with integral adhesive Ⓑ Qp Qh ⚕ A

IOM: 100-02, 15, 120

* **L8032** Nipple prosthesis, prefabricated, reusable, any type, each Ⓑ Qp Qh ⚕ A
* **L8033** Nipple prosthesis, custom fabricated, reusable, any material, any type, each A
⊛ **L8035** Custom breast prosthesis, post mastectomy, molded to patient model Ⓑ Qp Qh ♀ ⚕ A

IOM: 100-02, 15, 120

* **L8039** Breast prosthesis, not otherwise specified Ⓑ Qp Qh ♀ A

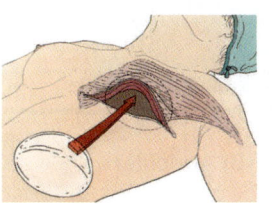

Figure 43 Implant breast prosthesis.

Nasal, Orbital, Auricular Prostherics

* **L8040** Nasal prosthesis, provided by a non-physician Ⓑ Qp Qh ♿ A
* **L8041** Midfacial prosthesis, provided by a non-physician Ⓑ Qp Qh ♿ A
* **L8042** Orbital prosthesis, provided by a non-physician Ⓑ Qp Qh ♿ A
* **L8043** Upper facial prosthesis, provided by a non-physician Ⓑ Qp Qh ♿ A
* **L8044** Hemi-facial prosthesis, provided by a non-physician Ⓑ Qp Qh ♿ A
* **L8045** Auricular prosthesis, provided by a non-physician Ⓑ Qp Qh ♿ A
* **L8046** Partial facial prosthesis, provided by a non-physician Ⓑ Qp Qh ♿ A
* **L8047** Nasal septal prosthesis, provided by a non-physician Ⓑ Qp Qh ♿ A
* **L8048** Unspecified maxillofacial prosthesis, by report, provided by a non-physician Ⓑ Qp Qh A
* **L8049** Repair or modification of maxillofacial prosthesis, labor component, 15 minute increments, provided by a non-physician Ⓑ Qp A

Trusses

○ **L8300** Truss, single with standard pad Ⓑ Qp Qh ♿ A
IOM: 100-02, 15, 120; 100-03, 4, 280.11; 100-03, 4, 280.12; 100-04, 4, 240

○ **L8310** Truss, double with standard pads Ⓑ Qp Qh ♿ A
IOM: 100-02, 15, 120; 100-03, 4, 280.11; 100-03, 4, 280.12; 100-04, 4, 240

○ **L8320** Truss, addition to standard pad, water pad Ⓑ Qp Qh ♿ A
IOM: 100-02, 15, 120; 100-03, 4, 280.11; 100-03, 4, 280.12; 100-04, 4, 240

○ **L8330** Truss, addition to standard pad, scrotal pad Ⓑ Qp Qh ♂ ♿ A
IOM: 100-02, 15, 120; 100-03, 4, 280.11; 100-03, 4, 280.12; 100-04, 4, 240

Prosthetic Socks

○ **L8400** Prosthetic sheath, below knee, each Ⓑ Qp ♿ A
IOM: 100-02, 15, 200

○ **L8410** Prosthetic sheath, above knee, each Ⓑ Qp ♿ A
IOM: 100-02, 15, 200

○ **L8415** Prosthetic sheath, upper limb, each Ⓑ Qp ♿ A
IOM: 100-02, 15, 200

* **L8417** Prosthetic sheath/sock, including a gel cushion layer, below knee or above knee, each Ⓑ Qp ♿ A

○ **L8420** Prosthetic sock, multiple ply, below knee, each Ⓑ Qp ♿ A
IOM: 100-02, 15, 200

○ **L8430** Prosthetic sock, multiple ply, above knee, each Ⓑ Qp ♿ A
IOM: 100-02, 15, 200

○ **L8435** Prosthetic sock, multiple ply, upper limb, each Ⓑ Qp ♿ A
IOM: 100-02, 15, 200

○ **L8440** Prosthetic shrinker, below knee, each Ⓑ Qp ♿ A
IOM: 100-02, 15, 200

○ **L8460** Prosthetic shrinker, above knee, each Ⓑ Qp ♿ A
IOM: 100-02, 15, 200

○ **L8465** Prosthetic shrinker, upper limb, each Ⓑ Qp ♿ A
IOM: 100-02, 15, 200

○ **L8470** Prosthetic sock, single ply, fitting, below knee, each Ⓑ Qp ♿ A
IOM: 100-02, 15, 200

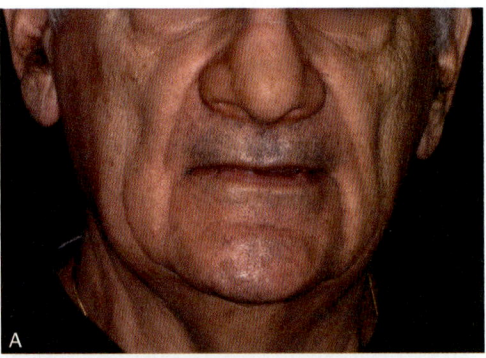
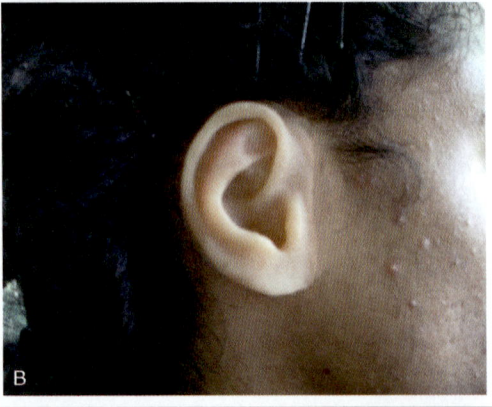

Figure 44 (A) Nasal prosthesis, (B) Auricular prosthesis.

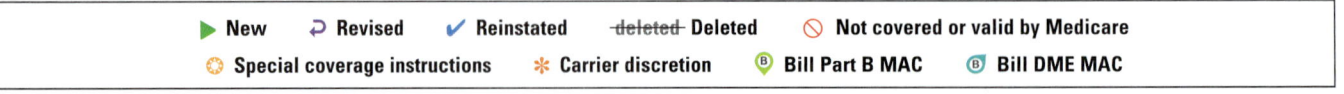

PROSTHETICS

- **L8480** Prosthetic sock, single ply, fitting, above knee, each ⓑ Qp ♿ A
  IOM: 100-02, 15, 200
- **L8485** Prosthetic sock, single ply, fitting, upper limb, each ⓑ Qp ♿ A
  IOM: 100-02, 15, 200

Unlisted

- **L8499** Unlisted procedure for miscellaneous prosthetic services ⓑ ⓑ A

Prosthetic Implants (L8500-L9900)

Larynx, Tracheoesophageal

- **L8500** Artificial larynx, any type ⓑ Qp Qh ♿ A
  IOM: 100-02, 15, 120; 100-03, 1, 50.2; 100-04, 4, 240
- **L8501** Tracheostomy speaking valve ⓑ Qp Qh ♿ A
  IOM: 100-03, 1, 50.4
- **L8505** Artificial larynx replacement battery/accessory, any type ⓑ A
- **L8507** Tracheo-esophageal voice prosthesis, patient inserted, any type, each ⓑ Qp Qh A
- **L8509** Tracheo-esophageal voice prosthesis, inserted by a licensed health care provider, any type ⓟ ⓑ Qp Qh ♿ A
- **L8510** Voice amplifier ⓑ Qp Qh ♿ A
  IOM: 100-03, 1, 50.2
- **L8511** Insert for indwelling tracheoesophageal prosthesis, with or without valve, replacement only, each ⓟ ⓑ Qp Qh ♿ A
- **L8512** Gelatin capsules or equivalent, for use with tracheoesophageal voice prosthesis, replacement only, per 10 ⓟ ⓑ ♿ A
- **L8513** Cleaning device used with tracheoesophageal voice prosthesis, pipet, brush, or equal, replacement only, each ⓟ ⓑ ♿ A
- **L8514** Tracheoesophageal puncture dilator, replacement only, each ⓟ ⓑ Qp Qh ♿ A
- **L8515** Gelatin capsule, application device for use with tracheoesophageal voice prosthesis, each ⓟ ⓑ Qp Qh ♿ A

Breast

- **L8600** Implantable breast prosthesis, silicone or equal ⓑ Qp Qh ♀ ♿ N1 N
  IOM: 100-02, 15, 120; 100-3, 2, 140.2

Bulking Agents

- **L8603** Injectable bulking agent, collagen implant, urinary tract, 2.5 ml syringe, includes shipping and necessary supplies ⓑ ♿ N1 N
  Bill on paper, acquisition cost invoice required
  IOM: 100-03, 4, 280.1
- **L8604** Injectable bulking agent, dextranomer/hyaluronic acid copolymer implant, urinary tract, 1 ml, includes shipping and necessary supplies ⓑ Qp Qh N1 N
- **L8605** Injectable bulking agent, dextranomer/hyaluronic acid copolymer implant, anal canal, 1 ml, includes shipping and necessary supplies ⓑ Qp Qh ♿ N1 N
- **L8606** Injectable bulking agent, synthetic implant, urinary tract, 1 ml syringe, includes shipping and necessary supplies ⓑ Qp Qh ♿ N1 N
  Bill on paper, acquisition cost invoice required
  IOM: 100-03, 4, 280.1
- **L8607** Injectable bulking agent for vocal cord medialization, 0.1 ml, includes shipping and necessary supplies ⓑ Qp Qh ♿ N1 N
  IOM: 100-03, 4, 280.1

Eye and Ear

- **L8608** Miscellaneous external component, supply or accessory for use with the Argus II retinal prosthesis system N
- **L8609** Artificial cornea ⓑ Qp Qh ♿ N1 N
- **L8610** Ocular implant ⓑ Qp Qh ♿ N1 N
  IOM: 100-02, 15, 120
- **L8612** Aqueous shunt ⓑ Qp Qh N1 N
  IOM: 100-02, 15, 120
  Cross Reference Q0074
- **L8613** Ossicula implant ⓑ Qp Qh ♿ N1 N
  IOM: 100-02, 15, 120
- **L8614** Cochlear device, includes all internal and external components ⓑ Qp Qh ♿ N1 N
  IOM: 100-02, 15, 120; 100-03, 1, 50.3
- **L8615** Headset/headpiece for use with cochlear implant device, replacement ⓑ Qp Qh ♿ A
  IOM: 100-03, 1, 50.3
- **L8616** Microphone for use with cochlear implant device, replacement ⓑ Qp Qh ♿ A
  IOM: 100-03, 1, 50.3

- **L8617** Transmitting coil for use with cochlear implant device, replacement ⓑ Qp Qh ♿ A
  IOM: 100-03, 1, 50.3

- **L8618** Transmitter cable for use with cochlear implant device or auditory osseointegrated device, replacement ⓑ Qp Qh ♿ A
  IOM: 100-03, 1, 50.3

- **L8619** Cochlear implant, external speech processor and controller, integrated system, replacement ⓑ Qp Qh ♿ A
  IOM: 100-03, 1, 50.3

- * **L8621** Zinc air battery for use with cochlear implant device and auditory osseointegrated sound processors, replacement, each ⓑ Qp Qh ♿ A

- * **L8622** Alkaline battery for use with cochlear implant device, any size, replacement, each ⓑ Qp Qh ♿ A

- * **L8623** Lithium ion battery for use with cochlear implant device speech processor, other than ear level, replacement, each ⓑ ♿ A

- * **L8624** Lithium ion battery for use with cochlear implant or auditory osseointegrated device speech processor, ear level, replacement, each ♿ A

- **L8625** External recharging system for battery for use with cochlear implant or auditory osseointegrated device, replacement only, each ♿ A
  IOM: 103-03, PART 1, 50.3

- **L8627** Cochlear implant, external speech processor, component, replacement ⓑ Qp Qh ♿ A
  IOM: 103-03, PART 1, 50.3

- **L8628** Cochlear implant, external controller component, replacement ⓑ Qp Qh ♿ A
  IOM: 103-03, PART 1, 50.3

- **L8629** Transmitting coil and cable, integrated, for use with cochlear implant device, replacement ⓑ Qp Qh ♿ A
  IOM: 103-03, PART 1, 50.3

Hand and Foot

- **L8630** Metacarpophalangeal joint implant ⓑ ♿ N1 N
  IOM: 100-02, 15, 120

- **L8631** Metacarpal phalangeal joint replacement, two or more pieces, metal (e.g., stainless steel or cobalt chrome), ceramic-like material (e.g., pyrocarbon), for surgical implantation (all sizes, includes entire system) ⓑ Qp Qh ♿ N1 N
  IOM: 100-02, 15, 120

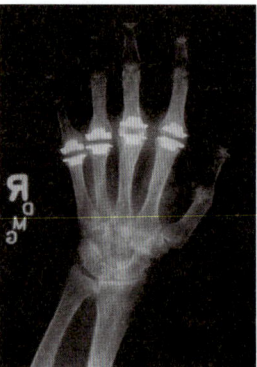

Figure 45 Metacarpophalangeal implant.

- **L8641** Metatarsal joint implant ⓑ Qp Qh ♿ N1 N
  IOM: 100-02, 15, 120

- **L8642** Hallux implant ⓑ Qp Qh ♿ N1 N
  May be billed by ambulatory surgical center or surgeon
  IOM: 100-02, 15, 120
  Cross Reference Q0073

- **L8658** Interphalangeal joint spacer, silicone or equal, each ⓑ Qp Qh ♿ N1 N
  IOM: 100-02, 15, 120

- **L8659** Interphalangeal finger joint replacement, 2 or more pieces, metal (e.g., stainless steel or cobalt chrome), ceramic-like material (e.g., pyrocarbon) for surgical implantation, any size ⓑ Qp Qh ♿ N1 N
  IOM: 100-02, 15, 120

Vascular

- **L8670** Vascular graft material, synthetic, implant ⓑ Qp Qh ♿ N1 N
  IOM: 100-02, 15, 120

Neurostimulator

- **L8678** Electrical stimulator supplies (external) for use with implantable neurostimulator, per month Qp Qh ♿ N

- **L8679** Implantable neurostimulator, pulse generator, any type ⓑ Qp Qh ♿ N1 N
  IOM: 100-03, 4, 280.4

- ⊘ **L8680** Implantable neurostimulator electrode, each ⓑ Qh E1
  Related CPT codes: 43647, 63650, 63655, 64553, 64555, 64560, 64561, 64565, 64573, 64575, 64577, 64580, 64581.

▶ New   ↻ Revised   ✓ Reinstated   ~~deleted~~ Deleted   ⊘ Not covered or valid by Medicare
⊛ Special coverage instructions   * Carrier discretion   ⓑ Bill Part B MAC   ⓑ Bill DME MAC

PROSTHETICS

○ **L8681** Patient programmer (external) for use with implantable programmable neurostimulator pulse generator, replacement only ⓑ Qp Qh ♿   A
IOM: 100-03, 4, 280.4

○ **L8682** Implantable neurostimulator radiofrequency receiver ⓑ Qp Qh ♿   N1   N
IOM: 100-03, 4, 280.4

○ **L8683** Radiofrequency transmitter (external) for use with implantable neurostimulator radiofrequency receiver ⓑ Qp Qh ♿   A
IOM: 100-03, 4, 280.4

○ **L8684** Radiofrequency transmitter (external) for use with implantable sacral root neurostimulator receiver for bowel and bladder management, replacement ⓑ Qp Qh ♿   A
IOM: 100-03, 4, 280.4

⊘ **L8685** Implantable neurostimulator pulse generator, single array, rechargeable, includes extension ⓑ Qp Qh   E1
Related CPT codes: 61885, 64590, 63685.

⊘ **L8686** Implantable neurostimulator pulse generator, single array, non-rechargeable, includes extension ⓑ Qp Qh   E1
Related CPT codes: 61885, 64590, 63685.

⊘ **L8687** Implantable neurostimulator pulse generator, dual array, rechargeable, includes extension ⓑ Qp Qh   E1
Related CPT codes: 64590, 63685, 61886.

⊘ **L8688** Implantable neurostimulator pulse generator, dual array, non-rechargeable, includes extension ⓑ Qp Qh   E1
Related CPT codes: 61885, 64590, 63685.

○ **L8689** External recharging system for battery (internal) for use with implantable neurostimulator, replacement only ⓑ Qp Qh ♿   A
IOM: 100-03, 4, 280.4

Miscellaneous Orthotic and Prosthetic Components, Services, and Supplies

* **L8690** Auditory osseointegrated device, includes all internal and external components ⓑ Qp Qh ♿   N1   N
Related CPT codes: 69714, 69715, 69717, 69718.

* **L8691** Auditory osseointegrated device, external sound processor, excludes transducer/actuator, replacement only, each ⓑ Qp Qh ♿   A

⊘ **L8692** Auditory osseointegrated device, external sound processor, used without osseointegration, body worn, includes headband or other means of external attachment ⓑ Qp Qh   E1
Medicare Statute 1862(a)(7)

* **L8693** Auditory osseointegrated device abutment, any length, replacement only ⓑ Qp Qh ♿   A

* **L8694** Auditory osseointegrated device, transducer/actuator, replacement only, each ♿   A

○ **L8695** External recharging system for battery (external) for use with implantable neurostimulator, replacement only ⓑ Qp Qh ♿   A
IOM: 100-03, 4, 280.4

○ **L8696** Antenna (external) for use with implantable diaphragmatic/phrenic nerve stimulation device, replacement, each ⓑ Qp Qh ♿   A

○ **L8698** Miscellaneous component, supply or accessory for use with total artificial heart system ⓑ   A

* **L8699** Prosthetic implant, not otherwise specified ⓑ   N1   N

* **L8701** Elbow, wrist, hand device, powered, with single or double upright(s), any type joint(s), includes microprocessor, sensors, all components and accessories ⓑ   A

* **L8702** Elbow, wrist, hand, finger device, powered, with single or double upright(s), any type joint(s), includes microprocessor, sensors, all components and accessories ⓑ   A

↺ **L8720** External lower extremity sensory prosthetic device, cutaneous stimulation of mechanoreceptors proximal to the ankle, per leg ⓑ   Y

     L8721 Receptor sole for use with L8720, replacement, each ⓑ   A

* **L9900** Orthotic and prosthetic supply, accessory, and/or service component of another HCPCS "L" code ⓑ ⓑ   N1   N

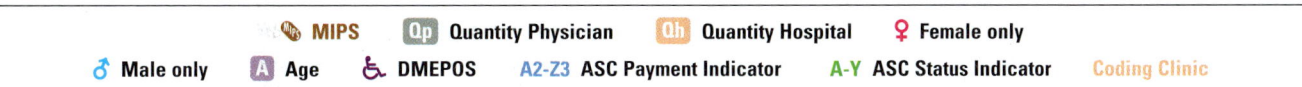

OTHER MEDICAL SERVICES (M0000-M0301)

- ✺ **M0001** Advancing cancer care MIPS value pathways **M**
- ✺ **M0002** Optimal care for kidney health MIPS value pathways **M**
- ~~M0003~~ ~~Optimal care for patients with episodic neurological conditions MIPS value pathways~~
- ↺ ✺ **M0004** Quality care for patients with neurological conditions MIPS value pathways **M**
- ✺ **M0005** Value in primary care MIPS value pathways **M**
- **M0010** Enhancing oncology model (EOM) monthly enhanced oncology services (MEOS) payment for EOM enhanced services **M**
- ⊘ **M0075** Cellular therapy ⓑ **E1**
- ⊘ **M0076** Prolotherapy ⓑ **E1**

  Prolotherapy stimulates production of new ligament tissue. Not covered by Medicare.
- ⊘ **M0100** Intragastric hypothermia using gastric freezing ⓑ **E1**
- ⊘ **M0201** Administration of pneumococcal, influenza, hepatitis b, and/or covid-19 vaccine inside a patient's home; reported only once per individual home per date of service when such vaccine administration(s) are performed at the patient's home **S**
- ~~M0222~~ ~~Intravenous injection, bebtelovimab, includes injection and post administration monitoring~~
- ~~M0223~~ ~~Intravenous injection, bebtelovimab, includes injection and post administration monitoring in the home or residence; this includes a beneficiary's home that has been made provider-based to the hospital during the covid 19 public health emergency~~
- ⊘ **M0224** Intravenous infusion, pemivibart, for the pre-exposure prophylaxis only, for certain adults and adolescents (12 years of age and older weighing at least 40 kg) with no known sars-cov-2 exposure, who either have moderate-to-severe immune compromise due to a medical condition or receipt of immunosuppressive medications or treatments, includes infusion and post administration monitoring **S**
- ▶ ⊘ **M0235** Intravenous infusion, monoclonal antibody products with an indication for post-exposure prophylaxis or treatment of Covid-19, for hospitalized adults and/or pediatric patients who are receiving systemic corticosteroids and require supplemental oxygen, non-invasive or invasive mechanical ventilation, or extracorporeal membrane oxygenation (ECMO) only, includes infusion and post administration monitoring, not otherwise classified, first dose **S**
- ▶ ⊘ **M0236** Intravenous infusion, monoclonal antibody products with an indication for post-exposure prophylaxis or treatment of Covid-19, for hospitalized adults and/or pediatric patients who are receiving systemic corticosteroids and require supplemental oxygen, non-invasive or invasive mechanical ventilation, or extracorporeal membrane oxygenation (ECMO) only, includes infusion and post administration monitoring, not otherwise classified, second dose **S**
- ▶ ⊘ **M0237** Intravenous infusion, tocilizumab-anoh, for hospitalized adult patients with Covid-19 who are receiving systemic corticosteroids and require supplemental oxygen, non-invasive or invasive mechanical ventilation, or extracorporeal membrane oxygenation (ECMO) only, includes infusion and post administration monitoring, first dose **S**
- ▶ ⊘ **M0238** Intravenous infusion, tocilizumab-anoh, for hospitalized adult patients with Covid-19 who are receiving systemic corticosteroids and require supplemental oxygen, non-invasive or invasive mechanical ventilation, or extracorporeal membrane oxygenation (ECMO) only, includes infusion and post administration monitoring, second dose **S**
- ~~M0240~~ ~~Intravenous infusion or subcutaneous injection, casirivimab and imdevimab includes infusion or injection, and post administration monitoring, subsequent repeat doses~~
- ~~M0241~~ ~~Intravenous infusion or subcutaneous injection, casirivimab and imdevimab includes infusion or injection, and post administration monitoring in the home or residence; this includes a beneficiary's home that has been made provider-based to the hospital during the covid 19 public health emergency, subsequent repeat doses~~
- ~~M0243~~ ~~Intravenous infusion or subcutaneous injection, casirivimab and imdevimab includes infusion and post administration monitoring~~

▶ New ↺ Revised ✓ Reinstated ~~deleted~~ Deleted ⊘ Not covered or valid by Medicare ✺ Special coverage instructions ✱ Carrier discretion ⓑ Bill Part B MAC ⓑ Bill DME MAC

OTHER MEDICAL SERVICES

- ~~M0244 Intravenous infusion or subcutaneous injection, casirivimab and imdevimab includes infusion or injection, and post administration monitoring in the home or residence; this includes a beneficiary's home that has been made provider-based to the hospital during the covid-19 public health emergency~~
- ~~M0245 Intravenous infusion, bamlanivimab and etesevimab, includes infusion and post administration monitoring~~
- ~~M0246 AIntravenous infusion, bamlanivimab and etesevimab, includes infusion and post administration monitoring in the home or residence; this includes a beneficiary's home that has been made provider based to the hospital during the covid 19 public health emergency~~
- ~~M0247 Intravenous infusion, sotrovimab, includes infusion and post administration monitoring~~
- ~~M0248 Intravenous infusion, sotrovimab, includes infusion and post administration monitoring in the home or residence; this includes a beneficiary's home that has been made provider-based to the hospital during the covid-19 public health emergency~~
- ⊘ M0249 Intravenous infusion, tocilizumab, for hospitalized adults and pediatric patients (2 years of age and older) with covid-19 who are receiving systemic corticosteroids and require supplemental oxygen, non-invasive or invasive mechanical ventilation, or extracorporeal membrane oxygenation (ecmo) only, includes infusion and post administration monitoring, first dose S
- ⊘ M0250 Intravenous infusion, tocilizumab, for hospitalized adults and pediatric patients (2 years of age and older) with covid-19 who are receiving systemic corticosteroids and require supplemental oxygen, non-invasive or invasive mechanical ventilation, or extracorporeal membrane oxygenation (ecmo) only, includes infusion and post administration monitoring, second dose S
- ⊘ M0300 IV chelation therapy (chemical endarterectomy) ⓑ E1
- ⊘ M0301 Fabric wrapping of abdominal aneurysm ⓑ E1

   Treatment for abdominal aneurysms that involves wrapping aneurysms with cellophane or fascia lata. Fabric wrapping of abdominal aneurysms is not a covered Medicare procedure.

- ✱ M1003 TB screening performed and results interpreted within twelve months prior to initiation of first-time biologic and/or immune response modifier therapy ⓑ M
- ✱ M1004 Documentation of medical reason for not screening for TB or interpreting results (i.e., patient positive for TB and documentation of past treatment; patient who has recently completed a course of anti-TB therapy) ⓑ M
- ✱ M1005 TB screening not performed or results not interpreted, reason not given ⓑ M
- ✱ M1006 Disease activity not assessed, reason not given ⓑ M
- ✱ M1007 >50% of total number of a patient's outpatient RA encounters assessed ⓑ M
- ✱ M1008 <50% of total number of a patient's outpatient RA encounters assessed ⓑ M
- ✱ M1009 Discharge/discontinuation of the episode of care documented in the medical record ⓑ M
- ✱ M1010 Discharge/discontinuation of the episode of care documented in the medical record ⓑ M
- ✱ M1011 Discharge/discontinuation of the episode of care documented in the medical record ⓑ M
- ✱ M1012 Discharge/discontinuation of the episode of care documented in the medical record ⓑ M
- ✱ M1013 Discharge/discontinuation of the episode of care documented in the medical record ⓑ M
- ✱ M1014 Discharge/discontinuation of the episode of care documented in the medical record ⓑ M
- ✱ M1016 Female patients unable to bear children ⓑ M
- ✱ M1018 Patients with an active diagnosis or history of cancer (except basal cell and squamous cell skin carcinoma), patients who are heavy tobacco smokers, lung cancer screening patients ⓑ M
- ✱ M1019 Adolescent patients 12 to 17 years of age with major depression or dysthymia who reached remission at twelve months as demonstrated by a twelve month (+/-60 days) PHQ-9 or PHQ-9m score of less than five ⓑ M
- ✱ M1020 Adolescent patients 12 to 17 years of age with major depression or dysthymia who did not reach remission at twelve months as demonstrated by a twelve month (+/-60 days) PHQ-9 or PHQ-9m score of less than 5. Either PHQ-9 or PHQ-9m score was not assessed or is greater than or equal to 5 ⓑ M
- ✱ M1021 Patient had only urgent care visits during the performance period ⓑ M
- ✱ M1027 Imaging of the head (CT or MRI) was obtained ⓑ M

| ✋ MIPS | Qp Quantity Physician | Qh Quantity Hospital | ♀ Female only |
| ♂ Male only | Ⓐ Age | ♿ DMEPOS | A2-Z3 ASC Payment Indicator | A-Y ASC Status Indicator | Coding Clinic |

361

* M1028	Documentation of patients with primary headache diagnosis and imaging other than CT or MRI obtained ⒷM
* M1029	Imaging of the head (CT or MRI) was not obtained, reason not given ⒷM
* M1032	Adults currently taking pharmacotherapy for OUD ⒷM
* M1034	Adults who have at least 180 days of continuous pharmacotherapy with a medication prescribed for OUD without a gap of more than seven days ⒷM
* M1035	Adults who are deliberately phased out of medication assisted treatment (MAT) prior to 180 days of continuous treatment ⒷM
* M1036	Adults who have not had at least 180 days of continuous pharmacotherapy with a medication prescribed for oud without a gap of more than seven days ⒷM
* M1037	Patients with a diagnosis of lumbar spine region cancer at the time of the procedure ⒷM
* M1038	Patients with a diagnosis of lumbar spine region fracture at the time of the procedure ⒷM
* M1039	Patients with a diagnosis of lumbar spine region infection at the time of the procedure ⒷM
* M1040	Patients with a diagnosis of lumbar idiopathic or congenital scoliosis ⒷM
* M1041	Patient had cancer, acute fracture or infection related to the lumbar spine or patient had neuromuscular, idiopathic or congenital lumbar scoliosis ⒷM
* M1043	Functional status was not measured by the Oswestry Disability Index (ODI version 2.1a) at one year (9 to 15 months) postoperatively ⒷM
* M1045	Functional status measured by the Oxford Knee Score (OKS) at one year (9 to 15 months) postoperatively was greater than or equal to 37 or knee injury and osteoarthritis outcome score joint replacement (Koos, jr.) was greater than or equal to 71 ⒷM
* M1046	Functional status the Oxford Knee Score (OKS) at one year (9 to 15 months) postoperatively was less than 37 or the knee injury and osteoarthritis outcome score joint replacement (Koos, jr.) was less than 71 postoperatively ⒷM
* M1049	Functional status was not measured by the Oswestry Disability Index (ODI version 2.1a) at three months (6 to 20 weeks) postoperatively ⒷM
* M1051	Patient had cancer, acute fracture or infection related to the lumbar spine or patient had neuromuscular, idiopathic or congenital lumbar scoliosis ⒷM
* M1052	Leg pain was not measured by the Visual Analog Scale (VAS) or numeric pain scale at one year (9 to 15 months) postoperatively ⒷM
* M1054	Patient had only urgent care visits during the performance period ⒷM
* M1055	Aspirin or another antiplatelet therapy used ⒷM
* M1056	Prescribed anticoagulant medication during the performance period, history of GI bleeding, history of intracranial bleeding, bleeding disorder and specific provider documented reasons: allergy to aspirin or anti-platelets, use of non-steroidal anti-inflammatory agents, drug-drug interaction, uncontrolled hypertension >180/110 mmhg or gastroesophageal reflux disease ⒷM
* M1057	Aspirin or another antiplatelet therapy not used, reason not given ⒷM
* M1058	Patient was a permanent nursing home resident at any time during the performance period ⒷM
* M1059	Patient was in hospice or receiving palliative care at any time during the performance period ⒷM
* M1060	Patient died prior to the end of the performance period ⒷM
* M1067	Hospice services for patient provided any time during the measurement period ⒷM
* M1068	Adults who are not ambulatory ⒷM
* M1069	Patient screened for future fall risk ⒷM
* M1070	Patient not screened for future fall risk, reason not given ⒷM
* M1072	Radiation therapy for anal cancer under the radiation oncology model, 90 day episode, professional component
* M1073	Radiation therapy for anal cancer under the radiation oncology model, 90 day episode, technical component
* M1074	Radiation therapy for bladder cancer under the radiation oncology model, 90 day episode, professional component
* M1075	Radiation therapy for bladder cancer under the radiation oncology model, 90 day episode, technical component
* M1076	Radiation therapy for bone metastases under the radiation oncology model, 90 day episode, professional component

▶ New ↻ Revised ✓ Reinstated ~~deleted~~ Deleted ⊘ Not covered or valid by Medicare
◉ Special coverage instructions * Carrier discretion Ⓑ Bill Part B MAC Ⓑ Bill DME MAC

OTHER MEDICAL SERVICES

* **M1077** Radiation therapy for bone metastases under the radiation oncology model, 90 day episode, technical component
* **M1078** Radiation therapy for brain metastases under the radiation oncology model, 90 day episode, professional component
* **M1079** Radiation therapy for brain metastases under the radiation oncology model, 90 day episode, technical component
* **M1080** Radiation therapy for breast cancer under the radiation oncology model, 90 day episode, professional componentt
* **M1081** Radiation therapy for breast cancer under the radiation oncology model, 90 day episode, technical component
* **M1082** Radiation therapy for cervical cancer under the radiation oncology model, 90 day episode, professional component
* **M1083** Radiation therapy for cervical cancer under the radiation oncology model, 90 day episode, technical component
* **M1084** Radiation therapy for cns tumors under the radiation oncology model, 90 day episode, professional component
* **M1085** Radiation therapy for cns tumors under the radiation oncology model, 90 day episode, technical component
* **M1086** Radiation therapy for colorectal cancer under the radiation oncology model, 90 day episode, professional component
* **M1087** Radiation therapy for colorectal cancer under the radiation oncology model, 90 day episode, technical component
* **M1088** Radiation therapy for head and neck cancer under the radiation oncology model, 90 day episode, professional component
* **M1089** Radiation therapy for head and neck cancer under the radiation oncology model, 90 day episode, technical component
* **M1094** Radiation therapy for lung cancer under the radiation oncology model, 90 day episode, professional component
* **M1095** Radiation therapy for lung cancer under the radiation oncology model, 90 day episode, technical component
* **M1096** Radiation therapy for lymphoma under the radiation oncology model, 90 day episode, professional component
* **M1097** Radiation therapy for lymphoma under the radiation oncology model, 90 day episode, technical component
* **M1098** Radiation therapy for pancreatic cancer under the radiation oncology model, 90 day episode, professional component
* **M1099** Radiation therapy for pancreatic cancer under the radiation oncology model, 90 day episode, technical component
* **M1100** Radiation therapy for prostate cancer under the radiation oncology model, 90 day episode, professional component
* **M1101** Radiation therapy for prostate cancer under the radiation oncology model, 90 day episode, technical component
* **M1102** Radiation therapy for upper GI cancer under the radiation oncology model, 90 day episode, professional componentt
* **M1103** Radiation therapy for upper GI cancer under the radiation oncology model, 90 day episode, technical component
* **M1104** Radiation therapy for uterine cancer under the radiation oncology model, 90 day episode, professional component
* **M1105** Radiation therapy for uterine cancer under the radiation oncology model, 90 day episode, technical component
* **M1106** The start of an episode of care documented in the medical record ⑧ M
* **M1107** Documentation stating patient has a diagnosis of a degenerative neurological condition such as ALS, MS, or Parkinson's diagnosed at any time before or during the episode of care ⑧ M
* **M1108** Ongoing care not clinically indicated because the patient needed a home program only, referred to another provider or facility, consultation only, as documented in the medical record ⑧ M
* **M1109** Ongoing care not medically possible because the patient was discharged early due to specific medical events, documented in the medical record, such as the patient became hospitalized or scheduled for surgery ⑧ M
* **M1110** Ongoing care not possible because the patient self-discharged early (e.g., financial or insurance reasons, transportation problems, or reason unknown) ⑧ M
* **M1111** The start of an episode of care documented in the medical record ⑧ M
* **M1112** Documentation stating patient has a diagnosis of a degenerative neurological condition such as ALS, MS, or Parkinson's diagnosed at any time before or during the episode of care ⑧ M

* **M1113** Ongoing care not clinically indicated because the patient needed a home program only, referred to another provider or facility, consultation only, as documented in the medical record Ⓑ M

* **M1114** Ongoing care not medically possible because the patient was discharged early due to specific medical events, documented in the medical record such as the patient becomes hospitalized or scheduled for surgery Ⓑ M

* **M1115** Ongoing care not possible because the patient self-discharged early (e.g., financial or insurance reasons, transportation problems, or reason unknown) Ⓑ M

* **M1116** The start of an episode of care documented in the medical record Ⓑ M

* **M1117** Documentation stating patient has a diagnosis of a degenerative neurological condition such as ALS, MS, or Parkinson's diagnosed at any time before or during the episode of care Ⓑ M

* **M1118** Ongoing care not clinically indicated because the patient needed a home program only, referred to another provider or facility, consultation only, as documented in the medical record Ⓑ M

* **M1119** Ongoing care not medically possible because the patient was discharged early due to specific medical events, documented in the medical record such as the patient becomes hospitalized or scheduled for surgery Ⓑ M

* **M1120** Ongoing care not possible because the patient self-discharged early (e.g., financial or insurance reasons, transportation problems, or reason unknown) Ⓑ M

* **M1121** The start of an episode of care documented in the medical record Ⓑ M

* **M1122** Documentation stating patient has a diagnosis of a degenerative neurological condition such as ALS, MS, or Parkinson's diagnosed at any time before or during the episode of care Ⓑ M

* **M1123** Ongoing care not clinically indicated because the patient needed a home program only, referred to another provider or facility, consultation only, as documented in the medical record M

* **M1124** Ongoing care not medically possible because the patient was discharged early due to specific medical events, documented in the medical record such as the patient becomes hospitalized or scheduled for surgery Ⓑ M

* **M1125** Ongoing care not possible because the patient self-discharged early (e.g., financial or insurance reasons, transportation problems, or reason unknown) Ⓑ M

* **M1126** The start of an episode of care documented in the medical record Ⓑ M

* **M1127** Documentation stating patient has a diagnosis of a degenerative neurological condition such as ALS, MS, or Parkinson's diagnosed at any time before or during the episode of care Ⓑ M

* **M1128** Ongoing care not clinically indicated because the patient needed a home program only, referred to another provider or facility, consultation only, as documented in the medical record Ⓑ M

* **M1129** Ongoing care not medically possible because the patient was discharged early due to specific medical events, documented in the medical record such as the patient becomes hospitalized or scheduled for surgery Ⓑ M

* **M1130** Ongoing care not possible because the patient self-discharged early (e.g., financial or insurance reasons, transportation problems, or reason unknown) Ⓑ M

* **M1131** Documentation stating patient has a diagnosis of a degenerative neurological condition such as ALS, MS, or Parkinson's diagnosed at any time before or during the episode of care Ⓑ M

* **M1132** Ongoing care not clinically indicated because the patient needed a home program only, referred to another provider or facility, consultation only, as documented in the medical record Ⓑ M

* **M1133** Ongoing care not due to specific medical events, documented in the medical record such as the patient becomes hospitalized or scheduled for surgery Ⓑ M

* **M1134** Ongoing care not possible because the patient self-discharged early (e.g., financial or insurance reasons, transportation problems, or reason unknown) Ⓑ M

OTHER MEDICAL SERVICES

* **M1135** The start of an episode of care documented in the medical record ⒷM

* **M1141** Functional status was not measured by the Oxford Knee Score (OKS) or the knee injury and osteoarthritis outcome score joint replacement (Koos, jr.) at one year (9 to 15 months) postoperatively ⒷM

* **M1142** Emergent cases ⒷM

* **M1143** Initiated episode of rehabilitation therapy, medical, or chiropractic care for neck impairment ⒷM

* **M1145** Most favored nation (MFN) model drug add-on amount, per dose, (do not bill with line items that have the JW modifier) K

* **M1146** Ongoing care not clinically indicated because the patient needed a home program only, referral to another provider or facility, or consultation only, as documented in the medical record M

* **M1147** Ongoing care not medically possible because the patient was discharged early due to specific medical events, documented in the medical record, such as the patient became hospitalized or scheduled for surgery M

* **M1148** Ongoing care not possible because the patient self-discharged early (e.g., financial or insurance reasons, transportation problems, or reason unknown) M

* **M1149** Patient unable to complete the neck fs prom at initial evaluation and/or discharge due to blindness, illiteracy, severe mental incapacity or language incompatibility, and an adequate proxy is not available M

↺ ○ **M1150** Current or prior left ventricular ejection fraction (LVEF) less than or equal to 40% or documentation of moderately or severely depressed left ventricular systolic function M

○ **M1151** Patients with a history of heart transplant or with a left ventricular assist device (LVAD) M

○ **M1152** Patients with a history of heart transplant or with a left ventricular assist device (LVAD) M

○ **M1153** Patient with diagnosis of osteoporosis on date of encounter M

~~M1154 Hospice services provided to patient any time during the measurement period~~

~~M1155 Patient had anaphylaxis due to the pneumococcal vaccine any time during or before the measurement period~~

○ **M1159** Hospice services provided to patient any time during the measurement period M

○ **M1160** Patient had anaphylaxis due to the meningococcal vaccine any time on or before the patient's 13th birthday M

○ **M1161** Patient had anaphylaxis due to the tetanus, diphtheria, or pertussis vaccine any time on or before the patient's 13th birthday M

○ **M1162** Patient had encephalitis due to the tetanus, diphtheria, or pertussis vaccine any time on or before the patient's 13th birthday M

○ **M1163** Patient had anaphylaxis due to the HPV vaccine any time on or before the patient's 13th birthday M

○ **M1164** Patients with dementia any time during the patient's history through the end of the measurement period M

○ **M1165** Patients who use hospice services any time during the measurement period M

○ **M1166** Pathology report for tissue specimens produced from wide local excisions or re-excisions M

○ **M1167** In hospice or using hospice services during the measurement period M

○ **M1168** Patient received an influenza vaccine on or between July 1 of the year prior to the measurement period and June 30 of the measurement period M

○ **M1169** Documentation of medical reason(s) for not administering influenza vaccine (e.g., prior anaphylaxis due to the influenza vaccine) M

○ **M1170** Patient did not receive an influenza vaccine on or between July 1 of the year prior to the measurement period and June 30 of the measurement period M

○ **M1171** Patient received at least one TD vaccine or one Tdap vaccine between nine years prior to the encounter and the end of the measurement period M

○ **M1172** Documentation of medical reason(s) for not administering TD or Tdap vaccine (e.g., prior anaphylaxis due to the TD or Tdap vaccine or history of encephalopathy within seven days after a previous dose of a TD-containing vaccine) M

○ **M1173** Patient did not receive at least one TD vaccine or one Tdap vaccine between nine years prior to the encounter and the end of the measurement period M

MIPS	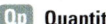 Quantity Physician	Quantity Hospital	♀ Female only
♂ Male only	Age	♿ DMEPOS	A2-Z3 ASC Payment Indicator	A-Y ASC Status Indicator	*Coding Clinic*

⊛ **M1174**	Patient received at least two doses of the herpes zoster recombinant vaccine (at least 28 days apart) anytime on or after the patient's 50th birthday before or during the measurement period M
⊛ **M1175**	Documentation of medical reason(s) for not administering zoster vaccine (e.g., prior anaphylaxis due to the zoster vaccine) M
⇌⊛ **M1176**	Patient did not receive two doses of the herpes zoster recombinant vaccine (at least 28 days apart) anytime on or after the patient's 50th birthday before or during the measurement period M
⇌⊛ **M1177**	Patient received any pneumococcal conjugate or polysaccharide vaccine on or after their 19th birthday and before the end of the measurement period M
⊛ **M1178**	Documentation of medical reason(s) for not administering pneumococcal vaccine (e.g., prior anaphylaxis due to the pneumococcal vaccine) M
⇌⊛ **M1179**	Patient did not receive any pneumococcal conjugate or polysaccharide vaccine, on or after their 19th birthday and before or during measurement period M
⊛ **M1180**	Patients on immune checkpoint inhibitor therapy M
⊛ **M1181**	Grade 2 or above diarrhea and/or grade 2 or above colitis M
⊛ **M1182**	Patients not eligible due to pre-existing inflammatory bowel disease (IBD) (e.g., ulcerative colitis, Crohn's disease) M
⊛ **M1183**	Documentation of immune checkpoint inhibitor therapy held and corticosteroids or immunosuppressants prescribed or administered M
⊛ **M1184**	Documentation of medical reason(s) for not prescribing or administering corticosteroid or immunosuppressant treatment (e.g., allergy, intolerance, infectious etiology, pancreatic insufficiency, hyperthyroidism, prior bowel surgical interventions, Celiac disease, receiving other medication, awaiting diagnostic workup results for alternative etiologies, other medical reasons/contraindication) M
⊛ **M1185**	Documentation of immune checkpoint inhibitor therapy not held and/or corticosteroids or immunosuppressants prescribed or administered was not performed, reason not given M
⊛ **M1186**	Patients who have an order for or are receiving hospice or palliative care M
⊛ **M1187**	Patients with a diagnosis of end stage renal disease (ESRD) M
⊛ **M1188**	Patients with a diagnosis of chronic kidney disease (CKD) stage 5 M
⊛ **M1189**	Documentation of a kidney health evaluation defined by an estimated glomerular filtration rate (EGFR) and urine albumin-creatinine ratio (UACR) performed M
⊛ **M1190**	Documentation of a kidney health evaluation was not performed or defined by an estimated glomerular filtration rate (EGFR) and urine albumin-creatinine ratio (UACR) M
⊛ **M1191**	Hospice services provided to patient any time during the measurement period M
⊛ **M1192**	Patients with an existing diagnosis of squamous cell carcinoma of the esophagus M
⊛ **M1193**	Surgical pathology reports that contain impression or conclusion of or recommendation for testing of MMR by immunohistochemistry, MSI by DNA-based testing status, or both M
⊛ **M1194**	Documentation of medical reason(s) surgical pathology reports did not contain impression or conclusion of or recommendation for testing of MMR by immunohistochemistry, MSI by DNA-based testing status, or both tests were not included (e.g., patient will not be treated with checkpoint inhibitor therapy, no residual carcinoma is present in the sample [tissue exhausted or status post neoadjuvant treatment], insufficient tumor for testing) M
⊛ **M1195**	Surgical pathology reports that do not contain impression or conclusion of or recommendation for testing of MMR by immunohistochemistry, MSI by DNA-based testing status, or both, reason not given M
⊛ **M1196**	Initial (index visit) numeric rating scale (NRS), visual rating scale (VRS), or itchyquant assessment score of greater than or equal to 4 M
⊛ **M1197**	Itch severity assessment score is reduced by 3 or more points from the initial (index) assessment score to the follow-up visit score M
⊛ **M1198**	Itch severity assessment score was not reduced by at least 3 points from initial (index) score to the follow-up visit score or assessment was not completed during the follow-up encounter M
⊛ **M1199**	Patients receiving RRT M
⊛ **M1200**	Ace inhibitor (ace-i) or ARB therapy prescribed during the measurement period M

▶ New ⇌ Revised ✓ Reinstated ~~deleted~~ Deleted ⊘ Not covered or valid by Medicare
⊛ Special coverage instructions ✱ Carrier discretion Ⓑ Bill Part B MAC Ⓑ Bill DME MAC

OTHER MEDICAL SERVICES

✪ **M1201** Documentation of medical reason(s) for not prescribing ace inhibitor (ace-i) or ARB therapy during the measurement period (e.g., pregnancy, history of angioedema to ace-i, other allergy to ace-i and ARB, hyperkalemia, or history of hyperkalemia while on ace-i or ARB therapy, acute kidney injury due to ace-i or ARB therapy), other medical reasons) M

✪ **M1202** Documentation of patient reason(s) for not prescribing ace inhibitor or ARB therapy during the measurement period, (e.g., patient declined, other patient reasons) M

✪ **M1203** Ace inhibitor or ARB therapy not prescribed during the measurement period, reason not given M

✪ **M1204** Initial (index visit) numeric rating scale (NRS), visual rating scale (VRS), or itchyquant assessment score of greater than or equal to 4 M

✪ **M1205** Itch severity assessment score is reduced by 3 or more points from the initial (index) assessment score to the follow-up visit score M

✪ **M1206** Itch severity assessment score was not reduced by at least 3 points from initial (index) score to the follow-up visit score or assessment was not completed during the follow-up encounter M

✪ **M1207** Patient is screened for food insecurity, housing instability, transportation needs, utility difficulties, and interpersonal safety M

✪ **M1208** Patient is not screened for food insecurity, housing instability, transportation needs, utility difficulties, and interpersonal safety M

✪ **M1209** At least two orders for high-risk medications from the same drug class, (table 4), not ordered M

✪ **M1210** At least two orders for high-risk medications from the same drug class, (table 4), not ordered M

↻ ✪ **M1211** Most recent glycemic status assessment (HBA1C or GMI) level >9.0% M

↻ ✪ **M1212** Glycemic status assessment (HBA1C or GMI) level is missing, or was not performed during the measurement period M

✪ **M1213** No history of spirometry results with confirmed airflow obstruction (fev1/fvc <70%) and present spirometry is >70% M

✪ **M1214** Spirometry results with confirmed airflow obstruction (fev1/fvc <70%) documented and reviewed M

✪ **M1215** Documentation of medical reason(s) for not documenting and reviewing spirometry results (e.g., patients with dementia or tracheostomy) M

✪ **M1216** No spirometry results with confirmed airflow obstruction (fev1/fvc <70%) documented and/or no spirometry performed with results documented during the encounter M

✪ **M1217** Documentation of system reason(s) for not documenting and reviewing spirometry results (e.g., spirometry equipment not available at the time of the encounter) M

✪ **M1218** Patient has COPD symptoms (e.g., dyspnea, cough/sputum, wheezing) M

~~M1219~~ ~~Anaphylaxis due to the vaccine on or before the date of the encounter~~

✪ **M1220** Dilated retinal eye exam with interpretation by an ophthalmologist or optometrist or artificial intelligence (ai) interpretation documented and reviewed; with evidence of retinopathy M

✪ **M1221** Dilated retinal eye exam with interpretation by an ophthalmologist or optometrist or artificial intelligence (AI) interpretation documented and reviewed; without evidence of retinopathy M

✪ **M1222** Glaucoma plan of care not documented; reason not otherwise specified M

✪ **M1223** Glaucoma plan of care documented M

✪ **M1224** Intraocular pressure (IOP) reduced by a value less than 20% from the pre-intervention level M

✪ **M1225** Intraocular pressure (IOP) reduced by a value of greater than or equal to 20% from the pre-intervention level M

✪ **M1226** IOP measurement not documented, reason not otherwise specified M

✪ **M1227** Evidence-based therapy was prescribed M

✪ **M1228** Patient, who has a reactive HCV antibody test, and has a follow up HCV viral test that detected HCV viremia, has HCV treatment initiated within 3 months of the reactive HCV antibody test M

✪ **M1229** Patient, who has a reactive HCV antibody test, and has a follow up HCV viral test that detected HCV viremia, is referred within 1 month of the reactive HCV antibody test to a clinician who treats HCV infection M

| 🗲 MIPS | Qp Quantity Physician | Qh Quantity Hospital | ♀ Female only |
| ♂ Male only | A Age | & DMEPOS | A2-Z3 ASC Payment Indicator | A-Y ASC Status Indicator | Coding Clinic |

- **M1230** Patient has a reactive HCV antibody test and does not have a follow up HCV viral test, or patient has a reactive HCV antibody test and has a follow up HCV viral test that detects HCV viremia and is not referred to a clinician who treats HCV infection within 1 month and does not have HCV treatment initiated within 3 months of the reactive HCV antibody test, reason not given M
- **M1231** Patient receives HCV antibody test with nonreactive result M
- **M1232** Patient receives HCV antibody test with reactive result M
- **M1233** Patient does not receive HCV antibody test or patient does receive HCV antibody test but results not documented, reason not given M
- **M1234** Patient has a reactive HCV antibody test, and has a follow up HCV viral test that does not detect HCV viremia M
- **M1235** Documentation or patient report of HCV antibody test or HCV MA test which occurred prior to the performance period M
- **M1236** Baseline MRS >2 M
- **M1237** Patient reason for not screening for food insecurity, housing instability, transportation needs, utility difficulties, and interpersonal safety (e.g., patient declined or other patient reasons) M
- **M1238** Documentation that administration of second recombinant zoster vaccine could not occur during the performance period due to the recommended 2-6 month interval between doses (i.e, first dose received after October 31) M
- **M1239** Patient did not respond to the question of patient felt heard and understood by this provider and team M
- **M1240** Patient did not respond to the question of patient felt this provider and team put my best interests first when making recommendations about my care M
- **M1241** Patient did not respond to the question of patient felt this provider and team saw me as a person, not just someone with a medical problem M
- **M1242** Patient did not respond to the question of patient felt this provider and team understood what is important to me in my life M
- **M1243** Patient provided a response other than "completely true" for the question of patient felt heard and understood by this provider and team M
- **M1244** Patient provided a response other than "completely true" for the question of patient felt this provider and team put my best interests first when making recommendations about my care M
- **M1245** Patient provided a response other than "completely true" for the question of patient felt this provider and team saw me as a person, not just someone with a medical problem M
- **M1246** Patient provided a response other than "completely true" for the question of patient felt this provider and team understood what is important to me in my life M
- **M1247** Patient responded "completely true" for the question of patient felt this provider and team put my best interests first when making recommendations about my care M
- **M1248** Patient responded "completely true" for the question of patient felt this provider and team saw me as a person, not just someone with a medical problem M
- **M1249** Patient responded "completely true" for the question of patient felt this provider and team understood what is important to me in my life M
- **M1250** Patient responded as "completely true" for the question of patient felt heard and understood by this provider and team M
- **M1251** Patients for whom a proxy completed the entire hu survey on their behalf for any reason (no patient involvement) M
- **M1252** Patients who did not complete at least one of the four patient experience hu survey items and return the hu survey within 60 days of the ambulatory palliative care visit M
- **M1253** Patients who respond on the patient experience hu survey that they did not receive care by the listed ambulatory palliative care provider in the last 60 days (disavowal) M
- **M1254** Patients who were deceased when the hu survey reached them M
- **M1255** Patients who have another reason for visiting the clinic [not prenatal or postpartum care] and have a positive pregnancy test but have not established the clinic as an OB provider (e.g., plan to terminate the pregnancy or seek prenatal services elsewhere) M
- **M1256** Prior history of known CVD M
- **M1257** CVD risk assessment not performed or incomplete (e.g., CVD risk assessment was not documented), reason not otherwise specified M

▶ New ↻ Revised ✓ Reinstated ~~deleted~~ Deleted ⊘ Not covered or valid by Medicare ✺ Special coverage instructions ∗ Carrier discretion Ⓑ Bill Part B MAC Ⓑ Bill DME MAC

OTHER MEDICAL SERVICES

✺ **M1258** CVD risk assessment performed, have a documented calculated risk score M

↺✺ **M1259** Patients status documented within the first year of initiating dialysis M

↺✺ **M1260** Patients status not documented within the first year of initiating dialysis M

✺ **M1261** Patients that were on the kidney or kidney-pancreas waitlist prior to initiation of dialysis M

✺ **M1262** Patients who had a transplant prior to initiation of dialysis M

✺ **M1263** Patients in hospice on their initiation of dialysis date or during the month of evaluation M

~~M1264~~ ~~Patients age 75 or older on their initiation of dialysis date~~

✺ **M1265** CMS medical evidence form 2728 for dialysis patients: initial form completed D

✺ **M1266** Patients admitted to a skilled nursing facility (SNF) M

↺✺ **M1267** Patients not observed in active status on any kidney or kidney-pancreas transplant waitlist as of the last day of each month during the measurement period M

↺✺ **M1268** Patients observed in active status on any kidney or kidney-pancreas transplant waitlist as of the last day of each month during the measurement period M

✺ **M1269** Receiving ESRD MCP dialysis services by the provider on the last day of the reporting month M

✺ **M1270** Patients not on any kidney or kidney-pancreas transplant waitlist as of the last day of each month during the measurement period M

✺ **M1271** Patients with dementia at any time prior to or during the month M

↺✺ **M1272** Patients observed on any kidney or kidney-pancreas transplant waitlist as of the last day of each month during the measurement period M

✺ **M1273** Patients who were admitted to a skilled nursing facility (SNF) within one year of dialysis initiation according to the CMS-2728 form M

✺ **M1274** Patients who were admitted to a skilled nursing facility (SNF) during the month of evaluation were excluded from that month M

✺ **M1275** Patients determined to be in hospice were excluded from month of evaluation and the remainder of reporting period M

✺ **M1276** BMI documented outside normal parameters, no follow-up plan documented, no reason given M

✺ **M1277** Colorectal cancer screening results documented and reviewed M

✺ **M1278** Elevated or hypertensive blood pressure reading documented, and the indicated follow-up is documented M

✺ **M1279** Elevated or hypertensive blood pressure reading documented, indicated follow-up not documented, reason not given M

✺ **M1280** Women who had a bilateral mastectomy or who have a history of a bilateral mastectomy or for whom there is evidence of a right and a left unilateral mastectomy M

✺ **M1281** Blood pressure reading not documented, reason not given M

✺ **M1282** Patient screened for tobacco use and identified as a tobacco non-user M

✺ **M1283** Patient screened for tobacco use and identified as a tobacco user M

✺ **M1284** Patients age 66 or older in institutional special needs plans (SNP) or residing in long term care with pos code 32, 33, 34, 54, or 56 for more than 90 consecutive days during the measurement period M

✺ **M1285** Screening, diagnostic, film, digital or digital breast tomosynthesis (3d) mammography results were not documented and reviewed, reason not otherwise specified M

✺ **M1286** BMI is documented as being outside of normal parameters, follow-up plan is not completed for documented medical reason M

✺ **M1287** BMI is documented below normal parameters and a follow-up plan is documented M

✺ **M1288** Documented reason for not screening or recommending a follow-up for high blood pressure M

✺ **M1289** Patient identified as tobacco user did not receive tobacco cessation intervention during the measurement period or in the six months prior to the measurement period (counseling and/or pharmacotherapy) M

✺ **M1290** Patient not eligible due to active diagnosis of hypertension M

✺ **M1291** Patients 66 years of age and older with at least one claim/encounter for frailty during the measurement period and a dispensed medication for dementia during the measurement period or the year prior to the measurement period M

| ✺ MIPS | Qp Quantity Physician | Qh Quantity Hospital | ♀ Female only |
| ♂ Male only | A Age | ♿ DMEPOS | A2-Z3 ASC Payment Indicator | A-Y ASC Status Indicator | Coding Clinic |

M1292	Patients 66 years of age and older with at least one claim/encounter for frailty during the measurement period and an advanced illness diagnosis during the measurement period or the year prior to the measurement period M
M1293	BMI is documented above normal parameters and a follow-up plan is documented M
M1294	Normal blood pressure reading documented, follow-up not required M
M1295	Patients with a diagnosis or past history of total colectomy or colorectal cancer M
M1296	BMI is documented within normal parameters and no follow-up plan is required M
M1297	BMI not documented due to medical reason or patient refusal of height or weight measurement M
M1298	Documentation of patient pregnancy anytime during the measurement period prior to and including the current encounter M
M1299	Influenza immunization administered or previously received M
M1300	Influenza immunization was not administered for reasons documented by clinician (e.g., patient allergy or other medical reasons, patient declined or other patient reasons, vaccine not available or other system reasons) M
M1301	Patient identified as a tobacco user received tobacco cessation intervention during the measurement period or in the six months prior to the measurement period (counseling and/or pharmacotherapy) M
M1302	Screening, diagnostic, film digital or digital breast tomosynthesis (3d) mammography results documented and reviewed M
M1303	Hospice services provided to patient any time during the measurement period M
M1304	Patient did not receive any pneumococcal conjugate or polysaccharide vaccine on or after their 19th birthday and before the end of the measurement period M
M1305	Patient received any pneumococcal conjugate or polysaccharide vaccine on or after their 19th birthday and before the end of the measurement period M
M1306	Patient had anaphylaxis due to the pneumococcal vaccine any time during or before the measurement period M
M1307	Documentation stating the patient has received or is currently receiving palliative or hospice care M
M1308	Influenza immunization was not administered, reason not given M
M1309	Palliative care services provided to patient any time during the measurement period M
M1310	Patient screened for tobacco use and received tobacco cessation intervention during the measurement period or in the six months prior to the measurement period (counseling, pharmacotherapy, or both), if identified as a tobacco user M
M1311	Anaphylaxis due to the vaccine on or before the date of the encounter M
M1312	Patient not screened for tobacco use M
M1313	Tobacco screening not performed or tobacco cessation intervention not provided during the measurement period or in the six months prior to the measurement period M
M1314	BMI not documented and no reason is given M
M1315	Colorectal cancer screening results were not documented and reviewed; reason not otherwise specified M
M1316	Current tobacco non-user M
M1317	Patients who are counseled on connection with a CSP and explicitly opt out M
M1318	Patients who did not have documented contact with a CSP for at least one of their screened positive HRSNS within 60 days after screening or documentation that there was no contact with a CSP M
M1319	Patients who had documented contact with a CSP for at least one of their screened positive HRSNS within 60 days after screening M
M1320	Patients who screened positive for at least 1 of the 5 HRSNS M
M1321	Patients who were not seen within 7 weeks following the date of injection for follow up or who did not have a documented IOP or no plan of care documented if the IOP was >25 mm hg M
M1322	Patients seen within 7 weeks following the date of injection and are screened for elevated intraocular pressure (IOP) with tonometry with documented IOP <25 mm hg for injected eye M

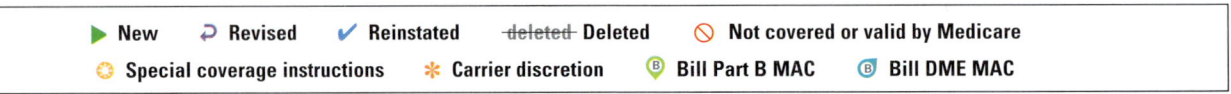

▶ New ⟲ Revised ✓ Reinstated ~~deleted~~ Deleted ⊘ Not covered or valid by Medicare
☼ Special coverage instructions ✳ Carrier discretion Ⓑ Bill Part B MAC Ⓑ Bill DME MAC

OTHER MEDICAL SERVICES

M1323 Patients seen within 7 weeks following the date of injection and are screened for elevated intraocular pressure (IOP) with tonometry with documented IOP >25 mm hg and a plan of care was documented M

M1324 Patients who had an intravitreal or periocular corticosteroid injection (e.g., triamcinolone, preservative-free triamcinolone, dexamethasone, dexamethasone intravitreal implant, or fluocinolone intravitreal implant) M

M1325 Patients who were not seen for reasons documented by clinician for patient or medical reasons (e.g., inadequate time for follow-up, patients who received a prior intravitreal or periocular steroid injection within the last six (6) months and had a subsequent IOP evaluation with IOP <25mm hg within seven (7) weeks of treatment) M

M1326 Patients with a diagnosis of hypotony M

M1327 Patients who were not appropriately evaluated during the initial exam and/or who were not re-evaluated within 8 weeks M

M1328 Patients with a diagnosis of acute vitreous hemorrhage M

M1329 Patients with a post-operative encounter of the eye with the acute PVD within 2 weeks before the initial encounter or 8 weeks after initial acute PVD encounter M

M1330 Documentation of patient reason(s) for not having a follow up exam (e.g., inadequate time for follow up) M

M1331 Patients who were appropriately evaluated during the initial exam and were re-evaluated no later than 8 weeks from initial exam M

M1332 Patients who were not appropriately evaluated during the initial exam and/or who were not re-evaluated within 2 weeks M

M1333 Acute vitreous hemorrhage M

M1334 Patients with a post-operative encounter of the eye with the acute PVD within 2 weeks before the initial encounter or 2 weeks after initial acute PVD encounter M

M1335 Documentation of patient reason(s) for not having a follow up exam (e.g., inadequate time for follow up) M

M1336 Patients who were appropriately evaluated during the initial exam and were re-evaluated no later than 2 weeks M

M1337 Acute PVD M

M1338 Patients who had follow-up assessment 30 to 180 days after the index assessment who did not demonstrate positive improvement or maintenance of functioning scores during the performance period M

M1339 Patients who had follow-up assessment 30 to 180 days after the index assessment who demonstrated positive improvement or maintenance of functioning scores during the performance period M

M1340 Index assessment completed using the 12-item WHODAS 2.0 or SDS during the denominator identification period M

M1341 Patients who did not have a follow-up assessment or did not have an assessment within 30 to 180 days after the index assessment during the performance period M

M1342 Patients who died during the performance period M

M1343 Patients who are at PAM level 4 at baseline or patients who are flagged with extreme straight line response sets on the PAM or with excessive missing responses M

M1344 Patients who did not have a baseline PAM score and/or a second score within 4 to 12 month of baseline score M

M1345 Patients who had a baseline PAM score and a second score within 4 to 12 month of baseline PAM score M

M1346 Patients who did not have a net increase in PAM score of at least 6 points within a 4 to 12 month period M

M1347 Patients who achieved a net increase in PAM score of at least 3 points in a 4 to 12 month period (passing) M

M1348 Patients who achieved a net increase in PAM score of at least 6-points in a 4 to 12 month period (excellent) M

M1349 Patients who did not have a net increase in PAM score of at least 3 points within 4 to 12 month period

M1350 Patients who had a completed suicide safety plan initiated, reviewed or updated in collaboration with their clinician (concurrent or within 24 hours) of the index clinical encounter M

⊛ **M1351**	Patients who had a suicide safety plan initiated, reviewed, or updated and reviewed and updated in collaboration with the patient and their clinician concurrent or within 24 hours of clinical encounter and within 120 days after initiation M
⊛ **M1352**	Suicidal ideation and/or behavior symptoms based on the C-SSRS or equivalent assessment M
⊛ **M1353**	Patients who did not have a completed suicide safety plan initiated, reviewed or updated in collaboration with their clinician (concurrent or within 24 hours) of the index clinical encounter M
⊛ **M1354**	Patients who did not have a suicide safety plan initiated, reviewed, or updated or reviewed and updated in collaboration with the patient and their clinician concurrent or within 24 hours of clinical encounter and within 120 days after initiation M
⊛ **M1355**	Suicide risk based on their clinician's evaluation or a clinician-rated tool M
⊛ **M1356**	Patients who died during the measurement period M
⊛ **M1357**	Patients who had a reduction in suicidal ideation and/or behavior upon follow-up assessment within 120 days of index assessment M
⊛ **M1358**	Patients who did not have a reduction in suicidal ideation and/or behavior upon follow-up assessment within 120 days of index assessment M
⊛ **M1359**	Index assessment during the denominator period when the suicidal ideation and/or behavior symptoms or increased suicide risk by clinician determination occurs and a non-zero C-SSRS score is obtained M
⊛ **M1360**	Suicidal ideation and/or behavior symptoms based on the C-SSRS M
⊛ **M1361**	Suicide risk based on their clinician's evaluation or a clinician-rated tool M
⊛ **M1362**	Patients who died during the measurement period M
⊛ **M1363**	Patients who did not have a follow-up assessment within 120 days of the index assessment M
⊛ **M1364**	Calculated 10-year ASCVD risk score of >20 percent during the performance period M
⊛ **M1365**	Patient encounter during the performance period with hospice and palliative care specialty code 17 M
⊛ **M1366**	Focusing on women's health MIPS value pathway M
⊛ **M1367**	Quality care for the treatment of ear, nose, and throat disorders MIPS value pathway M
⊛ **M1368**	Prevention and treatment of infectious disorders including hepatitis c and HIV MIPS value pathway M
⊛ **M1369**	Quality care in mental health and substance use disorders MIPS value pathway M
⊛ **M1370**	Rehabilitative support for musculoskeletal care MIPS value pathway M
▶ ⊛ **M1371**	Most recent glycemic status assessment (hba1c or GMI) level < 7.0% M
▶ ⊛ **M1372**	Most recent glycemic status assessment (hba1c or GMI) level >= 7.0% and < 8.0% M
▶ ⊛ **M1373**	Most recent glycemic status assessment (hba1c or GMI) level >= 8.0% and <= 9.0% M
▶ ⊛ **M1374**	An additional encounter with an RA diagnosis during the performance period or prior performance period that is at least 90 days before or after an encounter with an RA diagnosis during the performance period M
▶ ⊛ **M1375**	An additional encounter with an RA diagnosis during the performance period or prior performance period that is at least 90 days before or after an encounter with an RA diagnosis during the performance period M
▶ ⊛ **M1376**	An additional encounter with an RA diagnosis during the performance period or prior performance period that is at least 90 days before or after an encounter with an RA diagnosis during the performance period M
▶ ⊛ **M1377**	Recommended follow-up interval for repeat colonoscopy of 10 years documented in colonoscopy report and communicated with patient M
▶ ⊛ **M1378**	Documentation of medical reason(s) for not recommending a 10-year follow-up interval (e.g., inadequate prep, familial or personal history of colonic polyps, patient had no adenoma and age is >= 66 years old, or life expectancy < 10 years, other medical reasons) M
▶ ⊛ **M1379**	A 10-year follow-up interval for colonoscopy not recommended, reason not otherwise specified M

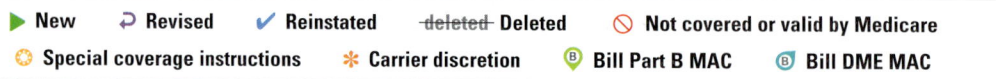

▶ New   ↻ Revised   ✔ Reinstated   ~~deleted~~ Deleted   ⊘ Not covered or valid by Medicare
⊛ Special coverage instructions   ✱ Carrier discretion   Ⓑ Bill Part B MAC   Ⓑ Bill DME MAC

OTHER MEDICAL SERVICES

▶ ✪ **M1380** Filled at least two prescriptions during the performance period for any combination of the qualifying oral antipsychotic medications listed under "denominator note" or the long-acting injectable antipsychotic medications listed under "denominator note" M

▶ ✪ **M1381** Patients with secondary stroke (e.g., a subsequent stroke that may occur with vasospasm in the setting of subarachnoid hemorrhage) within 5 days of the initial procedure M

▶ ✪ **M1382** Patient encounter during the performance period with place of service code 11 M

▶ ✪ **M1383** Acute PVD M

▶ ✪ **M1384** Patients who died during the performance period M

▶ ✪ **M1385** Documentation of patient reasons for patients who were not seen for the second pam survey (e.g., less than four months between baseline pam assessment and follow-up M

▶ ✪ **M1386** Patients with an excisional surgery for melanoma or melanoma in situ in the past 5 years with an initial AJCC staging of 0, I, or II at the start of the performance period M

▶ ✪ **M1387** Patients who died during the performance period M

▶ ✪ **M1388** Patients with documentation of an exam performed for recurrence of melanoma M

▶ ✪ **M1390** Patients who do not have a documented exam performed for recurrence of melanoma or no documentation within the performance period M

▶ ✪ **M1391** All patients who were diagnosed with recurrent melanoma during the current performance period M

▶ ✪ **M1392** Documentation of patient reasons for no examination, i.e., refusal of examination or lost to follow-up (documentation must include information that the clinician was unable to reach the patient by phone, mail or secure electronic mail - at least one method must be documented) M

▶ ✪ **M1393** Patients who were not diagnosed with recurrent melanoma during the current performance period M

▶ ✪ **M1394** Stages I-III breast cancer M

▶ ✪ **M1395** Patients receiving an initial chemotherapy regimen with a defined duration with the eligible clinician or group M

▶ ✪ **M1396** Patients on a therapeutic clinical trial M

▶ ✪ **M1397** Patients with recurrence/disease progression M

▶ ✪ **M1398** Patients with baseline and follow-up promis surveys documented in the medical record M

▶ ✪ **M1399** Patients who leave the practice during the follow-up period M

▶ ✪ **M1400** Patients who died during the follow-up period M

▶ ✪ **M1401** Stages I-III breast cancer M

▶ ✪ **M1402** Patients receiving an initial chemotherapy regimen with a defined duration with the eligible clinician or group M

▶ ✪ **M1403** Patients with baseline and follow-up promis surveys documented in the medical record M

▶ ✪ **M1404** Patients on a therapeutic clinical trial M

▶ ✪ **M1405** Patients with recurrence/disease progression M

▶ ✪ **M1406** Patients who leave the practice during the follow-up period M

▶ ✪ **M1407** Patients who died during the follow-up period M

▶ ✪ **M1408** Patients who have germline BRCA testing completed before diagnosis of epithelial ovarian, fallopian tube, or primary peritoneal cancer M

▶ ✪ **M1409** Patients who received germline testing for brca1 and brca2 or genetic counseling completed within 6 months of diagnosis M

▶ ✪ **M1410** Patients who did not have germline testing for brca1 and brca2 or genetic counseling completed within 6 months of diagnosis M

▶ ✪ **M1411** Currently on first-line immune checkpoint inhibitors without chemotherapy M

▶ ✪ **M1412** Patients with metastatic NSCLC with epidermal growth factor receptor (EGFR) mutations, ALK genomic tumor aberrations, or other targetable genomic abnormalities with approved first-line targeted therapy, such as NSCLC with ros1 rearrangement, BRAF v600e mutation, NTRK 1/2/3 gene fusion, met ex14 skipping mutation, and ret rearrangement M

▶ ✪ **M1413** Patients who had a positive pd-l1 biomarker expression test result prior to the initiation of first-line immune checkpoint inhibitor therapy M

▶ ✪ **M1414** Documentation of medical reason(s) for not performing the pd-l1 biomarker expression test prior to initiation of first-line immune checkpoint inhibitor therapy (e.g., patient is in an urgent or emergent situation where delay of treatment would jeopardize the patient's health status; other medical reasons/contraindication) M

▶ ✪ **M1415** Patients who did not have a positive pd-l1 biomarker expression test result prior to the initiation of first-line immune checkpoint inhibitor therapy M

▶ ✪ **M1416** Patient received hospice services any time during the performance period M

▶ ✪ **M1417** Patients who are up to date on their covid-19 vaccinations as defined by CDC recommendations on current vaccination M

▶ ✪ **M1418** Patients who are not up to date on their covid-19 vaccinations as defined by CDC recommendations on current vaccination because of a medical contraindication documented by clinician M

▶ ✪ **M1419** Patients who are not up to date on their covid-19 vaccinations as defined by CDC recommendations on current vaccination M

▶ ✪ **M1420** Complete ophthalmologic care MIPS value pathway M

▶ ✪ **M1421** Dermatological care MIPS value pathway M

▶ ✪ **M1422** Gastroenterology care MIPS value pathway M

▶ ✪ **M1423** Optimal care for patients with urologic conditions MIPS value pathway M

▶ ✪ **M1424** Pulmonology care MIPS value pathway M

▶ ✪ **M1425** Surgical care MIPS value pathway M

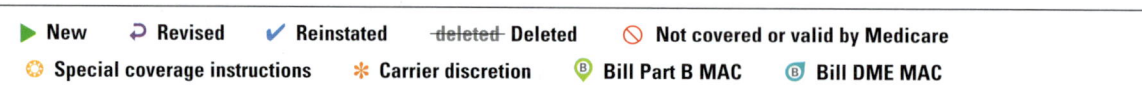

▶ New ⟲ Revised ✓ Reinstated ~~deleted~~ Deleted ⊘ Not covered or valid by Medicare ✪ Special coverage instructions ✱ Carrier discretion ⒷBill Part B MAC ⒷBill DME MAC

LABORATORY SERVICES

LABORATORY SERVICES (P0000-P9999)

Chemistry and Toxicology Tests

- **P2028** Cephalin floculation, blood ⓑ Qp Qh   A

  This code appears on a CMS list of codes that represent obsolete and unreliable tests and procedures. Verify before reporting.

  IOM: 100-03, 4, 300.1

- **P2029** Congo red, blood ⓑ Qp Qh   A

  This code appears on a CMS list of codes that represent obsolete and unreliable tests and procedures. Verify before reporting.

  IOM: 100-03, 4, 300.1

- ⊘ **P2031** Hair analysis (excluding arsenic) ⓑ   E1

  IOM: 100-03, 4, 300.1

- **P2033** Thymol turbidity, blood ⓑ Qp Qh   A

  This code appears on a CMS list of codes that represent obsolete and unreliable tests and procedures. Verify before reporting.

  IOM: 100-03, 4, 300.1

- **P2038** Mucoprotein, blood (seromucoid) (medical necessity procedure) ⓑ Qp Qh   A

  This code appears on a CMS list of codes that represent obsolete and unreliable tests and procedures. Verify before reporting.

  IOM: 100-03, 4, 300.1

Pathology Screening Tests

- **P3000** Screening Papanicolaou smear, cervical or vaginal, up to three smears, by technician under physician supervision ⓑ Qp Qh ♀   A

  Co-insurance and deductible waived

  Assign for Pap smear ordered for screening purposes only, conventional method, performed by technician

  IOM: 100-03, 3, 190.2

  Laboratory Certification: Cytology

- **P3001** Screening Papanicolaou smear, cervical or vaginal, up to three smears, requiring interpretation by physician ⓑ Qp Qh ♀   B

  Co-insurance and deductible waived

  Report professional component for Pap smears requiring physician interpretation. There are CPT codes assigned for diagnostic Paps, such as, 88141; HCPCS are for screening Paps.

  IOM: 100-03, 3, 190.2

  Laboratory Certification: Cytology

Microbiology Tests

- ⊘ **P7001** Culture, bacterial, urine; quantitative, sensitivity study ⓑ   E1

  Cross Reference CPT

  Laboratory Certification: Bacteriology

Miscellaneous Pathology

- **P9010** Blood (whole), for transfusion, per unit ⓑ Qp Qh   R

  Blood furnished on an outpatient basis, subject to Medicare Part B blood deductible; applicable to first 3 pints of whole blood or equivalent units of packed red cells in calendar year

  IOM: 100-01, 3, 20.5; 100-02, 1, 10

- **P9011** Blood, split unit ⓑ Qp Qh   R

  Reports all splitting activities of any blood component

  IOM: 100-01, 3, 20.5; 100-02, 1, 10

- **P9012** Cryoprecipitate, each unit ⓑ Qp Qh   R

  IOM: 100-01, 3, 20.5; 100-02, 1, 10

- **P9016** Red blood cells, leukocytes reduced, each unit ⓑ Qp Qh   R

  IOM: 100-01, 3, 20.5; 100-02, 1, 10

- **P9017** Fresh frozen plasma (single donor), frozen within 8 hours of collection, each unit ⓑ Qp Qh   R

  IOM: 100-01, 3, 20.5; 100-02, 1, 10

- **P9019** Platelets, each unit ⓑ Qp Qh   R

  IOM: 100-01, 3, 20.5; 100-02, 1, 10

- **P9020** Platelet rich plasma, each unit ⓑ Qp Qh   R

  IOM: 100-01, 3, 20.5; 100-02, 1, 10

- **P9021** Red blood cells, each unit ⓑ Qp Qh   R

  IOM: 100-01, 3, 20.5; 100-02, 1, 10

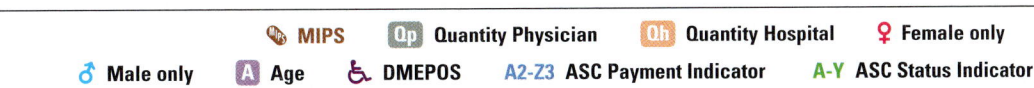

MIPS   Qp Quantity Physician   Qh Quantity Hospital   ♀ Female only   ♂ Male only   Ⓐ Age   &. DMEPOS   A2-Z3 ASC Payment Indicator   A-Y ASC Status Indicator   Coding Clinic

2026 HCPCS LEVEL II NATIONAL CODES

- ⊛ **P9022** Red blood cells, washed, each unit Ⓑ Qp Qh R
  IOM: 100-01, 3, 20.5; 100-02, 1, 10
- ⊛ **P9023** Plasma, pooled multiple donor, solvent/detergent treated, frozen, each unit Ⓑ Qp Qh R
  IOM: 100-01, 3, 20.5; 100-02, 1, 10
- ⊛ **P9025** Plasma, cryoprecipitate reduced, pathogen reduced, each unit R
- ⊛ **P9026** Cryoprecipitated fibrinogen complex, pathogen reduced, each unit R
- ⊛ **P9027** Red blood cells, leukocytes reduced, oxygen/carbon dioxide reduced, each unit R
- ⊛ **P9031** Platelets, leukocytes reduced, each unit Ⓑ Qp Qh R
  IOM: 100-01, 3, 20.5; 100-02, 1, 10
- ⊛ **P9032** Platelets, irradiated, each unit Ⓑ Qp Qh R
  IOM: 100-01, 3, 20.5; 100-02, 1, 10
- ⊛ **P9033** Platelets, leukocytes reduced, irradiated, each unit Ⓑ Qp Qh R
  IOM: 100-01, 3, 20.5; 100-02, 1, 10
- ⊛ **P9034** Platelets, pheresis, each unit Ⓑ Qp Qh R
  IOM: 100-01, 3, 20.5; 100-02, 1, 10
- ⊛ **P9035** Platelets, pheresis, leukocytes reduced, each unit Ⓑ Qp Qh R
  IOM: 100-01, 3, 20.5; 100-02, 1, 10
- ⊛ **P9036** Platelets, pheresis, irradiated, each unit Ⓑ Qp Qh R
  IOM: 100-01, 3, 20.5; 100-02, 1, 10
- ⊛ **P9037** Platelets, pheresis, leukocytes reduced, irradiated, each unit Ⓑ Qp Qh R
  IOM: 100-01, 3, 20.5; 100-02, 1, 10
- ⊛ **P9038** Red blood cells, irradiated, each unit Ⓑ Qp Qh R
  IOM: 100-01, 3, 20.5; 100-02, 1, 10
- ⊛ **P9039** Red blood cells, deglycerolized, each unit Ⓑ Qp Qh R
  IOM: 100-01, 3, 20.5; 100-02, 1, 10
- ⊛ **P9040** Red blood cells, leukocytes reduced, irradiated, each unit Ⓑ Qp Qh R
  IOM: 100-01, 3, 20.5; 100-02, 1, 10
- ✱ **P9041** Infusion, albumin (human), 5%, 50 ml Ⓑ Qp Qh K2 R
- **P9043** Infusion, plasma protein fraction (human), 5%, 50 ml Ⓑ Qp Qh R
  IOM: 100-01, 3, 20.5; 100-02, 1, 10
- ⊛ **P9044** Plasma, cryoprecipitate reduced, each unit Ⓑ Qp Qh R
  IOM: 100-01, 3, 20.5; 100-02, 1, 10
- ✱ **P9045** Infusion, albumin (human), 5%, 250 ml Ⓑ Qp Qh K2 K
- ✱ **P9046** Infusion, albumin (human), 25%, 20 ml Ⓑ Qp Qh K2 K
- ✱ **P9047** Infusion, albumin (human), 25%, 50 ml Ⓑ Qp Qh K2 R
- ✱ **P9048** Infusion, plasma protein fraction (human), 5%, 250 ml Ⓑ Qp Qh R
- ✱ **P9050** Granulocytes, pheresis, each unit Ⓑ Qp Qh E2
- ⊛ **P9051** Whole blood or red blood cells, leukocytes reduced, CMV-negative, each unit Ⓑ Qp Qh R
  Medicare Statute 1833(t)
- ⊛ **P9052** Platelets, HLA-matched leukocytes reduced, apheresis/pheresis, each unit Ⓑ Qp Qh R
  Medicare Statute 1833(t)
- ⊛ **P9053** Platelets, pheresis, leukocytes reduced, CMV-negative, irradiated, each unit Ⓑ Qp Qh R

  Freezing and thawing are reported separately, see Transmittal 1487 (Hospital outpatient)

  Medicare Statute 1833(t)
- ⊛ **P9054** Whole blood or red blood cells, leukocytes reduced, frozen, deglycerol, washed, each unit Ⓑ Qp Qh R
  Medicare Statute 1833(t)
- ⊛ **P9055** Platelets, leukocytes reduced, CMV-negative, apheresis/pheresis, each unit Ⓑ Qp Qh R
  Medicare Statute 1833(t)
- ⊛ **P9056** Whole blood, leukocytes reduced, irradiated, each unit Ⓑ Qp Qh R
  Medicare Statute 1833(t)
- ⊛ **P9057** Red blood cells, frozen/deglycerolized/washed, leukocytes reduced, irradiated, each unit Ⓑ Qp Qh R
  Medicare Statute 1833(t)
- ⊛ **P9058** Red blood cells, leukocytes reduced, CMV-negative, irradiated, each unit Ⓑ Qp Qh R
  Medicare Statute 1833(t)
- ⊛ **P9059** Fresh frozen plasma between 8-24 hours of collection, each unit Ⓑ Qp Qh R
  Medicare Statute 1833(t)

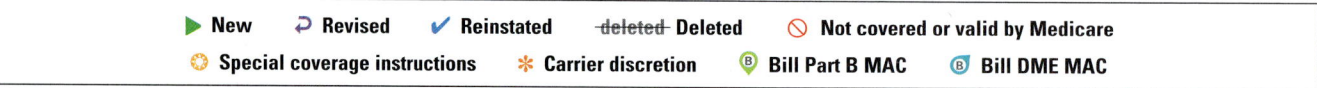

LABORATORY SERVICES

- **P9060** Fresh frozen plasma, donor retested, each unit ⓑ Qp Qh   R

  Medicare Statute 1833(t)

- **P9070** Plasma, pooled multiple donor, pathogen reduced, frozen, each unit ⓑ Qp Qh   R

  Medicare Statute 1833(T)

- **P9071** Plasma (single donor), pathogen reduced, frozen, each unit ⓑ Qp Qh   R

  IOM: 100-01, 3, 20.5; 100-02, 1, 10

  Medicare Statute 1833T

- **P9073** Platelets, pheresis, pathogen-reduced, each unit   R

  IOM: 100-01, 3, 20.5; 100-02, 1, 10

  Medicare Statute 1833T

- ∗ **P9099** Blood component or product not otherwise classified   R

- **P9100** Pathogen(s) test for platelets   S

  IOM: 100-03, 4, 300.1

Travel Allowance for Specimen Collection

- **P9603** Travel allowance one way in connection with medically necessary laboratory specimen collection drawn from home bound or nursing home bound patient; prorated miles actually traveled ⓑ Qp Qh   A

  Fee for clinical laboratory travel (P9603) is $1.025 per mile for CY2015.

  IOM: 100-04, 16, 60

- **P9604** Travel allowance one way in connection with medically necessary laboratory specimen collection drawn from home bound or nursing home bound patient; prorated trip charge ⓑ Qp Qh   A

  For CY2010, the fee for clinical laboratory travel is $10.30 per flat rate trip for CY2015.

  IOM: 100-04, 16, 60

Catheterization for Specimen Collection

- **P9612** Catheterization for collection of specimen, single patient, all places of service ⓑ Qp Qh   A

  NCCI edits indicate that when 51701 is comprehensive or is a Column 1 code, P9612 cannot be reported. When the catheter insertion is a component of another procedure, do not report straight catheterization separately.

  IOM: 100-04, 16, 60

  Coding Clinic: 2007, Q3, P7

- **P9615** Catheterization for collection of specimen(s) (multiple patients) ⓑ Qp Qh   N

  IOM: 100-04, 16, 60

| MIPS | Qp Quantity Physician | Qh Quantity Hospital | ♀ Female only |
| ♂ Male only | A Age | ♿ DMEPOS | A2-Z3 ASC Payment Indicator | A-Y ASC Status Indicator | Coding Clinic |

TEMPORARY CODES ASSIGNED BY CMS (Q0000-Q9999)

Cardiokymography

○ **Q0035** Cardiokymography ⓑ Qp Qh Q1

Report modifier 26 if professional component only

IOM: 100-03, 1, 20.24

Infusion Therapy

○ **Q0081** Infusion therapy, using other than chemotherapeutic drugs, per visit ⓑ Qh B

IV piggyback only assigned one time per patient encounter per day. Report for hydration or the intravenous administration of antibiotics, anti-emetics, or analgesics. Bill on paper. Requires a report.

IOM: 100-03, 4, 280.14

Coding Clinic: 2004, Q2, P11; Q1, P5, 8; 2002, Q2, P10; Q1, P7

Chemotherapy Administration

∗ **Q0083** Chemotherapy administration by other than infusion technique only (e.g., subcutaneous, intramuscular, push), per visit ⓑ Qh B

Coding Clinic: 2002, Q1, P7

○ **Q0084** Chemotherapy administration by infusion technique only, per visit ⓑ Qh B

IOM: 100-03, 4, 280.14

Coding Clinic: 2004, Q2, P11; 2002, Q1, P7

∗ **Q0085** Chemotherapy administration by both infusion technique and other technique(s) (e.g., subcutaneous, intramuscular, push), per visit ⓑ Qh B

Coding Clinic: 2002, Q1, P7

Smear Preparation

○ **Q0091** Screening Papanicolaou smear; obtaining, preparing and conveyance of cervical or vaginal smear to laboratory ⓑ Qp Qh ♀ S

Medicare does not cover comprehensive preventive medicine services; however, services described by G0101 and Q0091 (only for Medicare patients) are covered. Includes the services necessary to procure and transport the specimen to the laboratory.

IOM: 100-03, 3, 190.2

Coding Clinic: 2024, Q2, P35-36; 2002, Q4, P8

Portable X-ray Setup

○ **Q0092** Set-up portable x-ray equipment ⓑ N

IOM: 100-04, 13, 90

Miscellaneous Lab Services

∗ **Q0111** Wet mounts, including preparations of vaginal, cervical or skin specimens ⓑ Qp Qh A

Laboratory Certification: Bacteriology, Mycology, Parasitology

∗ **Q0112** All potassium hydroxide (KOH) preparations ⓑ Qp Qh A

Laboratory Certification: Mycology

∗ **Q0113** Pinworm examinations ⓑ Qp Qh A

Laboratory Certification: Parasitology

∗ **Q0114** Fern test ⓑ Qp Qh ♀ A

Laboratory Certification: Routine chemistry

∗ **Q0115** Post-coital direct, qualitative examinations of vaginal or cervical mucous ⓑ Qp Qh ♀ A

Laboratory Certification: Hematology

Drugs

∗ **Q0138** Injection, ferumoxytol, for treatment of iron deficiency anemia, 1 mg (non-ESRD use) ⓑ Qp Qh K2 K

Feraheme is FDA approved for chronic kidney disease.

Other: Feraheme

∗ **Q0139** Injection, ferumoxytol, for treatment of iron deficiency anemia, 1 mg (for ESRD on dialysis) ⓑ Qp Qh K2 K

Other: Feraheme

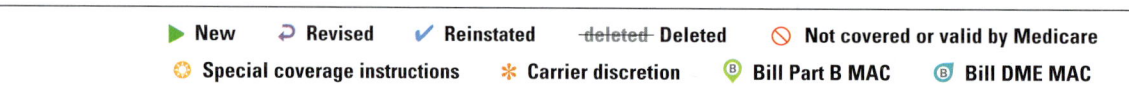

▶ New   ⟳ Revised   ✓ Reinstated   ~~deleted~~ Deleted   ⊘ Not covered or valid by Medicare
○ Special coverage instructions   ∗ Carrier discretion   ⓑ Bill Part B MAC   ⓑ Bill DME MAC

TEMPORARY CODES ASSIGNED BY CMS

- ⊘ **Q0144** Azithromycin dihydrate, oral, capsules/powder, 1 gm ⓑ Ⓑ Qp Qh E1

  Other: Zithromax, Zmax

- ▶ ✱ **Q0155** Dronabinol (syndros), 0.1 mg, oral, FDA approved prescription anti-emetic, for use as a complete therapeutic substitute for an IV anti-emetic at the time of chemotherapy treatment, not to exceed a 48 hour dosage regimen ⓑ Qp Qh N1 N

- ✳ **Q0161** Chlorpromazine hydrochloride, 5 mg, oral, FDA approved prescription anti-emetic, for use as a complete therapeutic substitute for an IV anti-emetic at the time of chemotherapy treatment, not to exceed a 48 hour dosage regimen ⓑ Qp Qh N1 N

- ✱ **Q0162** Ondansetron 1 mg, oral, FDA-approved prescription anti-emetic, for use as a complete therapeutic substitute for an iv anti-emetic at the time of chemotherapy treatment, not to exceed a 48 hour dosage regimen ⓑ Qp Qh N1 N

  Other: Zofran

  Medicare Statute 4557

  Coding Clinic: 2012, Q1, P9

- ✱ **Q0163** Diphenhydramine hydrochloride, 50 mg, oral, FDA approved prescription anti-emetic, for use as a complete therapeutic substitute for an IV anti-emetic at time of chemotherapy treatment not to exceed a 48 hour dosage regimen ⓑ Qp Qh N1 N

  Other: Alercap, Alertab, Allergy Relief Medicine, Allermax, Anti-Hist, Antihistamine, Banophen, Complete Allergy Medication, Complete Allergy medicine, Diphedryl, Diphenhist, Diphenhydramine, Dormin Sleep Aid, Genahist, Geridryl, Good Sense Antihistamine Allergy Relief, Good Sense Nighttime Sleep Aid, Mediphedryl, Night Time Sleep Aid, Nytol Quickcaps, Nytol Quickgels maximum strength, Quality Choice Sleep Aid, Quality Choice Rest Simply, Rapidpaq Dicopanol, Rite Aid Allergy, Serabrina La France, Siladryl Allergy, Silphen, Simply Sleep, Sleep Tabs, Sleepinal, Sominex, Twilite, Valu-Dryl Allergy

  Medicare Statute 4557

  Coding Clinic: 2012, Q2, P10

- ✱ **Q0164** Prochlorperazine maleate, 5 mg, oral, FDA approved prescription anti-emetic, for use as a complete therapeutic substitute for an IV anti-emetic at the time of chemotherapy treatment, not to exceed a 48 hour dosage regimen ⓑ Qp Qh N1 N

  Other: Compazine

  Medicare Statute 4557

  Coding Clinic: 2012, Q2, P10

- ✱ **Q0166** Granisetron hydrochloride, 1 mg, oral, FDA approved prescription anti-emetic, for use as a complete therapeutic substitute for an IV anti-emetic at the time of chemotherapy treatment, not to exceed a 24 hour dosage regimen ⓑ Qp Qh N1 N

  Other: Kytril

  Medicare Statute 4557

  Coding Clinic: 2012, Q2, P10

- ✱ **Q0167** Dronabinol, 2.5 mg, oral, FDA approved prescription anti-emetic, for use as a complete therapeutic substitute for an IV anti-emetic at the time of chemotherapy treatment, not to exceed a 48 hour dosage regimen ⓑ Qp Qh N1 N

  Other: Marinol

  Medicare Statute 4557

  Coding Clinic: 2012, Q2, P10

- ✱ **Q0169** Promethazine hydrochloride, 12.5 mg, oral, FDA approved prescription anti-emetic, for use as a complete therapeutic substitute for an IV anti-emetic at the time of chemotherapy treatment, not to exceed a 48 hour dosage regimen ⓑ Qp Qh N1 N

  Other: Anergan, Chlorpromazine, Hydroxyzine Pamoate, Phenazine, Phenergan, Prorex, Prothazine, V-Gan

  Medicare Statute 4557

  Coding Clinic: 2012, Q2, P10

- ✱ **Q0173** Trimethobenzamide hydrochloride, 250 mg, oral, FDA approved prescription anti-emetic, for use as a complete therapeutic substitute for an IV anti-emetic at the time of chemotherapy treatment, not to exceed a 48 hour dosage regimen ⓑ Qp Qh N1 E2

  Other: Arrestin, Ticon, Tigan, Tiject

  Medicare Statute 4557

  Coding Clinic: 2012, Q2, P10

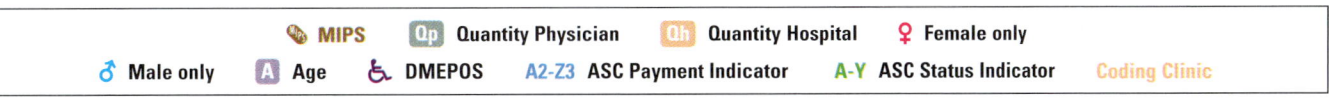

○ **Q0174** Thiethylperazine maleate, 10 mg, oral, FDA approved prescription anti-emetic, for use as a complete therapeutic substitute for an IV anti-emetic at the time of chemotherapy treatment, not to exceed a 48 hour dosage regimen ⑧ Qp Qh E2

Other: Torecan

Medicare Statute 4557

Coding Clinic: 2012, Q2, P10

○ **Q0175** Perphenazine, 4 mg, oral, FDA approved prescription anti-emetic, for use as a complete therapeutic substitute for an IV anti-emetic at the time of chemotherapy treatment, not to exceed a 48 hour dosage regimen ⑧ Qp Qh N1 N

Medicare Statute 4557

Coding Clinic: 2012, Q2, P10

○ **Q0177** Hydroxyzine pamoate, 25 mg, oral, FDA approved prescription anti-emetic, for use as a complete therapeutic substitute for an IV anti-emetic at the time of chemotherapy treatment, not to exceed a 48 hour dosage regimen ⑧ Qp Qh N1 N

Other: Vistaril

Medicare Statute 4557

Coding Clinic: 2012, Q2, P10

○ **Q0180** Dolasetron mesylate, 100 mg, oral, FDA approved prescription anti-emetic, for use as a complete therapeutic substitute for an IV anti-emetic at the time of chemotherapy treatment, not to exceed a 24 hour dosage regimen ⑧ Qp Qh N1 N

Other: Anzemet

Medicare Statute 4557

Coding Clinic: 2012, Q2, P10

○ **Q0181** Unspecified oral dosage form, FDA approved prescription anti-emetic, for use as a complete therapeutic substitute for a IV anti-emetic at the time of chemotherapy treatment, not to exceed a 48 hour dosage regimen ⑧ N1 N

Medicare Statute 4557

Coding Clinic: 2012, Q2, P10

~~Q0221 Injection, tixagevimab and cilgavimab, for the pre exposure prophylaxis only, for certain adults and pediatric individuals (12 years of age and older weighing at least 40kg) with no known sars-cov-2 exposure, who either have moderate to severely compromised immune systems or for whom vaccination with any available covid-19 vaccine is not recommended due to a history of severe adverse reaction to a covid-19 vaccine(s) and/or covid-19 vaccine component(s), 600 mg~~

~~Q0222 Injection, bebtelovimab, 175 mg~~

○ **Q0224** Injection, pemivibart, for the pre-exposure prophylaxis only, for certain adults and adolescents (12 years of age and older weighing at least 40 kg) with no known sars-cov-2 exposure, and who either have moderate-to-severe immune compromise due to a medical condition or receipt of immunosuppressive medications or treatments, and are unlikely to mount an adequate immune response to covid-19 vaccination, 4500 mg L

▶ ○ **Q0235** Injection, monoclonal antibody products with an indication for post-exposure prophylaxis or treatment of Covid-19, for hospitalized adults and/or pediatric patients who are receiving systemic corticosteroids and require supplemental oxygen, non-invasive or invasive mechanical ventilation, or extracorporeal membrane oxygenation (ECMO) only, not otherwise classified, 1 mg L

▶ ○ **Q0237** Injection, tocilizumab-anoh, for hospitalized adult patients with Covid-19 who are receiving systemic corticosteroids and require supplemental oxygen, non-invasive or invasive mechanical ventilation, or extracorporeal membrane oxygenation (ECMO) only, 1 mg L

~~Q0240 Injection, casirivimab and imdevimab, 600 mg~~

~~Q0243 Injection, Casirivimab and Imdevimab, 2400 mg~~

~~Q0244 Injection, casirivimab and imdevimab, 1200 mg~~

~~Q0245 Injection, bamlanivimab and etesevimab, 2100 mg~~

~~Q0247 Injection, sotrovimab, 500 mg~~

▶ New ↻ Revised ✓ Reinstated ~~deleted~~ Deleted ⊘ Not covered or valid by Medicare
○ Special coverage instructions ∗ Carrier discretion ⑧ Bill Part B MAC ⑧ Bill DME MAC

- **Q0249** Injection, tocilizumab, for hospitalized adults and pediatric patients (2 years of age and older) with covid-19 who are receiving systemic corticosteroids and require supplemental oxygen, non-invasive or invasive mechanical ventilation, or extracorporeal L1 L

Ventricular Assist Devices

- **Q0477** Power module patient cable for use with electric or electric/pneumatic ventricular assist device, replacement only A
- **Q0478** Power adapter for use with electric or electric/pneumatic ventricular assist device, vehicle type A

  CMS has determined the reasonable useful lifetime is one year. Add modifier RA to claims to report when battery is replaced because it was lost, stolen, or irreparably damaged.

- **Q0479** Power module for use with electric or electric/pneumatic ventricular assist device, replacemment only A

  CMS has determined the reasonable useful lifetime is one year. Add modifier RA in cases where the battery is being replaced because it was lost, stolen, or irreparably damaged.

- **Q0480** Driver for use with pneumatic ventricular assist device, replacement only A
- **Q0481** Microprocessor control unit for use with electric ventricular assist device, replacement only A
- **Q0482** Microprocessor control unit for use with electric/pneumatic combination ventricular assist device, replacement only A

- **Q0483** Monitor/display module for use with electric ventricular assist device, replacement only A
- **Q0484** Monitor/display module for use with electric or electric/pneumatic ventricular assist device, replacement only A
- **Q0485** Monitor control cable for use with electric ventricular assist device, replacement only A
- **Q0486** Monitor control cable for use with electric/pneumatic ventricular assist device, replacement only A
- **Q0487** Leads (pneumatic/electrical) for use with any type electric/pneumatic ventricular assist device, replacement only A
- **Q0488** Power pack base for use with electric ventricular assist device, replacement only A
- **Q0489** Power pack base for use with electric/pneumatic ventricular assist device, replacement only A
- **Q0490** Emergency power source for use with electric ventricular assist device, replacement only A
- **Q0491** Emergency power source for use with electric/pneumatic ventricular assist device, replacement only A
- **Q0492** Emergency power supply cable for use with electric ventricular assist device, replacement only A
- **Q0493** Emergency power supply cable for use with electric/pneumatic ventricular assist device, replacement only A
- **Q0494** Emergency hand pump for use with electric or electric/pneumatic ventricular assist device, replacement only A
- **Q0495** Battery/power pack charger for use with electric or electric/pneumatic ventricular assist device, replacement only A
- **Q0496** Battery, other than lithium-ion, for use with electric or electric/pneumatic ventricular assist device, replacement only A

  Reasonable useful lifetime is 6 months (CR3931).

- **Q0497** Battery clips for use with electric or electric/pneumatic ventricular assist device, replacement only A

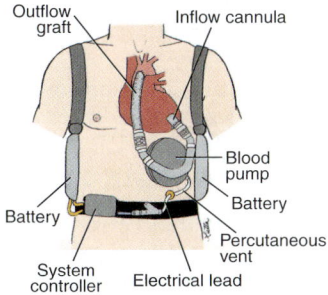

Figure 46 Ventricular assist device.

2026 HCPCS LEVEL II NATIONAL CODES

- ○ **Q0498** Holster for use with electric or electric/pneumatic ventricular assist device, replacement only ⓑ Qp Qh ♿ A
- ○ **Q0499** Belt/vest/bag for use to carry external peripheral components of any type ventricular assist device, replacement only ⓑ Qp Qh ♿ A
- ○ **Q0500** Filters for use with electric or electric/pneumatic ventricular assist device, replacement only ⓑ ♿ A
- ○ **Q0501** Shower cover for use with electric or electric/pneumatic ventricular assist device, replacement only ⓑ Qp Qh ♿ A
- ○ **Q0502** Mobility cart for pneumatic ventricular assist device, replacement only ⓑ Qp Qh ♿ A
- ○ **Q0503** Battery for pneumatic ventricular assist device, replacement only, each ⓑ Qp Qh ♿ A

  Reasonable useful lifetime is 6 months (CR3931).

- ○ **Q0504** Power adapter for pneumatic ventricular assist device, replacement only, vehicle type ⓑ Qp Qh ♿ A
- ○ **Q0506** Battery, lithium-ion, for use with electric or electric/pneumatic, ventricular assist device, replacement only ⓑ Qp Qh ♿ A

  Reasonable useful lifetime is 12 months. Add -RA for replacement if lost, stolen, or irreparable damage.

- ○ **Q0507** Miscellaneous supply or accessory for use with an external ventricular assist device ⓑ Qp Qh A
- ○ **Q0508** Miscellaneous supply or accessory for use with an implanted ventricular assist device ⓑ Qp Qh A
- ○ **Q0509** Miscellaneous supply or accessory for use with any implanted ventricular assist device for which payment was not made under Medicare Part A ⓑ Qp Qh A

Pharmacy: Supply and Dispensing Fee

- ○ **Q0510** Pharmacy supply fee for initial immunosuppressive drug(s), first month following transplant ⓑ Qp Qh M
- ○ **Q0511** Pharmacy supply fee for oral anti-cancer, oral anti-emetic or immunosuppressive drug(s); for the first prescription in a 30-day period ⓑ Qp Qh M
- ○ **Q0512** Pharmacy supply fee for oral anti-cancer, oral anti-emetic or immunosuppressive drug(s); for a subsequent prescription in a 30-day period ⓑ Qp Qh M
- ○ **Q0513** Pharmacy dispensing fee for inhalation drug(s); per 30 days ⓑ Qp Qh M
- ○ **Q0514** Pharmacy dispensing fee for inhalation drug(s); per 90 days ⓑ Qp Qh M

Sermorelin Acetate

- ○ **Q0515** Injection, sermorelin acetate, 1 mcg ⓑ Qp Qh E2

  IOM: 100-02, 15, 50

- ~~**Q0516** Pharmacy supplying fee for HIV pre-exposure prophylaxis FDA approved prescription oral drug, per 30 days~~
- ~~**Q0517** Pharmacy supplying fee for HIV pre-exposure prophylaxis FDA approved prescription oral drug, per 60 days~~
- ~~**Q0518** Pharmacy supplying fee for HIV pre-exposure prophylaxis FDA approved prescription oral drug, per 90 days~~
- ~~**Q0519** Pharmacy supplying fee for HIV pre-exposure prophylaxis FDA approved prescription injectable drug, per 30 days~~
- ~~**Q0520** Pharmacy supplying fee for HIV pre-exposure prophylaxis FDA approved prescription injectable drug, per 60 days~~
- ▶ ○ **Q0521** Pharmacy supplying fee for HIV pre-exposure prophylaxis FDA approved prescription ⓑ ⓑ M

New Technology: Intraocular Lens

- ○ **Q1004** New technology intraocular lens category 4 as defined in Federal Register notice ⓑ Qp Qh E1
- ○ **Q1005** New technology intraocular lens category 5 as defined in Federal Register notice ⓑ Qp Qh E1

Solutions and Drugs

- ○ **Q2004** Irrigation solution for treatment of bladder calculi, for example renacidin, per 500 ml ⓑ Qp Qh N1 N

  IOM: 100-02, 15, 50

  Medicare Statute 1861S2B

- ○ **Q2009** Injection, fosphenytoin, 50 mg phenytoin equivalent ⓑ Qp Qh K2 N

  IOM: 100-02, 15, 50

  Medicare Statute 1861S2B

▶ New   ⟲ Revised   ✓ Reinstated   ~~deleted~~ Deleted   ⊘ Not covered or valid by Medicare
○ Special coverage instructions   ✴ Carrier discretion   ⓑ Bill Part B MAC   ⓑ Bill DME MAC

TEMPORARY CODES ASSIGNED BY CMS

- ⊛ **Q2017** Injection, teniposide, 50 mg ⓑ Qp Qh   K2 E2
  IOM: 100-02, 15, 50
  Medicare Statute 1861S2B
- ⊛ **Q2026** Injection, radiesse, 0.1 ml ⓑ Qp Qh   K
  Coding Clinic: 2010, Q3, P8
- ⊛ **Q2028** Injection, sculptra, 0.5 mg ⓑ Qp Qh   K
- ⊛ **Q2034** Influenza virus vaccine, split virus, for intramuscular use (Agriflu) Sipuleucel-t, minimum of 50 million autologous CD54+ cells activated with PAP-GM-CSF, including leukapheresis and all other preparatory procedures, per infusion ⓑ Qp Qh   L1 L
  IOM: 100-02, 15, 50
- ⊛ **Q2035** Influenza virus vaccine, split virus, when administered to individuals 3 years of age and older, for intramuscular use (Afluria) ⓑ Qp Qh A   L1 L
  Preventive service; no deductible
  IOM: 100-02, 15, 50
  Coding Clinic: 2011, Q1, P7; 2010, Q4, P8-9
- ⊛ **Q2036** Influenza virus vaccine, split virus, when administered to individuals 3 years of age and older, for intramuscular use (Flulaval) ⓑ Qp Qh A   L1 L
  Preventive service; no deductible
  IOM: 100-02, 15, 50
  Coding Clinic: 2011, Q1, P7; 2010, Q4, P8-9
- ⊛ **Q2037** Influenza virus vaccine, split virus, when administered to individuals 3 years of age and older, for intramuscular use (Fluvirin) ⓑ Qp Qh A   L1 L
  Preventive service; no deductible
  IOM: 100-02, 15, 50
  Coding Clinic: 2011, Q1, P7; 2010, Q4, P8-9
- ⊛ **Q2038** Influenza virus vaccine, split virus, when administered to individuals 3 years of age or older, for intramuscular use (Fluzone) ⓑ Qp Qh A   L1 L
  Preventive service; no deductible
  IOM: 100-02, 15, 50
  Coding Clinic: 2011, Q1, P7; 2010, Q4, P8-9
- ⊛ **Q2039** Influenza virus vaccine, not otherwise specified ⓑ Qp Qh A   L1 L
  Preventive service; no deductible
  IOM: 100-02, 15, 50
  Coding Clinic: 2011, Q1, P7; 2010, Q4, P8-9
- ⊛ **Q2041** Axicabtagene ciloleucel, up to 200 million autologous anti-CD 19 CAR-positive viable T cells, including leukapheresis and dose preparation procedures, per therapeutic dose   K
- ⊛ **Q2042** Tisagenlecleucel, up to 600 million CAR-positive viable T cells, including leukapheresis and dose preparation procedures, per therapeutic dose ⓑ   K
- ⊛ **Q2043** Sipuleucel-T, minimum of 50 million autologous CD54+ cells activated with PAP-GM-CSF, including leukapheresis and all other preparatory procedures, per infusion ⓑ Qp Qh   K2 K
  Other: Provenge
  Coding Clinic: 2012, Q2, P7; Q1, P7, 9; 2011, Q3, P9
- ✱ **Q2049** Injection, doxorubicin hydrochloride, liposomal, imported lipodox, 10 mg ⓑ Qp Qh   K2 K
  Coding Clinic: 2012, Q3, P10
- ⊛ **Q2050** Injection, doxorubicin hydrochloride, liposomal, not otherwise specified, 10 mg ⓑ Qp Qh   K2 K
  Other: Doxil
  IOM: 100-02, 15, 50
- ⊛ **Q2052** Services, supplies and accessories used in the home for the administration of intravenous immune globulin (IVIG) ⓑ Qp Qh   A
  Coding Clinic: 2014, Q2, P6
- ⊛ **Q2053** Brexucabtagene autoleucel, up to 200 million autologous anti-cd19 car positive viable t cells, including leukapheresis and dose preparation procedures, per therapeutic dose   K
- ⊛ **Q2054** Lisocabtagene maraleucel, up to 110 million autologous anti-cd19 car-positive viable t cells, including leukapheresis and dose preparation procedures, per therapeutic dose   K
- ⊛ **Q2055** Idecabtagene vicleucel, up to 510 million autologous b-cell maturation antigen (bcma) directed car-positive t cells, including leukapheresis and dose preparation procedures, per therapeutic dose   K
- ⊛ **Q2056** Ciltacabtagene autoleucel, up to 100 million autologous B-cell maturation antigen (bcma) directed car-positive T cells, including leukapheresis and dose preparation procedures, per therapeutic dose   G
- ▶ ⊛ **Q2057** Afamitresgene autoleucel, including leukapheresis and dose preparation procedures, per therapeutic dose   G

| 🪙 MIPS | Qp Quantity Physician | Qh Quantity Hospital | ♀ Female only |
| ♂ Male only | A Age | ♿ DMEPOS | A2-Z3 ASC Payment Indicator | A-Y ASC Status Indicator | Coding Clinic |

2026 HCPCS LEVEL II NATIONAL CODES

▶ ⊙ **Q2058** Obecabtagene autoleucel, 10 up to 400 million cd19 car-positive viable t cells, including leukapheresis and dose preparation procedures, per infusion G

Brachytherapy Radioelements

⊙ **Q3001** Radioelements for brachytherapy, any type, each ⑧ B

IOM: 100-04, 12, 70; 100-04, 13, 20

Telehealth

∗ **Q3014** Telehealth originating site facility fee ⑧ Qp Qh A

Effective January of each year, the fee for telehealth services is increased by the Medicare Economic Index (MEI). The telehealth originating facility site fee (HCPCS code Q3014) for 2011 was 80 percent of the lesser of the actual charge or $24.10.

Drugs

⊙ **Q3027** Injection, interferon beta-1a, 1 mcg for intramuscular use ⑧ Qp Qh K2 K

Other: Avonex

IOM: 100-02, 15, 50

⊘ **Q3028** Injection, interferon beta-1a, 1 mcg for subcutaneous use ⑧ Qp Qh E1

Skin Test

⊙ **Q3031** Collagen skin test ⑧ Qp Qh N1 N

IOM: 100-03, 4, 280.1

Supplies: Cast

Q4001-Q4051: Payment on a reasonable charge basis is required for splints, casts by regulations contained in 42 CFR 405.501.

∗ **Q4001** Casting supplies, body cast adult, with or without head, plaster ⑧ Qp Qh A ♿ B

∗ **Q4002** Cast supplies, body cast adult, with or without head, fiberglass Qp Qh A ♿ B

∗ **Q4003** Cast supplies, shoulder cast, adult (11 years +), plaster ⑧ Qp Qh A ♿ B

∗ **Q4004** Cast supplies, shoulder cast, adult (11 years +), fiberglass ⑧ Qp Qh A ♿ B

∗ **Q4005** Cast supplies, long arm cast, adult (11 years +), plaster ⑧ A ♿ B

∗ **Q4006** Cast supplies, long arm cast, adult (11 years +), fiberglass ⑧ A ♿ B

∗ **Q4007** Cast supplies, long arm cast, pediatric (0-10 years), plaster ⑧ A ♿ B

∗ **Q4008** Cast supplies, long arm cast, pediatric (0-10 years), fiberglass ⑧ A ♿ B

∗ **Q4009** Cast supplies, short arm cast, adult (11 years +), plaster ⑧ A ♿ B

∗ **Q4010** Cast supplies, short arm cast, adult (11 years +), fiberglass ⑧ A ♿ B

∗ **Q4011** Cast supplies, short arm cast, pediatric (0-10 years), plaster ⑧ A ♿ B

∗ **Q4012** Cast supplies, short arm cast, pediatric (0-10 years), fiberglass ⑧ A ♿ B

∗ **Q4013** Cast supplies, gauntlet cast (includes lower forearm and hand), adult (11 years +), plaster ⑧ A ♿ B

∗ **Q4014** Cast supplies, gauntlet cast (includes lower forearm and hand), adult (11 years +), fiberglass ⑧ A ♿ B

∗ **Q4015** Cast supplies, gauntlet cast (includes lower forearm and hand), pediatric (0-10 years), plaster ⑧ A ♿ B

∗ **Q4016** Cast supplies, gauntlet cast (includes lower forearm and hand), pediatric (0-10 years), fiberglass ⑧ A ♿ B

∗ **Q4017** Cast supplies, long arm splint, adult (11 years +), plaster ⑧ A ♿ B

∗ **Q4018** Cast supplies, long arm splint, adult (11 years +), fiberglass ⑧ A ♿ B

∗ **Q4019** Cast supplies, long arm splint, pediatric (0-10 years), plaster ⑧ A ♿ B

∗ **Q4020** Cast supplies, long arm splint, pediatric (0-10 years), fiberglass ⑧ A ♿ B

∗ **Q4021** Cast supplies, short arm splint, adult (11 years +), plaster ⑧ A ♿ B

∗ **Q4022** Cast supplies, short arm splint, adult (11 years +), fiberglass ⑧ A ♿ B

∗ **Q4023** Cast supplies, short arm splint, pediatric (0-10 years), plaster ⑧ A ♿ B

∗ **Q4024** Cast supplies, short arm splint, pediatric (0-10 years), fiberglass ⑧ A ♿ B

∗ **Q4025** Cast supplies, hip spica (one or both legs), adult (11 years +), plaster ⑧ Qp Qh A ♿ B

∗ **Q4026** Cast supplies, hip spica (one or both legs), adult (11 years +), fiberglass ⑧ Qp Qh A ♿ B

∗ **Q4027** Cast supplies, hip spica (one or both legs), pediatric (0-10 years), plaster ⑧ Qp Qh A ♿ B

▶ New   ⤺ Revised   ✔ Reinstated   ~~deleted~~ Deleted   ⊘ Not covered or valid by Medicare
⊙ Special coverage instructions   ∗ Carrier discretion   ⑧ Bill Part B MAC   ⑧ Bill DME MAC

TEMPORARY CODES ASSIGNED BY CMS

* Q4028 Cast supplies, hip spica (one or both legs), pediatric (0-10 years), fiberglass ® Qp Qh A & B
* Q4029 Cast supplies, long leg cast, adult (11 years +), plaster ® A & B
* Q4030 Cast supplies, long leg cast, adult (11 years +), fiberglass ® A & B
* Q4031 Cast supplies, long leg cast, pediatric (0-10 years), plaster ® A & B
* Q4032 Cast supplies, long leg cast, pediatric (0-10 years), fiberglass ® A & B
* Q4033 Cast supplies, long leg cylinder cast, adult (11 years +), plaster ® A & B
* Q4034 Cast supplies, long leg cylinder cast, adult (11 years +), fiberglass ® A & B
* Q4035 Cast supplies, long leg cylinder cast, pediatric (0-10 years), plaster ® A & B
* Q4036 Cast supplies, long leg cylinder cast, pediatric (0-10 years), fiberglass ® A & B
* Q4037 Cast supplies, short leg cast, adult (11 years +), plaster ® A & B
* Q4038 Cast supplies, short leg cast, adult (11 years +), fiberglass ® A & B
* Q4039 Cast supplies, short leg cast, pediatric (0-10 years), plaster ® A & B
* Q4040 Cast supplies, short leg cast, pediatric (0-10 years), fiberglass ® A & B
* Q4041 Cast supplies, long leg splint, adult (11 years +), plaster ® A & B
* Q4042 Cast supplies, long leg splint, adult (11 years +), fiberglass ® A & B
* Q4043 Cast supplies, long leg splint, pediatric (0-10 years), plaster ® A & B
* Q4044 Cast supplies, long leg splint, pediatric (0-10 years), fiberglass ® A & B
* Q4045 Cast supplies, short leg splint, adult (11 years +), plaster ® A & B
* Q4046 Cast supplies, short leg splint, adult (11 years +), fiberglass ® A & B
* Q4047 Cast supplies, short leg splint, pediatric (0-10 years), plaster ® A & B
* Q4048 Cast supplies, short leg splint, pediatric (0-10 years), fiberglass ® A & B
* Q4049 Finger splint, static ® & B
* Q4050 Cast supplies, for unlisted types and materials of casts ® B
* Q4051 Splint supplies, miscellaneous (includes thermoplastics, strapping, fasteners, padding and other supplies) ® B

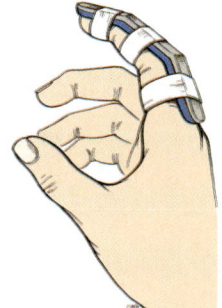

Figure 47 Finger splint.

Drugs

* Q4074 Iloprost, inhalation solution, FDA-approved final product, non-compounded, administered through DME, unit dose form, up to 20 mcg ® ® Qp Qh Y

   Other: Ventavis

⊛ Q4081 Injection, epoetin alfa, 100 units (for ESRD on dialysis) ® Qp Qh N

   Other: Epogen, Procrit

* Q4082 Drug or biological, not otherwise classified, Part B drug competitive acquisition program (CAP) ® B

Skin Substitutes

* Q4100 Skin substitute, not otherwise specified ® N1 N

   Coding Clinic: 2018, Q2, P3; 2012, Q2, P7

* Q4101 Apligraf, per square centimeter ® Qp Qh N1 N

   Coding Clinic: 2012, Q2, P7; 2011, Q1, P9

* Q4102 Oasis Wound Matrix, per square centimeter ® Qp Qh N1 N

   Coding Clinic: 2012, Q3, P8; Q2, P7; 2011, Q1, P9

* Q4103 Oasis Burn Matrix, per square centimeter ® Qp Qh N1 N

   Coding Clinic: 2012, Q2, P7; 2011, Q1, P9

* Q4104 Integra Bilayer Matrix Wound Dressing (BMWD), per square centimeter ® Qp Qh N1 N

   Coding Clinic: 2012, Q2, P7; 2011, Q1, P9; 2010, Q2, P8

* Q4105 Integra Dermal Regeneration Template (DRT) or integra omnigraft dermal regeneration matrix, per square centimeter ® Qp Qh N1 N

   Coding Clinic: 2012, Q2, P7; 2011, Q1, P9; 2010, Q2, P8

* Q4106 Dermagraft, per square centimeter ® Qp Qh N1 N

   Coding Clinic: 2012, Q2, P7; 2011, Q1, P9

 MIPS Qp Quantity Physician Qh Quantity Hospital ♀ Female only
 ♂ Male only A Age & DMEPOS A2-Z3 ASC Payment Indicator A-Y ASC Status Indicator Coding Clinic

* Q4107	Graftjacket, per square centimeter ⓑ Qp Qh	N1 N
	Coding Clinic: 2021, Q1, P9; 2012, Q2, P7; 2011, Q1, P9	
* Q4108	Integra Matrix, per square centimeter ⓑ Qp Qh	N1 N
	Coding Clinic: 2012, Q2, P7; 2011, Q1, P9; 2010, Q2, P8	
* Q4110	Primatrix, per square centimeter ⓑ Qp Qh	N1 N
	Coding Clinic: 2012, Q2, P7; 2011, Q1, P9	
* Q4111	GammaGraft, per square centimeter ⓑ Qp Qh	N1 N
	Coding Clinic: 2012, Q2, P7; 2011, Q1, P9	
* Q4112	Cymetra, injectable, 1 cc ⓑ Qp Qh	N1 N
	Coding Clinic: 2012, Q2, P7; 2011, Q1, P9	
* Q4113	GraftJacket Xpress, injectable, 1 cc Qp Qh	N1 N
	Coding Clinic: 2012, Q2, P7; 2011, Q1, P9	
* Q4114	Integra Flowable Wound Matrix, injectable, 1 cc Qp Qh	N1 N
	Coding Clinic: 2012, Q2, P7; 2010, Q2, P8	
* Q4115	Alloskin, per square centimeter ⓑ Qp Qh	N1 N
	Coding Clinic: 2012, Q2, P7; 2011, Q1, P9	
* Q4116	Alloderm, per square centimeter ⓑ Qp Qh	N1 N
	Coding Clinic: 2012, Q2, P7; 2011, Q1, P9	
* Q4117	Hyalomatrix, per square centimeter ⓑ Qp Qh	N1 N
	IOM: 100-02, 15, 50	
* Q4118	Matristem micromatrix, 1 mg ⓑ Qp Qh	N1 N
	Coding Clinic: 2013, Q4, P2; 2012, Q2, P7; 2011, Q1, P6	
* Q4121	Theraskin, per square centimeter ⓑ Qp Qh	N1 N
	Coding Clinic: 2012, Q2, P7; 2011, Q1, P6	
* Q4122	Dermacell, Dermacell AWM or Dermacell AWM Porous, per square centimeter ⓑ Qp Qh	N1 N
	Coding Clinic: 2012, Q2, P7; Q1, P8	
* Q4123	AlloSkin RT, per square centimeter ⓑ Qp Qh	N1 N
* Q4124	Oasis Ultra Tri-layer Wound Matrix, per square centimeter ⓑ Qp Qh	N1 N
	Coding Clinic: 2012, Q2, P7; Q1, P9	
* Q4125	Arthroflex, per square centimeter ⓑ Qp Qh	N1 N
* Q4126	Memoderm, dermaspan, tranzgraft or integuply, per square centimeter ⓑ Qp Qh	N1 N
* Q4127	Talymed, per square centimeter ⓑ Qp Qh	N1 N
* Q4128	FlexHD, Allopatch HD, per square centimeter ⓑ Qp Qh	N1 N
* Q4130	Strattice TM, per square centimeter ⓑ Qp Qh	N1 N
	Coding Clinic: 2012, Q2, P7	
* Q4132	Grafix core and GrafixPL core, per square centimeter ⓑ Qp Qh	N1 N
* Q4133	Grafix prime, GrafixPL prime, stravix and stravixpl, per square centimeter ⓑ Qp Qh	N1 N
* Q4134	Hmatrix, per square centimeter ⓑ Qp Qh	N1 N
* Q4135	Mediskin, per square centimeter ⓑ Qp Qh	N1 N
* Q4136	Ez-derm, per square centimeter ⓑ Qp Qh	N1 N
* Q4137	Amnioexcel, amnioexcel plus or biodexcel, per square centimeter ⓑ Qp Qh	N1 N
* Q4138	Biodfence dryflex, per square centimeter ⓑ Qp Qh	N1 N
* Q4139	Amniomatrix or biodmatrix, injectable, 1 cc ⓑ Qp Qh	N1 N
* Q4140	Biodfence, per square centimeter ⓑ Qp Qh	N1 N
* Q4141	Alloskin ac, per square centimeter ⓑ Qp Qh	N1 N
* Q4142	XCM biologic tissue matrix, per square centimeter ⓑ Qp Qh	N1 N
* Q4143	Repriza, per square centimeter ⓑ Qp Qh	N1 N
* Q4145	Epifix, injectable, 1 mg ⓑ Qp Qh	N1 N
* Q4146	Tensix, per square centimeter ⓑ Qp Qh	N1 N
* Q4147	Architect, architect PX, or architect FX, extracellular matrix, per square centimeter ⓑ Qp Qh	N1 N
* Q4148	Neox cord 1K, Neox cord RT, or Clarix cord 1K, per square centimeter ⓑ Qp Qh	N1 N
* Q4149	Excellagen, 0.1 cc ⓑ Qp Qh	N1 N
* Q4150	AlloWrap DS or dry, per square centimeter ⓑ Qp Qh	N1 N
* Q4151	Amnioband or guardian, per square centimeter ⓑ Qp Qh	N1 N
* Q4152	DermaPure, per square centimeter ⓑ Qp Qh	N1 N
* Q4153	Dermavest and Plurivest, per square centimeter ⓑ Qp Qh	N1 N
* Q4154	Biovance, per square centimeter Qp Qh	N1 N

▶ New ↻ Revised ✔ Reinstated ~~deleted~~ Deleted ⊘ Not covered or valid by Medicare
✳ Special coverage instructions * Carrier discretion ⓑ Bill Part B MAC ⒷBill DME MAC

TEMPORARY CODES ASSIGNED BY CMS

✱ Q4155	Neoxflo or clarixflo, 1 mg ⒷQpQh	N1 N
✱ Q4156	Neox 100 or Clarix 100, per square centimeter ⒷQpQh	N1 N
✱ Q4157	Revitalon, per square centimeter ⒷQpQh	N1 N
✱ Q4158	Kerecis Omega3, per square centimeter ⒷQpQh	N1 N
✱ Q4159	Affinity, per square centimeter ⒷQpQh	N1 N
✱ Q4160	Nushield, per square centimeter ⒷQpQh	N1 N
✱ Q4161	Bio-ConneKt Wound Matrix, per square centimeter ⒷQpQh	N1 N
✱ Q4162	Woundex flow, BioSkin flow 0.5 cc ⒷQpQh	N1 N
✱ Q4163	Woundex, BioSkin per square centimeter ⒷQpQh	N1 N
✱ Q4164	Helicoll, per square centimeter ⒷQpQh	N1 N
✱ Q4165	Keramatrix or kerasorb, per square centimeter ⒷQpQh	N1 N
✱ Q4166	Cytal, per square centimeter ⒷQpQh *Coding Clinic: 2017, Q1, P10*	N1 N
✱ Q4167	TruSkin, per square centimeter ⒷQpQh *Coding Clinic: 2017, Q1, P10*	N1 N
✱ Q4168	AmnioBand, 1 mg ⒷQpQh *Coding Clinic: 2017, Q1, P10*	N1 N
✱ Q4169	Artacent wound, per square centimeter ⒷQpQh *Coding Clinic: 2017, Q1, P10*	N1 N
✱ Q4170	Cygnus, per square centimeter ⒷQpQh *Coding Clinic: 2017, Q1, P10*	N1 N
✱ Q4171	Interfyl, 1 mg ⒷQpQh *Coding Clinic: 2017, Q1, P10*	N1 N
✱ Q4173	PalinGen or PalinGen XPlus, per square centimeter ⒷQpQh *Coding Clinic: 2017, Q1, P10*	N1 N
✱ Q4174	PalinGen or ProMatrX, 0.36 mg per 0.25 cc ⒷQpQh *Coding Clinic: 2017, Q1, P10*	N1 N
✱ Q4175	Miroderm, per square centimeter ⒷQpQh *Coding Clinic: 2017, Q1, P10*	N1 N
✱ Q4176	Neopatch or therion, per square centimeter Ⓑ	N1 N
✱ Q4177	Floweramnioflo, 0.1 cc Ⓑ	N1 N
✱ Q4178	Floweramniopatch, per square centimeter Ⓑ	N1 N
✱ Q4179	Flowerderm, per square centimeter Ⓑ	N1 N
✱ Q4180	Revita, per square centimeter Ⓑ	N1 N
✱ Q4181	Amnio wound, per square centimeter Ⓑ	N1 N
✱ Q4182	Transcyte, per square centimeter Ⓑ	N1 N
✱ Q4183	Surgigraft, per square centimeter Ⓑ	N
✱ Q4184	Cellesta or cellesta duo, per square centimeter Ⓑ	N
✱ Q4185	Cellesta flowable amnion (25 mg per cc); per 0.5 cc Ⓑ	N
✱ Q4186	Epifix, per square centimeter Ⓑ	N
✱ Q4187	Epicord, per square centimeter Ⓑ	N
✱ Q4188	Amnioarmor, per square centimeter Ⓑ	N
✱ Q4189	Artacent ac, 1 mg Ⓑ	N
✱ Q4190	Artacent ac, per square centimeter Ⓑ	N
✱ Q4191	Restorigin, per square centimeter Ⓑ	N
✱ Q4192	Restorigin, 1 cc Ⓑ	N
✱ Q4193	Coll-e-derm, per square centimeter Ⓑ	N
✱ Q4194	Novachor, per square centimeter Ⓑ	N
✱ Q4195	Puraply, per square centimeter Ⓑ	N
✱ Q4196	Puraply am, per square centimeter Ⓑ	N
✱ Q4197	Puraply xt, per square centimeter Ⓑ	N
✱ Q4198	Genesis amniotic membrane, per square centimeter Ⓑ	N
✱ Q4199	Cygnus matrix, per square centimeter	N
✱ Q4200	Skin te, per square centimeter Ⓑ	N
✱ Q4201	Matrion, per square centimeter Ⓑ	N
✱ Q4202	Keroxx (2.5g/cc), 1cc Ⓑ	N
✱ Q4203	Derma-gide, per square centimeter Ⓑ	N
✱ Q4204	Xwrap, per square centimeter Ⓑ	N
✱ Q4205	Membrane graft or membrane wrap, per square centimeter Ⓑ	N
✱ Q4206	Fluid flow or fluid Gf, 1 cc Ⓑ	N
✱ Q4208	Novafix, per square cenitmeter Ⓑ	N
✱ Q4209	Surgraft, per square centimeter Ⓑ	N
✱ Q4211	Amnion bio or axobiomembrane, per square centimeter Ⓑ	N
✱ Q4212	Allogen, per cc Ⓑ	N
✱ Q4213	Ascent, 0.5 mg Ⓑ	N
✱ Q4214	Cellesta cord, per square centimeter Ⓑ	N
✱ Q4215	Axolotl ambient or axolotl cryo, 0.1 mg Ⓑ	N
✱ Q4216	Artacent cord, per square centimeter Ⓑ	N

✋ MIPS   Qp Quantity Physician   Qh Quantity Hospital   ♀ Female only   ♂ Male only   Ⓐ Age   ♿ DMEPOS   A2-Z3 ASC Payment Indicator   A-Y ASC Status Indicator   *Coding Clinic*

* Q4217	Woundfix, BioWound, Woundfix Plus, BioWound Plus, Woundfix Xplus or BioWound Xplus, per square centimeter Ⓑ		N
* Q4218	Surgicord, per square centimeter Ⓑ		N
* Q4219	Surgigraft-dual, per square centimeter Ⓑ		N
* Q4220	BellaCell HD or Surederm, per square centimeter Ⓑ		N
* Q4221	Amniowrap2, per square centimeter Ⓑ		N
* Q4222	Progenamatrix, per square centimeter Ⓑ		N
* Q4225	Amniobind or dermabind TL, per square centimeter Ⓑ		N
* Q4226	MyOwn skin, includes harvesting and preparation procedures, per square centimeter Ⓑ		N
* Q4227	Amniocore, per square centimeter	N1	N
* Q4229	Cogenex amniotic membrane, per square centimeter	N1	N
* Q4230	Cogenex flowable amnion, per 0.5 cc	N1	N
~~Q4231~~	~~Corplex P, per cc~~		
* Q4232	Corplex, per square centimeter	N1	N
* Q4233	Surfactor or Nudyn, per 0.5 cc	N1	N
* Q4234	Xcellerate, per square centimeter	N1	N
* Q4235	Amniorepair or Altiply, per square centimeter	N1	N
* Q4237	Cryo-cord, per square centimeter	N1	N
* Q4238	Derm-maxx, per square centimeter	N1	N
* Q4239	Amnio-maxx or amnio-maxx lite, per square centimeter	N1	N
* Q4240	Corecyte, for topical use only, per 0.5 cc	N1	N
* Q4241	Polycyte, for topical use only, per 0.5 cc	N1	N
* Q4242	Amniocyte plus, per 0.5 cc	N1	N
* Q4245	Amniotext, per cc	N1	N
* Q4246	Coretext or Protext, per cc	N1	N
* Q4248	Dermacyte amniotic membrane allograft, per square centimeter	N1	N
* Q4249	Amniply, for topical use only, per square centimeter		N
* Q4950	Amnioamp-MP, per square centimeter		N
* Q4251	Vim, per square centimeter		N
* Q4252	Vendaje, per square centimeter		N
* Q4253	Zenith amniotic membrane, per square centimeter		N
* Q4254	Novafix DL, per square centimeter		N
* Q4255	Reguard, for topical use only, per square centimeter	N
⊛ Q4259	Celera dual layer or celera dual membrane, per square centimeter	N
⊛ Q4260	Signature apatch, per square centimeter	N
⊛ Q4261	Tag, per square centimeter	N
⊛ Q4262	Dual layer impax membrane, per square centimeter	N
⊛ Q4263	Surgraft tl, per square centimeter	N
⊛ Q4264	Cocoon membrane, per square centimeter	N
⊛ Q4265	Neostim tl, per square centimeter	N
⊛ Q4266	Neostim membrane, per square centimeter	N
⊛ Q4267	Neostim dl, per square centimeter	N
⊛ Q4268	Surgraft ft, per square centimeter	N
⊛ Q4269	Surgraft xt, per square centimeter	N
⊛ Q4270	Complete sl, per square centimeter	N
⊛ Q4271	Complete ft, per square centimeter	N
⊛ Q4272	Esano a, per square centimeter	N
⊛ Q4273	Esano aaa, per square centimeter	N
⊛ Q4274	Esano ac, per square centimeter	N
⊛ Q4275	Esano aca, per square centimeter	N
⊛ Q4276	Orion, per square centimeter	N
⊛ Q4278	Epieffect, per square centimeter	N
⊛ Q4279	Vendaje ac, per square centimeter	N
⊛ Q4280	Xcell amnio matrix, per square centimeter	N
⊛ Q4281	Barrera sl or barrera dl, per square centimeter	N
⊛ Q4282	Cygnus dual, per square centimeter	N
⊛ Q4283	Biovance tri-layer or biovance 3l, per square centimeter	N
⊛ Q4284	Dermabind sl, per square centimeter	N
⊛ Q4285	Nudyn dl or nudyn dl mesh, per square centimeter	N
⊛ Q4286	Nudyn sl or nudyn slw, per square centimeter	N
⊛ Q4287	Dermabind dl, per square centimeter	N
⊛ Q4288	Dermabind ch, per square centimeter	N
⊛ Q4289	Revoshield + amniotic barrier, per square centimeter	N
⊛ Q4290	Membrane wrap-hydro, per square centimeter	N
⊛ Q4291	Lamellas xt, per square centimeter	N
⊛ Q4292	Lamellas, per square centimeter	N
⊛ Q4293	Acesso dl, per square centimeter	N

▶ New   ⤺ Revised   ✓ Reinstated   ~~deleted~~ Deleted   ⊘ Not covered or valid by Medicare
⊛ Special coverage instructions   * Carrier discretion   Ⓑ Bill Part B MAC   Ⓑ Bill DME MAC

TEMPORARY CODES ASSIGNED BY CMS

✪ Q4294	Amnio quad-core, per square centimeter	N
✪ Q4295	Amnio tri-core amniotic, per square centimeter	N
✪ Q4296	Rebound matrix, per square centimeter	N
✪ Q4297	Emerge matrix, per square centimeter	N
✪ Q4298	Amnicore pro, per square centimeter	N
✪ Q4299	Amnicore pro+, per square centimeter	N
✪ Q4300	Acesso tl, per square centimeter	N
✪ Q4301	Activate matrix, per square centimeter	N
✪ Q4302	Complete aca, per square centimeter	N
✪ Q4303	Complete aa, per square centimeter	N
✪ Q4304	Grafix plus, per square centimeter	N
✪ Q4305	American amnion ac tri-layer, per square centimeter	N
✪ Q4306	American amnion ac, per square centimeter	N
✪ Q4307	American amnion, per square centimeter	N
✪ Q4308	Sanopellis, per square centimeter	N
✪ Q4309	Via matrix, per square centimeter	N
✪ Q4310	Procenta, per 100 mg	N
✪ Q4311	Acesso, per square centimeter	N
✪ Q4312	Acesso ac, per square centimeter	N
✪ Q4313	Dermabind fm, per square centimeter	N
✪ Q4314	Reeva ft, per square cenitmeter	N
✪ Q4315	Regenelink amniotic membrane allograft, per square centimeter	N
✪ Q4316	Amchoplast, per square centimeter	N
✪ Q4317	Vitograft, per square centimeter	N
✪ Q4318	E-graft, per square centimeter	N
✪ Q4319	Sanograft, per square centimeter	N
✪ Q4320	Pellograft, per square centimeter	N
✪ Q4321	Renograft, per square centimeter	N
✪ Q4322	Caregraft, per square centimeter	N
✪ Q4323	Alloply, per square centimeter	N
✪ Q4324	Amniotx, per square centimeter	N
✪ Q4325	Acapatch, per square centimeter	N
✪ Q4326	Woundplus, per square centimeter	N
✪ Q4327	Duoamnion, per square centimeter	N
✪ Q4328	Most, per square centimeter	N
✪ Q4329	Singlay, per square centimeter	N
✪ Q4330	Total, per square centimeter	N
✪ Q4331	Axolotl graft, per square centimeter	N
✪ Q4332	Axolotl dualgraft, per square centimeter	N
✪ Q4333	Ardeograft, per square centimeter	N
✪ Q4334	Amnioplast 1, per square centimeter	N
✪ Q4335	Amnioplast 2, per square centimeter	N
✪ Q4336	Artacent c, per square centimeter	N
✪ Q4337	Artacent trident, per square centimeter	N
✪ Q4338	Artacent velos, per square centimeter	N
✪ Q4339	Artacent vericlen, per square centimeter	N
✪ Q4340	Simpligraft, per square centimeter	N
✪ Q4341	Simplimax, per square centimeter	N
✪ Q4342	Theramend, per square centimeter	N
✪ Q4343	Dermacyte ac matrix amniotic membrane allograft, per square centimeter	N
✪ Q4344	Tri-membrane wrap, per square centimeter	N
✪ Q4335	Matrix hd allograft dermis, per square centimeter	N
▶ ✴ Q4346	Shelter DM matrix, per square centimeter	N
▶ ✴ Q4347	Rampart DL matrix, per square centimeter	N
▶ ✴ Q4348	Sentry SL matrix, per square centimeter	N
▶ ✴ Q4349	Mantle DL matrix, per square centimeter	N
▶ ✴ Q4350	Palisade DM matrix, per square centimeter	N
▶ ✴ Q4351	Enclose TL matrix, per square centimeter	N
▶ ✴ Q4352	Overlay SL matrix, per square centimeter	N
▶ ✴ Q4353	Xceed TL matrix, per square centimeter	N
▶ ✴ Q4354	Palingen dual-layer membrane, per square centimeter	N
▶ ✴ Q4355	Abiomend xplus membrane and abiomend xplus hydromembrane, per square centimeter	N
▶ ✴ Q4356	Abiomend membrane and abiomend hydromembrane, per square centimeter	N
▶ ✴ Q4357	Xwrap plus, per square centimeter	N
▶ ✴ Q4358	Xwrap dual, per square centimeter	N
▶ ✴ Q4359	Choriply, per square centimeter	N
▶ ✴ Q4360	Amchoplast fd, per square centimeter	N
▶ ✴ Q4361	Epixpress, per square centimeter	N

MIPS ◆ Quantity Physician ◆ Quantity Hospital ◆ Female only ♀
♂ Male only ◆ Age ◆ DMEPOS ◆ A2-Z3 ASC Payment Indicator ◆ A-Y ASC Status Indicator ◆ Coding Clinic

▶ * Q4362	Cygnus disk, per square centimeter	N
▶ * Q4363	Amnio burgeon membrane and hydromembrane, per square centimeter	N
▶ * Q4364	Amnio burgeon xplus membrane and xplus hydromembrane, per square centimeter	N
▶ * Q4365	Amnio burgeon dual-layer membrane, per square centimeter	N
▶ * Q4366	Dual layer amnio burgeon x-membrane, per square centimeter	N
▶ * Q4367	Amniocore sl, per square centimeter	N
▶ * Q4368	Amchothick, per square centimeter	N
▶ * Q4369	Amnioplast 3, per square centimeter	N
▶ * Q4370	Aeroguard, per square centimeter	N
▶ * Q4371	Neoguard, per square centimeter	N
▶ * Q4372	Amchoplast excel, per square centimeter	N
▶ * Q4373	Membrane wrap lite, per square centimeter	N
▶ * Q4375	Duograft ac, per square centimeter	N
▶ * Q4376	Duograft aa, per square centimeter	N
▶ * Q4377	Trigraft ft, per square centimeter	N
▶ * Q4378	Renew ft matrix, per square centimeter	N
▶ * Q4379	Amniodefend ft matrix, per square centimeter	N
▶ * Q4380	Advograft one, per square centimeter	N
▶ * Q4382	Advograft dual, per square centimeter	N
▶ * Q4383	Axolotl graft ultra, per square centimeter	N
▶ * Q4384	Axolotl dualgraft ultra, per square centimeter	N
▶ * Q4385	Apollo ft, per square centimeter	N
▶ * Q4386	Acesso trifaca, per square centimeter	N
▶ * Q4387	Neothelium ft, per square centimeter	N
▶ * Q4388	Neothelium 4l, per square centimeter	N
▶ * Q4389	Neothelium 4l+, per square centimeter	N
▶ * Q4390	Ascendion, per square centimeter	N
▶ * Q4391	Amnioplast double, per square centimeter	N
▶ * Q4392	Grafix duo, per square centimeter	N
▶ * Q4393	Surgraft ac, per square centimeter	N
▶ * Q4394	Surgraft aca, per square centimeter	N
▶ * Q4395	Acelagraft, per square centimeter	N
▶ * Q4396	Natalin, per square centimeter	N
▶ * Q4397	Summit aaa, per square centimeter	N

Hospice Care

⊛ Q5001	Hospice or home health care provided in patient's home/residence Ⓑ	B
⊛ Q5002	Hospice or home health care provided in assisted living facility Ⓑ	B
⊛ Q5003	Hospice care provided in nursing long term care facility (LTC) or non-skilled nursing facility (NF) Ⓑ	B
⊛ Q5004	Hospice care provided in skilled nursing facility (SNF) Ⓑ	B
⊛ Q5005	Hospice care provided in inpatient hospital Ⓑ	B
⊛ Q5006	Hospice care provided in inpatient hospice facility Ⓑ	B

Hospice care provided in an inpatient hospice facility. These are residential facilities, which are places for patients to live while receiving routine home care or continuous home care. These hospice residential facilities are not certified by Medicare or Medicaid for provision of General Inpatient (GIP) or respite care, and regulations at 42 CFR 418.202(e) do not allow provision of GIP or respite care at hospice residential facilities.

⊛ Q5007	Hospice care provided in long term care facility Ⓑ	B
⊛ Q5008	Hospice care provided in inpatient psychiatric facility Ⓑ	B
⊛ Q5009	Hospice or home health care provided in place not otherwise specified (NOS) Ⓑ	B
⊛ Q5010	Hospice home care provided in a hospice facility Ⓑ	B

Biosimilar Drugs

▶ ⊛ Q5098	Injection, ustekinumab-srlf (imuldosa), biosimilar, 1 mg	E2
▶ ⊛ Q5099	Injection, ustekinumab-stba (steqeyma), biosimilar, 1 mg	K
▶ ⊛ Q5100	Injection, ustekinumab-kfce (yesintek), biosimilar, 1 mg	G
⊛ Q5101	Injection, filgrastim-sndz, biosimilar, (zarxio), 1 mcg Ⓑ Ⓑ Qp Qh	K2 N
	Other: Zarxio	
⊛ Q5103	Injection, infliximab-dyyb, biosimilar, (inflectra), 10 mg Ⓑ Ⓑ	G
	Other: Remicade, Inflectra, Renflexis	
⊛ Q5104	Injection, infliximab-abda, biosimilar, (renflexis), 10 mgn Ⓑ Ⓑ	K2 G
	Other: Remicade	

▶ New   ⮂ Revised   ✓ Reinstated   ~~deleted~~ Deleted   ⊘ Not covered or valid by Medicare
⊛ Special coverage instructions   * Carrier discretion   Ⓑ Bill Part B MAC   Ⓑ Bill DME MAC

TEMPORARY CODES ASSIGNED BY CMS

Code	Description	Indicator
⊛ Q5105	Injection, epoetin alfa-epbx, biosimilar, (retacrit) (for ESRD on dialysis), 100 units ⓑ Ⓑ	K2 G
	Other: Retacrit	
⊛ Q5106	Injection, epoetin alfa-epbx, biosimilar (retacrit) (for non-ESRD use), 1000 units ⓑ Ⓑ	G
	Other: Retacrit	
⊛ Q5107	Injection, bevacizumab-awwb, biosimilar (mvasi), 10 mg ⓑ Ⓑ	K
	Other: Avastin	
⊛ Q5108	Injection, pegfilgrastim-jmdb, (fulphila), biosimilar 0.5 mg ⓑ Ⓑ	K
	Other: Neulasta	
⊛ Q5109	Injection, infliximab-qbtx, biosimilar (ixifi), 10 mg ⓑ Ⓑ	E2
	Other: Remicade, Inflectra, Renflexis	
⊛ Q5110	Injection, filgrastim-aafi, biosimilar (nivestym), 1 mcg ⓑ Ⓑ	K
	Other: Nivestym	
Q5111	Injection, pegfilgrastim-cbqv (udenyca), biosimilar, 0.5 mg ⓑ Ⓑ	K
✱ Q5112	Injection, trastuzumab-dttb, biosimilar (ontruzant), 10 mg ⓑ Ⓑ	E2
✱ Q5113	Injection, trastuzumab-pkrb, biosimilar (herzuma), 10 mg ⓑ Ⓑ	E2
✱ Q5114	Injection, trastuzumab-dkst, biosimilar (ogivri), 10 mg ⓑ Ⓑ	E2
⊛ Q5115	Injection, rituximab-abbs, biosimilar (truxima), 10 mg ⓑ Ⓑ	E2
✱ Q5116	Injection, trastuzumab-qyyp, biosimilar (trazimera), 10 mg ⓑ Ⓑ	E2
✱ Q5117	Injection, trastuzumab-anns, biosimilar (kanjinti), 10 mg ⓑ Ⓑ	K2 K
✱ Q5118	Injection, bevacizumab-bvzr, biosimilar (zirabev), 10 mg ⓑ Ⓑ	E2
✱ Q5119	Injection, rituximab-pvvr, biosimilar (ruxience), 10 mg ⓑ Ⓑ	G
✱ Q5120	Injection, pegfilgrastim-bmez, (ziextenzo), biosimilar 0.5 mg ⓑ Ⓑ	K2 G
✱ Q5121	Injection, infliximab-axxq, (avsola), biosimilar 10 mg ⓑ Ⓑ	K2 G
✱ Q5122	Injection, pegfilgrastim-apgf, (nyvepria), biosimilar, 0.5 mg ⓑ Ⓑ	K5 E1
✱ Q5123	Injection, rituximab-arrx, biosimilar, (riabni), 10 mg ⓑ Ⓑ	K2 G
✱ Q5125	Injection, filgrastim-ayow, biosimilar, (releuko), 1 mcg ⓑ Ⓑ	K2 G
⊛ Q5126	Injection, bevacizumab-maly, biosimilar, (alymsys), 10 mg ⓑ Ⓑ	G
⊛ Q5127	Injection, pegfilgrastim-fpgk (stimufend), biosimilar, 0.5 mg ⓑ Ⓑ	G
⊛ Q5128	Injection, ranibizumab-eqrn (cimerli), biosimilar, 0.1 mg ⓑ Ⓑ	
⊛ Q5129	Injection, bevacizumab-adcd (vegzelma), biosimilar, 10 mg ⓑ Ⓑ	G
⊛ Q5130	Injection, pegfilgrastim-pbbk (fylnetra), biosimilar, 0.5 mg ⓑ Ⓑ	G
~~Q5131~~	~~Injection, adalimumab-aacf (idacio), biosimilar, 20 mg~~	
~~Q5132~~	~~Injection, adalimumab-afzb (abrilada), biosimilar, 10 mg~~	
Q5133	Injection, tocilizumab-bavi (tofidence), biosimilar, 1 mg ⓑ Ⓑ	G
Q5134	Injection, natalizumab-sztn (tyruko), biosimilar, 1 mg ⓑ Ⓑ	E2
✱ Q5135	Injection, tocilizumab-aazg (tyenne), biosimilar, 1 mg ⓑ Ⓑ	G
✱ Q5136	Injection, denosumab-bbdz (jubbonti/wyost), biosimilar, 1 mg ⓑ Ⓑ	G
✱ Q5137	Injection, ustekinumab-auub (wezlana), biosimilar, subcutaneous, 1 mg	G
✱ Q5138	Injection, ustekinumab-auub (wezlana), biosimilar, intravenous, 1 mg	G
▶ ✱ Q5139	Injection, eculizumab-aeeb (bkemv), biosimilar, 10 mg	K
▶ Q5140	Injection, adalimumab-fkjp, biosimilar, 1 mg	K
▶ ✱ Q5141	Injection, adalimumab-aaty, biosimilar, 1 mg	K
▶ ✱ Q5142	Injection, adalimumab-ryvk biosimilar, 1 mg	K
▶ ✱ Q5143	Injection, adalimumab-adbm, biosimilar, 1 mg	K
▶ ✱ Q5144	Injection, adalimumab-aacf (idacio), biosimilar, 1 mg	K
▶ ✱ Q5145	Injection, adalimumab-afzb (abrilada), biosimilar, 1 mg	K
▶ ✱ Q5146	Injection, trastuzumab-strf (hercessi), biosimilar, 10 mg	K
▶ ✱ Q5147	Injection, aflibercept-ayyh (pavblu), biosimilar, 1 mg	G
▶ ✱ Q5148	Injection, filgrastim-txid (nypozi), biosimilar, 1 microgram	G
▶ ✱ Q5149	Injection, aflibercept-abzv (enzeevu), biosimilar, 1 mg	E2
▶ ✱ Q5150	Injection, aflibercept-mrbb (ahzantive), biosimilar, 1 mg	E2
▶ ✱ Q5151	Injection, eculizumab-aagh (epysqli), biosimilar, 2 mg	G

2026 HCPCS LEVEL II NATIONAL CODES

▶ * **Q5152** Injection, eculizumab-aeeb (bkemv), biosimilar, 2 mg   G

▶ * **Q5153** Injection, aflibercept-yszy (opuviz), biosimilar, 1 mg   E2

▶ * **Q5154** Injection, omalizumab-igec (omlyclo), biosimilar, 5 mg   E2

▶ * **Q5155** Injection, aflibercept-jbvf (yesafili), biosimilar, 1 mg   E2

▶ * **Q5156** Injection, tocilizumab-anoh (avtozma), biosimilar, 1 mg   E2

▶ * **Q5157** Injection, denosumab-bmwo (stoboclo/osenvelt), biosimilar, 1 mg   K

▶ * **Q5158** Injection, denosumab-bnht (bomyntra/conexxence), biosimilar, 1 mg   K

▶ * **Q5159** Injection, denosumab-dssb (ospomyv/xbryk), biosimilar, 1 mg   E2

Veteran Services Chaplain

* **Q9001** Assessment by chaplain services   B

* **Q9002** Counseling, individual, by chaplain services   B

* **Q9003** Counseling, group, by chaplain services   B

* **Q9004** Department of veterans affairs whole health partner services   E1

Contrast Agents

* **Q9950** Injection, sulfur hexafluoride lipid microspheres, per ml   B Qp Qh   N1 N

Other: Lumason

⊛ **Q9951** Low osmolar contrast material, 400 or greater mg/ml iodine concentration, per ml   B Qp Qh   N1 N

IOM: 100-04, 12, 70; 100-04, 13, 20; 100-04, 13, 90

Coding Clinic: 2012, Q3, P8

⊛ **Q9953** Injection, iron-based magnetic resonance contrast agent, per ml   B Qp Qh   N1 N

IOM: 100-04, 12, 70; 100-04, 13, 20; 100-04, 13, 90

Coding Clinic: 2012, Q3, P8

⊛ **Q9954** Oral magnetic resonance contrast agent, per 100 ml   B Qp Qh   N1 N

IOM: 100-04, 12, 70; 100-04, 13, 20; 100-04, 13, 90

Coding Clinic: 2012, Q3, P8

* **Q9955** Injection, perflexane lipid microspheres, per ml   B Qp Qh   N1 N

Coding Clinic: 2012, Q3, P8

* **Q9956** Injection, octafluoropropane microspheres, per ml   B Qp Qh   N1 N

Other: Optison

Coding Clinic: 2012, Q3, P8

* **Q9957** Injection, perflutren lipid microspheres, per ml   B Qp Qh   N1 N

Other: Definity

Coding Clinic: 2012, Q3, P8

⊛ **Q9958** High osmolar contrast material, up to 149 mg/ml iodine concentration, per ml   B Qp Qh   N1 N

Other: Conray 30, Cysto-Conray II, Cystografin

IOM: 100-04, 12, 70; 100-04, 13, 20; 100-04, 13, 90

Coding Clinic: 2012, Q3, P8; 2007, Q1, P6

⊛ **Q9959** High osmolar contrast material, 150-199 mg/ml iodine concentration, per ml   B Qp Qh   N1 N

IOM: 100-04, 12, 70; 100-04, 13, 20; 100-04, 13, 90

Coding Clinic: 2012, Q3, P8; 2007, Q1, P6

⊛ **Q9960** High osmolar contrast material, 200-249 mg/mliodine concentration, per ml   B Qp Qh   N1 N

Other: Conray 43

IOM: 100-04, 12, 70; 100-04, 13, 20; 100-04, 13, 90

Coding Clinic: 2012, Q3, P8; 2007, Q1, P6

⊛ **Q9961** High osmolar contrast material, 250-299 mg/mliodine concentration, per ml   B Qp Qh   N1 N

Other: Conray, Cholografin Meglumine

IOM: 100-04, 12, 70; 100-04, 13, 20; 100-04, 13, 90

Coding Clinic: 2012, Q3, P8; 2007, Q1, P6

⊛ **Q9962** High osmolar contrast material, 300-349 mg/ml iodine concentration, per ml   B Qp Qh   N1 N

IOM: 100-04, 12, 70; 100-04, 13, 20; 100-04, 13, 90

Coding Clinic: 2012, Q3, P8; 2007, Q1, P6

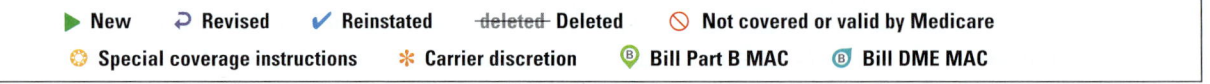

▶ New   ⟳ Revised   ✓ Reinstated   ~~deleted~~ Deleted   ⊘ Not covered or valid by Medicare   ⊛ Special coverage instructions   * Carrier discretion   B Bill Part B MAC   B Bill DME MAC

TEMPORARY CODES ASSIGNED BY CMS

✪ **Q9963** High osmolar contrast material, 350-399 mg/ml iodine concentration, per ml Ⓑ Qp Qh N1 N

Other: Gastrografin, MD-76R, MD Gastroview, Sinografin

IOM: 100-04, 12, 70; 100-04, 13, 20; 100-04, 13, 90

Coding Clinic: 2012, Q3, P8; 2007, Q1, P6

✪ **Q9964** High osmolar contrast material, 400 or greater mg/ml iodine concentration, per ml Ⓑ Qp Qh N1 N

IOM: 100-04, 12, 70; 100-04, 13, 20; 100-04, 13, 90

Coding Clinic: 2012, Q3, P8; 2007, Q1, P6

✪ **Q9965** Low osmolar contrast material, 100-199 mg/ml iodine concentration, per ml Ⓑ N1 N

Other: Omnipaque

IOM: 100-04, 12, 70; 100-04, 13, 20; 100-04, 13, 90

Coding Clinic: 2012, Q3, P8

✪ **Q9966** Low osmolar contrast material, 200-299 mg/ml iodine concentration, per ml Ⓑ Qp Qh N1 N

Other: Isovue, Omnipaque, Optiray, Ultravist 240, Visipaque

IOM: 100-04, 12, 70; 100-04, 13, 20; 100-04, 13, 90

Coding Clinic: 2012, Q3, P8

✪ **Q9967** Low osmolar contrast material, 300-399 mg/ml iodine concentration, per ml Ⓑ Qp Qh N1 N

Other: Hexabrix 320, Isovue, Omnipaque, Optiray, Oxilan, Ultravist, Vispaque

IOM: 100-04, 12, 70; 100-04, 13, 20; 100-04, 13, 90

Coding Clinic: 2012, Q3, P8

✳ **Q9968** Injection, non-radioactive, non-contrast, visualization adjunct (e.g., Methylene Blue, Isosulfan Blue), 1 mg Ⓑ K2 K

✪ **Q9969** Tc-99m from non-highly enriched uranium source, full cost recovery add-on, per study dose Ⓑ Qp Qh K

Radiopharmaceuticals

✪ **Q9982** Flutemetamol F18, diagnostic, per study dose, up to 5 millicuries Ⓑ Qp Qh K2 G

Other: Vizamyl

✪ **Q9983** Florbetaben F18, diagnostic, per study dose, up to 8.1 millicuries Ⓑ Qp Qh K2 G

Other: Neuraceq

✳ **Q9991** Injection, buprenorphine extended-release (sublocade), less than or equal to 100 mg Ⓑ Ⓑ G

Other: Subutex, Buprenex, Belbuca, Probuphine, Butrans

✳ **Q9992** Injection, buprenorphine extended-release (sublocade), greater than 100 mg Ⓑ Ⓑ G

Other: Subutex, Buprenex, Belbuca, Probuphine, Butrans

▶ ✳ **Q9996** Injection, ustekinumab-ttwe (pyzchiva), subcutaneous, 1 mg N

▶ ✳ **Q9997** Injection, ustekinumab-ttwe (pyzchiva), intravenous, 1 mg N

▶ ✳ **Q9998** Injection, ustekinumab-aekn (selarsdi), biosimilar, 1 mg K

▶ ✳ **Q9999** Injection, ustekinumab-aauz (otulfi), biosimilar, 1 mg G

🪙 MIPS Qp Quantity Physician Qh Quantity Hospital ♀ Female only ♂ Male only Ⓐ Age ♿ DMEPOS A2-Z3 ASC Payment Indicator A-Y ASC Status Indicator Coding Clinic

DIAGNOSTIC RADIOLOGY SERVICES (R0000-R9999)

Transportation/Setup of Portable Equipment

R0070 Transportation of portable x-ray equipment and personnel to home or nursing home, per trip to facility or location, one patient seen ⓑ Qp Qh B

CMS Transmittal B03-049; specific instructions to contractors on pricing

IOM: 100-04, 13, 90; 100-04, 13, 90.3

R0075 Transportation of portable x-ray equipment and personnel to home or nursing home, per trip to facility or location, more than one patient seen ⓑ Qp Qh B

This code would not apply to the x-ray equipment if stored at the location where the x-ray was performed (e.g., a nursing home).

IOM: 100-04, 13, 90; 100-04, 13, 90.3

R0076 Transportation of portable ECG to facility or location, per patient ⓑ Qp Qh B

EKG procedure code 93000 or 93005 must be submitted on same claim as transportation code. Bundled status on physician fee schedule

IOM: 100-01, 5, 90.2; 100-02, 15, 80; 100-03, 1, 20.15; 100-04, 13, 90; 100-04, 16, 10; 100-04, 16, 110.4

TEMPORARY NATIONAL CODES ESTABLISHED BY PRIVATE PAYERS (S0000-S9999)

NOTE: Medicare and other federal payers do not recognize "S" codes; however, S codes may be useful for claims to some private insurers.

Non-Medicare Drugs

⊘	S0012	Butorphanol tartrate, nasal spray, 25 mg
⊘	S0013	Esketamine, nasal spray, 1 mg
⊘	S0014	Tacrine hydrochloride, 10 mg
	S0017	Injection, aminocaproic acid, 5 grams
⊘	S0021	Injection, cefoperazone sodium, 1 gram
⊘	S0023	Injection, cimetidine hydrochloride, 300 mg
⊘	S0028	Injection, famotidine, 20 mg
⊘	S0032	Injection, nafcillin sodium, 2 grams
⊘	S0034	Injection, ofloxacin, 400 mg
⊘	S0039	Injection, sulfamethoxazole and trimethoprim, 10 ml
⊘	S0040	Injection, ticarcillin disodium and clavulanate potassium, 3.1 grams
	S0074	Injection, cefotetan disodium, 500 mg
⊘	S0077	Injection, clindamycin phosphate, 300 mg
⊘	S0078	Injection, fosphenytoin sodium, 750 mg
⊘	S0080	Injection, pentamidine isethionate, 300 mg
⊘	S0081	Injection, piperacillin sodium, 500 mg
⊘	S0088	Imatinib, 100 mg
⊘	S0090	Sildenafil citrate, 25 mg
⊘	S0091	Granisetron hydrochloride, 1 mg (for circumstances falling under the Medicare Statute, use Q0166)
⊘	S0092	Injection, hydromorphone hydrochloride, 250 mg (loading dose for infusion pump)
⊘	S0093	Injection, morphine sulfate, 500 mg (loading dose for infusion pump)
⊘	S0104	Zidovudine, oral, 100 mg
⊘	S0106	Bupropion HCl sustained release tablet, 150 mg, per bottle of 60 tablets
⊘	S0108	Mercaptopurine, oral, 50 mg
⊘	S0109	Methadone, oral, 5 mg
⊘	S0117	Tretinoin, topical, 5 grams
⊘	S0119	Ondansetron, oral, 4 mg (for circumstances falling under the Medicare statute, use HCPCS Q code)
⊘	S0122	Injection, menotropins, 75 IU
⊘	S0126	Injection, follitropin alfa, 75 IU
	S0128	Injection, follitropin beta, 75 IU
	S0132	Injection, ganirelix acetate, 250 mcg
⊘	S0136	Clozapine, 25 mg
⊘	S0137	Didanosine (DDI), 25 mg
⊘	S0138	Finasteride, 5 mg
	S0139	Minoxidil, 10 mg
⊘	S0140	Saquinavir, 200 mg
⊘	S0142	Colistimethate sodium, inhalation solution administered through DME, concentrated form, per mg
⊘	S0145	Injection, pegylated interferon alfa-2a, 180 mcg per ml
⊘	S0148	Injection, pegylated interferon ALFA-2b, 10 mcg
⊘	S0155	Sterile dilutant for epoprostenol, 50 ml
⊘	S0156	Exemestane, 25 mg
⊘	S0157	Becaplermin gel 0.01%, 0.5 gm
⊘	S0160	Dextroamphetamine sulfate, 5 mg
⊘	S0169	Calcitrol, 0.25 mcg
⊘	S0170	Anastrozole, oral, 1 mg
⊘	S0172	Chlorambucil, oral, 2 mg
⊘	S0174	Dolasetron mesylate, oral 50 mg (for circumstances falling under the Medicare Statute, use Q0180)
⊘	S0175	Flutamide, oral, 125 mg
⊘	S0176	Hydroxyurea, oral, 500 mg
⊘	S0178	Lomustine, oral, 10 mg
⊘	S0179	Megestrol acetate, oral, 20 mg
⊘	S0182	Procarbazine hydrochloride, oral, 50 mg
⊘	S0183	Prochlorperazine maleate, oral, 5 mg (for circumstances falling under the Medicare Statute, use Q0164)
⊘	S0187	Tamoxifen citrate, oral, 10 mg
⊘	S0189	Testosterone pellet, 75 mg

MIPS	Qp Quantity Physician	Qh Quantity Hospital	♀ Female only
♂ Male only	Age	DMEPOS	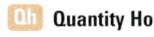 ASC Payment Indicator	A-Y ASC Status Indicator	Coding Clinic

⊘ S0190	Mifepristone, oral, 200 mg
⊘ S0191	Misoprostol, oral 200 mcg
⊘ S0194	Dialysis/stress vitamin supplement, oral, 100 capsules
⊘ S0197	Prenatal vitamins, 30-day supply ♀

Provider Services

⊘ S0199	Medically induced abortion by oral ingestion of medication including all associated services and supplies (e.g., patient counseling, office visits, confirmation of pregnancy by HCG, ultrasound to confirm duration of pregnancy, ultrasound to confirm completion of abortion) except drugs ♀
⊘ S0201	Partial hospitalization services, less than 24 hours, per diem
⊘ S0207	Paramedic intercept, non-hospital-based ALS service (non-voluntary), non-transport
⊘ S0208	Paramedic intercept, hospital-based ALS service (non-voluntary), non-transport
⊘ S0209	Wheelchair van, mileage, per mile
⊘ S0215	Non-emergency transportation; mileage per mile
⊘ S0220	Medical conference by a physician with interdisciplinary team of health professionals or representatives of community agencies to coordinate activities of patient care (patient is present); approximately 30 minutes
⊘ S0221	Medical conference by a physician with interdisciplinary team of health professionals or representatives of community agencies to coordinate activities of patient care (patient is present); approximately 60 minutes
⊘ S0250	Comprehensive geriatric assessment and treatment planning performed by assessment team A
⊘ S0255	Hospice referral visit (advising patient and family of care options) performed by nurse, social worker, or other designated staff
⊘ S0257	Counseling and discussion regarding advance directives or end of life care planning and decisions, with patient and/or surrogate (list separately in addition to code for appropriate evaluation and management service)
⊘ S0260	History and physical (outpatient or office) related to surgical procedure (list separately in addition to code for appropriate evaluation and management service)
⊘ S0265	Genetic counseling, under physician supervision, each 15 minutes
⊘ S0270	Physician management of patient home care, standard monthly case rate (per 30 days)
⊘ S0271	Physician management of patient home care, hospice monthly case rate (per 30 days)
⊘ S0272	Physician management of patient home care, episodic care monthly case rate (per 30 days)
⊘ S0273	Physician visit at member's home, outside of a capitation arrangement
⊘ S0274	Nurse practitioner visit at member's home, outside of a capitation arrangement
⊘ S0280	Medical home program, comprehensive care coordination and planning, initial plan
⊘ S0281	Medical home program, comprehensive care coordination and planning, maintenance of plan
⊘ S0285	Colonoscopy consultation performed prior to a screening colonoscopy procedure
⊘ S0302	Completed Early Periodic Screening Diagnosis and Treatment (EPSDT) service (list in addition to code for appropriate evaluation and management service) A
⊘ S0310	Hospitalist services (list separately in addition to code for appropriate evaluation and management service)
⊘ S0311	Comprehensive management and care coordination for advanced illness, per calendar month
⊘ S0315	Disease management program; initial assessment and initiation of the program
⊘ S0316	Disease management program; follow-up/reassessment
⊘ S0317	Disease management program; per diem
⊘ S0320	Telephone calls by a registered nurse to a disease management program member for monitoring purposes; per month
⊘ S0340	Lifestyle modification program for management of coronary artery disease, including all supportive services; first quarter/stage

▶ New ⟳ Revised ✔ Reinstated ~~deleted~~ Deleted ⊘ Not covered or valid by Medicare
✪ Special coverage instructions ✳ Carrier discretion Ⓑ Bill Part B MAC Ⓑ Bill DME MAC

TEMPORARY NATIONAL CODES ESTABLISHED BY PRIVATE PAYERS

- ⊘ **S0341** Lifestyle modification program for management of coronary artery disease, including all supportive services; second or third quarter/stage
- ⊘ **S0342** Lifestyle modification program for management of coronary artery disease, including all supportive services; fourth quarter/stage
- ⊘ **S0353** Treatment planning and care coordination management for cancer, initial treatment
- ⊘ **S0354** Treatment planning and care coordination management for cancer, established patient with a change of regimen
- ⊘ **S0390** Routine foot care; removal and/or trimming of corns, calluses and/or nails and preventive maintenance in specific medical conditions (e.g., diabetes), per visit
- ⊘ **S0395** Impression casting of a foot performed by a practitioner other than the manufacturer of the orthotic
- ⊘ **S0400** Global fee for extracorporeal shock wave lithotripsy treatment of kidney stone(s)

Vision Supplies

- ⊘ **S0500** Disposable contact lens, per lens
- ⊘ **S0504** Single vision prescription lens (safety, athletic, or sunglass), per lens
- ⊘ **S0506** Bifocal vision prescription lens (safety, athletic, or sunglass), per lens
- ⊘ **S0508** Trifocal vision prescription lens (safety, athletic, or sunglass), per lens
- ⊘ **S0510** Non-prescription lens (safety, athletic, or sunglass), per lens
- ⊘ **S0512** Daily wear specialty contact lens, per lens
- ⊘ **S0514** Color contact lens, per lens
- ⊘ **S0515** Scleral lens, liquid bandage device, per lens
- ⊘ **S0516** Safety eyeglass frames
- ⊘ **S0518** Sunglasses frames
- ⊘ **S0580** Polycarbonate lens (list this code in addition to the basic code for the lens)
- ⊘ **S0581** Nonstandard lens (list this code in addition to the basic code for the lens)
- ⊘ **S0590** Integral lens service, miscellaneous services reported separately
- ⊘ **S0592** Comprehensive contact lens evaluation
- ⊘ **S0595** Dispensing new spectacle lenses for patient supplied frame
- ⊘ **S0596** Phakic intraocular lens for correction of refractive error

Screening and Examinations

- ⊘ **S0601** Screening proctoscopy
- ⊘ **S0610** Annual gynecological examination, new patient ♀
- ⊘ **S0612** Annual gynecological examination, established patient ♀
- ⊘ **S0613** Annual gynecological examination; clinical breast examination without pelvic evaluation ♀
- ⊘ **S0618** Audiometry for hearing aid evaluation to determine the level and degree of hearing loss
- ⊘ **S0620** Routine ophthalmological examination including refraction; new patient

  Many non-Medicare vision plans may require code for routine encounter, no complaints

- ⊘ **S0621** Routine ophthalmological examination including refraction; established patient

  Many non-Medicare vision plans may require code for routine encounter, no complaints

- ⊘ **S0622** Physical exam for college, new or established patient (list separately) in addition to appropriate evaluation and management code [A]

Provider Services and Supplies

- ⊘ **S0630** Removal of sutures; by a physician other than the physician who originally closed the wound
- ⊘ **S0800** Laser in situ keratomileusis (LASIK)

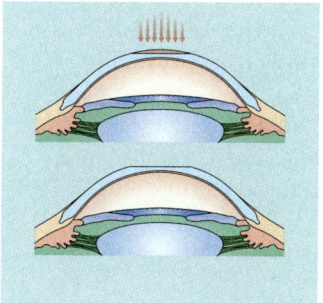

Figure 48 Phototherapeutic keratectomy (PRK).

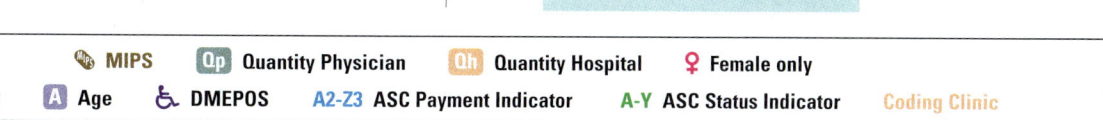

⊘ S0810	Photorefractive keratectomy (PRK)
⊘ S0812	Phototherapeutic keratectomy (PTK)
⊘ S1001	Deluxe item, patient aware (list in addition to code for basic item)
⊘ S1002	Customized item (list in addition to code for basic item)
⊘ S1015	IV tubing extension set
⊘ S1016	Non-PVC (polyvinyl chloride) intravenous administration set, for use with drugs that are not stable in PVC (e.g., paclitaxel)
⊘ S1030	Continuous noninvasive glucose monitoring device, purchase (for physician interpretation of data, use CPT code)
⊘ S1031	Continuous noninvasive glucose monitoring device, rental, including sensor, sensor replacement, and download to monitor (for physician interpretation of data, use CPT code)
⊘ S1034	Artificial pancreas device system (e.g., low glucose suspend (LGS) feature) including continuous glucose monitor, blood glucose device, insulin pump and computer algorithm that communicates with all of the devices
⊘ S1035	Sensor; invasive (e.g., subcutaneous), disposable, for use with artificial pancreas device system
⊘ S1036	Transmitter; external, for use with artificial pancreas device system
⊘ S1037	Receiver (monitor); external, for use with artificial pancreas device system
⊘ S1040	Cranial remolding orthosis, pediatric, rigid, with soft interface material, custom fabricated, includes fitting and adjustment(s) A
⊘ S1091	Stent, non-coronary, temporary, with delivery system (propel)
⊘ S2053	Transplantation of small intestine and liver allografts
⊘ S2054	Transplantation of multivisceral organs
⊘ S2055	Harvesting of donor multivisceral organs, with preparation and maintenance of allografts; from cadaver donor
⊘ S2060	Lobar lung transplantation
⊘ S2061	Donor lobectomy (lung) for transplantation, living donor
⊘ S2065	Simultaneous pancreas kidney transplantation

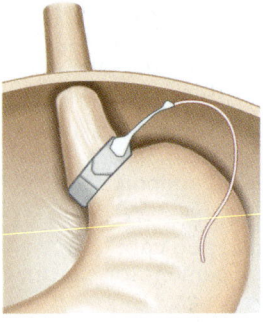

Figure 49 Gastric band.

⊘ S2066	Breast reconstruction with gluteal artery perforator (GAP) flap, including harvesting of the flap, microvascular transfer, closure of donor site and shaping the flap into a breast, unilateral ♀
⊘ S2067	Breast reconstruction of a single breast with "stacked" deep inferior epigastric perforator (DIEP) flap(s) and/or gluteal artery perforator (GAP) flap(s), including harvesting of the flap(s), microvascular transfer, closure of donor site(s) and shaping the flap into a breast, unilateral ♀
⊘ S2068	Breast reconstruction with deep inferior epigastric perforator (DIEP) flap, or superficial inferior epigastric artery (SIEA) flap, including harvesting of the flap, microvascular transfer, closure of donor site and shaping the flap into a breast, unilateral ♀
⊘ S2070	Cystourethroscopy, with ureteroscopy and/or pyeloscopy; with endoscopic laser treatment of ureteral calculi (includes ureteral catheterization)
⊘ S2079	Laparoscopic esophagomyotomy (Heller type)
⊘ S2080	Laser-assisted uvulopalatoplasty (LAUP)
⊘ S2083	Adjustment of gastric band diameter via subcutaneous port by injection or aspiration of saline
⊘ S2095	Transcatheter occlusion or embolization for tumor destruction, percutaneous, any method, using yttrium-90 microspheres
⊘ S2102	Islet cell tissue transplant from pancreas; allogeneic
⊘ S2103	Adrenal tissue transplant to brain
⊘ S2107	Adoptive immunotherapy i.e. development of specific anti-tumor reactivity (e.g., tumor-infiltrating lymphocyte therapy) per course of treatment

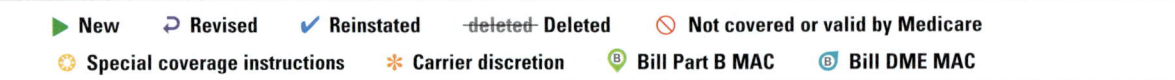

TEMPORARY NATIONAL CODES ESTABLISHED BY PRIVATE PAYERS

⊘ S2112	Arthroscopy, knee, surgical for harvesting of cartilage (chondrocyte cells)
⊘ S2115	Osteotomy, periacetabular, with internal fixation
⊘ S2117	Arthroereisis, subtalar
⊘ S2118	Metal-on-metal total hip resurfacing, including acetabular and femoral components
⊘ S2120	Low density lipoprotein (LDL) apheresis using heparin-induced extracorporeal LDL precipitation
⊘ S2140	Cord blood harvesting for transplantation, allogeneic
⊘ S2142	Cord blood-derived stem cell transplantation, allogeneic
⊘ S2150	Bone marrow or blood-derived stem cells (peripheral or umbilical), allogeneic or autologous, harvesting, transplantation, and related complications; including: pheresis and cell preparation/storage; marrow ablative therapy; drugs, supplies, hospitalization with outpatient follow-up; medical/surgical, diagnostic, emergency, and rehabilitative services; and the number of days of pre- and post-transplant care in the global definition
⊘ S2152	Solid organ(s), complete or segmental, single organ or combination of organs; deceased or living donor(s), procurement, transplantation, and related complications; including: drugs; supplies; hospitalization with outpatient follow-up; medical/surgical, diagnostic, emergency, and rehabilitative services, and the number of days of pre- and post-transplant care in the global definition
⊘ S2202	Echosclerotherapy
🎖⊘ S2205	Minimally invasive direct coronary artery bypass surgery involving mini-thoracotomy or mini-sternotomy surgery, performed under direct vision; using arterial graft(s), single coronary arterial graft
🎖⊘ S2206	Minimally invasive direct coronary artery bypass surgery involving mini-thoracotomy or mini-sternotomy surgery, performed under direct vision; using arterial graft(s), two coronary arterial grafts
🎖⊘ S2207	Minimally invasive direct coronary artery bypass surgery involving mini-thoracotomy or mini-sternotomy surgery, performed under direct vision; using venous graft only, single coronary venous graft
🎖⊘ S2208	Minimally invasive direct coronary artery bypass surgery involving mini-thoracotomy or mini-sternotomy surgery, performed under direct vision; using single arterial and venous graft(s), single venous graft
🎖⊘ S2209	Minimally invasive direct coronary artery bypass surgery involving mini-thoracotomy or mini-sternotomy surgery, performed under direct vision; using two arterial grafts and single venous graft
⊘ S2225	Myringotomy, laser-assisted
⊘ S2230	Implantation of magnetic component of semi-implantable hearing device on ossicles in middle ear
⊘ S2235	Implantation of auditory brain stem implant
⊘ S2260	Induced abortion, 17 to 24 weeks ♀
⊘ S2265	Induced abortion, 25 to 28 weeks ♀
⊘ S2266	Induced abortion, 29 to 31 weeks ♀
⊘ S2267	Induced abortion, 32 weeks or greater ♀
⊘ S2300	Arthroscopy, shoulder, surgical; with thermally-induced capsulorrhaphy
⊘ S2325	Hip core decompression
	Coding Clinic: 2017, Q3, P1
⊘ S2340	Chemodenervation of abductor muscle(s) of vocal cord
⊘ S2341	Chemodenervation of adductor muscle(s) of vocal cord
⊘ S2342	Nasal endoscopy for post-operative debridement following functional endoscopic sinus surgery, nasal and/or sinus cavity(s), unilateral or bilateral
⊘ S2348	Decompression procedure, percutaneous, of nucleus pulpous of intervertebral disc, using radiofrequency energy, single or multiple levels, lumbar
⊘ S2350	Diskectomy, anterior, with decompression of spinal cord and/or nerve root(s), including osteophytectomy; lumbar, single interspace

---

🎖 MIPS   **Qp** Quantity Physician   **Qh** Quantity Hospital   ♀ Female only
♂ Male only   **A** Age   ♿ DMEPOS   A2-Z3 ASC Payment Indicator   A-Y ASC Status Indicator   *Coding Clinic*

⊘	**S2351**	Diskectomy, anterior, with decompression of spinal cord and/or nerve root(s) including osteophytectomy; lumbar, each additional interspace (list separately in addition to code for primary procedure)		
⊘	**S2400**	Repair, congenital diaphragmatic hernia in the fetus using temporary tracheal occlusion, procedure performed in utero ♀ Ⓐ		
⊘	**S2401**	Repair, urinary tract obstruction in the fetus, procedure performed in utero ♀ Ⓐ		
⊘	**S2402**	Repair, congenital cystic adenomatoid malformation in the fetus, procedure performed in utero ♀ Ⓐ		
⊘	**S2403**	Repair, extralobar pulmonary sequestration in the fetus, procedure performed in utero ♀ Ⓐ		
⊘	**S2404**	Repair, myelomeningocele in the fetus, procedure performed in utero ♀ Ⓐ		
⊘	**S2405**	Repair of sacrococcygeal teratoma in the fetus, procedure performed in utero ♀ Ⓐ		
⊘	**S2409**	Repair, congenital malformation of fetus, procedure performed in utero, not otherwise classified ♀ Ⓐ		
⊘	**S2411**	Fetoscopic laser therapy for treatment of twin-to-twin transfusion syndrome Ⓐ		
⊘	**S2900**	Surgical techniques requiring use of robotic surgical system (list separately in addition to code for primary procedure)		
		Coding Clinic: 2010, Q2, P6		
⊘	**S3000**	Diabetic indicator; retinal eye exam, dilated, bilateral		
⊘	**S3005**	Performance measurement, evaluation of patient self assessment, depression		
⊘	**S3600**	STAT laboratory request (situations other than S3601)		
⊘	**S3601**	Emergency STAT laboratory charge for patient who is homebound or residing in a nursing facility		
✳	**S3620**	Newborn metabolic screening panel, includes test kit, postage and the laboratory tests specified by the state for inclusion in this panel (e.g., galactose; hemoglobin, electrophoresis; hydroxyprogesterone, 17-D; phenylalanine (PKU); and thyroxine, total) Ⓐ		
⊘	**S3630**	Eosinophil count, blood, direct		
⊘	**S3645**	HIV-1 antibody testing of oral mucosal transudate		
⊘	**S3650**	Saliva test, hormone level; during menopause ♀		
⊘	**S3652**	Saliva test, hormone level; to assess preterm labor risk ♀		
⊘	**S3655**	Antisperm antibodies test (immunobead) ♀		
⊘	**S3708**	Gastrointestinal fat absorption study		
⊘	**S3722**	Dose optimization by area under the curve (AUC) analysis, for infusional 5-fluorouracil		

Genetic Testing

⊘	**S3800**	Genetic testing for amyotrophic lateral sclerosis (ALS)
⊘	**S3840**	DNA analysis for germline mutations of the RET proto-oncogene for susceptibility to multiple endocrine neoplasia type 2
⊘	**S3841**	Genetic testing for retinoblastoma
⊘	**S3842**	Genetic testing for von Hippel-Lindau disease
⊘	**S3844**	DNA analysis of the connexin 26 gene (GJB2) for susceptibility to congenital, profound deafness
⊘	**S3845**	Genetic testing for alpha-thalassemia
⊘	**S3846**	Genetic testing for hemoglobin E beta-thalassemia
⊘	**S3849**	Genetic testing for Niemann-Pick disease
⊘	**S3850**	Genetic testing for sickle cell anemia
⊘	**S3852**	DNA analysis for APOE epilson 4 allele for susceptibility to Alzheimer's disease
⊘	**S3853**	Genetic testing for myotonic muscular dystrophy
⊘	**S3854**	Gene expression profiling panel for use in the management of breast cancer treatment ♀
⊘	**S3861**	Genetic testing, sodium channel, voltage-gated, type V, alpha subunit (SCN5A) and variants for suspected Brugada syndrome
⊘	**S3865**	Comprehensive gene sequence analysis for hypertrophic cardiomyopathy
⊘	**S3866**	Genetic analysis for a specific gene mutation for hypertrophic cardiomyopathy (HCM) in an individual with a known HCM mutation in the family
⊘	**S3870**	Comparative genomic hybridization (CGH) microarray testing for developmental delay, autism spectrum disorder and/or intellectual disability

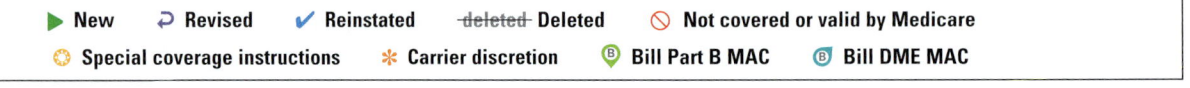

▶ New ↺ Revised ✓ Reinstated ~~deleted~~ Deleted ⊘ Not covered or valid by Medicare
✳ Special coverage instructions ✱ Carrier discretion Ⓑ Bill Part B MAC Ⓑ Bill DME MAC

TEMPORARY NATIONAL CODES ESTABLISHED BY PRIVATE PAYERS

Other Tests

- ⊘ **S3900** Surface electromyography (EMG)
- ⊘ **S3902** Ballistrocardiogram
- ⊘ **S3904** Masters two step
  Bill on paper. Requires a report.

Obstetric and Fertility Services

- ⊘ **S4005** Interim labor facility global (labor occurring but not resulting in delivery) ♀
- ⊘ **S4011** In vitro fertilization; including but not limited to identification and incubation of mature oocytes, fertilization with sperm, incubation of embryo(s), and subsequent visualization for determination of development ♀
- ⊘ **S4013** Complete cycle, gamete intrafallopian transfer (GIFT), case rate ♀
- ⊘ **S4014** Complete cycle, zygote intrafallopian transfer (ZIFT), case rate ♀
- ⊘ **S4015** Complete in vitro fertilization cycle, not otherwise specified, case rate ♀
- ⊘ **S4016** Frozen in vitro fertilization cycle, case rate ♀
- ⊘ **S4017** Incomplete cycle, treatment cancelled prior to stimulation, case rate ♀
- ⊘ **S4018** Frozen embryo transfer procedure cancelled before transfer, case rate ♀
- ⊘ **S4020** In vitro fertilization procedure cancelled before aspiration, case rate ♀
- ⊘ **S4021** In vitro fertilization procedure cancelled after aspiration, case rate ♀
- ⊘ **S4022** Assisted oocyte fertilization, case rate ♀
- ⊘ **S4023** Donor egg cycle, incomplete, case rate ♀
- ▶ ⊘ **S4024** Air polymer-type a intrauterine foam, per study dose ♀
- ⊘ **S4025** Donor services for in vitro fertilization (sperm or embryo), case rate
- ⊘ **S4026** Procurement of donor sperm from sperm bank ♂
- ⊘ **S4027** Storage of previously frozen embryos ♀
- ⊘ **S4028** Microsurgical epididymal sperm aspiration (MESA) ♂
- ⊘ **S4030** Sperm procurement and cryopreservation services; initial visit ♂
- ⊘ **S4031** Sperm procurement and cryopreservation services; subsequent visit ♂

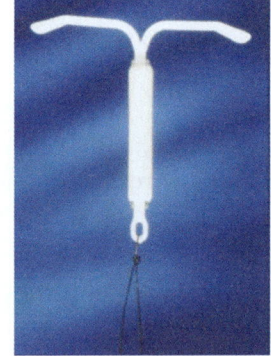

Figure 50 IUD.

- ⊘ **S4035** Stimulated intrauterine insemination (IUI), case rate ♀
- ⊘ **S4037** Cryopreserved embryo transfer, case rate ♀
- ⊘ **S4040** Monitoring and storage of cryopreserved embryos, per 30 days ♀
- ⊘ **S4042** Management of ovulation induction (interpretation of diagnostic tests and studies, non-face-to-face medical management of the patient), per cycle ♀
- ⊘ **S4981** Insertion of levonorgestrel-releasing intrauterine system ♀
- ~~S4988~~ ~~Penile contracture device, manual, greater than 3 lbs traction force~~
- ⊘ **S4989** Contraceptive intrauterine device (e.g., Progestasert IUD), including implants and supplies ♀

Therapeutic Substances and Medications

- ⊘ **S4990** Nicotine patches, legend
- ⊘ **S4991** Nicotine patches, non-legend
- ⊘ **S4993** Contraceptive pills for birth control ♀
  Only billed by Family Planning Clinics
- ⊘ **S4995** Smoking cessation gum
- ⊘ **S5000** Prescription drug, generic
- ⊘ **S5001** Prescription drug, brand name
- ⊘ **S5010** 5% dextrose and 0.45% normal saline, 1000 ml
- ⊘ **S5012** 5% dextrose with potassium chloride, 1000 ml
- ⊘ **S5013** 5% dextrose/0.45% normal saline with potassium chloride and magnesium sulfate, 1000 ml
- ⊘ **S5014** 5% dextrose/0.45% normal saline with potassium chloride and magnesium sulfate, 1500 ml

---

MIPS | **Qp** Quantity Physician | **Qh** Quantity Hospital | ♀ Female only
♂ Male only | **A** Age | & DMEPOS | A2-Z3 ASC Payment Indicator | A-Y ASC Status Indicator | Coding Clinic

Home Care Services

- ⊘ **S5035** Home infusion therapy, routine service of infusion device (e.g., pump maintenance)
- ⊘ **S5036** Home infusion therapy, repair of infusion device (e.g., pump repair)
- ⊘ **S5100** Day care services, adult; per 15 minutes Ⓐ
- ⊘ **S5101** Day care services, adult; per half day Ⓐ
- ⊘ **S5102** Day care services, adult; per diem Ⓐ
- ⊘ **S5105** Day care services, center-based; services not included in program fee, per diem
- ⊘ **S5108** Home care training to home care client, per 15 minutes
- ⊘ **S5109** Home care training to home care client, per session
- ⊘ **S5110** Home care training, family; per 15 minutes
- ⊘ **S5111** Home care training, family; per session
- ⊘ **S5115** Home care training, non-family; per 15 minutes
- ⊘ **S5116** Home care training, non-family; per session
- ⊘ **S5120** Chore services; per 15 minutes
- ⊘ **S5121** Chore services; per diem
- ⊘ **S5125** Attendant care services; per 15 minutes
- ⊘ **S5126** Attendant care services; per diem
- ⊘ **S5130** Homemaker service, NOS; per 15 minutes
- ⊘ **S5131** Homemaker service, NOS; per diem
- ⊘ **S5135** Companion care, adult (e.g., IADL/ADL); per 15 minutes Ⓐ
- ⊘ **S5136** Companion care, adult (e.g., IADL/ADL); per diem Ⓐ
- ⊘ **S5140** Foster care, adult; per diem Ⓐ
- ⊘ **S5141** Foster care, adult; per month Ⓐ
- ⊘ **S5145** Foster care, therapeutic, child; per diem Ⓐ
- ⊘ **S5146** Foster care, therapeutic, child; per month Ⓐ
- ⊘ **S5150** Unskilled respite care, not hospice; per 15 minutes
- ⊘ **S5151** Unskilled respite care, not hospice; per diem
- ⊘ **S5160** Emergency response system; installation and testing
- ⊘ **S5161** Emergency response system; service fee, per month (excludes installation and testing)
- ⊘ **S5162** Emergency response system; purchase only
- ⊘ **S5165** Home modifications; per service
- ⊘ **S5170** Home delivered meals, including preparation; per meal
- ⊘ **S5175** Laundry service, external, professional; per order
- ⊘ **S5180** Home health respiratory therapy, initial evaluation
- ⊘ **S5181** Home health respiratory therapy, NOS, per diem
- ⊘ **S5185** Medication reminder service, non-face-to-face; per month
- ⊘ **S5190** Wellness assessment, performed by non-physician
- ⊘ **S5199** Personal care item, NOS, each

Home Infusion Therapy

- ⊘ **S5497** Home infusion therapy, catheter care/maintenance, not otherwise classified; includes administrative services, professional pharmacy services, care coordination, and all necessary supplies and equipment (drugs and nursing visits coded separately), per diem
- ⊘ **S5498** Home infusion therapy, catheter care/maintenance, simple (single lumen), includes administrative services, professional pharmacy services, care coordination and all necessary supplies and equipment, (drugs and nursing visits coded separately), per diem
- ⊘ **S5501** Home infusion therapy, catheter care/maintenance, complex (more than one lumen), includes administrative services, professional pharmacy services, care coordination, and all necessary supplies and equipment (drugs and nursing visits coded separately), per diem
- ⊘ **S5502** Home infusion therapy, catheter care/maintenance, implanted access device, includes administrative services, professional pharmacy services, care coordination, and all necessary supplies and equipment, (drugs and nursing visits coded separately), per diem (use this code for interim maintenance of vascular access not currently in use)
- ⊘ **S5517** Home infusion therapy, all supplies necessary for restoration of catheter patency or declotting
- ⊘ **S5518** Home infusion therapy, all supplies necessary for catheter repair

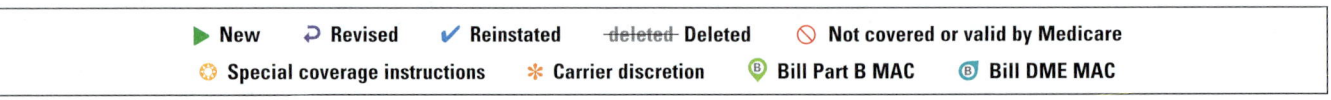

TEMPORARY NATIONAL CODES ESTABLISHED BY PRIVATE PAYERS

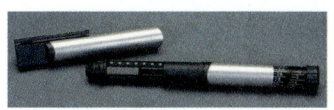

Figure 51 Nova pen.

⊘ S5520 Home infusion therapy, all supplies (including catheter) necessary for a peripherally inserted central venous catheter (PICC) line insertion
Bill on paper. Requires a report.

⊘ S5521 Home infusion therapy, all supplies (including catheter) necessary for a midline catheter insertion

⊘ S5522 Home infusion therapy, insertion of peripherally inserted central venous catheter (PICC), nursing services only (no supplies or catheter included)

⊘ S5523 Home infusion therapy, insertion of midline central venous catheter, nursing services only (no supplies or catheter included)

Insulin Services

⊘ S5550 Insulin, rapid onset, 5 units
⊘ S5551 Insulin, most rapid onset (Lispro or Aspart); 5 units
⊘ S5552 Insulin, intermediate acting (NPH or Lente); 5 units
⊘ S5553 Insulin, long acting; 5 units
⊘ S5560 Insulin delivery device, reusable pen; 1.5 ml size
⊘ S5561 Insulin delivery device, reusable pen; 3 ml size
⊘ S5565 Insulin cartridge for use in insulin delivery device other than pump; 150 units
⊘ S5566 Insulin cartridge for use in insulin delivery device other than pump; 300 units
⊘ S5570 Insulin delivery device, disposable pen (including insulin); 1.5 ml size
⊘ S5571 Insulin delivery device, disposable pen (including insulin); 3 ml size

Imaging

⊘ S8030 Scleral application of tantalum ring(s) for localization of lesions for proton beam therapy
⊘ S8035 Magnetic source imaging
⊘ S8037 Magnetic resonance cholangiopancreatography (MRCP)
⊘ S8040 Topographic brain mapping
⊘ S8042 Magnetic resonance imaging (MRI), low-field
⊘ S8055 Ultrasound guidance for multifetal pregnancy reduction(s), technical component (only to be used when the physician doing the reduction procedure does not perform the ultrasound, guidance is included in the CPT code for multifetal pregnancy reduction - 59866) ♀
⊘ S8080 Scintimammography (radioimmunoscintigraphy of the breast), unilateral, including supply of radiopharmaceutical ♀
⊘ S8085 Fluorine-18 fluorodeoxyglucose (F-18 FDG) imaging using dual-head coincidence detection system (non-dedicated PET scan)
⊘ S8092 Electron beam computed tomography (also known as ultrafast CT, cine CT)

Assistive Breathing Supplies

⊘ S8096 Portable peak flow meter
⊘ S8097 Asthma kit (including but not limited to portable peak expiratory flow meter, instructional video, brochure, and/or spacer)
⊘ S8100 Holding chamber or spacer for use with an inhaler or nebulizer; without mask
⊘ S8101 Holding chamber or spacer for use with an inhaler or nebulizer; with mask
⊘ S8110 Peak expiratory flow rate (physician services)
⊘ S8120 Oxygen contents, gaseous, 1 unit equals 1 cubic foot
⊘ S8121 Oxygen contents, liquid, 1 unit equals 1 pound
⊘ S8130 Interferential current stimulator, 2 channel
⊘ S8131 Interferential current stimulator, 4 channel
⊘ S8185 Flutter device
⊘ S8186 Swivel adapter
⊘ S8189 Tracheostomy supply, not otherwise classified
⊘ S8210 Mucus trap

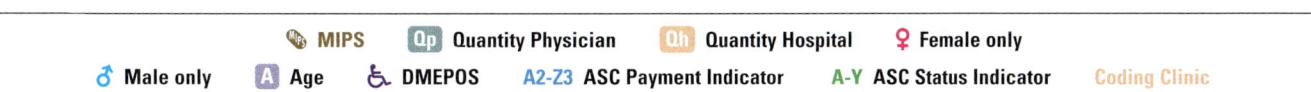

Miscellaneous Supplies and Services

- ⊘ **S8265** Haberman feeder for cleft lip/palate
- ⊘ **S8270** Enuresis alarm, using auditory buzzer and/or vibration device
- ⊘ **S8301** Infection control supplies, not otherwise specified
- ⊘ **S8415** Supplies for home delivery of infant [A]
- ⊘ **S8420** Gradient pressure aid (sleeve and glove combination), custom made
- ⊘ **S8421** Gradient pressure aid (sleeve and glove combination), ready made
- ⊘ **S8422** Gradient pressure aid (sleeve), custom made, medium weight
- ⊘ **S8423** Gradient pressure aid (sleeve), custom made, heavy weight
- ⊘ **S8424** Gradient pressure aid (sleeve), ready made
- ⊘ **S8425** Gradient pressure aid (glove), custom made, medium weight
- ⊘ **S8426** Gradient pressure aid (glove), custom made, heavy weight
- ⊘ **S8427** Gradient pressure aid (glove), ready made
- ⊘ **S8428** Gradient pressure aid (gauntlet), ready made
- ⊘ **S8429** Gradient pressure exterior wrap
- ⊘ **S8430** Padding for compression bandage, roll
- ⊘ **S8431** Compression bandage, roll
- ⊘ **S8450** Splint, prefabricated, digit (specify digit by use of modifier)
- ⊘ **S8451** Splint, prefabricated, wrist or ankle
- ⊘ **S8452** Splint, prefabricated, elbow
- ⊘ **S8460** Camisole, post-mastectomy
- ⊘ **S8490** Insulin syringes (100 syringes, any size)
- ⊘ **S8930** Electrical stimulation of auricular acupuncture points; each 15 minutes of personal one-on-one contact with the patient
- ⊘ **S8940** Equestrian/Hippotherapy, per session
- ⊘ **S8948** Application of a modality (requiring constant provider attendance) to one or more areas; low-level laser; each 15 minutes
- ⊘ **S8950** Complex lymphedema therapy, each 15 minutes
- ⊘ **S8990** Physical or manipulative therapy performed for maintenance rather than restoration
- ⊘ **S8999** Resuscitation bag (for use by patient on artificial respiration during power failure or other catastrophic event)
- ⊘ **S9001** Home uterine monitor with or without associated nursing services ♀
- ⊘ **S9002** Intra-vaginal motion sensor system, provides biofeedback for pelvic floor muscle rehabilitation device
- ⊘ **S9007** Ultrafiltration monitor
- ⊘ **S9024** Paranasal sinus ultrasound
- ⊘ **S9025** Omnicardiogram/cardiointegram
- ⊘ **S9034** Extracorporeal shockwave lithotripsy for gall stones (if performed with ERCP, use 43265)
- ⊘ **S9055** Procuren or other growth factor preparation to promote wound healing
- ⊘ **S9056** Coma stimulation per diem
- ⊘ **S9061** Home administration of aerosolized drug therapy (e.g., pentamidine); administrative services, professional pharmacy services, care coordination, all necessary supplies and equipment (drugs and nursing visits coded separately), per diem
- ⊘ **S9083** Global fee urgent care centers
- ⊘ **S9088** Services provided in an urgent care center (list in addition to code for service)
- ⊘ **S9090** Vertebral axial decompression, per session
- ⊘ **S9097** Home visit for wound care
- ⊘ **S9098** Home visit, phototherapy services (e.g., Bili-Lite), including equipment rental, nursing services, blood draw, supplies, and other services, per diem
- ⊘ **S9110** Telemonitoring of patient in their home, including all necessary equipment; computer system, connections, and software; maintenance; patient education and support; per month
- ⊘ **S9117** Back school, per visit
- ⊘ **S9122** Home health aide or certified nurse assistant, providing care in the home; per hour
- ⊘ **S9123** Nursing care, in the home; by registered nurse, per hour (use for general nursing care only, not to be used when CPT codes 99500-99602 can be used)
- ⊘ **S9124** Nursing care, in the home; by licensed practical nurse, per hour
- ⊘ **S9125** Respite care, in the home, per diem
- ⊘ **S9126** Hospice care, in the home, per diem
- ⊘ **S9127** Social work visit, in the home, per diem
- ⊘ **S9128** Speech therapy, in the home, per diem

▶ New   ⮂ Revised   ✔ Reinstated   ~~deleted~~ Deleted   ⊘ Not covered or valid by Medicare
✴ Special coverage instructions   ∗ Carrier discretion   🅑 Bill Part B MAC   🅑 Bill DME MAC

TEMPORARY NATIONAL CODES ESTABLISHED BY PRIVATE PAYERS

⊘ S9129 Occupational therapy, in the home, per diem

⊘ S9131 Physical therapy; in the home, per diem

⊘ S9140 Diabetic management program, follow-up visit to non-MD provider

⊘ S9141 Diabetic management program, follow-up visit to MD provider

⊘ S9145 Insulin pump initiation, instruction in initial use of pump (pump not included)

⊘ S9150 Evaluation by ocularist

⊘ S9152 Speech therapy, re-evaluation

Home Management of Pregnancy

⊘ S9208 Home management of preterm labor, including administrative services, professional pharmacy services, care coordination, and all necessary supplies or equipment (drugs and nursing visits coded separately), per diem (do not use this code with any home infusion per diem code) ♀

⊘ S9209 Home management of preterm premature rupture of membranes (PPROM), including administrative services, professional pharmacy services, care coordination, and all necessary supplies or equipment (drugs and nursing visits coded separately), per diem (do not use this code with any home infusion per diem code) ♀

⊘ S9211 Home management of gestational hypertension, includes administrative services, professional pharmacy services, care coordination, and all necessary supplies and equipment (drugs and nursing visits coded separately); per diem (do not use this code with any home infusion per diem code) ♀

⊘ S9212 Home management of postpartum hypertension, includes administrative services, professional pharmacy services, care coordination, and all necessary supplies and equipment (drugs and nursing visits coded separately); per diem (do not use this code with any home infusion per diem code) ♀

⊘ S9213 Home management of preeclampsia, includes administrative services, professional pharmacy services, care coordination, and all necessary supplies and equipment (drugs and nursing services coded separately); per diem (do not use this code with any home infusion per diem code) ♀

⊘ S9214 Home management of gestational diabetes, includes administrative services, professional pharmacy services, care coordination, and all necessary supplies and equipment (drugs and nursing visits coded separately); per diem (do not use this code with any home infusion per diem code) ♀

Home Infusion Therapy

⊘ S9325 Home infusion therapy, pain management infusion; administrative services, professional pharmacy services, care coordination, and all necessary supplies and equipment, (drugs and nursing visits coded separately), per diem (do not use this code with S9326, S9327 or S9328)

⊘ S9326 Home infusion therapy, continuous (twenty-four hours or more) pain management infusion; administrative services, professional pharmacy services, care coordination, and all necessary supplies and equipment (drugs and nursing visits coded separately), per diem

⊘ S9327 Home infusion therapy, intermittent (less than twenty-four hours) pain management infusion; administrative services, professional pharmacy services, care coordination, and all necessary supplies and equipment (drugs and nursing visits coded separately), per diem

⊘ S9328 Home infusion therapy, implanted pump pain management infusion; administrative services, professional pharmacy services, care coordination, and all necessary supplies and equipment (drugs and nursing visits coded separately), per diem

⊘ S9329 Home infusion therapy, chemotherapy infusion; administrative services, professional pharmacy services, care coordination, and all necessary supplies and equipment (drugs and nursing visits coded separately), per diem (do not use this code with S9330 or S9331)

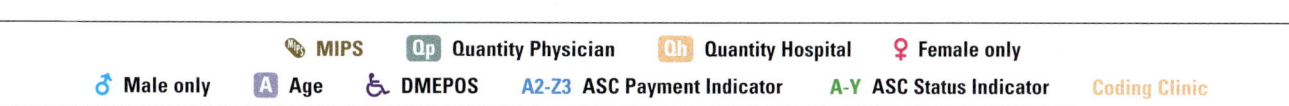

⊘	**S9330**	Home infusion therapy, continuous (twenty-four hours or more) chemotherapy infusion; administrative services, professional pharmacy services, care coordination, and all necessary supplies and equipment (drugs and nursing visits coded separately), per diem		

⊘ **S9330** Home infusion therapy, continuous (twenty-four hours or more) chemotherapy infusion; administrative services, professional pharmacy services, care coordination, and all necessary supplies and equipment (drugs and nursing visits coded separately), per diem

⊘ **S9331** Home infusion therapy, intermittent (less than twenty-four hours) chemotherapy infusion; administrative services, professional pharmacy services, care coordination, and all necessary supplies and equipment (drugs and nursing visits coded separately), per diem

⊘ **S9335** Home therapy, hemodialysis; administrative services, professional pharmacy services, care coordination, and all necessary supplies and equipment (drugs and nursing services coded separately), per diem

⊘ **S9336** Home infusion therapy, continuous anticoagulant infusion therapy (e.g., heparin), administrative services, professional pharmacy services, care coordination, and all necessary supplies and equipment (drugs and nursing visits coded separately), per diem

⊘ **S9338** Home infusion therapy, immunotherapy, administrative services, professional pharmacy services, care coordination, and all necessary supplies and equipment (drug and nursing visits coded separately), per diem

⊘ **S9339** Home therapy; peritoneal dialysis, administrative services, professional pharmacy services, care coordination and all necessary supplies and equipment (drugs and nursing visits coded separately), per diem

⊘ **S9340** Home therapy; enteral nutrition; administrative services, professional pharmacy services, care coordination, and all necessary supplies and equipment (enteral formula and nursing visits coded separately), per diem

⊘ **S9341** Home therapy; enteral nutrition via gravity; administrative services, professional pharmacy services, care coordination, and all necessary supplies and equipment (enteral formula and nursing visits coded separately), per diem

⊘ **S9342** Home therapy; enteral nutrition via pump; administrative services, professional pharmacy services, care coordination, and all necessary supplies and equipment (enteral formula and nursing visits coded separately), per diem

⊘ **S9343** Home therapy; enteral nutrition via bolus; administrative services, professional pharmacy services, care coordination, and all necessary supplies and equipment (enteral formula and nursing visits coded separately), per diem

⊘ **S9345** Home infusion therapy, anti-hemophilic agent infusion therapy (e.g., Factor VIII); administrative services, professional pharmacy services, care coordination, and all necessary supplies and equipment (drugs and nursing visits coded separately), per diem

⊘ **S9346** Home infusion therapy, alpha-1-proteinase inhibitor (e.g., Prolastin); administrative services, professional pharmacy services, care coordination, and all necessary supplies and equipment (drugs and nursing visits coded separately), per diem

⊘ **S9347** Home infusion therapy, uninterrupted, long-term, controlled rate intravenous or subcutaneous infusion therapy (e.g., Epoprostenol); administrative services, professional pharmacy services, care coordination, and all necessary supplies and equipment (drugs and nursing visits coded separately), per diem

⊘ **S9348** Home infusion therapy, sympathomimetic/inotropic agent infusion therapy (e.g., Dobutamine); administrative services, professional pharmacy services, care coordination, all necessary supplies and equipment (drugs and nursing visits coded separately), per diem

⊘ **S9349** Home infusion therapy, tocolytic infusion therapy; administrative services, professional pharmacy services, care coordination, and all necessary supplies and equipment (drugs and nursing visits coded separately), per diem

⊘ **S9351** Home infusion therapy, continuous or intermittent anti-emetic infusion therapy; administrative services, professional pharmacy services, care coordination, and all necessary supplies and equipment (drugs and visits coded separately), per diem

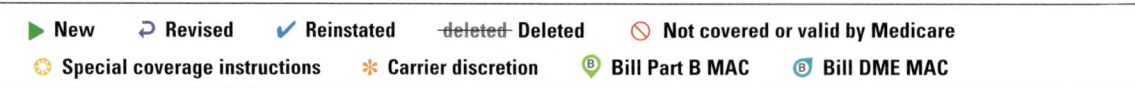

▶ New   ⮂ Revised   ✔ Reinstated   ~~deleted~~ Deleted   ⊘ Not covered or valid by Medicare   ✦ Special coverage instructions   ∗ Carrier discretion   🅱 Bill Part B MAC   🅱 Bill DME MAC

TEMPORARY NATIONAL CODES ESTABLISHED BY PRIVATE PAYERS

⊘ **S9353** Home infusion therapy, continuous insulin infusion therapy; administrative services, professional pharmacy services, care coordination, and all necessary supplies and equipment (drugs and nursing visits coded separately), per diem

⊘ **S9355** Home infusion therapy, chelation therapy; administrative services, professional pharmacy services, care coordination, and all necessary supplies and equipment (drugs and nursing visits coded separately), per diem

⊘ **S9357** Home infusion therapy, enzyme replacement intravenous therapy (e.g., Imiglucerase); administrative services, professional pharmacy services, care coordination, and all necessary supplies and equipment (drugs and nursing visits coded separately), per diem

⊘ **S9359** Home infusion therapy, anti-tumor necrosis factor intravenous therapy (e.g., Infliximab); administrative services, professional pharmacy services, care coordination, and all necessary supplies and equipment (drugs and nursing visits coded separately), per diem

⊘ **S9361** Home infusion therapy, diuretic intravenous therapy; administrative services, professional pharmacy services, care coordination, and all necessary supplies and equipment (drugs and nursing visits coded separately), per diem

⊘ **S9363** Home infusion therapy, anti-spasmotic therapy; administrative services, professional pharmacy services, care coordination, and all necessary supplies and equipment (drugs and nursing visits coded separately), per diem

⊘ **S9364** Home infusion therapy, total parenteral nutrition (TPN); administrative services, professional pharmacy services, care coordination, and all necessary supplies and equipment including standard TPN formula (lipids, specialty amino acid formulas, drugs other than in standard formula, and nursing visits coded separately) per diem (do not use with home infusion codes S9365-S9368 using daily volume scales)

⊘ **S9365** Home infusion therapy, total parenteral nutrition (TPN); one liter per day, administrative services, professional pharmacy services, care coordination, and all necessary supplies and equipment including standard TPN formula (lipids, specialty amino acid formulas, drugs other than in standard formula and nursing visits coded separately), per diem

⊘ **S9366** Home infusion therapy, total parenteral nutrition (TPN); more than one liter but no more than two liters per day, administrative services, professional pharmacy services, care coordination, and all necessary supplies and equipment including standard TPN formula (lipids, specialty amino acid formulas, drugs other than in standard formula and nursing visits coded separately), per diem

⊘ **S9367** Home infusion therapy, total parenteral nutrition (TPN); more than two liters but no more than three liters per day, administrative services, professional pharmacy services, care coordination, and all necessary supplies and equipment including standard TPN formula (lipids, specialty amino acid formulas, drugs other than in standard formula and nursing visits coded separately), per diem

⊘ **S9368** Home infusion therapy, total parenteral nutrition (TPN); more than three liters per day, administrative services, professional pharmacy services, care coordination, and all necessary supplies and equipment (including standard TPN formula; lipids, specialty amino acid formulas, drugs other than in standard formula and nursing visits coded separately), per diem

⊘ **S9370** Home therapy, intermittent anti-emetic injection therapy; administrative services, professional pharmacy services, care coordination, and all necessary supplies and equipment (drugs and nursing visits coded separately), per diem

⊘ **S9372** Home therapy; intermittent anticoagulant injection therapy (e.g., heparin); administrative services, professional pharmacy services, care coordination, and all necessary supplies and equipment (drugs and nursing visits coded separately), per diem (do not use this code for flushing of infusion devices with heparin to maintain patency)

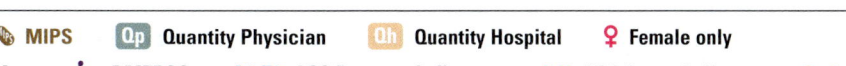

🍥 MIPS Qp Quantity Physician Qh Quantity Hospital ♀ Female only
♂ Male only A Age ♿ DMEPOS A2-Z3 ASC Payment Indicator A-Y ASC Status Indicator Coding Clinic

⊘ S9373	Home infusion therapy, hydration therapy; administrative services, professional pharmacy services, care coordination, and all necessary supplies and equipment (drugs and nursing visits coded separately), per diem (do not use with hydration therapy codes S9374-S9377 using daily volume scales)
⊘ S9374	Home infusion therapy, hydration therapy; one liter per day, administrative services, professional pharmacy services, care coordination, and all necessary supplies and equipment (drugs and nursing visits coded separately), per diem
⊘ S9375	Home infusion therapy, hydration therapy; more than one liter but no more than two liters per day, administrative services, professional pharmacy services, care coordination, and all necessary supplies and equipment (drugs and nursing visits coded separately), per diem
⊘ S9376	Home infusion therapy, hydration therapy; more than two liters but no more than three liters per day, administrative services, professional pharmacy services, care coordination, and all necessary supplies and equipment (drugs and nursing visits coded separately), per diem
⊘ S9377	Home infusion therapy, hydration therapy; more than three liters per day, administrative services, professional pharmacy services, care coordination, and all necessary supplies (drugs and nursing visits coded separately), per diem
⊘ S9379	Home infusion therapy, infusion therapy, not otherwise classified; administrative services, professional pharmacy services, care coordination, and all necessary supplies and equipment (drugs and nursing visits coded separately), per diem

Miscellaneous Supplies and Services

⊘ S9381	Delivery or service to high risk areas requiring escort or extra protection, per visit
⊘ S9401	Anticoagulation clinic, inclusive of all services except laboratory tests, per session
⊘ S9430	Pharmacy compounding and dispensing services
⊘ S9432	Medical foods for non-inborn errors of metabolism
⊘ S9433	Medical food nutritionally complete, administered orally, providing 100% of nutritional intake
⊘ S9434	Modified solid food supplements for inborn errors of metabolism
⊘ S9435	Medical foods for inborn errors of metabolism
⊘ S9436	Childbirth preparation/Lamaze classes, non-physician provider, per session ♀
⊘ S9437	Childbirth refresher classes, non-physician provider, per session ♀
⊘ S9438	Cesarean birth classes, non-physician provider, per session ♀
⊘ S9439	VBAC (vaginal birth after cesarean) classes, non-physician provider, per session ♀
⊘ S9441	Asthma education, non-physician provider, per session
⊘ S9442	Birthing classes, non-physician provider, per session ♀
⊘ S9443	Lactation classes, non-physician provider, per session ♀
⊘ S9444	Parenting classes, non-physician provider, per session
⊘ S9445	Patient education, not otherwise classified, non-physician provider, individual, per session
⊘ S9446	Patient education, not otherwise classified, non-physician provider, group, per session
⊘ S9447	Infant safety (including CPR) classes, non-physician provider, per session
⊘ S9449	Weight management classes, non-physician provider, per session
⊘ S9451	Exercise classes, non-physician provider, per session
⊘ S9452	Nutrition classes, non-physician provider, per session
⊘ S9453	Smoking cessation classes, non-physician provider, per session
⊘ S9454	Stress management classes, non-physician provider, per session
⊘ S9455	Diabetic management program, group session
⊘ S9460	Diabetic management program, nurse visit
⊘ S9465	Diabetic management program, dietitian visit
⊘ S9470	Nutritional counseling, dietitian visit
⊘ S9472	Cardiac rehabilitation program, non-physician provider, per diem
⊘ S9473	Pulmonary rehabilitation program, non-physician provider, per diem

▶ New ⟲ Revised ✔ Reinstated ~~deleted~~ Deleted ⊘ Not covered or valid by Medicare
◉ Special coverage instructions ✱ Carrier discretion Ⓑ Bill Part B MAC Ⓓ Bill DME MAC

TEMPORARY NATIONAL CODES ESTABLISHED BY PRIVATE PAYERS

⊘ **S9474** Enterostomal therapy by a registered nurse certified in enterostomal therapy, per diem

⊘ **S9475** Ambulatory setting substance abuse treatment or detoxification services, per diem

⊘ **S9476** Vestibular rehabilitation program, non-physician provider, per diem

⊘ **S9480** Intensive outpatient psychiatric services, per diem

⊘ **S9482** Family stabilization services, per 15 minutes

⊘ **S9484** Crisis intervention mental health services, per hour

⊘ **S9485** Crisis intervention mental health services, per diem

Home Therapy Services

⊘ **S9490** Home infusion therapy, corticosteroid infusion; administrative services, professional pharmacy services, care coordination, and all necessary supplies and equipment (drugs and nursing visits coded separately), per diem

⊘ **S9494** Home infusion therapy, antibiotic, antiviral, or antifungal therapy; administrative services, professional pharmacy services, care coordination, and all necessary supplies and equipment (drugs and nursing visits coded separately) per diem (do not use this code with home infusion codes for hourly dosing schedules S9497-S9504)

⊘ **S9497** Home infusion therapy, antibiotic, antiviral, or antifungal therapy; once every 3 hours; administrative services, professional pharmacy services, care coordination, and all necessary supplies and equipment (drugs and nursing visits coded separately), per diem

⊘ **S9500** Home infusion therapy, antibiotic, antiviral, or antifungal therapy; once every 24 hours; administrative services, professional pharmacy services, care coordination, and all necessary supplies and equipment (drugs and nursing visits coded separately), per diem

⊘ **S9501** Home infusion therapy, antibiotic, antiviral, or antifungal therapy; once every 12 hours; administrative services, professional pharmacy services, care coordination, and all necessary supplies and equipment (drugs and nursing visits coded separately), per diem

⊘ **S9502** Home infusion therapy, antibiotic, antiviral, or antifungal therapy; once every 8 hours, administrative services, professional pharmacy services, care coordination, and all necessary supplies and equipment (drugs and nursing visits coded separately), per diem

⊘ **S9503** Home infusion therapy, antibiotic, antiviral, or antifungal; once every 6 hours; administrative services, professional pharmacy services, care coordination, and all necessary supplies and equipment (drugs and nursing visits coded separately), per diem

⊘ **S9504** Home infusion therapy, antibiotic, antiviral, or antifungal; once every 4 hours; administrative services, professional pharmacy services, care coordination, and all necessary supplies and equipment (drugs and nursing visits coded separately), per diem

⊘ **S9529** Routine venipuncture for collection of specimen(s), single home bound, nursing home, or skilled nursing facility patient

⊘ **S9537** Home therapy; hematopoietic hormone injection therapy (e.g., erythropoietin, G-CSF, GM-CSF); administrative services, professional pharmacy services, care coordination, and all necessary supplies and equipment (drugs and nursing visits coded separately), per diem

⊘ **S9538** Home transfusion of blood product(s); administrative services, professional pharmacy services, care coordination, and all necessary supplies and equipment (blood products, drugs, and nursing visits coded separately), per diem

⊘ **S9542** Home injectable therapy; not otherwise classified, including administrative services, professional pharmacy services, care coordination, and all necessary supplies and equipment (drugs and nursing visits coded separately), per diem

⊘ **S9558** Home injectable therapy; growth hormone, including administrative services, professional pharmacy services, care coordination, and all necessary supplies and equipment (drugs and nursing visits coded separately), per diem

⊘ S9559	Home injectable therapy; interferon, including administrative services, professional pharmacy services, care coordination, and all necessary supplies and equipment (drugs and nursing visits coded separately), per diem
⊘ S9560	Home injectable therapy; hormonal therapy (e.g., Leuprolide, Goserelin), including administrative services, professional pharmacy services, care coordination, and all necessary supplies and equipment (drugs and nursing visits coded separately), per diem
⊘ S9562	Home injectable therapy, palivizumab, or other monoclonal antibody for rsv, including administrative services, professional pharmacy services, care coordination, and all necessary supplies and equipment (drugs and nursing visits coded separately), per diem
⊘ S9563	Home injectable therapy, immunotherapy, including administrative services, professional pharmacy services, care coordination, and all necessary supplies and equipment (drugs and nursing visits coded separately), per diem
⊘ S9590	Home therapy, irrigation therapy (e.g., sterile irrigation of an organ or anatomical cavity); including administrative services, professional pharmacy services, care coordination, and all necessary supplies and equipment (drugs and nursing visits coded separately), per diem
⊘ S9810	Home therapy; professional pharmacy services for provision of infusion, specialty drug administration, and/or disease state management, not otherwise classified, per hour (do not use this code with any per diem code)

Other Services and Fees

⊘ S9900	Services by journal-listed Christian Science Practitioner for the purpose of healing, per diem
⊘ S9901	Services by a journal-listed Christian Science nurse, per hour
⊘ S9960	Ambulance service, conventional air service, nonemergency transport, one way (fixed wing)
⊘ S9961	Ambulance service, conventional air service, nonemergency transport, one way (rotary wing)
⊘ S9970	Health club membership, annual
⊘ S9975	Transplant related lodging, meals and transportation, per diem
⊘ S9976	Lodging, per diem, not otherwise classified
⊘ S9977	Meals, per diem, not otherwise specified
⊘ S9981	Medical records copying fee, administrative
⊘ S9982	Medical records copying fee, per page
⊘ S9986	Not medically necessary service (patient is aware that service not medically necessary)
⊘ S9988	Services provided as part of a Phase I clinical trial
⊘ S9989	Services provided outside of the United States of America (list in addition to code(s) for services(s))
⊘ S9990	Services provided as part of a Phase II clinical trial
⊘ S9991	Services provided as part of a Phase III clinical trial
⊘ S9992	Transportation costs to and from trial location and local transportation costs (e.g., fares for taxicab or bus) for clinical trial participant and one caregiver/companion
⊘ S9994	Lodging costs (e.g., hotel charges) for clinical trial participant and one caregiver/companion
⊘ S9996	Meals for clinical trial participant and one caregiver/companion
⊘ S9999	Sales tax

▶ New   ⤴ Revised   ✔ Reinstated   ~~deleted~~ Deleted   ⊘ Not covered or valid by Medicare
✦ Special coverage instructions   ✱ Carrier discretion   Ⓑ Bill Part B MAC   Ⓑ Bill DME MAC

TEMPORARY NATIONAL CODES ESTABLISHED BY MEDICAID (T1000-T9999)

Not Valid For Medicare

- ⊘ **T1000** Private duty/independent nursing service(s) - licensed, up to 15 minutes
- ⊘ **T1001** Nursing assessment/evaluation
- ⊘ **T1002** RN services, up to 15 minutes
- ⊘ **T1003** LPN/LVN services, up to 15 minutes
- ⊘ **T1004** Services of a qualified nursing aide, up to 15 minutes
- ⊘ **T1005** Respite care services, up to 15 minutes
- ⊘ **T1006** Alcohol and/or substance abuse services, family/couple counseling
- ⊘ **T1007** Alcohol and/or substance abuse services, treatment plan development and/or modification
- ⊘ **T1009** Child sitting services for children of the individual receiving alcohol and/or substance abuse services Ⓐ
- ⊘ **T1010** Meals for individuals receiving alcohol and/or substance abuse services (when meals not included in the program)
- ⊘ **T1012** Alcohol and/or substance abuse services, skills development
- ⊘ **T1013** Sign language or oral interpretive services, per 15 minutes
- ⊘ **T1014** Telehealth transmission, per minute, professional services bill separately
- ⊘ **T1015** Clinic visit/encounter, all-inclusive
- ⊘ **T1016** Case Management, each 15 minutes
- ⊘ **T1017** Targeted Case Management, each 15 minutes
- ⊘ **T1018** School-based individualized education program (IEP) services, bundled
- ⊘ **T1019** Personal care services, per 15 minutes, not for an inpatient or resident of a hospital, nursing facility, ICF/MR or IMD, part of the individualized plan of treatment (code may not be used to identify services provided by home health aide or certified nurse assistant)
- ⊘ **T1020** Personal care services, per diem, not for an inpatient or resident of a hospital, nursing facility, ICF/MR or IMD, part of the individualized plan of treatment (code may not be used to identify services provided by home health aide or certified nurse assistant)
- ⊘ **T1021** Home health aide or certified nurse assistant, per visit
- ⊘ **T1022** Contracted home health agency services, all services provided under contract, per day
- ⊘ **T1023** Screening to determine the appropriateness of consideration of an individual for participation in a specified program, project or treatment protocol, per encounter
- ⊘ **T1024** Evaluation and treatment by an integrated, specialty team contracted to provide coordinated care to multiple or severely handicapped children, per encounter Ⓐ
- ⊘ **T1025** Intensive, extended multidisciplinary services provided in a clinic setting to children with complex medical, physical, mental and psychosocial impairments, per diem Ⓐ
- ⊘ **T1026** Intensive, extended multidisciplinary services provided in a clinic setting to children with complex medical, physical, mental and psychosocial impairments, per hour Ⓐ
- ⊘ **T1027** Family training and counseling for child development, per 15 minutes Ⓐ
- ⊘ **T1028** Assessment of home, physical and family environment, to determine suitability to meet patient's medical needs
- ⊘ **T1029** Comprehensive environmental lead investigation, not including laboratory analysis, per dwelling
- ⊘ **T1030** Nursing care, in the home, by registered nurse, per diem
- ⊘ **T1031** Nursing care, in the home, by licensed practical nurse, per diem
- ⊘ **T1032** Services performed by a doula birth worker, per 15 minutes
- ⊘ **T1033** Services performed by a doula birth worker, per diem
- ⊘ **T1040** Medicaid certified community behavioral health clinic services, per diem
- ⊘ **T1041** Medicaid certified community behavioral health clinic services, per month
- ⊘ **T1502** Administration of oral, intramuscular and/or subcutaneous medication by health care agency/professional, per visit
- ⊘ **T1503** Administration of medication, other than oral and/or injectable, by a health care agency/professional, per visit

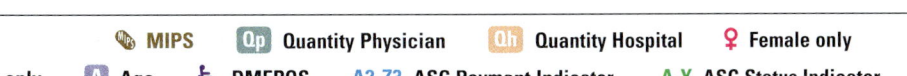

⊘ **T1505**	Electronic medication compliance management device, includes all components and accessories, not otherwise classified
⊘ **T1999**	Miscellaneous therapeutic items and supplies, retail purchases, not otherwise classified; identify product in "remarks"
⊘ **T2001**	Non-emergency transportation; patient attendant/escort
⊘ **T2002**	Non-emergency transportation; per diem
⊘ **T2003**	Non-emergency transportation; encounter/trip
⊘ **T2004**	Non-emergency transport; commercial carrier, multi-pass
⊘ **T2005**	Non-emergency transportation: stretcher van
⊘ **T2007**	Transportation waiting time, air ambulance and non-emergency vehicle, one-half (1/2) hour increments
⊘ **T2010**	Preadmission screening and resident review (PASRR) level I identification screening, per screen
⊘ **T2011**	Preadmission screening and resident review (PASRR) level II evaluation, per evaluation
⊘ **T2012**	Habilitation, educational, waiver; per diem
⊘ **T2013**	Habilitation, educational, waiver; per hour
⊘ **T2014**	Habilitation, prevocational, waiver; per diem
⊘ **T2015**	Habilitation, prevocational, waiver; per hour
⊘ **T2016**	Habilitation, residential, waiver; per diem
⊘ **T2017**	Habilitation, residential, waiver; 15 minutes
⊘ **T2018**	Habilitation, supported employment, waiver; per diem
⊘ **T2019**	Habilitation, supported employment, waiver; per 15 minutes
⊘ **T2020**	Day habilitation, waiver; per diem
⊘ **T2021**	Day habilitation, waiver; per 15 minutes
⊘ **T2022**	Case management, per month
⊘ **T2023**	Targeted case management; per month
⊘ **T2024**	Service assessment/plan of care development, waiver
⊘ **T2025**	Waiver services; not otherwise specified (NOS)
⊘ **T2026**	Specialized childcare, waiver; per diem
⊘ **T2027**	Specialized childcare, waiver; per 15 minutes
⊘ **T2028**	Specialized supply, not otherwise specified, waiver
⊘ **T2029**	Specialized medical equipment, not otherwise specified, waiver
⊘ **T2030**	Assisted living, waiver; per month
⊘ **T2031**	Assisted living; waiver, per diem
⊘ **T2032**	Residential care, not otherwise specified (NOS), waiver; per month
⊘ **T2033**	Residential care, not otherwise specified (NOS), waiver; per diem
⊘ **T2034**	Crisis intervention, waiver; per diem
⊘ **T2035**	Utility services to support medical equipment and assistive technology/devices, waiver
⊘ **T2036**	Therapeutic camping, overnight, waiver; each session
⊘ **T2037**	Therapeutic camping, day, waiver; each session
⊘ **T2038**	Community transition, waiver; per service
⊘ **T2039**	Vehicle modifications, waiver; per service
⊘ **T2040**	Financial management, self-directed, waiver; per 15 minutes
⊘ **T2041**	Supports brokerage, self-directed, waiver; per 15 minutes
⊘ **T2042**	Hospice routine home care; per diem
⊘ **T2043**	Hospice continuous home care; per hour
⊘ **T2044**	Hospice inpatient respite care; per diem
⊘ **T2045**	Hospice general inpatient care; per diem
⊘ **T2046**	Hospice long term care, room and board only; per diem
⊘ **T2047**	Habilitation, prevocational, waiver; per 15 minutes
⊘ **T2048**	Behavioral health; long-term care residential (non-acute care in a residential treatment program where stay is typically longer than 30 days), with room and board, per diem
⊘ **T2049**	Non-emergency transportation; stretcher van, mileage; per mile
⊘ **T2101**	Human breast milk processing, storage and distribution only ♀
⊘ **T4521**	Adult sized disposable incontinence product, brief/diaper, small, each Ⓐ
	IOM: 100-03, 4, 280.1

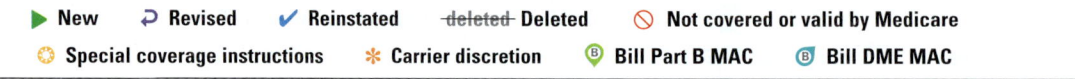

⊘	T4522	Adult sized disposable incontinence product, brief/diaper, medium, each [A]		

⊘ **T4522** Adult sized disposable incontinence product, brief/diaper, medium, each [A]
IOM: 100-03, 4, 280.1

⊘ **T4523** Adult sized disposable incontinence product, brief/diaper, large, each [A]
IOM: 100-03, 4, 280.1

⊘ **T4524** Adult sized disposable incontinence product, brief/diaper, extra large, each [A]
IOM: 100-03, 4, 280.1

⊘ **T4525** Adult sized disposable incontinence product, protective underwear/pull-on, small size, each [A]
IOM: 100-03, 4, 280.1

⊘ **T4526** Adult sized disposable incontinence product, protective underwear/pull-on, medium size, each [A]
IOM: 100-03, 4, 280.1

⊘ **T4527** Adult sized disposable incontinence product, protective underwear/pull-on, large size, each [A]
IOM: 100-03, 4, 280.1

⊘ **T4528** Adult sized disposable incontinence product, protective underwear/pull-on, extra large size, each [A]
IOM: 100-03, 4, 280.1

⊘ **T4529** Pediatric sized disposable incontinence product, brief/diaper, small/medium size, each [A]
IOM: 100-03, 4, 280.1

⊘ **T4530** Pediatric sized disposable incontinence product, brief/diaper, large size, each [A]
IOM: 100-03, 4, 280.1

⊘ **T4531** Pediatric sized disposable incontinence product, protective underwear/pull-on, small/medium size, each [A]
IOM: 100-03, 4, 280.1

⊘ **T4532** Pediatric sized disposable incontinence product, protective underwear/pull-on, large size, each [A]
IOM: 100-03, 4, 280.1

⊘ **T4533** Youth sized disposable incontinence product, brief/diaper, each [A]
IOM: 100-03, 4, 280.1

⊘ **T4534** Youth sized disposable incontinence product, protective underwear/pull-on, each [A]
IOM: 100-03, 4, 280.1

⊘ **T4535** Disposable liner/shield/guard/pad/undergarment, for incontinence, each
IOM: 100-03, 4, 280.1

⊘ **T4536** Incontinence product, protective underwear/pull-on, reusable, any size, each
IOM: 100-03, 4, 280.1

⊘ **T4537** Incontinence product, protective underpad, reusable, bed size, each
IOM: 100-03, 4, 280.1

⊘ **T4538** Diaper service, reusable diaper, each diaper
IOM: 100-03, 4, 280.1

⊘ **T4539** Incontinence product, diaper/brief, reusable, any size, each
IOM: 100-03, 4, 280.1

⊘ **T4540** Incontinence product, protective underpad, reusable, chair size, each
IOM: 100-03, 4, 280.1

⊘ **T4541** Incontinence product, disposable underpad, large, each

⊘ **T4542** Incontinence product, disposable underpad, small size, each

⊘ **T4543** Adult sized disposable incontinence product, protective brief/diaper, above extra large, each [A]
IOM: 100-03, 4, 280.1

⊘ **T4544** Adult sized disposable incontinence product, protective underwear/pull-on, above extra large, each [A]
IOM: 100-03, 4, 280.1

⊘ **T4545** Incontinence product, disposable, penile wrap, each ♂

⊘ **T5001** Positioning seat for persons with special orthopedic needs, supply, not otherwise specified

⊘ **T5999** Supply, not otherwise specified

♂ Male only   [A] Age   ♿ DMEPOS   A2-Z3 ASC Payment Indicator   🖐 MIPS   Qp Quantity Physician   Qh Quantity Hospital   ♀ Female only   A-Y ASC Status Indicator   Coding Clinic

CORONAVIRUS DIAGNOSTIC PANEL (U0001-U0002)

U0001 CDC 2019 novel coronavirus (2019-nCoV) real-time RT-PCR diagnostic panel   A

U0002 2019-nCoV coronavirus, SARS-CoV-2/2019-nCoV (COVID-19), any technique, multiple types or subtypes (includes all targets), non-CDC   A

VISION SERVICES

VISION SERVICES (V0000-V2999)

Frames

- ⊛ **V2020** Frames, purchases ⓑ Qp Qh ♿ A

  Includes cost of frame/replacement and dispensing fee. One unit of service represents one pair of eyeglass frames.

  IOM: 100-02, 15, 120

- ⊘ **V2025** Deluxe frame ⓑ Qp Qh E1

  Not a benefit. Billing deluxe frames-submit V2020 on one line; V2025 on second line.

  IOM: 100-04, 1, 30.3.5

If a CPT procedure code for supply of spectacles or a permanent prosthesis is reported, recode with the specific lens type listed below.

Single Vision Lenses

- ✱ **V2100** Sphere, single vision, plano to plus or minus 4.00, per lens ⓑ Qp Qh ♿ A
- ✱ **V2101** Sphere, single vision, plus or minus 4.12 to plus or minus 7.00d, per lens ⓑ Qp Qh ♿ A
- ✱ **V2102** Sphere, single vision, plus or minus 7.12 to plus or minus 20.00d, per lens ⓑ Qp Qh ♿ A
- ✱ **V2103** Spherocylinder, single vision, plano to plus or minus 4.00d sphere, .12 to 2.00d cylinder, per lens ⓑ Qp Qh ♿ A
- ✱ **V2104** Spherocylinder, single vision, plano to plus or minus 4.00d sphere, 2.12 to 4.00d cylinder, per lens ⓑ Qp Qh ♿ A
- ✱ **V2105** Spherocylinder, single vision, plano to plus or minus 4.00d sphere, 4.25 to 6.00d cylinder, per lens ⓑ Qp Qh ♿ A
- ✱ **V2106** Spherocylinder, single vision, plano to plus or minus 4.00d sphere, over 6.00d cylinder, per lens ⓑ Qp Qh ♿ A
- ✱ **V2107** Spherocylinder, single vision, plus or minus 4.25 to plus or minus 7.00 sphere, .12 to 2.00d cylinder, per lens ⓑ Qp Qh ♿ A
- ✱ **V2108** Spherocylinder, single vision, plus or minus 4.25d to plus or minus 7.00d sphere, 2.12 to 4.00d cylinder, per lens ⓑ Qp Qh ♿ A
- ✱ **V2109** Spherocylinder, single vision, plus or minus 4.25 to plus or minus 7.00 sphere, 4.25 to 6.00d cylinder, per lens ⓑ Qp Qh ♿ A

- ✱ **V2110** Sperocylinder, single vision, plus or minus 4.25 to 7.00d sphere, over 6.00d cylinder, per lens ⓑ Qp Qh ♿ A
- ✱ **V2111** Spherocylinder, single vision, plus or minus 7.25 to plus or minus 12.00d sphere, .25 to 2.25d cylinder, per lens ⓑ Qp Qh ♿ A
- ✱ **V2112** Spherocylinder, single vision, plus or minus 7.25 to plus or minus 12.00d sphere, 2.25d to 4.00d cylinder, per lens ⓑ Qp Qh ♿ A
- ✱ **V2113** Spherocylinder, single vision, plus or minus 7.25 to plus or minus 12.00d sphere, 4.25 to 6.00d cylinder, per lens ⓑ Qp Qh ♿ A
- ✱ **V2114** Spherocylinder, single vision, sphere over plus or minus 12.00d, per lens ⓑ Qp Qh ♿ A
- ✱ **V2115** Lenticular, (myodisc), per lens, single vision ⓑ Qp Qh ♿ A
- ✱ **V2118** Aniseikonic lens, single vision ⓑ Qp Qh ♿ A
- ⊛ **V2121** Lenticular lens, per lens, single ⓑ Qp Qh ♿ A

  IOM: 100-02, 15, 120; 100-04, 3, 10.4

- ✱ **V2199** Not otherwise classified, single vision lens ⓑ Qp Qh A

  Bill on paper. Requires report of type of single vision lens and optical lab invoice.

Bifocal Lenses

- ✱ **V2200** Sphere, bifocal, plano to plus or minus 4.00d, per lens ⓑ Qp Qh ♿ A
- ✱ **V2201** Sphere, bifocal, plus or minus 4.12 to plus or minus 7.00d, per lens ⓑ Qp Qh ♿ A
- ✱ **V2202** Sphere, bifocal, plus or minus 7.12 to plus or minus 20.00d, per lens ⓑ Qp Qh ♿ A
- ✱ **V2203** Spherocylinder, bifocal, plano to plus or minus 4.00d sphere, .12 to 2.00d cylinder, per lens ⓑ Qp Qh ♿ A
- ✱ **V2204** Spherocylinder, bifocal, plano to plus or minus 4.00d sphere, 2.12 to 4.00d cylinder, per lens ⓑ Qp Qh ♿ A
- ✱ **V2205** Spherocylinder, bifocal, plano to plus or minus 4.00d sphere, 4.25 to 6.00d cylinder, per lens ⓑ Qp Qh ♿ A
- ✱ **V2206** Spherocylinder, bifocal, plano to plus or minus 4.00d sphere, over 6.00d cylinder, per lens ⓑ Qp Qh ♿ A

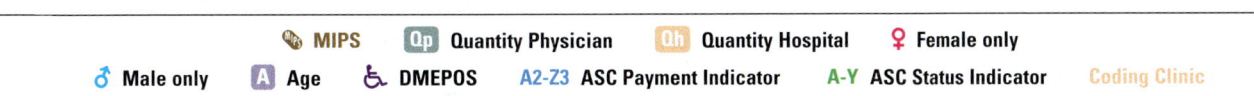

♦ MIPS   Qp Quantity Physician   Qh Quantity Hospital   ♀ Female only
♂ Male only   A Age   ♿ DMEPOS   A2-Z3 ASC Payment Indicator   A-Y ASC Status Indicator   Coding Clinic

* **V2207**	Spherocylinder, bifocal, plus or minus 4.25 to plus or minus 7.00d sphere, .12 to 2.00d cylinder, per lens Ⓑ Qp Qh ♿	A
* **V2208**	Spherocylinder, bifocal, plus or minus 4.25 to plus or minus 7.00d sphere, 2.12 to 4.00d cylinder, per lens Ⓑ Qp Qh ♿	A
* **V2209**	Spherocylinder, bifocal, plus or minus 4.25 to plus or minus 7.00d sphere, 4.25 to 6.00d cylinder, per lens Ⓑ Qp Qh ♿	A
* **V2210**	Spherocylinder, bifocal, plus or minus 4.25 to plus or minus 7.00d sphere, over 6.00d cylinder, per lens Ⓑ Qp Qh ♿	A
* **V2211**	Spherocylinder, bifocal, plus or minus 7.25 to plus or minus 12.00d sphere, .25 to 2.25d cylinder, per lens Ⓑ Qp Qh ♿	A
* **V2212**	Spherocylinder, bifocal, plus or minus 7.25 to plus or minus 12.00d sphere, 2.25 to 4.00d cylinder, per lens Ⓑ Qp Qh ♿	A
* **V2213**	Spherocylinder, bifocal, plus or minus 7.25 to plus or minus 12.00d sphere, 4.25 to 6.00d cylinder, per lens Ⓑ Qp Qh ♿	A
* **V2214**	Spherocylinder, bifocal, sphere over plus or minus 12.00d, per lens Ⓑ Qp Qh ♿	A
* **V2215**	Lenticular (myodisc), per lens, bifocal Ⓑ Qp Qh ♿	A
* **V2218**	Aniseikonic, per lens, bifocal Ⓑ Qp Qh ♿	A
* **V2219**	Bifocal seg width over 28 mm Ⓑ Qp Qh ♿	A
* **V2220**	Bifocal add over 3.25d Ⓑ Qp Qh ♿	A
◉ **V2221**	Lenticular lens, per lens, bifocal Ⓑ Qp Qh ♿	A
	IOM: 100-02, 15, 120; 100-04, 3, 10.4	
* **V2299**	Specialty bifocal (by report) Ⓑ Qp Qh	A
	Bill on paper. Requires report of type of specialty bifocal lens and optical lab invoice.	

Trifocal Lenses

* **V2300**	Sphere, trifocal, plano to plus or minus 4.00d, per lens Ⓑ Qp Qh ♿	A
* **V2301**	Sphere, trifocal, plus or minus 4.12 to plus or minus 7.00d per lens Ⓑ Qp Qh ♿	A
* **V2302**	Sphere, trifocal, plus or minus 7.12 to plus or minus 20.00, per lens Ⓑ Qp Qh ♿	A
* **V2303**	Spherocylinder, trifocal, plano to plus or minus 4.00d sphere, .12 to 2.00d cylinder, per lens Ⓑ Qp Qh ♿	A
* **V2304**	Spherocylinder, trifocal, plano to plus or minus 4.00d sphere, 2.25-4.00d cylinder, per lens Ⓑ Qp Qh ♿	A
* **V2305**	Spherocylinder, trifocal, plano to plus or minus 4.00d sphere, 4.25 to 6.00 cylinder, per lens Ⓑ Qp Qh ♿	A
* **V2306**	Spherocylinder, trifocal, plano to plus or minus 4.00d sphere, over 6.00d cylinder, per lens Ⓑ Qp Qh ♿	A
* **V2307**	Spherocylinder, trifocal, plus or minus 4.25 to plus or minus 7.00d sphere, .12 to 2.00d cylinder, per lens Ⓑ Qp Qh ♿	A
* **V2308**	Spherocylinder, trifocal, plus or minus 4.25 to plus or minus 7.00d sphere, 2.12 to 4.00d cylinder, per lens Ⓑ Qp Qh ♿	A
* **V2309**	Spherocylinder, trifocal, plus or minus 4.25 to plus or minus 7.00d sphere, 4.25 to 6.00d cylinder, per lens Ⓑ Qp Qh ♿	A
* **V2310**	Spherocylinder, trifocal, plus or minus 4.25 to plus or minus 7.00d sphere, over 6.00d cylinder, per lens Ⓑ Qp Qh ♿	A
* **V2311**	Spherocylinder, trifocal, plus or minus 7.25 to plus or minus 12.00d sphere, .25 to 2.25d cylinder, per lens Ⓑ Qp Qh ♿	A
* **V2312**	Spherocylinder, trifocal, plus or minus 7.25 to plus or minus 12.00d sphere, 2.25 to 4.00d cylinder, per lens Ⓑ Qp Qh ♿	A
* **V2313**	Spherocylinder, trifocal, plus or minus 7.25 to plus or minus 12.00d sphere, 4.25 to 6.00d cylinder, per lens Ⓑ Qp Qh ♿	A
* **V2314**	Spherocylinder, trifocal, sphere over plus or minus 12.00d, per lens Ⓑ Qp Qh ♿	A
* **V2315**	Lenticular, (myodisc), per lens, trifocal Ⓑ Qp Qh ♿	A
* **V2318**	Aniseikonic lens, trifocal Ⓑ Qp Qh ♿	A
* **V2319**	Trifocal seg width over 28 mm Ⓑ Qp Qh ♿	A
* **V2320**	Trifocal add over 3.25d Ⓑ Qp Qh ♿ A

▶ New ⮂ Revised ✓ Reinstated ~~deleted~~ Deleted ⊘ Not covered or valid by Medicare
◉ Special coverage instructions * Carrier discretion Ⓑ Bill Part B MAC Ⓑ Bill DME MAC

VISION SERVICES

○ **V2321** Lenticular lens, per lens, trifocal Ⓑ Qp Qh ♿ A

   IOM: 100-02, 15, 120; 100-04, 3, 10.4

✱ **V2399** Specialty trifocal (by report) Ⓑ Qp Qh A

   Bill on paper. Requires report of type of trifocal lens and optical lab invoice.

Variable Asphericity/Sphericity Lenses

✱ **V2410** Variable asphericity lens, single vision, full field, glass or plastic, per lens Ⓑ Qp Qh ♿ A

✱ **V2430** Variable asphericity lens, bifocal, full field, glass or plastic, per lens Ⓑ Qp Qh ♿ A

✱ **V2499** Variable sphericity lens, other type Ⓑ Qp Qh A

   Bill on paper. Requires report of other ptical lab invoice.

Contact Lenses

If a CPT procedure code for supply of contact lens is reported, recode with specific lens type listed below (per lens).

✱ **V2500** Contact lens, PMMA, spherical, per lens Ⓑ Qp Qh ♿ A

   Requires prior authorization for patients under age 21.

✱ **V2501** Contact lens, PMMA, toric or prism ballast, per lens Ⓑ Qp Qh ♿ A

   Requires prior authorization for clients under age 21.

✱ **V2502** Contact lens, PMMA, bifocal, per lens Ⓑ Qp Qh ♿ A

   Requires prior authorization for clients under age 21. Bill on paper. Requires optical lab invoice.

✱ **V2503** Contact lens PMMA, color vision deficiency, per lens Ⓑ Qp Qh ♿ A

   Requires prior authorization for clients under age 21. Bill on paper. Requires optical lab invoice.

✱ **V2510** Contact lens, gas permeable, spherical, per lens Ⓑ Qp Qh ♿ A

   Requires prior authorization for clients under age 21.

✱ **V2511** Contact lens, gas permeable, toric, prism ballast, per lens Ⓑ Qp Qh ♿ A

   Requires prior authorization for clients under age 21.

✱ **V2512** Contact lens, gas permeable, bifocal, per lens Ⓑ Qp Qh A

   Requires prior authorization for clients under age 21.

✱ **V2513** Contact lens, gas permeable, extended wear, per lens Ⓑ Qp Qh ♿ A

   Requires prior authorization for clients under age 21.

○ **V2520** Contact lens, hydrophilic, spherical, per lens ⓠ Ⓑ Qp Qh ♿ A

   Requires prior authorization for clients under age 21.

   IOM: 100-03, 1, 80.1; 100-03, 1, 80.4

○ **V2521** Contact lens, hydrophilic, toric, or prism ballast, per lens Ⓑ Ⓑ Qp Qh ♿ A

   Requires prior authorization for clients under age 21.

   IOM: 100-03, 1, 80.1; 100-03, 1, 80.4

○ **V2522** Contact lens, hydrophilic, bifocal, per lens Ⓑ Ⓑ Qp Qh ♿ A

   Requires prior authorization for clients under age 21.

   IOM: 100-03, 1, 80.1; 100-03, 1, 80.4

○ **V2523** Contact lens, hydrophilic, extended wear, per lens Ⓑ Ⓑ Qp Qh ♿ A

   Requires prior authorization for clients under age 21.

   IOM: 100-03, 1, 80.1; 100-03, 1, 80.4

○ **V2524** Contact lens, hydrophilic, spherical, photochromic additive, per lens ♿ A

V2526 Contact lens, hydrophilic, with blue-violet filter, per lens E1

✱ **V2530** Contact lens, scleral, gas impermeable, per lens (for contact lens modification, see 92325) Ⓑ Qp Qh ♿ A

   Requires prior authorization for clients under age 21.

○ **V2531** Contact lens, scleral, gas permeable, per lens (for contact lens modification, see 92325) Ⓑ Qp Qh ♿ A

   Requires prior authorization for clients under age 21. Bill on paper. Requires optical lab invoice.

   IOM: 100-03, 1, 80.5

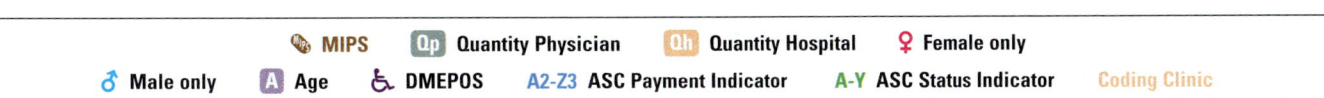

* **V2599** Contact lens, other type Ⓑ Ⓑ Qp Qh A
    Requires prior authorization for clients under age 21. Bill on paper. Requires report of other type of contact lens and optical invoice.

Low Vision Aids

If a CPT procedure code for supply of low vision aid is reported, recode with specific systems listed below.

* **V2600** Hand held low vision aids and other nonspectacle mounted aids Ⓑ Qp Qh A
    Requires prior authorization.

* **V2610** Single lens spectacle mounted low vision aids Ⓑ Qp Qh A
    Requires prior authorization.

* **V2615** Telescopic and other compound lens system, including distance vision telescopic, near vision telescopes and compound microscopic lens system Ⓑ Qp Qh A
    Requires prior authorization. Bill on paper. Requires optical lab invoice.

Prosthetic Eye

◎ **V2623** Prosthetic eye, plastic, custom Ⓑ Qp Qh ♿ A
    DME regional carrier. Requires prior authorization. Bill on paper. Requires optical lab invoice.

* **V2624** Polishing/resurfacing of ocular prosthesis Ⓑ Qp Qh ♿ A
    Requires prior authorization. Bill on paper. Requires optical lab invoice.

* **V2625** Enlargement of ocular prosthesis Ⓑ Qp Qh ♿ A
    Requires prior authorization. Bill on paper. Requires optical lab invoice.

* **V2626** Reduction of ocular prosthesis Ⓑ Qp Qh ♿ A
    Requires prior authorization. Bill on paper. Requires optical lab invoice.

◎ **V2627** Scleral cover shell Ⓑ Qp Qh ♿ A
    DME regional carrier
    Requires prior authorization. Bill on paper. Requires optical lab invoice.
    IOM: 100-03, 4, 280.2

* **V2628** Fabrication and fitting of ocular conformer Ⓑ Qp Qh ♿ A
    Requires prior authorization. Bill on paper. Requires optical lab invoice.

* **V2629** Prosthetic eye, other type Ⓑ Qp Qh A
    Requires prior authorization. Bill on paper. Requires optical lab invoice.

Intraocular Lenses

◎ **V2630** Anterior chamber intraocular lens Ⓑ Qp Qh ♿ N1 N
    IOM: 100-02, 15, 120

◎ **V2631** Iris supported intraocular lens Ⓑ Qp Qh ♿ N1 N
    IOM: 100-02, 15, 120

◎ **V2632** Posterior chamber intraocular lens Ⓑ Qp Qh ♿ N1 N
    IOM: 100-02, 15, 120

Figure 52 Posterior intraocular lens.

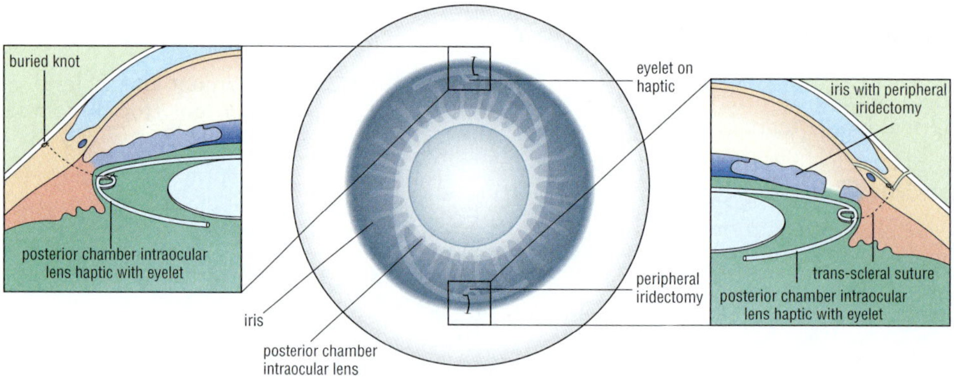

▶ New   ↻ Revised   ✓ Reinstated   ~~deleted~~ Deleted   ⊘ Not covered or valid by Medicare
◎ Special coverage instructions   * Carrier discretion   Ⓑ Bill Part B MAC   Ⓑ Bill DME MAC

VISION SERVICES

Miscellaneous Vision Services

* **V2700** Balance lens, per lens A
* ⊘ **V2702** Deluxe lens feature E1
  IOM: 100-02, 15, 120; 100-04, 3, 10.4
* **V2710** Slab off prism, glass or plastic, per lens A
* **V2715** Prism, per lens A
* **V2718** Press-on lens, Fresnel prism, per lens A
* **V2730** Special base curve, glass or plastic, per lens A
* ✺ **V2744** Tint, photochromatic, per lens A
  Requires prior authorization.
  IOM: 100-02, 15, 120; 100-04, 3, 10.4
* ✺ **V2745** Addition to lens, tint, any color, solid, gradient or equal, excludes photochroatic, any lens material, per lens A
  Includes photochromatic lenses (V2744) used as sunglasses, which are prescribed in addition to regular prosthetic lenses for aphakic patient will be denied as not medically necessary.
  IOM: 100-02, 15, 120; 100-04, 3, 10.4
* ✺ **V2750** Anti-reflective coating, per lens A
  Requires prior authorization.
  IOM: 100-02, 15, 120; 100-04, 3, 10.4
* ✺ **V2755** U-V lens, per lens A
  IOM: 100-02, 15, 120; 100-04, 3, 10.4
* * **V2756** Eye glass case E1
* * **V2760** Scratch resistant coating, per lens E1
* ✺ **V2761** Mirror coating, any type, solid, gradient or equal, any lens material, per lens B
  IOM: 100-02, 15, 120; 100-04, 3, 10.4
* * **V2762** Polarization, any lens material, per lens E1
  IOM: 100-02, 15, 120; 100-04, 3, 10.4
* * **V2770** Occluder lens, per lens A
  Requires prior authorization.
* * **V2780** Oversize lens, per lens A
  Requires prior authorization.
* * **V2781** Progressive lens, per lens B
  Requires prior authorization.

* ✺ **V2782** Lens, index 1.54 to 1.65 plastic or 1.60 to 1.79 glass, excludes polycarbonate, per lens A
  Do not bill in addition to V2784
  IOM: 100-02, 15, 120; 100-04, 3, 10.4
* ✺ **V2783** Lens, index greater than or equal to 1.66 plastic or greater than or equal to 1.80 glass, excludes polycarbonate, per lens A
  Do not bill in addition to V2784
  IOM: 100-02, 15, 120; 100-04, 3, 10.4
* ✺ **V2784** Lens, polycarbonate or equal, any index, per lens A
  Covered only for patients with functional vision in one eye-in this situation, an impact-resistant material is covered for both lenses if eyeglasses are covered. Claims with V2784 that do not meet this coverage criterion will be denied as not medically necessary.
  IOM: 100-02, 15, 120; 100-04, 3, 10.4
* * **V2785** Processing, preserving and transporting corneal tissue F4 F
  For ASC, bill on paper. Must attach eye bank invoice to claim.
  For Hospitals, bill charges for corneal tissue to receive cost based reimbursement.
  IOM: 100-04, 4, 200.1
* ✺ **V2786** Specialty occupational multifocal lens, per lens E1
  IOM: 100-02, 15, 120; 100-04, 3, 10.4
* ⊘ **V2787** Astigmatism correcting function of intraocular lens E1
  Medicare Statute 1862(a)(7)
* ⊘ **V2788** Presbyopia correcting function of intraocular lens E1
  Medicare Statute 1862a7
* * **V2790** Amniotic membrane for surgical reconstruction, per procedure N1 N
* * **V2797** Vision supply, accessory and/or service component of another HCPCS vision code E1
* * **V2799** Vision item or service, miscellaneous A
  Bill on paper. Requires report of miscellaneous service and optical lab invoice.

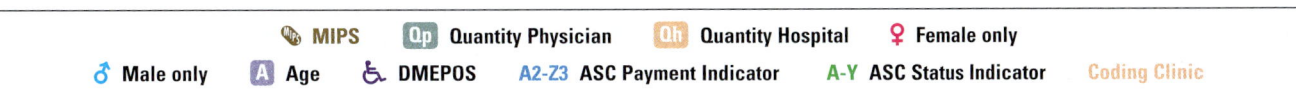

MIPS | Qp Quantity Physician | Qh Quantity Hospital | ♀ Female only
♂ Male only | A Age | DMEPOS | A2-Z3 ASC Payment Indicator | A-Y ASC Status Indicator | Coding Clinic

HEARING SERVICES (V5000-V5999)

These codes are for non-physician services.

Assessments and Evaluations

- ⊘ **V5008** Hearing screening Ⓑ Qp Qh E1
  IOM: 100-02, 16, 90
- ⊘ **V5010** Assessment for hearing aid Ⓑ Qp Qh E1
  Medicare Statute 1862a7
- ⊘ **V5011** Fitting/orientation/checking of hearing aid Ⓑ Qp Qh E1
  Medicare Statute 1862a7
- ⊘ **V5014** Repair/modification of a hearing aid Ⓑ E1
  Medicare Statute 1862a7
- ⊘ **V5020** Conformity evaluation Ⓑ E1
  Medicare Statute 1862a7

Monaural Hearing Aid

- ⊘ **V5030** Hearing aid, monaural, body worn, air conduction Ⓑ E1
  Medicare Statute 1862a7
- ⊘ **V5040** Hearing aid, monaural, body worn, bone conduction Ⓑ E1
  Medicare Statute 1862a7
- ⊘ **V5050** Hearing aid, monaural, in the ear Ⓑ E1
  Medicare Statute 1862a7
- ⊘ **V5060** Hearing aid, monaural, behind the ear Ⓑ E1
  Medicare Statute 1862a7

Miscellaneous Services and Supplies

- ⊘ **V5070** Glasses, air conduction Ⓑ E1
  Medicare Statute 1862a7
- ⊘ **V5080** Glasses, bone conduction Ⓑ E1
  Medicare Statute 1862a7
- ⊘ **V5090** Dispensing fee, unspecified hearing aid Ⓑ E1
  Medicare Statute 1862a7
- ⊘ **V5095** Semi-implantable middle ear hearing prosthesis Ⓑ E1
  Medicare Statute 1862a7

- ⊘ **V5100** Hearing aid, bilateral, body worn Ⓑ E1
  Medicare Statute 1862a7
- ⊘ **V5110** Dispensing fee, bilateral Ⓑ E1
  Medicare Statute 1862a7

Hearing Aids

- ⊘ **V5120** Binaural, body Ⓑ E1
  Medicare Statute 1862a7
- ⊘ **V5130** Binaural, in the ear Ⓑ E1
  Medicare Statute 1862a7
- ⊘ **V5140** Binaural, behind the ear Ⓑ E1
  Medicare Statute 1862a7
- ⊘ **V5150** Binaural, glasses Ⓑ E1
  Medicare Statute 1862a7
- ⊘ **V5160** Dispensing fee, binaural Ⓑ E1
  Medicare Statute 1862a7
- ⊘ **V5171** Hearing aid, contralateral routing device, monaural, in the ear (ITE) E1
  Medicare Statute 1862a7
- ⊘ **V5172** Hearing aid, contralateral routing device, monaural, in the canal (ITC) E1
  Medicare Statute 1862a7
- ⊘ **V5181** Hearing aid, contralateral routing device, monaural, behind the ear (BTE) E1
  Medicare Statute 1862a7
- ⊘ **V5190** Hearing aid, contralateral routing, monaural, glasses Ⓑ E1
  Medicare Statute 1862a7
- ⊘ **V5200** Dispensing fee, contralateral, monaural Ⓑ E1
  Medicare Statute 1862a7
- ⊘ **V5211** Hearing aid, contralateral routing system, binaural, ITE/ITE E1
  Medicare Statute 1862a7
- ⊘ **V5212** Hearing aid, contralateral routing system, binaural, ITE/ITC E1
  Medicare Statute 1862a7
- ⊘ **V5213** Hearing aid, contralateral routing system, binaural, ITE/BTE E1
  Medicare Statute 1862a7
- ⊘ **V5214** Hearing aid, contralateral routing system, binaural, ITC/ITC E1
  Medicare Statute 1862a7

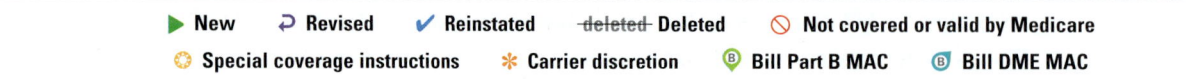

▶ New　⤾ Revised　✓ Reinstated　deleted Deleted　⊘ Not covered or valid by Medicare　✦ Special coverage instructions　✱ Carrier discretion　Ⓑ Bill Part B MAC　Ⓑ Bill DME MAC

HEARING SERVICES

⊘ **V5215** Hearing aid, contralateral routing system, binaural, ITC/BTE E1
Medicare Statute 1862a7

⊘ **V5221** Hearing aid, contralateral routing system, binaural, BTE/BTE E1
Medicare Statute 1862a7

⊘ **V5230** Hearing aid, contralateral routing system, binaural, glasses ⓑ E1
Medicare Statute 1862a7

⊘ **V5240** Dispensing fee, contralateral routing system, binaural ⓑ E1
Medicare Statute 1862a7

⊘ **V5241** Dispensing fee, monaural hearing aid, any type ⓑ E1
Medicare Statute 1862a7

⊘ **V5242** Hearing aid, analog, monaural, CIC (completely in the ear canal) ⓑ E1
Medicare Statute 1862a7

⊘ **V5243** Hearing aid, analog, monaural, ITC (in the canal) ⓑ E1
Medicare Statute 1862a9

⊘ **V5244** Hearing aid, digitally programmable analog, monaural, CIC ⓑ E1
Medicare Statute 1862a7

⊘ **V5245** Hearing aid, digitally programmable, analog, monaural, ITC ⓑ E1
Medicare Statute 1862a7

⊘ **V5246** Hearing aid, digitally programmable analog, monaural, ITE (in the ear) ⓑ E1
Medicare Statute 1862a7

⊘ **V5247** Hearing aid, digitally programmable analog, monaural, BTE (behind the ear) ⓑ E1
Medicare Statute 1862a7

⊘ **V5248** Hearing aid, analog, binaural, CIC ⓑ E1
Medicare Statute 1862a7

⊘ **V5249** Hearing aid, analog, binaural, ITC ⓑ E1
Medicare Statute 1862a7

⊘ **V5250** Hearing aid, digitally programmable analog, binaural, CIC ⓑ E1
Medicare Statute 1862a7

⊘ **V5251** Hearing aid, digitally programmable analog, binaural, ITC ⓑ E1
Medicare Statute 1862a7

⊘ **V5252** Hearing aid, digitally programmable, binaural, ITE ⓑ E1
Medicare Statute 1862a7

⊘ **V5253** Hearing aid, digitally programmable, binaural, BTE ⓑ E1
Medicare Statute 1862a7

⊘ **V5254** Hearing aid, digital, monaural, CIC ⓑ E1
Medicare Statute 1862a7

⊘ **V5255** Hearing aid, digital, monaural, ITC ⓑ E1
Medicare Statute 1862a7

⊘ **V5256** Hearing aid, digital, monaural, ITE ⓑ E1
Medicare Statute 1862a7

⊘ **V5257** Hearing aid, digital, monaural, BTE ⓑ E1
Medicare Statute 1862a7

⊘ **V5258** Hearing aid, digital, binaural, CIC ⓑ E1
Medicare Statute 1862a7

⊘ **V5259** Hearing aid, digital, binaural, ITC ⓑ E1
Medicare Statute 1862a7

⊘ **V5260** Hearing aid, digital, binaural, ITE ⓑ E1
Medicare Statute 1862a7

⊘ **V5261** Hearing aid, digital, binaural, BTE ⓑ E1
Medicare Statute 1862a7

⊘ **V5262** Hearing aid, disposable, any type, monaural ⓑ E1
Medicare Statute 1862a7

⊘ **V5263** Hearing aid, disposable, any type, binaural ⓑ E1
Medicare Statute 1862a7

⊘ **V5264** Ear mold/insert, not disposable, any type ⓑ E1
Medicare Statute 1862a7

⊘ **V5265** Ear mold/insert, disposable, any type ⓑ E1
Medicare Statute 1862a7

⊘ **V5266** Battery for use in hearing device ⓑ E1
Medicare Statute 1862a7

⊘ **V5267** Hearing aid or assistive listening device/supplies/accessories, not otherwise specified ⓑ E1
Medicare Statute 1862a7

Assistive Listening Devices

⊘ **V5268** Assistive listening device, telephone amplifier, any type ⓑ E1
Medicare Statute 1862a7

⊘ **V5269** Assistive listening device, alerting, any type ⓑ E1
Medicare Statute 1862a7

2026 HCPCS LEVEL II NATIONAL CODES

⊘ **V5270** Assistive listening device, television amplifier, any type ⓑ　　E1
　　Medicare Statute 1862a7

⊘ **V5271** Assistive listening device, television caption decoder ⓑ　　E1
　　Medicare Statute 1862a7

⊘ **V5272** Assistive listening device, TDD ⓑ　　E1
　　Medicare Statute 1862a7

⊘ **V5273** Assistive listening device, for use with cochlear implant ⓑ　　E1
　　Medicare Statute 1862a7

⊘ **V5274** Assistive listening device, not otherwise specified ⓑ Qp Qh　　E1
　　Medicare Statute 1862a7

⊘ **V5275** Ear impression, each ⓑ　　E1
　　Medicare Statute 1862a7

⊘ **V5281** Assistive listening device, personal FM/DM system, monaural (1 receiver, transmitter, microphone), any type ⓑ Qp Qh　　E1
　　Medicare Statute 1862a7

⊘ **V5282** Assistive listening device, personal FM/DM system, binaural (2 receivers, transmitter, microphone), any type ⓑ Qp Qh　　E1
　　Medicare Statute 1862a7

⊘ **V5283** Assistive listening device, personal FM/DM neck, loop induction receiver ⓑ Qp Qh　　E1
　　Medicare Statute 1862a7

⊘ **V5284** Assistive listening device, personal FM/DM, ear level receiver ⓑ Qp Qh　E1
　　Medicare Statute 1862a7

⊘ **V5285** Assistive listening device, personal FM/DM, direct audio input receiver ⓑ Qp Qh　　E1
　　Medicare Statute 1862a7

⊘ **V5286** Assistive listening device, personal Bluetooth FM/DM receiver ⓑ Qp Qh　E1
　　Medicare Statute 1862a7

⊘ **V5287** Assistive listening device, personal FM/DM receiver, not otherwise specified ⓑ Qp Qh　　E1
　　Medicare Statute 1862a7

⊘ **V5288** Assistive listening device, personal FM/DM transmitter assistive listening device ⓑ Qp Qh　　E1
　　Medicare Statute 1862a7

⊘ **V5289** Assistive listening device, personal FM/DM adapter/boot coupling device for receiver, any type ⓑ Qp Qh　　E1
　　Medicare Statute 1862a7

⊘ **V5290** Assistive listening device, transmitter microphone, any type ⓑ Qp Qh　　E1
　　Medicare Statute 1862a7

Other Supllies and Miscellaneous Services

⊘ **V5298** Hearing aid, not otherwise classified ⓑ　　E1
　　Medicare Statute 1862a7

✱ **V5299** Hearing service, miscellaneous ⓑ　　B
　　IOM: 100-02, 16, 90

Repair/Modification

⊘ **V5336** Repair/modification of augmentative communicative system or device (excludes adaptive hearing aid) ⓑ　　E1
　　Medicare Statute 1862a7

Speech, Language, and Pathology Screening

These codes are for non-physician services.

⊘ **V5362** Speech screening ⓑ　　E1
　　Medicare Statute 1862a7

⊘ **V5363** Language screening ⓑ　　E1
　　Medicare Statute 1862a7

⊘ **V5364** Dysphagia screening ⓑ　　E1
　　Medicare Statute 1862a7

▶ New　↻ Revised　✓ Reinstated　~~deleted~~ Deleted　⊘ Not covered or valid by Medicare
✱ Special coverage instructions　＊ Carrier discretion　ⓑ Bill Part B MAC　ⓓ Bill DME MAC

APPENDIX A

Jurisdiction List for DMEPOS HCPCS Codes

Deleted codes are valid for dates of service on or before the date of deletion. The jurisdiction list includes codes that are not payable by Medicare. Please consult the Medicare contractor in whose jurisdiction a claim would be filed in order to determine coverage under Medicare.

NOTE: All Local Carrier language has been changed to Part B MAC

HCPCS	DESCRIPTION	JURISDICTION
A4206 - A4209	Medical, Surgical, and Self-Administered Injection, Supplies	Part B MAC if incident to a physician's service (not separately payable). If other, DME MAC.
A4210	Needle Free Injection Device	DME MAC
A4211	Medical, Surgical, and Self-Administered Injection Supplies	Part B MAC if incident to a physician's service (not separately payable). If other, DME MAC.
A4213 - A4215	Medical, Surgical, and Self-Administered Injection Supplies	Part B MAC if incident to a physician's service (not separately payable). If other, DME MAC.
A4216 - A4218	Saline	Part B MAC if incident to a physician's service (not separately payable). If other, DME MAC.
A4221 - A4239	Self-Administered Injection and Diabetic Supplies	DME MAC
A4244 - A4250	Medical, Surgical, and Self-Administered Injection Supplies	Part B MAC if incident to a physician's service (not separately payable). If other, DME MAC.
A4252 - A4259; A4271	Diabetic Supplies	DME MAC
A4265	Paraffin	Part B MAC if incident to a physician's service (not separately payable). If other, DME MAC.
A4280	Accessory for Breast Prosthesis	DME MAC
A4281 - A4288	Accessory for Breast Pump	DME MAC
A4305 - A4306	Disposable Drug Delivery System	Part B MAC if incident to a physician's service (not separately payable). If other, DME MAC.
A4310 - A4340	Incontinence Supplies/ Urinary Supplies	Part B MAC if incident to a physician's service. If other, DME MAC.
A4341-A4342	Urinary Supplies	DME MAC
A4344 - A4358	Incontinence Supplies/ Urinary Supplies	Part B MAC if incident to a physician's service. If other, DME MAC.
A4360 - A4437	Urinary Supplies	Part B MAC if incident to a physician's service. If other, DME MAC
A4450 - A4452	Tape; Adhesive Remover	Part B MAC if incident to a physician's service (not separately payable), or if supply for implanted prosthetic device. If other, DME MAC.
A4453	Rectal Catheter	DME MAC
A4455 - A4456	Tape; Adhesive Remover	Part B MAC if incident to a physician's service (not separately payable), or if supply for implanted prosthetic device. If other, DME MAC.
A4457	Enema tube	Part B MAC if a supply for or inserted by a licensed healthcare provider. If other, DME MAC.
A4458 - A4459	Bowel Management	DME MAC
A4461 - A4463	Surgical Dressing Holders	Part B MAC if incident to a physician's service (not separately payable). If other, DME MAC.
A4465 - A4468	Non-elastic Binder and Garment, Strap, Covering, Exsufflation Belt	DME MAC
A4481	Tracheostomy Supply	Part B MAC if incident to a physician's service (not separately payable). If other, DME MAC.
A4483	Moisture Exchanger	DME MAC
A4490 - A4510	Surgical Stockings	DME MAC
A4520	Diapers	DME MAC
A4540 - A4545	Stimulator and Supplies	DME MAC
A4553 - A4554	Underpads	DME MAC
A4555 - A4558	Electrodes; Lead Wires; Conductive Paste	Part B MAC if incident to a physician's service (not separately payable). If other, DME MAC.
A4560	Disposable	DME MAC
A4559	Coupling Gel	Part B MAC if incident to a physician's service (not separately payable). If other, DME MAC.
A4575	Topical Hyperbaric Oxygen Chamber, Disposable	DME MAC
A4593-A4594	Stimulator and Supplies	DME MAC
A4595	TENS Supplies	Part B MAC if incident to a physician's service (not separately payable). If other, DME MAC.
A4596	Electrical Stimulator Supplies	DME MAC
A4600	Sleeve for Intermittent Limb Compression Device	DME MAC
A4601 - A4602	Lithium Replacement Batteries	DME MAC
A4604	Tubing for Positive Airway Pressure Device	DME MAC

2026 HCPCS: LEVEL II NATIONAL CODES

HCPCS	DESCRIPTION	JURISDICTION
A4605	Tracheal Suction Catheter	DME MAC
A4606	Oxygen Probe for Oximeter	DME MAC
A4608	Transtracheal Oxygen Catheter	DME MAC
A4611 - A4613	Oxygen Equipment Batteries and Supplies	DME MAC
A4614	Peak Flow Rate Meter	Part B MAC if incident to a physician's service (not separately payable). If other, DME MAC.
A4615 - A4629	Oxygen & Tracheostomy Supplies	Part B MAC if incident to a physician's service (not separately payable). If other, DME MAC.
A4630 - A4640	DME Supplies	DME MAC
A4649	Miscellaneous Surgical Supplies	Part B MAC if incident to a physician's service (not separately payable), or if supply for implanted prosthetic device or implanted DME. If other, DME MAC.
A4651 - A4932	Supplies for ESRD	DME MAC (not separately payable)
A5051 - A5093	Additional Ostomy Supplies	Part B MAC if incident to a physician's service. If other, DME MAC
A5102 - A5200	Additional Incontinence and Ostomy Supplies	Part B MAC if incident to a physician's service. If other, DME MAC
A5500 - A5514	Therapeutic Shoes	DME MAC
A6000	Non-Contact Wound Warming Cover	DME MAC
A6010-A6024	Surgical Dressing	Part B MAC if incident to a physician's service (not separately payable) or if supply for implanted prosthetic device or implanted DME. If other, DME MAC.
A6025	Silicone Gel Sheet	Part B MAC if incident to a physician's service (not separately payable) or if supply for implanted prosthetic device or implanted DME. If other, DME MAC.
A6154 - A6411	Surgical Dressing	Part B MAC if incident to a physician's service (not separately payable) or if supply for implanted prosthetic device or implanted DME. If other, DME MAC.
A6412	Eye Patch	Part B MAC if incident to a physician's service (not separately payable) or if supply for implanted prosthetic device or implanted DME. If other, DME MAC.
A6413	Adhesive Bandage	Part B MAC if incident to a physician's service (not separately payable) or if supply for implanted prosthetic device or implanted DME. If other, DME MAC.
A6441 - A6457	Surgical Dressing	Part B MAC if incident to a physician's service (not separately payable) or if supply for implanted prosthetic device or implanted DME. If other, DME MAC.

HCPCS	DESCRIPTION	JURISDICTION
A6501 - A6512	Surgical Dressing	Part B MAC if incident to a physician's service (not separately payable) or if supply for implanted prosthetic device or implanted DME. If other, DME MAC.
A6513; A6515-A6519	Compression Burn Mask, Lymphedema Compression Treatment Items	DME MAC
A6520 - A6549	Gradient Compression Garments	DME MAC
A6550	Supplies for Negative Pressure Wound Therapy Electrical Pump	DME MAC
A6552 - A6589	Lymphedema Compression Items	DME MAC
A6590 - A6591	Accessories for Suction Pumps	DME MAC
A6593 - A6611	Lymphedema Compression Items Aspirators and Ventilators	DME MAC
A7000 - A7002	Accessories for Suction Pumps	DME MAC
A7003 - A7039	Accessories for Nebulizers, Aspirators and Ventilators	DME MAC
A7044 - A7047	Respiratory Accessories	DME MAC
A7049	Respiratory Item	DME MAC
A7501-A7527	Tracheostomy Supplies	DME MAC
A8000-A8004	Protective Helmets	DME MAC
A9156; A9268-A9269	Mucoadhesive and Programmable oral capsule	DME MAC
A9270	Noncovered Items or Services	DME MAC
A9272	Disposable Wound Suction Pump	DME MAC
A9273	Hot Water Bottles, Ice Caps or Collars, and Heat and/or Cold Wraps	DME MAC
A9274 - A9278	Glucose Monitoring	DME MAC
A9279	Monitoring Feature/ Device	DME MAC
A9280	Alarm Device	DME MAC
A9281	Reaching/Grabbing Device	DME MAC
A9282	Wig	DME MAC
A9283	Foot Off Loading Device	DME MAC
A9284- A9286	Non-electric Spirometer, Inversion Devices and Hygienic Items	DME MAC
A9300	Exercise Equipment	DME MAC
A9900	Miscellaneous DME Supply or Accessory	Part B MAC if used with implanted DME. If other, DME MAC.
A9901	Delivery	DME MAC

APPENDIX A

HCPCS	DESCRIPTION	JURISDICTION
A9999	Miscellaneous DME Supply or Accessory	Part B MAC if used with implanted DME. If other, DME MAC.
B4034 - B9999	Enteral and Parenteral Therapy	DME MAC
E0100 - E0105	Canes	DME MAC
E0110 - E0118	Crutches	DME MAC
E0130 - E0159	Walkers	DME MAC
E0160 - E0175	Commodes	DME MAC
E0181 - E0199	Decubitus Care Equipment	DME MAC
E0200 - E0239	Heat/Cold Applications	DME MAC
E0240 - E0248	Bath and Toilet Aids	DME MAC
E0249	Pad for Heating Unit	DME MAC
E0250 - E0304	Hospital Beds	DME MAC
E0305 - E0326	Hospital Bed Accessories	DME MAC
E0328 - E0329	Pediatric Hospital Beds	DME MAC
E0350 - E0352	Electronic Bowel Irrigation System	DME MAC
E0370	Heel Pad	DME MAC
E0371 - E0373	Decubitus Care Equipment	DME MAC
E0424 - E0484	Oxygen and Related Respiratory Equipment	DME MAC
E0485 - E0486	Oral Device to Reduce Airway Collapsibility	DME MAC
E0487	Electric Spirometer	DME MAC
E0490 - E0493	Oral Neuromuscular Stimulator	DME MAC
E0500	IPPB Machine	DME MAC
E0530	Electric Sleep Apnea Treatment	DME MAC
E0550 - E0585	Compressors/Nebulizers	DME MAC
E0600	Suction Pump	DME MAC
E0601	CPAP Device	DME MAC
E0602 - E0604	Breast Pump	DME MAC
E0605	Vaporizer	DME MAC
E0606	Drainage Board	DME MAC
E0607	Home Blood Glucose Monitor	DME MAC
E0610 - E0615	Pacemaker Monitor	DME MAC
E0617	External Defibrillator	DME MAC
E0618 - E0619	Apnea Monitor	DME MAC
E0620	Skin Piercing Device	DME MAC
E0621 - E0636	Patient Lifts	DME MAC
E0637 - E0642	Standing Devices/Lifts	DME MAC
E0650 - E0683	Pneumatic/Non-Pneumatic Devices and Appliances	DME MAC
E0691 - E0694	Ultraviolet Light Therapy Systems	DME MAC
E0700	Safety Equipment	DME MAC
E0705	Transfer Board	DME MAC
E0710 - E0716	Restraints/Enclosures; Pelvic Device	DME MAC
E0720 - E0745	Electrical Nerve Stimulators; Rehab system	DME MAC
E0747 - E0748	Osteogenic Stimulators	DME MAC
E0755- E0770	Stimulation Devices	DME MAC
E0776	IV Pole	DME MAC
E0779 - E0780	External Infusion Pumps	DME MAC
E0781	Ambulatory Infusion Pump	DME MAC
E0784	Infusion Pumps, insulin	DME MAC
E0791	Parenteral Infusion Pump	DME MAC
E0830	Ambulatory Traction Device	DME MAC
E0840 - E0900	Traction Equipment	DME MAC
E0910 - E0930	Trapeze/Fracture Frame	DME MAC
E0935 - E0936	Passive Motion Exercise Device	DME MAC
E0940	Trapeze Equipment	DME MAC
E0941	Traction Equipment	DME MAC
E0942 - E0945	Orthopedic Devices	DME MAC
E0946 - E0948	Fracture Frame	DME MAC
E0950 - E1298	Wheelchairs	DME MAC
E1300 - E1310	Whirlpool Equipment	DME MAC
E1352 - E1392	Additional Oxygen Related Equipment	DME MAC
E1399	Miscellaneous DME	Part B MAC if implanted DME. If other, DME MAC.
E1405 - E1406	Additional Oxygen Equipment	DME MAC
E1500 - E1625	Artificial Kidney Machines and Accessories	DME MAC (not separately payable)
E1630 - E1699	Artifical Kidney Machines and Accessories	DME MAC (not separately payable)
E1700 - E1702	TMJ Device and Supplies	DME MAC
E1800 - E1841	Dynamic Flexion Devices	DME MAC
E1902	Communication Board	DME MAC
E1905	CBT Device	DME MAC
E2000 - E2001	Suction Pump	DME MAC
E2100 - E2104	Blood Glucose Monitors with Special Features; Continuous Glucose Monitor	DME MAC
E2120	Pulse Generator for Tympanic Treatment of Inner Ear	DME MAC
E2201 - E2299	Wheelchair Accessories	DME MAC

425

2026 HCPCS: LEVEL II NATIONAL CODES

HCPCS	DESCRIPTION	JURISDICTION
E2301 - E2398	Wheelchair Accessories	DME MAC
E2402	Negative Pressure Wound Therapy Pump	DME MAC
E2500 - E2599	Speech Generating Device	DME MAC
E2601 - E2633	Wheelchair Cushions and Accessories	DME MAC
E3000 - E3200	Devices	DME MAC
E8000 - E8002	Gait Trainers	DME MAC
G0333	Dispensing Fee	DME MAC
J0120 - J0134	Injection	Part B MAC if incident to a physician's service or used in an implanted infusion pump. If other, DME MAC.
J0136 - J0567	Injection	Part B MAC if incident to a physician's service or used in an implanted infusion pump. If other, DME MAC.
J0571 - J0575	Injection	Part B MAC if incident to a physician's service or used in an implanted infusion pump. If other, DME MAC.
J0577 - J0600	Injection	Part B MAC if incident to a physician's service or used in an implanted infusion pump. If other, DME MAC.
J0610 - J0614	Injection	Part B MAC if incident to a physician's service or used in an implanted infusion pump. If other, DME MAC.
J0618 - J0738	Injection	Part B MAC if incident to a physician's service, Part B pharmacy supplier, or used in an implanted infusion pump. If other, DME MAC.
J0739	Injection	Part B MAC if incident to a physician's service, Part B pharmacy supplier, or used in an implanted infusion pump. If other, DME MAC.
J0740 - J0749	Injection	Part B MAC if incident to a physician's service or used in an implanted infusion pump. If other, DME MAC.
J0750 - J0752	Oral	Part B MAC or DME MAC
J0752 - J0798	Injection	Part B MAC if incident to a physician's service or used in an implanted infusion pump. If other, DME MAC.
J0799	NOC Drugs	Part B MAC or DME MAC
J0800 - J0900	Injection	Part B MAC if incident to a physician's service or used in an implanted infusion pump. If other, DME MAC.
J0902 - J0910	Injection	Part B MAC if incident to a physician's service or used in an implanted infusion pump. If other, DME MAC.
J0912 - J1019	Injection	Part B MAC if incident to a physician's service or used in an implanted infusion pump. If other, DME MAC.
J1021 - J1029	Injection	Part B MAC if incident to a physician's service or used in an implanted infusion pump. If other, DME MAC.
J1031 - J1039	Injection	Part B MAC if incident to a physician's service or used in an implanted infusion pump. If other, DME MAC.
J1041 - J1093	Injection	Part B MAC if incident to a physician's service or used in an implanted infusion pump. If other, DME MAC.
J1100 - J1104	Injection	Part B MAC if incident to a physician's service or used in an implanted infusion pump. If other, DME MAC.
J1105	Oral	Part B MAC if incident to a physician's service. If other, DME MAC.
J1106 - J1169	Injection	Part B MAC if incident to a physician's service or used in an implanted infusion pump. If other, DME MAC.
J1171 - J1299	Injection	Part B MAC if incident to a physician's service or used in an implanted infusion pump. If other, DME MAC.
J1301 - J1809	Injection	Part B MAC if incident to a physician's service or used in an implanted infusion pump. If other, DME MAC.
J1811 - J1839	Injection	Part B MAC if incident to a physician's service or used in an implanted infusion pump. If other, DME MAC.
J1841 - J1849	Injection	Part B MAC if incident to a physician's service or used in an implanted infusion pump. If other, DME MAC.
J1851 - J1889	Injection	Part B MAC if incident to a physician's service or used in an implanted infusion pump. If other, DME MAC.
J1891 - J1939	Injection	Part B MAC if incident to a physician's service or used in an implanted infusion pump. If other, DME MAC.
J1941 - J1960	Injection	Part B MAC if incident to a physician's service or used in an implanted infusion pump. If other, DME MAC.
J1961	Injection	Part B MAC if incident to a physician's service, Part B pharmacy supplier, or used in an implanted infusion pump. If other, DME MAC.
J1962 - J2000	Injection	Part B MAC if incident to a physician's service or used in an implanted infusion pump. If other, DME MAC.
J2002 - J2100	Injection	Part B MAC if incident to a physician's service or used in an implanted infusion pump. If other, DME MAC.

APPENDIX A

HCPCS	DESCRIPTION	JURISDICTION
J2151 - J2305	Injection	Part B MAC if incident to a physician's service or used in an implanted infusion pump. If other, DME MAC.
J2312 - J2402	Injection	Part B MAC if incident to a physician's service or used in an implanted infusion pump. If other, DME MAC.
J2403	Miscellaneous Drug and Solutions	Part B MAC if incident to a physician's service or used in an implanted infusion pump. If other, DME MAC.
J2404 - J2502	Injection	Part B MAC if incident to a physician's service or used in an implanted infusion pump. If other, DME MAC.
J2504 - J2779	Injection	Part B MAC if incident to a physician's service or used in an implanted infusion pump. If other, DME MAC.
J2781 - J2786	Injection	Part B MAC if incident to a physician's service or used in an implanted infusion pump. If other, DME MAC.
J2788 - J2795	Injection	Part B MAC if incident to a physician's service or used in an implanted infusion pump. If other, DME MAC.
J2797-J2805	Injection	Part B MAC if incident to a physician's service or used in an implanted infusion pump. If other, DME MAC.
J2807 - J2919	Injection	Part B MAC if incident to a physician's service or used in an implanted infusion pump. If other, DME MAC.
J2921 - J2929	Injection	Part B MAC if incident to a physician's service or used in an implanted infusion pump. If other, DME MAC.
J2931 - J3356	Injection	Part B MAC if incident to a physician's service or used in an implanted infusion pump. If other, DME MAC.
J3360 - J3365	Injection	Part B MAC if incident to a physician's service or used in an implanted infusion pump. If other, DME MAC.
J3373 - J3400	Injection	Part B MAC if incident to a physician's service or used in an implanted infusion pump. If other, DME MAC.
J3401	Topical	Part B MAC if incident to a physician's service If other, DME MAC.
J3402	Injection	Part B MAC if incident to a physician's service or used in an implanted infusion pump. If other, DME MAC.
J3410 - J3570	Injection	Part B MAC if incident to a physician's service or used in an implanted infusion pump. If other, DME MAC.

HCPCS	DESCRIPTION	JURISDICTION
J7030 - J7131	Miscellaneous Drugs and Solutions	Part B MAC if incident to a physician's service or used in an implanted infusion pump. If other, DME MAC.
J7165	Injection	Part B MAC if incident to a physician's service or used in an implanted infusion pump. If other, DME MAC.
J7171 - J7172	Injection	Part B MAC if incident to a physician's service or used in an implanted infusion pump. If other, DME MAC.
J7340	Carbidopa/Levodopa	Part B MAC if incident to a physician's service or used in an implanted infusion pump. If other, DME MAC.
J7356	Injection	Part B MAC if incident to a physician's service or used in an implanted infusion pump. If other, DME MAC.
J7500 - J7599	Immunosuppressive Drugs	Part B MAC if incident to a physician's service or used in an implanted infusion pump. If other, DME MAC.
J7601	Inhalation Suspension	Part B MAC if incident to a physician's service. If other, DME MAC.
J7604 - J7699	Inhalation Solutions	Part B MAC if incident to a physician's service. If other, DME MAC.
J7799 - J7999	NOC Drugs, Other than Inhalation Drugs	Part B MAC if incident to a physician's service or used in an implanted infusion pump. If other, DME MAC.
J8498	Anti-emetic Drug	DME MAC
J8499	Prescription Drug, Oral, Non Chemotherapeutic	Part B MAC if incident to a physician's service. If other, DME MAC.
J8501 - J8519	Oral Anti-Cancer Drugs	DME MAC
J8522 - J8999	Oral Anti-Cancer Drugs	DME MAC
J9000 - J9036	Chemotherapy Drugs	Part B MAC if incident to a physician's service or used in an implanted infusion pump. If other, DME MAC.
J9038 - J9057	Chemotherapy Drugs	Part B MAC if incident to a physician's service or used in an implanted infusion pump. If other, DME MAC
J9060 - J9065	Chemotherapy Drugs	Part B MAC if incident to a physician's service or used in an implanted infusion pump. If other, DME MAC
J9071 - J9046	Chemotherapy Drugs	Part B MAC if incident to a physician's service or used in an implanted infusion pump. If other, DME MAC.
J9248 - J9249	Chemotherapy Drugs	Part B MAC if incident to a physician's service or used in an implanted infusion pump. If other, DME MAC

2026 HCPCS: LEVEL II NATIONAL CODES

HCPCS	DESCRIPTION	JURISDICTION
J9251- J9257	Chemotherapy Drugs	Part B MAC if incident to a physician's service or used in an implanted infusion pump. If other, DME MAC.
J9260 - J9334	Chemotherapy Drugs	Part B MAC if incident to a physician's service or used in an implanted infusion pump. If other, DME MAC.
J9341 - J9370	Chemotherapy Drugs	Part B MAC if incident to a physician's service or used in an implanted infusion pump. If other, DME MAC.
J9372- J9999	Chemotherapy Drugs	Part B MAC if incident to a physician's service or used in an implanted infusion pump. If other, DME MAC.
K0001 - K0108	Wheelchairs	DME MAC
K0195	Elevating Leg Rests	DME MAC
K0455	Infusion Pump used for Uninterrupted Administration of Epoprostenal	DME MAC
K0462	Loaner Equipment	DME MAC
K0552	External Infusion Pump Supplies	DME MAC
K0555-K0605	External Infusion Pump Supplies	DME MAC
K0606 - K0609	Defibrillator Accessories	DME MAC
K0669	Wheelchair Cushion	DME MAC
K0672	Soft Interface for Orthosis	DME MAC
K0730	Inhalation Drug Delivery System	DME MAC
K0733	Power Wheelchair Accessory	DME MAC
K0738	Oxygen Equipment	DME MAC
K0739	Repair or Nonroutine Service for DME	Part B MAC if implanted DME. If other, DME MAC.
K0740	Repair or Nonroutine Service for Oxygen Equipment	DME MAC
K0743 - K0746	Suction Pump and Dressings	DME MAC
K0800 - K0899	Power Mobility Devices	DME MAC
K0900	Custom DME, other than Wheelchair	DME MAC
K1004	Devices	DME MAC when the supplier considers the item DMEPOS. Part B MAC if the supplier considers the item something other than DMEPOS (e.g., supplies furnished incident to the professional service of a physician)
K1007	Devices	DME MAC
K1027	Devices	DME MAC when the supplier considers the item DMEPOS. Part B MAC if the supplier considers the item something other than DMEPOS (e.g., supplies furnished incident to the professional service of a physician).
K1035 - K1037	Devices	DME MAC
L0112 - L4631	Orthotics & Devices	DME MAC
L5000 - L5999	Lower Limb Prosthetics	DME MAC
L6000 - L7499	Upper Limb Prosthetics	DME MAC
L7510 - L7520	Repair of Prosthetic Device	Part B MAC if repair of implanted prosthetic device. If other, DME MAC.
L7600 - L8009	Prosthetics	DME MAC
L8011 - L8485	Prosthetics	DME MAC
L8499	Unlisted Procedure for Miscellaneous Prosthetic Services	Part B MAC if implanted prosthetic device. If other, DME MAC.
L8500 - L8501	Artificial Larynx; Tracheostomy Speaking Valve	DME MAC
L8505	Artificial Larynx Accessory	DME MAC
L8507	Voice Prosthesis, Patient Inserted	DME MAC
L8509	Voice Prosthesis, Inserted by a Licensed Health Care Provider	Part B MAC for dates of service on or after 10/01/2010. DME MAC for dates of service prior to 10/01/2010.
L8510	Voice Prosthesis	DME MAC
L8511 - L8515	Voice Prosthesis	Part B MAC if used with tracheoesophageal voice prostheses inserted by a licensed health care provider. If other, DME MAC.
L8701 - L8721	Devices	DME MAC
L9900	Miscellaneous Orthotic or Prosthetic Component or Accessory	Part B MAC if used with implanted prosthetic device. If other, DME MAC.
Q0144	Azithromycin Dihydrate	Part B MAC if incident to a physician's service. If other, DME MAC.
Q0155	Anti-emetic	DME MAC
Q0161 - Q0181	Anti-emetic	DME MAC
Q0510 - Q0514	Drug Dispensing Fees	DME MAC
Q0516-Q0520	Supply fee HIV prep	Part B MAC if incident to a physician's Service or Part B Pharmacy Supplier, If other, DME MAC
Q0521	Supply fee HIV prep	Part B MAC if incident to a physician's Service or Part B Pharmacy Supplier, If other, DME MAC.
Q2049 -Q2050	Doxorubicin	Part B MAC if incident to a physician's service or used in an implanted infusion pump. If other, DME MAC.
Q2052	IVIG	DME MAC

APPENDIX A

HCPCS	DESCRIPTION	JURISDICTION
Q2058	Injection	Part B MAC if incident to a physician's service or used in an implanted infusion pump. If other, DME MAC.
Q4074	Inhalation Drug	Part B MAC if incident to a physician's service. If other, DME MAC.
Q5101 - Q5130	Injection	Part B MAC if incident to a physician's service or used in an implanted infusion pump. If other, DME MAC.
Q5133 - Q5136	Injection	Part B MAC if incident to a physician's service or used in an implanted infusion pump. If other, DME MAC.
Q5140 - Q5153	Injection	Part B MAC if incident to a physician's service or used in an implanted infusion pump. If other, DME MAC.
Q5155 - Q5156	Injection	Part B MAC if incident to a physician's service or used in an implanted infusion pump. If other, DME MAC.
Q9991 - Q9992	Injection	Part B MAC if incident to a physician's service or used in an implanted infusion pump. If other, DME MAC.
V2020 - V2025	Frames	DME MAC

HCPCS	DESCRIPTION	JURISDICTION
V2100 - V2513	Lenses	DME MAC
V2520 - V2523	Hydrophilic Contact Lenses	Part B MAC if incident to a physician's service. If other, DME MAC.
V2524 - V2526	Hydrophilic Contact Lenses	DME MAC
V2530 - V2531	Contact Lenses, Scleral	DME MAC
V2599	Contact Lens, Other Type	Part B MAC if incident to a physician's service. If other, DME MAC.
V2600 - V2615	Low Vision Aids	DME MAC
V2623 - V2629	Prosthetic Eyes	DME MAC
V2700 - V2780	Miscellaneous Vision Service	DME MAC
V2781	Progressive Lens	DME MAC
V2782 - V2784	Lenses	DME MAC
V2786	Lens	DME MAC
V2797	Vision Supply	DME MAC
V2799	Miscellaneous Vision Service	Part B MAC if supply for an implanted prosthetic device. If other, DME MAC.
V5336	Repair/Modification of Augmentative Communicative System or Device	DME MAC

APPENDIX B

CHAPTER I
GENERAL CORRECT CODING POLICIES
MEDICARE NATIONAL CORRECT CODING INITIATIVE POLICY MANUAL

Revised January 1, 2025

Current Procedural Terminology (CPT) codes, descriptions and other data only are copyright 2024 American Medical Association. All rights reserved.

CPT® is a registered trademark of the American Medical Association.

Applicable FARS\DFARS Restrictions Apply to Government Use.

Fee schedules, relative value units, conversion factors and/or related components aren't assigned by the AMA, aren't part of CPT, and the AMA isn't recommending their use. The AMA doesn't directly or indirectly practice medicine or dispense medical services. The AMA assumes no liability for the data contained or not contained herein.

CMS issues the Hospital Outpatient Prospective Payment System (OPPS) and Ambulatory Surgical Center (ASC) Payment System.

Chapter I
Revision Date 02/28/2025

GENERAL CORRECT CODING POLICIES

A. Introduction

Healthcare providers/suppliers use Healthcare Common Procedure Coding System/Current Procedural Terminology (HCPCS/CPT) codes to report medical and surgical services performed on patients to Medicare Administrative Contractors (MACs). Healthcare Common Procedure Coding System (HCPCS) consists of Level I CPT (Current Procedural Terminology) codes and Level II codes. CPT codes are defined in the American Medical Association's (AMA's) CPT Professional *codebook*, which is updated and published annually. HCPCS Level II codes are defined by the Centers for Medicare & Medicaid Services (CMS) and are updated throughout the year as necessary. Changes in CPT codes are approved by the AMA CPT Editorial Panel, which meets 3 times per year.

HCPCS Level II *and CPT* codes define medical and surgical procedures performed on patients. Some procedure codes are very specific in defining a single service (e.g., CPT code 93000 (electrocardiogram)), while other codes define procedures consisting of many services (e.g., CPT code 58263 (Vaginal hysterectomy, for uterus 250 g or less; with removal of tube(s) and/or ovary(s), with repair of enterocele)). Because many procedures can be performed via different approaches, different methods, or in combination with other procedures, there are often multiple HCPCS/CPT codes defining similar or related procedures.

HCPCS Level II *and CPT* code descriptors usually do not define all services included in a procedure. There are often services inherent in a procedure or group of procedures. For example, anesthesia services include certain preparation and monitoring services.

The CMS developed the National Correct Coding Initiative (NCCI) program to prevent inappropriate payment of services that should not be reported together. Prior to April 1, 2012, NCCI Procedure-to-Procedure (PTP) edits were placed into either the "Column One/Column Two Correct Coding Edit Table" or the "Mutually Exclusive Edit Table." However, on April 1, 2012, the edits in the "Mutually Exclusive Edit Table" were moved to the "Column One/Column Two Correct Coding Edit Table" so that all NCCI PTP edits are currently contained in this single table. Combining the 2 tables simplifies researching NCCI PTP edits and online use of the NCCI tables.

Each edit table contains edits which are pairs of HCPCS/CPT codes that in general should not be reported together. Each edit has a Column One and Column Two HCPCS/CPT code. If a provider/supplier reports the 2 codes of an edit pair, the Column Two code is denied, and the Column One code is eligible for payment. However, if it is clinically appropriate to use an NCCI PTP-associated modifier, both the Column One and Column Two codes are eligible for payment. (NCCI PTP-associated modifiers and their appropriate use are discussed elsewhere in this chapter.)

When the NCCI program was first established and during its early years, the "Column One/Column Two Correct Coding Edit Table" was termed the "Comprehensive/Component Edit Table." This latter terminology was a misnomer. Although the Column Two code is often a component of a more comprehensive Column One code, this relationship is not true for many edits. In the latter type of edit, the code pair edit simply represents 2 codes that should not be reported together. For example, a provider/supplier shall not report a vaginal hysterectomy code and total abdominal hysterectomy code together.

In this chapter, Sections B–Q address various issues relating to NCCI PTP edits.

Medically Unlikely Edits (MUEs) prevent payment for a potentially inappropriate number/quantity of the same service on a single day. An MUE is the maximum units of service (UOS) reported for a HCPCS/CPT code on the vast majority of appropriately reported claims by the same provider/supplier for the same beneficiary on the same date of service. For more information concerning MUEs, see Section V of this chapter.

In this Manual, many policies are described using the term "physician." Unless otherwise indicated, the use of this term does not restrict the application of policies to physicians only. Rather, the policies apply to all practitioners, hospitals, providers, or suppliers eligible to bill the relevant HCPCS/CPT codes pursuant to applicable portions of the Social Security Act (SSA) of 1965, the Code of Federal Regulations (CFR), and Medicare rules. In some sections of this Manual, the term "physician" would not include some of these entities because specific rules do not apply to them. For example, Anesthesia

Rules, CMS Internet-Only Manual (IOM), Publication 100-04 Medicare Claims Processing Manual (MCPM), Chapter 12 (Physician/Nonphysician Practitioners), Section 50 (Payment for Anesthesiology Services) and Global Surgery Rules [e.g., CMS IOM, Publication 100-04 MCPM, Chapter 12 (Physician/Nonphysician Practitioners), Section 40 (Surgeons and Global Surgery)] do not apply to hospitals.

Providers/suppliers reporting services under Medicare's hospital Outpatient Prospective Payment System (OPPS) shall report all services in accordance with appropriate Medicare "IOM" instructions.

Providers/suppliers must report services correctly. This manual discusses general coding principles in Chapter I, and principles more relevant to other specific groups of HCPCS/CPT codes in the other chapters. There are certain types of improper coding that providers/suppliers must avoid.

Procedures shall be reported with the most comprehensive HCPCS/CPT code that describes the services performed. Providers/suppliers must not unbundle the services described by a HCPCS/CPT code. Some examples follow:

- A provider/supplier shall not report multiple HCPCS/CPT codes when a single comprehensive HCPCS/CPT code describes these services. For example, if a physician performs a vaginal hysterectomy on a uterus weighing less than 250 grams with bilateral salpingo-oophorectomy, the provider/supplier shall report CPT code 58262 (Vaginal hysterectomy, for uterus 250 g or less; with removal of tube(s), and/or ovary(s)). The provider/supplier shall not report CPT code 58260 (Vaginal hysterectomy, for uterus 250 g or less;) plus CPT code 58720 (Salpingo-oophorectomy, complete or partial, unilateral, or bilateral (separate procedure)).
- A physician shall not fragment a procedure into component parts. For example, if a physician performs an anal endoscopy with biopsy, the provider/supplier shall report CPT code 46606 (Anoscopy; with biopsy, single or multiple). It is improper to unbundle this procedure and report CPT code 46600 (Anoscopy; diagnostic...) plus CPT code 45100 (Biopsy of anorectal wall, anal approach...). The latter code is not intended to be used with an endoscopic procedure code.
- A provider/supplier shall not unbundle a bilateral procedure code into 2 unilateral procedure codes. For example, if a physician performs bilateral mammography, the provider/supplier shall report CPT code 77066 (Diagnostic mammography... bilateral). The provider/supplier shall not report CPT code 77065 (Diagnostic mammography...unilateral) with 2 UOS or 77065 LT plus 77065 RT.
- A provider/supplier shall not unbundle services that are integral to a more comprehensive procedure. For example, surgical access is integral to a surgical procedure. A provider/supplier shall not report CPT code 49000 (Exploratory laparotomy...) when performing an open abdominal procedure such as a total abdominal colectomy (e.g., CPT code 44150).
- Providers/suppliers shall only report a biopsy separately when pathologic examination results in a decision to immediately proceed with a more extensive procedure (e.g., excision, destruction, removal) on the same lesion; or when performed on a separate lesion.
- Providers/suppliers shall not report a biopsy separately when it is to assess resection margins or to verify resectability; or when performed and submitted for pathologic evaluation completed after performing the more extensive procedure.

Providers/suppliers must avoid downcoding. If a HCPCS/CPT code exists that describes the services performed, the providers/suppliers must report this code rather than report a less comprehensive code with other codes describing the services not included in the less comprehensive code. For example, if a physician performs a unilateral partial mastectomy with axillary lymphadenectomy, the provider/supplier shall report CPT code 19302 (Mastectomy, partial...; with axillary lymphadenectomy). A provider/supplier shall not report CPT code 19301 (Mastectomy, partial...) plus CPT code 38745 (Axillary lymphadenectomy; complete).

Providers/suppliers must avoid upcoding. A HCPCS/CPT code may be reported only if all services described by that code have been performed. For example, if a physician performs a superficial axillary lymphadenectomy (CPT code 38740), the provider/supplier shall not report CPT code 38745 (Axillary lymphadenectomy; complete).

Providers/suppliers must report UOS correctly. Each HCPCS/CPT code has a defined unit of service for reporting purposes. A provider/supplier shall not report UOS for a HCPCS/CPT code using a criterion that differs from the code's defined unit of service. For example, some therapy codes are reported in fifteen-minute increments (e.g., CPT codes 97110-97124). Others are reported per session (e.g., CPT codes 92507, 92508). A provider/supplier shall not report a per session code using fifteen-minute increments. CPT code 92507 or 92508 should be reported with one unit of service on a single date of service.

The MUE values and NCCI PTP edits are based on services provided by the same physician to the same beneficiary on the same date of service. Physicians shall not inconvenience beneficiaries nor increase risks to beneficiaries by performing services on different dates of service to avoid MUE or NCCI PTP edits.

In 2010, the *CPT* Professional *codebook* modified the numbering of codes so that the sequence of codes as they appear in the *CPT* Professional *codebook* does not necessarily correspond to a sequential numbering of codes. In the Medicare NCCI Policy Manual, use of a numerical range of codes reflects all codes that numerically fall within the range regardless of their sequential order in the *CPT* Professional *codebook*.

This chapter addresses general coding principles, issues, and policies. Many of these principles, issues, and policies are addressed further in subsequent chapters dealing with specific groups of HCPCS/CPT codes. In this chapter, examples are often used to clarify principles, issues, or policies. The examples do not represent the only codes to which the principles, issues, or policies apply.

B. Coding Based on Standards of Medical/Surgical Practice

Most HCPCS/CPT code defined procedures include services that are integral to them. Some of these integral services have specific CPT codes for reporting the service when not performed as an integral part of another procedure. (For example, CPT code 36000 (Introduction of needle or intracatheter, vein) is integral to all nuclear medicine procedures requiring injection of a radiopharmaceutical into a vein. CPT code 36000 is not separately reportable with these types of nuclear medicine procedures. However, CPT code 36000 may be reported alone if the only service provided is the introduction of a needle into a vein. Other integral services do not have specific CPT codes. (For example, wound irrigation is integral to the treatment of all wounds and does not have a HCPCS/CPT code.) Services integral to HCPCS/CPT code defined procedures are included in those procedures based upon the standards of medical/surgical practice. It is inappropriate to separately report services that are integral to another procedure with that procedure.

Many NCCI PTP edits are based upon the standards of medical/surgical practice. Services that are integral to another service are component parts of the more comprehensive service. When integral component services have their own HCPCS/CPT codes, NCCI PTP edits place the comprehensive service in Column One and the component service in Column Two. Since a component service integral to a comprehensive service is not separately reportable, the Column Two code is not separately reportable with the Column One code.

Some services are integral to large numbers of procedures. Other services are integral to a more limited number of procedures. Examples of services integral to a large number of procedures include:

- Cleansing, shaving and prepping of skin
- Draping and positioning of patient
- Insertion of intravenous access for medication administration;
- Insertion of urinary catheter
- Sedative administration by the physician performing a procedure (see Chapter II, Anesthesia Services)
- Local, topical or regional anesthesia administered by the physician performing the procedure
- Surgical approach including identification of anatomical landmarks, incision, evaluation of the surgical field, debridement of traumatized tissue, lysis of adhesions, and isolation of structures limiting access to the surgical field such as bone, blood vessels, nerve, and muscles including stimulation for identification or monitoring
- Surgical cultures
- Wound irrigation
- Insertion and removal of drains, suction devices, and pumps into same site
- Surgical closure and dressings
- Application, management, and removal of postoperative dressings and analgesic devices (peri-incisional)
- Application of TENS unit
- Institution of Patient Controlled Anesthesia
- Preoperative, intraoperative and postoperative documentation, including photographs, drawings, dictation, or transcription as necessary to document the services provided
- Imaging and/or ultrasound guidance
- Surgical supplies, except for specific situations where CMS policy permits separate payment.

Although other chapters in this Manual further address issues related to the standards of medical/surgical practice for the procedures covered by that chapter, it is not possible to discuss all NCCI PTP edits based upon the principle of the standards of medical/surgical practice due to space limitations. However, there are several general principles that can be applied to the edits, as follows:

1. The component service is an accepted standard of care when performing the comprehensive service.
2. The component service is usually necessary to complete the comprehensive service.
3. The component service is not a separately distinguishable procedure when performed with the comprehensive service.

Specific examples of services that are not separately reportable because they are components of more comprehensive services follow:

Medical Examples

1. Because interpretation of cardiac rhythm is an integral component of the interpretation of an electrocardiogram, a rhythm strip is not separately reportable.
2. Because determination of ankle/brachial indices requires both upper and lower extremity Doppler studies, an upper extremity Doppler study is not separately reportable.
3. Because a cardiac stress test includes multiple electrocardiograms, an electrocardiogram is not separately reportable.

Surgical Examples

1. Because a myringotomy requires access to the tympanic membrane through the external auditory canal, removal of impacted cerumen from the external auditory canal is not separately reportable.
2. A "scout" bronchoscopy to assess the surgical field, anatomic landmarks, extent of disease, etc., is not separately reportable with an open pulmonary procedure such as a pulmonary lobectomy. By contrast, an initial diagnostic bronchoscopy is separately reportable. If the diagnostic bronchoscopy is performed at the same patient encounter as the open pulmonary procedure and does not duplicate an earlier diagnostic bronchoscopy by the same or another physician, the diagnostic bronchoscopy may be reported with modifier 58 appended to the open pulmonary procedure code to indicate a staged procedure. A cursory examination of the upper airway during a bronchoscopy with the bronchoscope shall not be reported separately as a laryngoscopy. However, separate endoscopies of anatomically distinct areas with different endoscopes may be reported separately (e.g., thoracoscopy and mediastinoscopy).
3. If an endoscopic procedure is performed at the same patient encounter as a nonendoscopic procedure to ensure no intraoperative injury occurred or verify the procedure was performed correctly, the endoscopic procedure is not separately reportable with the nonendoscopic procedure.
4. Because a colectomy requires exposure of the colon, the laparotomy and adhesiolysis to expose the colon are not separately reportable.

Medical/Surgical Package

Most medical and surgical procedures include pre-procedure, intra-procedure, and postprocedure work. When multiple procedures are performed at the same patient encounter, there is often overlap of the pre-procedure and post-procedure work. Payment methodologies for surgical procedures account for the overlap of the pre-procedure and post-procedure work.

The component elements of the pre-procedure and post-procedure work for each procedure are included component services of that procedure as a standard of medical/surgical practice. Some general guidelines follow:

1. Many invasive procedures require vascular and/or airway access. The work associated with obtaining the required access is included in the pre-procedure or intra-procedure work. The work associated with returning a patient to the appropriate post-procedure state is included in the post-procedure work.

Airway access is necessary for general anesthesia and is not separately reportable. There is no CPT code for elective endotracheal intubation. CPT code 31500 describes an emergency endotracheal intubation and shall not be reported for elective endotracheal intubation. Visualization of the airway is a component part of an endotracheal intubation, and CPT codes describing procedures that visualize the airway (e.g., nasal endoscopy, laryngoscopy, bronchoscopy) shall not be reported with an endotracheal intubation. These CPT codes describe diagnostic and therapeutic endoscopies, and it is a misuse of these codes to report visualization of the airway for endotracheal intubation.

Intravenous access (e.g., CPT codes 36000, 36400, 36410) is not separately reportable when performed with many types of procedures (e.g., surgical procedures, anesthesia procedures, radiological procedures requiring intravenous contrast, nuclear medicine procedures requiring intravenous radiopharmaceutical).

After vascular access is achieved, the access must be maintained by a slow infusion (e.g., saline) or injection of heparin or saline into a "lock." Since these services are necessary for maintenance of the vascular access, they are not separately reportable with the vascular access CPT codes or procedures requiring vascular access as a standard of medical/surgical practice. CPT codes 37211-37214 (Transcatheter therapy with infusion for thrombolysis) shall not be reported for use of an anticoagulant to maintain vascular access.

The global surgical package includes the administration of fluids and drugs during the operative procedure. CPT codes 96360-96379 shall not be reported separately for that operative procedure. Under OPPS, the administration of fluids and drugs during or for an operative procedure are included services and are not separately reportable (e.g., CPT codes 96360-96379).

When a procedure requires more invasive vascular access services (e.g., central venous access, pulmonary artery access), the more invasive vascular service is separately reportable if it is not typical of the procedure and the work of the more invasive vascular service has not been included in the valuation of the procedure.

Insertion of a central venous access device (e.g., central venous catheter, pulmonary artery catheter) requires passage of a catheter through central venous vessels and, in the case of a pulmonary artery catheter, through the right atrium and ventricle. These services often require the use of fluoroscopic guidance. Separate reporting of CPT codes for right heart catheterization, selective venous catheterization, or pulmonary artery catheterization is not appropriate when reporting a CPT code for insertion of a central venous access device. Since CPT code 77001 describes fluoroscopic guidance for central venous access device procedures, CPT codes for more general fluoroscopy (e.g., 76000, 77002) shall not be reported separately. (CPT code 76001 was deleted January 1, 2019.)

2. Medicare Anesthesia Rules prevent separate payment for anesthesia services by the same physician performing a surgical or medical procedure. The physician performing a surgical or medical procedure shall not report CPT codes 96360-96379 for the administration of anesthetic agents during the procedure. If it is medically reasonable and necessary that a separate provider/supplier (anesthesia practitioner) perform anesthesia services (e.g., monitored anesthesia care) for a surgical or medical procedure, a separate anesthesia service may be reported by the second provider/supplier.

Under the OPPS, anesthesia for a surgical procedure is an included service and is not separately reportable. For example, a provider/supplier shall not report CPT codes 96360-96379 for anesthesia services.

When anesthesia services are not separately reportable, providers/suppliers shall not unbundle components of anesthesia and report them in lieu of an anesthesia code.

3. If an endoscopic procedure is performed at the same patient encounter as a nonendoscopic procedure to ensure that no intraoperative injury occurred or to verify that the procedure was performed correctly, the endoscopic procedure is not separately reportable with the non-endoscopic procedure.
4. Many procedures require cardiopulmonary monitoring, either by the physician performing the procedure or an anesthesia practitioner. Since these services are integral to the procedure, they are not separately reportable. Examples of these services include cardiac monitoring, pulse oximetry, and ventilation management (e.g., 93000-93010, 93040-93042, 94760, 94761).
5. For more information regarding biopsies, see Section A, Introduction.
6. Exposure and exploration of the surgical field is integral to an operative procedure and is not separately reportable. For example, an exploratory laparotomy (CPT code 49000) is not separately reportable with an intra-abdominal procedure. If exploration of the surgical field results in additional procedures other than the primary procedure, the additional procedures may generally be reported separately. However, a procedure designated by the CPT code descriptor as a "separate procedure" is not separately reportable if performed in a region anatomically related to the other procedure(s) through the same skin incision, orifice, or surgical approach.
7. If a definitive surgical procedure requires access through diseased tissue (e.g., necrotic skin, abscess, hematoma, seroma), a separate service for this access (e.g., debridement, incision, and drainage) is not separately reportable. Types of procedures to which this principle applies include, but are not limited to, -ectomy, -otomy, excision, resection, -plasty, insertion, revision, replacement, relocation, removal, or closure. For example, debridement of skin and subcutaneous tissue at the site of an abdominal incision made to perform an intra-abdominal procedure is not separately reportable. (See Chapter IV, Section I (General Policy Statements), Subsection 11 for guidance on reporting debridement with open fractures and dislocations.)
8. If removal, destruction, or other form of elimination of a lesion requires coincidental elimination of other pathology, only the primary procedure may be reported. For example, if an area of pilonidal disease contains an abscess, incision, and drainage of the abscess during the procedure to excise the area of pilonidal disease is not separately reportable.
9. An excision and removal (-ectomy) includes the incision and opening (-otomy) of the organ. A HCPCS/CPT code for an –otomy procedure shall not be reported with an –ectomy code for the same organ.
10. Multiple approaches to the same procedure are mutually exclusive of one another and shall not be reported separately. For example, both a vaginal hysterectomy and abdominal hysterectomy shall not be reported separately.
11. If a procedure using one approach fails and is converted to a procedure using a different approach, only the completed procedure may be reported. For example, if a

laparoscopic hysterectomy is converted to an open hysterectomy, only the open hysterectomy procedure code may be reported.

12. If a laparoscopic procedure fails and is converted to an open procedure, the physician shall not report a diagnostic laparoscopy in lieu of the failed laparoscopic procedure. For example, if a laparoscopic cholecystectomy is converted to an open cholecystectomy, the physician shall not report the failed laparoscopic cholecystectomy nor a diagnostic laparoscopy.

13. If a diagnostic endoscopy is the basis for and precedes an open procedure, the diagnostic endoscopy may be reported with modifier 58 appended to the open procedure code. However, the medical record must document the medical reasonableness and necessity for the diagnostic endoscopy. A scout endoscopy to assess anatomic landmarks and extent of disease is not separately reportable with an open procedure. When an endoscopic procedure fails and is converted to another surgical procedure, only the completed surgical procedure may be reported. The endoscopic procedure is not separately reportable with the completed surgical procedure.

14. Treatment of complications of primary surgical procedures is separately reportable with some limitations. The global surgical package for an operative procedure includes all intra-operative services that are normally a usual and necessary part of the procedure. Additionally, the global surgical package includes all medical and surgical services required of the surgeon during the postoperative period of the surgery to treat complications that do not require return to the operating room. Thus, treatment of a complication of a primary surgical procedure is not separately reportable:
    (1) if it represents usual and necessary care in the operating room during the procedure; or
    (2) if it occurs postoperatively and does not require return to the operating room. For example, control of hemorrhage is a usual and necessary component of a surgical procedure in the operating room and is not separately reportable. Control of postoperative hemorrhage is also not separately reportable unless the patient must be returned to the operating room for treatment. In the latter case, the control of hemorrhage may be separately reportable with modifier 78.

D. Evaluation & Management (E&M) Services

Medicare Global Surgery Rules define the rules for reporting Evaluation & Management (E&M) services with procedures covered by these rules. This section summarizes some of the rules.

All procedures on the Medicare Physician Fee Schedule are assigned a global period of 000, 010, 090, XXX, YYY, ZZZ, or MMM. The global concept does not apply to XXX procedures. The global period for YYY procedures is defined by the MAC. All procedures with a global period of ZZZ are related to another procedure, and the applicable global period for the ZZZ code is determined by the related procedure. Procedures with a global period of MMM are maternity procedures.

Since NCCI PTP edits are applied to same-day services by the same provider/supplier to the same beneficiary, certain Global Surgery Rules are applicable to the NCCI program. An E&M service is separately reportable on the same date of service as a procedure with a global period of 000, 010, or 090 under limited circumstances.

If a procedure has a global period of 090 days, it is defined as a major surgical procedure. If an E&M service is performed on the same date of service as a major surgical procedure to decide whether to perform this surgical procedure, the E&M service is separately reportable with modifier 57. Other preoperative E&M services on the same date of service as a major surgical procedure are included in the global payment for the procedure and are not separately reportable. NCCI does not contain edits based on this rule because MACs have separate edits.

If a procedure has a global period of 000 or 010 days, it is defined as a minor surgical procedure. In general, E&M services performed on the same date of service as a minor surgical procedure are included in the payment for the procedure. The decision to perform a minor surgical procedure is included in the payment for the minor surgical procedure and shall not be reported separately as an E&M service. However, a significant and separately identifiable E&M service unrelated to the decision to perform the minor surgical procedure is separately reportable with modifier 25. The E&M service and minor surgical procedure do not require different diagnoses. If a minor surgical procedure is performed on a new patient, the same rules for reporting E&M services apply. The fact that the patient is "new" to the provider/supplier is not sufficient alone to justify reporting an E&M service on the same date of service as a minor surgical procedure. *The* NCCI *program* contains many, but not all, possible edits based on these principles.

For major and minor surgical procedures, postoperative E&M services related to recovery from the surgical procedure during the postoperative period are included in the global surgical package as are E&M services related to complications of the surgery. Postoperative visits unrelated to the diagnosis for which the surgical procedure was performed, unless related to a complication of surgery, may be reported separately on the same day as a surgical procedure with modifier 24 ("Unrelated Evaluation and Management Service by the Same Physician or Other Qualified Health Care Professional During a Postoperative Period").

Procedures with a global surgery indicator of "XXX" are not covered by these rules. Many of these "XXX" procedures are performed by physicians and have inherent pre-procedure, intraprocedure, and post-procedure work usually performed each time the procedure is completed. This work shall **not** be reported as a separate E&M code. Other "XXX" procedures are not usually performed by a physician and have no physician work relative value units associated with them. A physician shall **not** report a separate E&M code with these procedures for the supervision of others performing the procedure or for the interpretation of the procedure. With most "XXX" procedures, the physician may, however, perform a significant and separately identifiable E&M *service that is above and beyond usual pre- and post-operative work of the procedure* on the same date of service which may be reported by appending modifier 25 to the E&M code. This E&M service may be related to the same diagnosis necessitating performance of the "XXX" procedure but cannot include any work inherent in the "XXX" procedure, supervision of others performing the "XXX" procedure, or time for interpreting the result of the "XXX" procedure. Appending modifier 25 to a significant, separately identifiable E&M service when performed on the same date of service as an "XXX" procedure *may be appropriate in some instances.*

E. Modifiers and Modifier Indicators

The AMA *CPT* Professional *codebook* and the CMS define modifiers that may be appended to HCPCS/CPT codes to provide additional information about the services rendered. Modifiers consist of 2 alphanumeric characters.

Modifiers may be appended to HCPCS/CPT codes only if the clinical circumstances justify the use of the modifier. A modifier shall not be appended to a HCPCS/CPT code solely to bypass an NCCI PTP edit if the clinical circumstances do not justify its use. If the Medicare program imposes restrictions on the use of a modifier, the modifier may only be used to bypass an NCCI PTP edit if the Medicare restrictions are fulfilled. Modifiers that may be used under appropriate clinical circumstances to bypass an NCCI PTP edit include:

Anatomic modifiers: E1-E4, FA, F1-F9, TA, T1-T9, LT, RT, LC, LD, RC, LM, RI

Global surgery modifiers: 24, 25, 57, 58, 78, 79

Other modifiers: 27, 59, 91, XE, XS, XP, XU

These modifiers are referred to as NCCI PTP-associated modifiers. Modifiers 22 *("Increased Procedural Services"),* 76 ("Repeat Procedure or Service by Same Physician *or Other Qualified Health Care Professional*") and 77 ("Repeat Procedure by Another Physician *or Other Qualified Health Care Professional*") are not NCCI PTP-associated modifiers. *The use* of **modifiers 22, 76, or 77** does not bypass an NCCI PTP edit.

Each NCCI PTP edit has an assigned Correct Coding Modifier Indicator (CCMI). A CCMI of "0" indicates that NCCI PTP-associated modifiers cannot be used to bypass the edit. A CCMI of "1" indicates that NCCI PTP-associated modifiers may be used to bypass an edit under appropriate circumstances. A modifier indicator of "9" indicates that the use of NCCI PTP-associated modifiers is not specified. This indicator is used for all code pairs that have a deletion date that is the same as the effective date. This indicator prevents blank spaces from appearing in the indicator field.

It is very important that NCCI PTP-associated modifiers only be used when appropriate. In general, these circumstances relate to separate patient encounters, separate anatomic sites, or separate specimens. (See subsequent discussion of modifiers in this section.) Most edits involving paired organs or structures (e.g., eyes, ears, extremities, lungs, kidneys) have NCCI PTP modifier indicators of "1" because the 2 codes of the code pair edit may be reported if performed on the contralateral organs or structures. Most of these code pairs should not be reported with NCCI PTPassociated modifiers when performed on the ipsilateral organ or structure unless there is a specific coding rationale to bypass the edit. The existence of the NCCI PTP edit indicates that the 2 codes generally cannot be reported together unless the 2 corresponding procedures are performed at 2 separate patient encounters or 2 separate anatomic locations. However, if the 2 corresponding procedures are performed at the same patient encounter and in contiguous structures in the same organ or anatomic region, NCCI PTP-associated modifiers generally should not be used.

The appropriate use of most of these modifiers is straightforward. However, further explanation is provided regarding modifiers 25, 58, *59, XE, XP, XS,* and *XU*. Although modifier 22 is not a modifier that bypasses an NCCI PTP edit, its use is occasionally relevant to an NCCI PTP edit and is discussed below.

a) **Modifier 22**: *The CPT* Professional *codebook defines modifier 22* as "Increased Procedural Services." This modifier shall not be reported unless the service(s) performed is (are) substantially more extensive than the usual service(s) included in the procedure described by the HCPCS/CPT code reported.

When an NCCI PTP edit allows use of NCCI PTP-associated modifiers to bypass the edit and the clinical circumstances justify use of one of these modifiers, both services may be reported with the NCCI PTP-associated modifier. However, if the NCCI PTP edit does not allow use of NCCI PTP-associated modifiers to bypass it and the procedure qualifies as an unusual procedural service, the physician may report the Column One HCPCS/CPT code of the NCCI PTP edit with modifier 22. The MAC may then evaluate the unusual procedural service to determine whether additional payment is justified.

For example, CMS limits payment for CPT code 69990 (Microsurgical techniques, requiring use of operating microscope...) to procedures listed in the IOM, Publication 100-04 MCPM Chapter 12 Section 20.4.5. If a physician reports CPT code 69990 with 2 other CPT codes and 1 of the codes is not on this list, an NCCI PTP edit with the code not on the list will prevent payment for CPT code 69990. Claims processing systems do not determine which procedure is linked with CPT code 69990. In situations such as this, the physician may submit their claim to the local MAC for readjudication appending modifier 22 to the CPT code. Although MAC cannot override an NCCI PTP edit that does not allow use of NCCI PTP-associated modifiers, the MAC has discretion to adjust payment to include use of the operating microscope based on modifier 22.

b) **Modifier 25**: The *CPT* Professional *codebook* defines modifier 25 as a "Significant, Separately Identifiable Evaluation and Management Service by the Same Physician or Other Qualified Health Care Professional on the Same Day of the Procedure or Other Service." Modifier 25 may be appended to an evaluation and management (E&M) CPT code to indicate that the E&M service is significant and separately identifiable from other services reported on the same date of service. The E&M service may be related to the same or different diagnosis as the other procedure(s).

Modifier 25 may be appended to E&M services reported with minor surgical procedures (with global periods of 000 or 010 days) or procedures not covered by Global Surgery Rules (with a global indicator of XXX). Since minor surgical procedures and XXX procedures include preprocedure, intra-procedure, and post-procedure work inherent in the procedure, the provider/supplier shall not report an E&M service for this work. Furthermore, Medicare Global Surgery Rules prevent the reporting of a separate E&M service for the work associated with the decision to perform a minor surgical procedure regardless of whether the patient is a new or established patient.

c) **Modifier 58**: *The CPT* Professional *codebook defines modifier 58* as a "Staged or Related Procedure or Service by the Same Physician or Other Qualified Health Care Professional During the Postoperative Period." It may be used to indicate that a procedure was followed by a second procedure during the post-operative period of the first procedure. This situation may occur because the second procedure was planned prospectively, was more extensive than the first procedure, or was therapy after a diagnostic surgical service. Use of modifier 58 will bypass NCCI PTP edits that allow use of NCCI PTP-associated modifiers.

If a diagnostic endoscopic procedure results in the decision to perform an open procedure, both procedures may be reported with modifier 58 appended to the HCPCS/CPT code for the open procedure. However, if the endoscopic procedure preceding an open procedure is a "scout" procedure to assess anatomic landmarks and/or extent of disease, it is not separately reportable.

Diagnostic endoscopy is never separately reportable with another endoscopic procedure of the same organ(s) or anatomic region when performed at the same patient encounter. Similarly, diagnostic laparoscopy is never separately reportable with a surgical laparoscopic procedure of the same body cavity when performed at the same patient encounter.

If a planned laparoscopic procedure fails and is converted to an open procedure, only the open procedure may be reported. The failed laparoscopic procedure is not separately reportable. The NCCI program contains many, but not all, edits bundling laparoscopic procedures into open procedures. Since the number of possible code combinations bundling a laparoscopic procedure into an open procedure is much greater than the number of such edits in the NCCI program, the principle stated in this paragraph is applicable regardless of whether the selected code pair combination is included in the NCCI tables. A provider/supplier shall not select laparoscopic and open HCPCS/CPT codes to report because the combination is not included in the NCCI tables.

d) **Modifier 59:** Modifier 59 is an important NCCI PTP-associated modifier that is often used incorrectly. For the NCCI program, its primary purpose is to indicate that 2 or more procedures are performed at different anatomic sites or different patient encounters. One function of NCCI PTP edits is to prevent payment for codes that report overlapping services, except in those instances where the services are "separate and distinct." Modifier 59 shall only be used if no other modifier more appropriately describes the relationships of the 2 or more procedure codes (see Section E for modifiers XE, XP, XS, XU). The *CPT* Professional *codebook* defines modifier 59 as follows:

Modifier 59: Distinct Procedural Service: Under certain circumstances, it may be necessary to indicate that a procedure or service was distinct or independent from other non-E/M services performed on the same day. Modifier 59 is used to identify procedures/services, other than E/M services, that are not normally reported together, but are appropriate under the circumstances. Documentation must support a different session, different procedure or surgery, different site or organ system, separate incision/excision, separate lesion, or separate injury (or area of injury in extensive injuries) not ordinarily encountered or performed on the same day by the same individual. However, when another already established modifier is appropriate, it should be used rather than modifier 59. Only if no more descriptive modifier is available, and the use of modifier 59 best explains the circumstances, should modifier 59 be used. Note: Modifier 59 should not be appended to an E/M service. To report a separate and distinct E/M service with a nonE/M service performed on the same date, see modifier 25*".*

Modifier 59 and other NCCI-associated modifiers should *not* be used to bypass a PTP edit unless the proper criteria for use of the modifier are met. Documentation in the medical record must satisfy the criteria required by any NCCI-associated modifier that is used. Modifier "-59" shall not be used with code 77427 Radiation treatment management, 5 treatments.

NCCI PTP edits define when 2 procedure HCPCS/CPT codes may not be reported together, except under special circumstances. If an edit allows use of NCCI PTP-associated modifiers, the 2 procedure codes may be reported together when the 2 procedures are performed at different anatomic sites or different patient encounters. MAC processing systems use NCCI PTP associated modifiers to allow payment of both codes of an edit. Modifiers 59 or XE, XP, XS, XU and other NCCI PTP-associated modifiers shall NOT be used to bypass an NCCI PTP edit unless the proper criteria for use of the modifier are met. Documentation in the medical record must satisfy the criteria required by any NCCI PTP-associated modifier used. Some examples of the appropriate use of modifiers 59 or XE, XP, XS, XU are contained in the individual chapter policies.

One of the common misuses of modifier 59 is related to the portion of the definition of modifier 59 allowing its use to describe "different procedure or surgery." The code descriptors of the 2 codes of a code pair edit usually represent different procedures or surgeries. The edit indicates that the 2 procedures/surgeries cannot be reported together if performed at the same anatomic site and same patient encounter. The provider/supplier cannot use modifier 59 for such an edit based on the 2 codes being different procedures/surgeries. However, if the 2 procedures/surgeries are performed at separate anatomic sites or at separate patient encounters on the same date of service, modifiers 59 or XE or XS may be appended to indicate that they are different procedures/surgeries on that date of service.

Modifier 59 or XS is used appropriately for different anatomic sites during the same encounter only when procedures which are not ordinarily performed or encountered on the same day are performed on different organs, or different anatomic regions, or in limited situations on different, non-contiguous lesions in different anatomic regions of the same organ.

There are several exceptions to this general principle about misuse of modifiers 59 or XE, XP, XS, XU that apply to some code pair edits for procedures performed at the same patient encounter.

(1) When a diagnostic procedure precedes a surgical or non-surgical therapeutic procedure and is the basis on which the decision to perform the surgical or non-surgical therapeutic procedure is made, that diagnostic procedure may be considered to be a separate and distinct procedure as long as (a) it occurs before the therapeutic procedure and is not interspersed with services that are required for the therapeutic intervention; (b) it clearly provides the information needed to decide whether to proceed with the therapeutic procedure; and (c) it does not constitute a service that would have otherwise been required during the therapeutic intervention. If the diagnostic procedure is an inherent component of the surgical or non-surgical therapeutic procedure, it shall not be reported separately.

(2) When a diagnostic procedure follows a surgical procedure or non-surgical therapeutic procedure, that diagnostic procedure may be considered to be a separate and distinct procedure as long as (a) it occurs after the completion of the therapeutic procedure and is not interspersed with or otherwise commingled with services

that are only required for the therapeutic intervention, and (b) it does not constitute a service that would have otherwise been required during the therapeutic intervention. If the postprocedure diagnostic procedure is an inherent component or otherwise included (or not separately payable) post-procedure service of the surgical procedure or non-surgical therapeutic procedure, it shall not be reported separately.

(3) There is an appropriate use for modifiers 59 or XE or XS that is applicable only to codes for which the unit of service is a measure of time (e.g., per 15 minutes, per hour). If 2 separate and distinct timed services are provided in separate and distinct time blocks, modifier 59 may be used to identify the services. The separate and distinct time blocks for the 2 services may be sequential to one another or split. When the 2 services are split, the time block for 1 service may be followed by a time block for the second service followed by another time block for the first service. All Medicare rules for reporting timed services are applicable. For example, the total time is calculated for all related timed services performed. The number of reportable UOS is based on the total time, and these UOS are allocated between the HCPCS/CPT codes for the individual services performed. The practitioner is not permitted to perform multiple services, each for the minimal reportable time, and report each of these as separate UOS.

Use of modifiers 59 or XE or XS to indicate different procedures/surgeries does not require a different diagnosis for each HCPCS/CPT coded procedure/surgery. Additionally, different diagnoses are not adequate criteria for use of modifiers 59 or XE, *or* XS. The HCPCS/CPT codes remain bundled unless the procedures/surgeries are performed at different anatomic sites or separate patient encounters.

From an NCCI program perspective, the definition of different anatomic sites includes different organs, different anatomic regions, or different lesions in the same organ. It does not include treatment of contiguous structures in the same organ or anatomic region. For example, treatment of the nail, nail bed, and adjacent soft tissue constitutes treatment of a single anatomic site. Treatment of posterior segment structures in the ipsilateral eye constitutes treatment of a single anatomic site.

If the same procedure is performed at different anatomic sites, it does not necessarily imply that a HCPCS/CPT code may be reported with more than one unit of service for the procedure. Determining whether additional UOS may be reported depends in part upon the HCPCS/CPT code descriptor including the definition of the code's unit of service when present.

Example 1

The Column One/Column Two code edit with Column One CPT code 38221 (Diagnostic bone marrow biopsy(ies)) and Column Two CPT code 38220 (Diagnostic bone marrow, aspiration) includes two distinct procedures when performed at separate anatomic sites (e.g., contralateral iliac bones) or separate patient encounters. In these circumstances, it would be acceptable to use modifier 59. However, if both 38221 and 38220 are performed on the same iliac bone at the same patient encounter which is the usual practice, modifier 59 shall NOT be used. Although CMS does not allow separate payment for CPT code 38220 with CPT code 38221 when bone marrow aspiration and biopsy are performed on the same iliac bone at a single patient encounter, a physician may report CPT code 38222 (Diagnostic bone marrow; biopsy(ies) and aspiration(s)).

Example 2

The Column One/Column Two code edit with Column One CPT code 11055 (Paring or cutting of benign hyperkeratotic lesion (eg, corn or callus); single lesion) and Column Two CPT code 11720 (Debridement of nail(s) by any method(s); 1 to 5) should not be reported together for services performed on skin distal to and including the skin overlying the distal interphalangeal joint of the same toe. Modifiers 59 or XE, XP, XS, XU should not be used if a nail is debrided on the same toe on which a hyperkeratotic lesion of the skin on or distal to the distal interphalangeal joint is pared. Modifiers 59 or XS may be reported with code 11720 if 1 to 5 nails are debrided, and a hyperkeratotic lesion is pared on a toe other than 1 with a debrided toenail or the hyperkeratotic lesion is proximal to the skin overlying the distal interphalangeal joint of a toe on which a nail is debrided.

e) **Modifiers XE, XS, XP, XU:** These modifiers were effective January 1, 2015. These modifiers were developed to provide greater reporting specificity in situations where modifier 59 was previously reported and may be used in lieu of modifier 59 whenever possible. The modifiers are defined as follows:

XE – "Separate Encounter, A service that is distinct because it occurred during a separate encounter." This modifier shall only be used to describe separate encounters on the same date of service.
XS – "Separate Structure, A service that is distinct because it was performed on a separate organ/structure"
XP – "Separate Practitioner, A service that is distinct because it was performed by a different practitioner"
XU – "Unusual Non-Overlapping Service, the use of a service that is distinct because it does not overlap usual components of the main service"

F. Standard Preparation/Monitoring Services for Anesthesia

With few exceptions, anesthesia HCPCS/CPT codes do not specify the mode of anesthesia for a particular procedure. Regardless of the mode of anesthesia, preparation and monitoring services are not separately reportable with anesthesia service HCPCS/CPT codes when performed in association with the anesthesia service. However, if the provider/supplier of the anesthesia service performs 1 or more of these services prior to and unrelated to the anticipated anesthesia service or after the patient is released from the anesthesia practitioner's postoperative care, the service may be separately reportable with modifiers 59 or XE or XU. *Refer to Chapter 2 for additional information concerning anesthesia coding.*

G. Anesthesia Service Included in the Surgical Procedure

Under the CMS Anesthesia Rules, with limited exceptions, Medicare does not allow separate payment for anesthesia services performed by the physician who also furnishes the medical or surgical service. In this case, payment for the anesthesia service is included in the payment for the medical or surgical procedure. Likewise, under OPPS, payment for the anesthesia service is generally included in the payment for the medical or surgical procedure. For example, separate payment is not allowed for the physician's performance of local, regional, or most other anesthesia including nerve blocks if the physician also performs the medical or surgical procedure. Medicare generally allows separate reporting for moderate conscious sedation services (CPT codes 99151-99153) when provided by the same physician performing a medical or surgical procedure except when the anesthesia service is bundled into the procedure, e.g., radiation treatment management.

CPT codes describing anesthesia services (00100-01999) or services that are bundled into anesthesia shall not be reported in addition to the surgical or medical procedure requiring the anesthesia services if performed by the same physician. Examples of improperly reported services that are bundled into the anesthesia service when anesthesia is provided by the physician performing the medical or surgical procedure include introduction of needle or intracatheter into a vein (CPT code 36000), venipuncture (CPT code 36410), intravenous infusion/injection (CPT codes 96360-96368, 96374-96377) or cardiac assessment (e.g., CPT codes 93000-93010, 9304093042). However, if these services are not related to the delivery of an anesthetic agent or are not an inherent component of the procedure or global service, they may be reported separately.

The physician performing a surgical or medical procedure shall not report an epidural/subarachnoid injection (CPT codes 62320-62327) or nerve block (CPT codes 6440064530) for anesthesia for that procedure.

H. HCPCS/CPT Procedure Code Definition

The HCPCS/CPT code descriptors of 2 codes are often the basis of an NCCI PTP edit. If 2 HCPCS/CPT codes describe redundant services, they shall not be reported separately. Several general principles follow:

1. A family of CPT codes may include a CPT code followed by one or more indented CPT codes. The first CPT code descriptor includes a semicolon. The portion of the descriptor of the first code in the family preceding the semicolon is a common part of the descriptor for each subsequent code of the family. For example:

   CPT code 70120   Radiologic examination, mastoids; less than 3 views per side

   CPT code 70130   complete, minimum of 3 views per side

   The portion of the descriptor preceding the semicolon ("Radiologic examination, mastoids") is common to both CPT codes 70120 and 70130. The difference between the 2 codes is the portion of the descriptors following the semicolon. Often, as in this case, 2 codes from a family may not be reported separately. A physician cannot report CPT codes 70120 and 70130 for a procedure performed on ipsilateral mastoids at the same patient encounter. It is important to recognize, however, that there are numerous circumstances when it may be appropriate to report more than one code from a family of codes. For example, CPT codes 70120 and 70130 may be reported separately if the 2 procedures are performed on contralateral mastoids or at 2 separate patient encounters on the same date of service.

2. If a HCPCS/CPT code is reported, it includes all components of the procedure defined by the descriptor. For example, CPT code 58291 includes a vaginal hysterectomy with "removal of tube(s) and/or ovary(s)." A physician cannot report a salpingo-oophorectomy (CPT code 58720) separately with CPT code 58291.

3. CPT code descriptors often define correct coding relationships where 2 codes may not be reported separately with one another at the same anatomic site and/or same patient encounter. A few examples follow:
   a) A "partial" procedure is not separately reportable with a "complete" procedure.
   b) A "partial" procedure is not separately reportable with a "total" procedure.
   c) A "unilateral" procedure is not separately reportable with a "bilateral" procedure.
   d) A "single" procedure is not separately reportable with a "multiple" procedure.
   e) A "with" procedure is not separately reportable with a "without" procedure.
   f) An "initial" procedure is not separately reportable with a "subsequent" procedure.

I. CPT Professional *Codebook* and CMS Coding Manual Instructions

The CMS often publishes coding instructions in its rules, manuals, and notices. Physicians must use these instructions when reporting services rendered to Medicare patients.

The CPT Professional *codebook* also includes coding instructions which may be found in the "Introduction," individual chapters, and appendices. In individual chapters, the instructions may appear at the beginning of a chapter, at the beginning of a subsection of the chapter, or after specific CPT codes. Physicians should follow CPT Professional *codebook* instructions unless the CMS has provided different coding or reporting instructions.

The American Medical Association publishes "CPT Assistant" which contains coding guidelines. The CMS does not review or approve the information in this publication. *As a result, CMS may adopt NCCI edits that are not consistent with CPT Assistant.* If a physician uses information from "CPT Assistant" to report services rendered to Medicare patients, it is possible that MACs may use different criteria to process claims.

J. CPT "Separate Procedure" Definition

If a CPT code descriptor includes the term "separate procedure," the CPT code may not be reported separately with a related procedure. The CMS interprets this designation to prohibit the separate reporting of a "separate procedure" when performed with another procedure in an anatomically related region often through the same skin incision, orifice, or surgical approach.

A CPT code with the "separate procedure" designation may be reported with another procedure if it is performed at a separate patient encounter on the same date of service or at the same patient encounter in an anatomically unrelated area often through a separate skin incision, orifice, or surgical approach. Modifiers 59 or XE or XS (or a more specific modifier, e.g., anatomic modifier) may be appended to the "separate procedure" CPT code to indicate that it qualifies as a separately reportable service.

K. Family of Codes

The *CPT* Professional *codebook* often contains a group of codes that describe related procedures that may be performed in various combinations. Some codes describe limited component services, and other codes describe various combinations of component services. Physicians must use several principles in selecting the correct code to report:

1. A HCPCS/CPT code may be reported if and only if all services described by the code are performed.
2. The *most comprehensive* HCPCS/CPT code describing the services performed shall be reported. A physician shall not report multiple codes corresponding to component services if a single comprehensive code describes the services performed. There are limited exceptions to this rule which are specifically identified in this Manual.
3. HCPCS/CPT code(s) corresponding to component service(s) of other more comprehensive HCPCS/CPT code(s) shall not be reported separately with the more comprehensive HCPCS/CPT code(s) that include the component service(s).
4. If the HCPCS/CPT codes do not correctly describe the procedure(s) performed, the physician shall report a "not otherwise specified" CPT code rather than a HCPCS/CPT code that most closely describes the procedure(s) performed.

L. More Extensive Procedure

The *CPT* Professional *codebook* often describes groups of similar codes differing in the complexity of the service. Unless services are performed at separate patient encounters or at separate anatomic sites, the less complex service is included in the more complex service and is not separately reportable. Several examples of this principle follow:

1. If 2 procedures only differ in that 1 is described as a "simple" procedure and the other as a "complex" procedure, the "simple" procedure is included in the "complex" procedure and is not separately reportable unless the 2 procedures are performed at separate patient encounters or at separate anatomic sites.
2. If 2 procedures only differ in that 1 is described as a "simple" procedure and the other as a "complicated" procedure, the "simple" procedure is included in the "complicated" procedure and is not separately reportable unless the 2 procedures are performed at separate patient encounters or at separate anatomic sites.
3. If 2 procedures only differ in that 1 is described as a "limited" procedure and the other as a "complete" procedure, the "limited" procedure is included in the "complete" procedure and is not separately reportable unless the 2 procedures are performed at separate patient encounters or at separate anatomic sites.
4. If 2 procedures only differ in that 1 is described as an "intermediate" procedure and the other as a "comprehensive" procedure, the "intermediate" procedure is included in the "comprehensive" procedure and is not separately reportable unless the 2 procedures are performed at separate patient encounters or at separate anatomic sites.
5. If 2 procedures only differ in that 1 is described as a "superficial" procedure and the other as a "deep" procedure, the "superficial" procedure is included in the "deep" procedure and is not separately reportable unless the 2 procedures are performed at separate patient encounters or at separate anatomic sites.
6. If 2 procedures only differ in that 1 is described as an "incomplete" procedure and the other as a "complete" procedure, the "incomplete" procedure is included in the "complete" procedure and is not separately reportable unless the 2 procedures are performed at separate patient encounters or at separate anatomic sites.
7. If 2 procedures only differ in that 1 is described as an "external" procedure and the other as an "internal" procedure, the "external" procedure is included in the "internal" procedure and is not separately reportable unless the 2 procedures are performed at separate patient encounters or at separate anatomic sites.

M. Sequential Procedure

Some surgical procedures may be performed by different surgical approaches. If an initial surgical approach to a procedure fails and a second surgical approach is used at the same patient encounter, only the HCPCS/CPT code corresponding to the second surgical approach may be reported. If there are different HCPCS/CPT codes for the 2 different surgical approaches, the 2 procedures are considered "sequential," and only the HCPCS/CPT code corresponding to the second surgical approach may be reported. For example, a physician may begin a cholecystectomy procedure using a laparoscopic approach and have to convert the procedure to an open abdominal approach. Only the CPT code for the open cholecystectomy may be reported. The CPT code for the failed laparoscopic cholecystectomy is not separately reportable.

N. Laboratory Panel

The *CPT* Professional *codebook* defines organ and disease specific panels of laboratory tests. If a laboratory performs all tests included in one of these panels, the laboratory shall report the CPT code for the panel. If the laboratory repeats 1 of these component tests as a medically reasonable and necessary service on the same date of service, the CPT code corresponding to the repeat laboratory test may be reported with modifier 91 appended (See Chapter X, Section C, Organ or Disease Oriented Panels).

O. Misuse of Column Two Column Code with Column One Code (Misuse of Code Edit Rationale)

The CMS manuals and instructions often describe groups of HCPCS/CPT codes that should not be reported together for the Medicare program. Edits based on these instructions are often included as misuse of a Column Two code with a Column One code.

A HCPCS/CPT code descriptor does not include exhaustive information about the code. Physicians who are not familiar with a HCPCS/CPT code may incorrectly report the code in a context different than intended. The NCCI program has identified HCPCS/CPT codes that are incorrectly reported with other HCPCS/CPT codes as a result of the misuse of the Column

Two code with the Column One code. If these edits allow use of NCCI PTP-associated modifiers (modifier indicator of "1"), there are limited circumstances when the Column Two code may be reported on the same date of service as the Column One code. Two examples follow:

1. Three or more HCPCS/CPT codes may be reported on the same date of service. Although the Column Two code is misused if reported as a service associated with the Column One code, the Column Two code may be appropriately reported with a third HCPCS/CPT code reported on the same date of service. For example, the CMS limits separate payment for use of the operating microscope for microsurgical techniques (CPT code 69990) to a group of procedures listed in the online "Claims Processing Manual" (Chapter 12, Section 20.4.5 (Allowable Adjustments)). The NCCI program has edits with Column One codes of surgical procedures not listed in this section of the manual and Column Two CPT code of 69990. Some of these edits allow use of NCCI PTP-associated modifiers because the 2 services listed in the edit may be performed at the same patient encounter as a third procedure for which CPT code 69990 is separately reportable.
2. There may be limited circumstances when the Column Two code is separately reportable with the Column One code. For example, the NCCI program has an edit with Column One CPT code of 47600 (Cholecystectomy) and Column Two CPT code of 12035 (Repair, intermediate, wounds of scalp, axillae, trunk and/or extremities (excluding hands and feet); 12.6 cm to 20.0 cm). If the patient has an abdominal wound in addition to and separate from the cholecystectomy surgical incision, then it may be separately reportable with CPT code 12035 using an NCCI PTP-associated modifier to bypass the edit. 47600 includes repair of the cholecystectomy surgical incision.

Misuse of code as an edit rationale may be applied to PTP edits where the Column Two code is not separately reportable with the Column One code based on the nature of the Column One coded procedure. This edit rationale may also be applied to code pairs where use of the Column Two code with the Column One code is deemed to be a coding error.

P. Mutually Exclusive Procedures

Many procedure codes cannot be reported together because they are mutually exclusive of each other. Mutually exclusive procedures cannot reasonably be performed at the same anatomic site or same patient encounter. An example of a mutually exclusive situation is the repair of an organ that can be performed by 2 different methods. Only one method can be chosen to repair the organ. A second example is a service that can be reported as an "initial" service or a "subsequent" service.

Pairs of HCPCS/CPT codes that are mutually exclusive of one another based either on the HCPCS/CPT code descriptors or the medical impossibility/improbability that the 2 procedures could be performed at the same patient encounter are included in the NCCI PTP edit tables. Many of these edits allow the use of NCCI PTP-associated modifiers. For example, the 2 procedures of a code pair edit may be performed at different anatomic sites (e.g., contralateral eyes) or separate patient encounters on the same date of service.

Q. Reserved for future use

R. Add-on Codes

Some codes in the CPT Professional *codebook* are identified as "Add-on" Codes (AOCs), which describe a service that can only be reported in addition to a primary procedure. CPT Professional *codebook* instructions specify the primary procedure code(s) for most AOCs. For other AOCs, the primary procedure code(s) is (are) not specified. When the CPT Professional *codebook* identifies specific primary codes, the AOCs shall not be reported as a supplemental service for other HCPCS/CPT codes not listed as a primary code.

AOCs permit the reporting of significant supplemental services commonly performed in addition to the primary procedure. By contrast, incidental services that are necessary to accomplish the primary procedure (e.g., lysis of adhesions in the course of an open cholecystectomy) are not separately reportable with an AOC. Similarly, complications inherent in an invasive procedure occurring during the procedure are not separately reportable. For example, control of bleeding during an invasive procedure is considered part of the procedure and is not separately reportable.

In general, NCCI PTP edits do not include edits with most AOCs because edits related to the primary procedure(s) are adequate to prevent inappropriate payment for an add-on coded procedure (i.e., if an edit prevents payment of the primary procedure code, the AOC shall not be paid). However, the NCCI program does include edits for some AOCs when coding edits related to the primary procedures must be supplemented. Examples include edits with add-on HCPCS/CPT codes 69990 (Microsurgical techniques requiring use of operating microscope) and 95940/95941/G0453 (Intraoperative neurophysiology testing).

HCPCS/CPT codes that are not designated as AOCs shall not be misused as an AOC to report a supplemental service. A HCPCS/CPT code may be reported if and only if all services described by the CPT code are performed. A HCPCS/CPT code shall not be reported with another service because a portion of the service described by the HCPCS/CPT code was performed with the other procedure. For example, if an ejection fraction is estimated from an echocardiogram study, it would be inappropriate to additionally report CPT code 78472 (Cardiac blood pool imaging gated equilibrium; planar, single study at rest or stress (exercise and/or pharmacologic), wall motion study plus ejection fraction, with or without additional quantitative processing) with the echocardiography (e.g., CPT code 93307). Although the procedure described by CPT code 78472 includes an ejection fraction, it is measured by gated equilibrium with a radionuclide which is not used in echocardiography.

S. Excluded Service

The NCCI program does not generally address issues related to HCPCS/CPT codes describing services that are excluded from Medicare coverage or are not otherwise recognized for payment under the Medicare program.

T. Unlisted Procedure Codes

The CPT Professional *codebook* includes codes to identify services or procedures not described by other HCPCS/CPT codes. These unlisted procedure codes are generally identified as XXX99 or XXXX9 codes and are located at the end of each section or subsection of the Manual. If a physician provides a service that is not accurately described by other HCPCS/CPT codes, the service shall be reported using an unlisted procedure code. A physician shall not report a CPT code for a specific procedure if it does not accurately describe the service performed. It is inappropriate to report the best fit HCPCS/CPT code unless it accurately describes the service performed, and all components of the HCPCS/CPT code were performed. Since unlisted procedure codes may be reported for a very diverse group of services, the NCCI program generally does not include edits with these codes.

U. Modified, Deleted, and Added Code Pairs/Edits – Information moved to Introduction chapter, Section (Purpose), Page Intro-5 of this Manual

V. Medically Unlikely Edits (MUEs)

To lower the Medicare Fee-For-Service Paid Claims Error Rate, the CMS has established units of service edits referred to as Medically Unlikely Edit(s)(MUEs).

An MUE is the maximum UOS reported for a HCPCS/CPT code on the vast majority of appropriately reported claims by the same provider/supplier for the same beneficiary on the same date of service.

All claims submitted to MACs and Durable Medical Equipment (DME) MACs, and outpatient facility services claims (e.g., Type of Bill 13X, 14X, 85X, 87X) are tested against MUEs.

Prior to April 1, 2013, each line of a claim was adjudicated separately against the MUE value for the HCPCS/CPT code reported on that claim line. If the UOS on that claim line exceeded the MUE value, the entire claim line was denied.

In the April 1, 2013, version of MUEs, the CMS began introducing date of service (DOS) MUEs. Over time the CMS will convert many, but not all, MUEs to DOS MUEs. Since April 1, 2013, MUEs are adjudicated either as claim line edits or DOS edits. If the MUE is adjudicated as a claim line edit, the UOS on each claim line are compared to the MUE value for the HCPCS/CPT code on that claim line. If the UOS exceed the MUE value, all UOS on that claim line are denied. If the MUE is adjudicated as a DOS MUE, all UOS on each claim line for the same date of service for the same HCPCS/CPT code are summed, and the sum is compared to the MUE value. If the summed UOS exceed the MUE value, all UOS for the HCPCS/CPT code for that date of service are denied. Denials due to claim line MUEs or DOS MUEs may be appealed to the local claims processing contractor. DOS MUEs are used for HCPCS/CPT codes where it would be extremely unlikely that more UOS than the MUE value would ever be performed on the same date of service for the same patient.

The MUE files on the CMS NCCI website display an "MUE Adjudication Indicator" (MAI) for each HCPCS/CPT code. An MAI of "1" indicates that the edit is a claim line MUE. An MAI of "2" or "3" indicates that the edit is a DOS MUE.

If a HCPCS/CPT code has an MUE that is adjudicated as a claim line edit, (i.e., MAI equal to "1") appropriate use of CPT modifiers (i.e., 59 or XE, XP, XS, XU; 76, 77, 91, anatomic) may be used to report the same HCPCS/CPT code on separate lines of a claim. Each line of the claim with that HCPCS/CPT code will be separately adjudicated against the MUE value for that HCPCS/CPT code. Claims processing contractors have rules limiting use of these modifiers with some HCPCS/CPT codes.

MUEs for HCPCS codes with an MAI of "2" are absolute date of service edits. These are "per day edits based on policy." HCPCS codes with an MAI of "2" have been rigorously reviewed and vetted within CMS and obtain this MAI designation because UOS on the same date of service (DOS) in excess of the MUE value would be considered impossible because it was contrary to statute, regulation, or subregulatory guidance. This subregulatory guidance includes clear correct coding policy that is binding on both providers/suppliers and CMS claims processing contractors. Limitations created by anatomical, or coding limitations are incorporated in correct coding policy, both in the HIPAA mandated coding descriptors and CMS-approved coding guidance as well as specific guidance in the CMS and NCCI manuals. For example, it would be contrary to correct coding policy to report more than one unit of service for CPT 94002 (Ventilation assist and management . . . initial day) because such use could not accurately describe 2 initial days of management occurring on the same date of service as would be required by the code descriptor. As a result, claims processing contractors are instructed that an MAI of "2" denotes a claims processing restriction for which override during processing, reopening, or redetermination would be contrary to CMS policy.

MUEs for HCPCS codes with an MAI of "3" are "per day edits based on clinical benchmarks." MUEs assigned an MAI of "3" are based on criteria (e.g., nature of service, prescribing information) combined with data such that it would be possible but medically highly unlikely that higher values would represent correctly reported medically necessary services. If contractors have evidence (e.g., medical review) that UOS in excess of the MUE value were actually provided, were correctly coded and were medically necessary, the contractor may bypass the MUE for a HCPCS code with an MAI of "3" during claim processing, reopening, or redetermination, or in response to effectuation instructions from a reconsideration or higher-level appeal.

An MUE or the lack of an MUE, does not necessarily indicate coverage status of a HCPCS/CPT code. The NCCI program does not establish medical necessity or payment policy.

Both the MAI and MUE value for each HCPCS/CPT code are based on one or more of the following criteria:

(1) Anatomic considerations may limit UOS based on anatomic structures. For example:
  a) The MUE value for an appendectomy is "1" since there is only 1 appendix.
  b) The MUE for a knee brace is "2" because there are 2 knees and Medicare policy does not cover back-up equipment.
  c) The MUE value for a lumbar spine procedure reported per lumbar vertebra or per lumbar interspace cannot exceed "5" since there are only 5 lumbar vertebrae or interspaces.

d) The MUE value for a procedure reported per lung lobe cannot exceed "5" since there are only 5 lung lobes (3 in right lung and 2 in left lung).

(2) CPT code descriptors/CPT coding instructions in the *CPT Professional codebook* may limit UOS. For example:
  a) A procedure described as the "initial 30 minutes" would have an MUE value of "1" because of the use of the term "initial." A different code may be reported for additional time.
  b) If a code descriptor uses the plural form of the procedure, it must not be reported with multiple UOS. For example, if the code descriptor states "biopsies," the code is reported with "1" unit of service regardless of the number of biopsies performed.
  c) The MUE value for a procedure with "per day," "per week," or "per month" in its code descriptor is "1" because MUEs are based on number of services per day of service.
  d) The MUE value of a code for a procedure described as "unilateral" is "1" if there is a different code for the procedure described as "bilateral."
  e) The code descriptors of a family of codes may define different levels of service, each having an MUE of "1." For example, CPT codes 78102-78104 describe bone marrow imaging. CPT code 78102 is reported for imaging a "limited area." CPT code 78103 is reported for imaging "multiple areas." CPT code 78104 is reported for imaging the "whole body."
  f) The MUE value for CPT code 86021 (Antibody identification; leukocyte antibodies) is "1" because the code descriptor is plural including testing for any and all leukocyte antibodies. On a single date of service only one specimen from a patient would be tested for leukocyte antibodies.
  g) When reporting codes, it is important to assure the accuracy of coding and the correct UOS by selecting a code that accurately identifies the service performed based on factors including but not limited to, the route of administration. For example, for intravitreal injection of bevacizumab, select an intravitreal code (e.g., C9257) rather than an intravenous code (e.g., J9035).

(3) Edits based on established CMS policies may limit UOS. For example:
  a) The MUE value for a surgical or diagnostic procedure may be based on the bilateral surgery indicator on the Medicare Physician Fee Schedule Database (MPFSDB).
    i. If the bilateral surgery indicator is "0," a bilateral procedure must be reported with "1" unit of service. There is no additional payment for the code if reported as a unilateral or bilateral procedure because of anatomy or physiology. Alternatively, the code descriptor may specifically state that the procedure is a unilateral procedure, and there is a separate code for a bilateral procedure.
    ii. If the bilateral surgery indicator is "1," a bilateral surgical procedure must be reported with "1" unit of service and modifier 50 (bilateral modifier). A bilateral diagnostic procedure may be reported with "1" unit of service and modifier 50 on 1 claim line, or "1" unit of service with modifier RT on 1 claim line plus "1" unit of service and modifier LT on a second claim line.
    iii. If the bilateral surgery indicator is "2," a bilateral procedure must be reported with "1" unit of service. The procedure is priced as a bilateral procedure because (1) the code descriptor defines the procedure as bilateral; (2) the code descriptor states that the procedure is performed unilaterally or bilaterally; or (3) the procedure is usually performed as a bilateral procedure.
    iv. If the bilateral surgery indicator is "3," a bilateral surgical procedure must be reported with "1" unit of service and modifier 50 (bilateral modifier). A bilateral diagnostic procedure may be reported with "2" UOS on 1 claim line, "1" unit of service and modifier 50 on 1 claim line, or 1 unit of service with modifier RT on 1 claim line plus "1" unit of service and modifier LT on a second claim line.
  b) The MUE value for a code may be "1" where the code descriptor does not specify a unit of service and the CMS considers the default UOS to be "per day." c) The MUE value for a code may be "0" because the code is listed as invalid, not covered, bundled, not separately payable, statutorily excluded, not reasonable and necessary, etc. based on:
    i. The Medicare Physician Fee Schedule Database
    ii. OPPS Addendum B
    iii. Alpha-Numeric HCPCS Code File
    iv. DMEPOS Jurisdiction List
    v. Medicare "Internet-Only Manual ("IOM")

(4) The nature of an analyte may limit UOS and is in general determined by:
  a) The nature of the specimen may limit the UOS. For example, CPT code 82575 describes a creatinine clearance test and has an MUE of "1" because the test requires a twenty-four-hour urine collection; or
  b) The physiology, pathophysiology, or clinical application of the analyte is such that a maximum unit of service for a single date of service can be determined. For example, the MUE for CPT code 82747 (RBC folic acid) is "1" because the test result would not be expected to change during a single day, and thus it is not necessary to perform the test more than once on a single date of service.

(5) The nature of a procedure/service may limit UOS and is in general determined by the amount of time required to perform a procedure/service (e.g., overnight sleep studies) or clinical application of a procedure/service (e.g., motion analysis tests).
  a) The MUE for many surgical or medical procedures is "1" because the procedure is rarely, if ever, performed more than 1 time per day (e.g., colonoscopy, motion analysis tests).
  b) The MUE value for a procedure is "1" because of the amount of time required to perform the procedure (e.g., overnight sleep study).

(6) The nature of equipment may limit UOS and is in general determined by the number of items of equipment that would be used. For example, the MUE value for a wheelchair code is "1" because only 1 wheelchair is used at 1 time and Medicare policy does not cover back-up equipment.

(7) Although clinical judgment considerations and determinations based on input from numerous physicians and certified coders are sometimes initially used to establish some MUE values, these values are subsequently validated or changed based on submitted and/or paid claims data.

(8) Prescribing information is based on FDA labeling as well as off-label information published in CMS-approved drug compendia. See below for additional information about how prescribing information is used in determining the MUE values.

(9) Submitted and paid claims data (100%) from a six-month period is used to ascertain the distribution pattern of UOS typically reported for a given HCPCS/CPT code.

(10) Published policies of the Durable Medical Equipment (DME) Medicare Administrative Contractors (MACs) may limit UOS for some durable medical equipment, prosthetics, orthotics, and supplies (DMEPOS). For example:
  a) The MUE values for many ostomy and urological supply codes, nebulizer codes, and CPAP accessory codes are typically based on a three-month supply of items.
  b) The MUE values for surgical dressings, parenteral and enteral nutrition, immunosuppressive drugs, and oral anti-cancer drugs are typically based on a one-month supply.
  c) The MUE values take into account the requirement for reporting certain codes with date spans.
  d) The MUE value of a code may be "0" if the item is noncovered, not medically necessary, or not separately payable.
  e) The MUE value of a code may be "0" if the code is invalid for claim submission to the DME MAC.

UOS denied based on an MUE may be appealed. Because a denial of services due to an MUE is a coding denial, not a medical necessity denial, the presence of an Advanced Beneficiary Notice of Noncoverage (ABN) shall not shift liability to the beneficiary for UOS denied based on an MUE. If during reopening or redetermination medical records are provided with respect to an MUE denial for an edit with an MAI of "3," contractors will review the records to determine if the provider actually furnished units in excess of the MUE, if the codes were used correctly, and whether the services were medically reasonable and necessary. If the units were actually provided but one of the other conditions is not met, a change in denial reason may be warranted (for example, a change from the MUE denial based on incorrect coding to a determination that the item/service is not reasonable and necessary under section 1862(a)(1)). This may also be true for certain edits with an MAI of "1." The CMS interprets the notice delivery requirements under §1879 of the Social Security Act (the Act) as applying to situations in which a provider expects the initial claim determination to be a reasonable and necessary denial. Consistent with NCCI guidance, denials resulting from MUEs are not based on any of the statutory provisions that give liability protection to beneficiaries under Section 1879 of the Act. Thus, ABN issuance based on an MUE is NOT appropriate. A provider/supplier may not issue an ABN in connection with services denied due to an MUE and cannot bill the beneficiary for UOS denied based on an MUE.

HCPCS J-code and drug related C and Q-code MUEs are based on prescribing information, how product is supplied, and/or 100% claims data for a six-month period of time. Using the prescribing information, the highest total daily dose for each drug was determined. This dose and its corresponding UOS were evaluated against paid and submitted claims data. Some of the guiding principles used in developing these edits are as follows:

(1) If the prescribing information defined a maximum daily dose, this value was used to determine the MUE value. For some drugs there is an absolute maximum daily dose. For others there is a maximum "recommended" or "usual" dose. In the latter 2 cases, the daily dose calculation was evaluated against claims data.

(2) If the maximum daily dose calculation is based on actual body weight, a dose based on a weight range of 110-150 kg was evaluated against the claims data. If the maximum daily dose calculation is based on ideal body weight, a dose based on a weight range of 90-110 kg was evaluated against claims data. If the maximum daily dose calculation is based on body surface area (BSA), a dose based on a BSA range of 2.4-3.0 square meters was evaluated against claims data.

(3) For drugs where the maximum daily dose is based on patient response or need, prescribing information and claims data were used to establish the MUE values.

(4) Published off-label use of a drug was considered for the maximum daily dose calculation.

(5) The MUE values for some drug codes are set to "0." The rationale for such values include but are not limited to: discontinued manufacture of drug, non-FDA-approved compounded drug, practitioner MUE values for oral anti-neoplastic, oral anti-emetic, and oral immune suppressive drugs which should be billed to the DME MACs, outpatient hospital MUE values for inhalation drugs which should be billed to the DME MACs, and Practitioner/ASC MUE values for HCPCS C codes describing medications that would not be related to a procedure performed in an ASC.

Non-drug-related HCPCS/CPT codes may be assigned an MUE of "0" for a variety of reasons including, but not limited to, outpatient hospital MUE value for a surgical procedure only performed as an inpatient procedure, noncovered service, bundled service, DME MUE value for implanted devices and items related to implanted devices which should not be billed to the DME MACs, or packaged service.

The MUE files on the *CMS Medicare NCCI Medically Unlikely Edits (MUEs) webpage* display an "Edit Rationale" for each HCPCS/CPT code. Although an MUE may be based on several rationales, only one is displayed on the website. One of the listed rationales is "Data." This rationale indicates that 100% claims data from a six-month period of time was the major factor in determining the MUE value. If a physician appeals an MUE denial for a HCPCS/CPT code where the MUE is based on "Data," the reviewer will usually confirm that (1) the correct code is reported; (2) the correct UOS are used; (3) the number of reported UOS were performed; and (4) all UOS were medically reasonable and necessary.

The first MUEs were implemented January 1, 2007. Additional MUEs are added on a quarterly basis on the same schedule as NCCI PTP updates. Prior to implementation proposed MUEs are sent to numerous national healthcare organizations for a 60-day review and comment period.

Many surgical procedures may be performed bilaterally. Instructions in the CMS IOM (Publication 100-04 MCPM Chapter 12 (Physicians/Nonphysician Practitioners), Section 40.7.B. and Chapter 4 (Part B Hospital (Including Inpatient Hospital Part B and OPPS)), Section 20.6.2 require that bilateral surgical procedures be reported using modifier 50 with one unit of service unless the code descriptor defines the procedure as "bilateral." If the code descriptor defines the procedure as a "bilateral" procedure, it shall be reported with one unit of service without modifier 50. If a bilateral surgical procedure is performed at different sites bilaterally, one unit of service may be reported for each site. That is, the HCPCS/CPT code may be reported with modifier 50 and one unit of service for each site at which it was performed bilaterally.

Some A/B MACs allow providers/suppliers to report repetitive services performed over a range of dates on a single line of a claim with multiple UOS. If a provider/supplier reports services in this fashion, the provider/supplier should report the "from date" and "to date" on the claim line. Contractors are instructed to divide the UOS reported on the claim line by the number of days in the date span and round to the nearest whole number. This number is compared to the MUE value for the code on the claim line.

Providers/Suppliers billing services to the DME MACs typically report some HCPCS codes for supply items for a period exceeding a single day. The DME MACs have billing rules for these codes. For some codes the DME MACs require that the "from date" and "to date" be reported. The MUEs for these codes are based on the maximum number of UOS that may be reported for a single date of service. For other codes the DME MACs permit multiple days' supply items to be reported on a single claim line where the "from date" and "to date" are the same. The DME MACs have rules allowing supply items for a maximum number of days to be reported at one time for each of these types of codes. The MUE values for these codes are based on the maximum number of days that may be reported at one time. As with all MUEs, the MUE value does not represent a utilization guideline. Providers/suppliers shall not assume that they may report UOS up to the MUE value on each date of service. Providers/suppliers may only report supply items that are medically reasonable and necessary.

Most MUE values are set so that a provider or supplier would only very occasionally have a claim line denied. If a provider/supplier encounters a code with frequent denials due to the MUE or frequent use of a CPT modifier to bypass the MUE, the provider or supplier should consider the following: (1) Is the HCPCS/CPT code being used correctly? (2) Is the unit of service being counted correctly? (3) Are all reported services medically reasonable and necessary? and (4) Why does the provider's or supplier's practice differ from national patterns? A provider or supplier may choose to discuss these questions with the local Medicare contractor or a national healthcare organization whose members frequently perform the procedure.

Most MUE values are published on the CMS MUE webpage. However, some MUE values are not published and are confidential. These values shall not be published in oral or written form by any party that acquires one or more of them.

MUEs are not utilization edits. Although the MUE value for some codes may represent the commonly reported UOS (e.g., MUE of "1" for appendectomy), the usual UOS for many HCPCS/CPT codes is less than the MUE value. Claims reporting UOS less than the MUE value may be subject to review by claims processing contractors, Unified Program Integrity Contractor (UPICS), Recovery Audit Contractors (RACs), and Department of Justice (DOJ).

Since MUEs are coding edits, rather than medical necessity edits, claims processing contractors may have UOS edits that are more restrictive than MUEs. In such cases, the more restrictive claims processing contractor edit would be applied to the claim. Similarly, if the MUE is more restrictive than a claims processing contractor edit, the more restrictive MUE would apply.

W. Add-on Code Edits

Add-on Codes (AOCs) are discussed in Chapter I, Section R (Add-on Codes). CMS publishes a text file of AOCs and their primary codes annually prior to January 1. CMS updates the file quarterly based on the AMA's "CPT Errata" documents or implementation of new HCPCS/CPT add-on codes. The CMS identifies AOCs and their primary codes based on *CPT Professional codebook* instructions, CMS interpretation of HCPCS/CPT codes, and CMS coding instructions.

An AOC is a HCPCS/CPT code that describes a service that, with rare exception, is performed in conjunction with another primary service by the same practitioner. An AOC is rarely eligible for payment if it is the only procedure reported by a practitioner.

For Type 1 AOCs edits, the *CPT Professional codebook* or HCPCS files define all acceptable primary codes. MACs should not allow other primary codes with Type I AOCs. CPT code 99292 (Critical care, evaluation, and management of the critically ill or critically injured patient; each additional 30 minutes (List separately in addition to code for primary service)) is included as a Type I AOC since its only primary code is CPT code 99291 (Critical care, evaluation, and management of the critically ill or critically injured patient; first 30-74 minutes). For Medicare purposes, CPT code 99292 may be eligible for payment to a physician without CPT code 99291 if another physician of the same specialty and physician group reports and is paid for CPT code 99291.

For Type 2 AOCs edits, the *CPT Professional codebook* and HCPCS files do not define any primary codes. MACs should develop their own lists of acceptable primary codes.

For Type 3 AOCs edits, the *CPT Professional codebook* or HCPCS files define some, but not all, acceptable primary codes. MACs should allow the listed primary codes for these AOCs but may develop their own lists of additional acceptable primary codes.

Although the AOC and primary code are normally reported for the same date of service, there are unusual circumstances where the 2 services may be reported for different dates of service (e.g., CPT codes 99291 and 99292).

CMS updates the complete file of AOC edits with their primary procedure codes on an annual basis on or by January 1 every year based on changes to the *CPT Professional codebook* or HCPCS Level II Manual. CMS posts quarterly updates as a complete file of AOC edits, if necessary, on April 1, July 1, and October 1 of each year. If no changes occur in the AOC edits, no quarterly update will be posted.

FIGURE CREDITS

1. From Little J, et al: *Dental Management of the Medically Compromised Patient*, ed 9, St. Louis, 2017, Mosby. *(Courtesy Medtronic, Minneapolis)*
2. From Franklin I, Dawson P, Rodway A: *Essentials of Clinical Surgery*, ed 2, St. Louis, 2012, Saunders.
3. Modified from Grosfeld J, et al: *Pediatric Surgery*, ed 7, Philadelphia, 2012, Mosby.
4. Modified from Hsu J, Michael J, Fisk J: *AAOS Atlas of Orthoses and Assistive Devices*, ed 4, Philadelphia, 2008, Mosby.
5. From Wold G: *Basic Geriatric Nursing*, ed 5, St. Louis, 2011, Mosby.
6. Modified from Roberts J, Hedges J: *Clinical Procedures in Emergency Medicine*, ed 6, St. Louis, 2013, Saunders.
7. From Auerbach P: *Wilderness Medicine*, ed 7, Philadelphia, 2016, Mosby. *(Courtesy Black Diamond Equipment, Ltd.)*
8. (Original to book).
9. Modified from Abeloff M, et al: *Clinical Oncology*, ed 5, Philadelphia, 2013, Churchill Livingstone.
10. (Original to book).
11. Modified from Duthie E, Katz P, Malone M: *Practice of Geriatrics*, ed 4, Philadelphia, 2007, Saunders.
12. Modified from Roberts J, Hedges J: *Clinical Procedures in Emergency Medicine*, ed 6, St. Louis, 2013, Saunders.
13. From Young A, Proctor D: *Kinn's The Medical Assistant*, ed 13, St. Louis, 2016, Saunders.
14. From Bonewit-West K: *Clinical Procedures for Medical Assistants*, ed 9, Philadelphia, 2015, WB Saunders.
15. From Roberts J, Hedges J: *Clinical Procedures in Emergency Medicine*, ed 6, St. Louis, 2013, Saunders.
16. From Yeo: *Shackelford's Surgery of the Alimentary Tract*, ed 7, Philadelphia, 2012, Saunders.
17. Redrawn from Bragg D, Rubin P, Hricak H: *Oncologic Imaging*, ed 2, 2002, Saunders.
18. From Roberts J, Hedges J: *Clinical Procedures in Emergency Medicine*, ed 6, St. Louis, 2013, Saunders. *(Courtesy Atrium Medical Corp., Hudson, NH 03051)*
19. **A** From Auerbach P: *Wilderness Medicine*, ed 7, Philadelphia, 2016, Mosby. **B** Modified from Hsu J, Michael J, Fisk J: *AAOS Atlas of Orthoses and Assistive Devices*, ed 4, Philadelphia, 2008, Mosby.
20. Modified from Lusardi M, Nielsen C: *Orthotics and Prosthetics in Rehabilitation*, ed 3, St. Louis, 2013, Butterworth-Heinemann.
21. Modified from Lusardi M, Nielsen C: *Orthotics and Prosthetics in Rehabilitation*, ed 3, St. Louis, 2013, Butterworth-Heinemann.
22. Modified from Lusardi M, Nielsen C: *Orthotics and Prosthetics in Rehabilitation*, ed 3, St. Louis, 2013, Butterworth-Heinemann.
23. From Elsevier: *Buck's The Next Step: Advanced Medical Coding and Auditing, 2025/2026 Edition*, 2025 St. Louis, 2025, Elsevier.
24. From Jardins T: *Clinical Manifestations and Assessment of Respiratory Disease*, ed 7, St. Louis, 2015, Elsevier.
25. From Hsu J, Michael J, Fisk J: *AAOS Atlas of Orthoses and Assistive Devices*, ed 4, Philadelphia, 2008, Mosby.
26. Modified from Hsu J, Michael J, Fisk J: *AAOS Atlas of Orthoses and Assistive Devices*, ed 4, Philadelphia, 2008, Mosby.
27. Modified from Hsu J, Michael J, Fisk J: *AAOS Atlas of Orthoses and Assistive Devices*, ed 4, Philadelphia, 2008, Mosby.
28. From Didomenico L, Gatlyak N: "End-Stage Ankle Arthritis." *Clinics in Podiatric Medicine and Surgery* 29.3 (2012): 391-412.
29. Cameron M, Monroe L: *Physical Rehabilitation for the Physical Therapist Assistant*, ed 1, St. Louis, 2011, Saunders.
30. From Rowe D, Jadhav A: "Care of the Adolescent with Spina Bifida." *Pediatric Clinics of North America* 55.6 (2008): 1359-374.
31. Modified from Lusardi M, Nielsen C: *Orthotics and Prosthetics in Rehabilitation*, ed 3, St. Louis, 2013, Butterworth-Heinemann.
32. From Hsu J, Michael J, Fisk J: *AAOS Atlas of Orthoses and Assistive Devices*, ed 4, Philadelphia, 2008, Mosby.
33. (Original to book.)
34. From Hochberg M: *Rheumatology*, ed 5, Philadelphia, 2011, Mosby.
35. Modified from Hsu J, Michael J, Fisk J: *AAOS Atlas of Orthoses and Assistive Devices*, ed 4, Philadelphia, 2008, Mosby.
36. From Coughlin M, Mann R, Saltzman C: *Surgery of the Foot and Ankle*, ed 9, Philadelphia, 2013, Mosby.
37. From Canale S: *Campbell's Operative Orthopaedics*, ed 12, St. Louis, 2012, Mosby.
38. From Sorrentino S, Gorek B: *Mosby's Textbook for Long-term Care Nursing Assistants*, ed 7, St. Louis, 2014, Mosby.
39. From Pedretti L, Pendleton H, Schultz-Krohn W: *Pedretti's Occupational Therapy: Practice Skills for Physical Dysfunction*, ed 7, St. Louis, 2013, Elsevier.
40. From Skirven T: *Rehabilitation of the Hand and Upper Extremity*, ed 6, Philadelphia, 2010, Mosby.
41. From Lusardi M, Nielsen C: *Orthotics and Prosthetics in Rehabilitation*, ed 3, St. Louis, 2013, Butterworth-Heinemann. *(Courtesy Michael Curtain)*
42. Schickendantz M: "Diagnosis and Treatment of Elbow Disorders in the Overhead Athlete." *Hand Clinics* 18.1 (2002): 65-75.
43. Modified from Bland K, Copeland E: *The Breast: Comprehensive Management of Benign and Malignant Disorders*, ed 4, St. Louis, 2009, Saunders.
44. From Shah J, Patel S, Singh B, Shah J: *Jatin Shah's Head and Neck Surgery and Oncology*, ed 4, Philadelphia, 2012, Mosby, 2012. From Subburaj K, Nair C, Rajesh S, Ravi B: "Rapid Development of Auricular Prosthesis Using CAD and Rapid Prototyping Technologies." *International Journal of Oral and Maxillofacial Surgery* 36.10 (2007): 938-43.
45. From Weinzweig J: *Plastic Surgery Secrets*, ed 2, Philadelphia, 2010, Hanley & Belfus, p 543.
46. Modified from Mann D: *Heart Failure: A Companion to Braunwald's Heart Disease*, ed 3, Philadelphia, 2015, Saunders.
47. Modified from Roberts J, Hedges J: *Clinical Procedures in Emergency Medicine*, ed 6, Philadelphia, 2013, Saunders.
48. From Yanoff M, Duker J: *Ophthalmology*, ed 4, St. Louis, 2014, Mosby.
49. From Feldman M, Friedman L, Brandt L: *Sleisenger and Fordtran's Gastrointestinal and Liver Disease*, ed 10, Philadelphia, 2015, Saunders.
50. From Katz V, et al: *Comprehensive Gynecology*, ed 7, Philadelphia, 2016, Mosby.
51. From Young A, Proctor D: *Kinn's The Medical Assistant*, ed 13, St. Louis, 2016, Saunders.
52. From Yanoff M, Duker J: *Ophthalmology*, ed 4, St. Louis, 2014, Mosby.

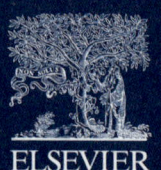

Trust Elsevier to support you every step of your coding career!

From beginning to advanced, from the classroom to the workplace, from application to certification, Elsevier coding solutions are your guide to greater opportunities and successful career advancement.

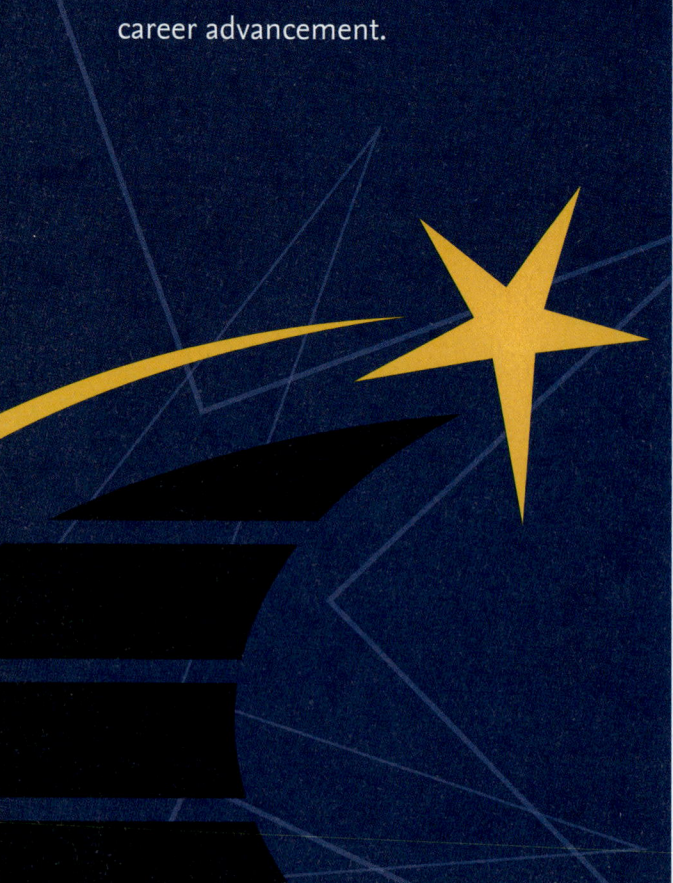

Step One: Learn

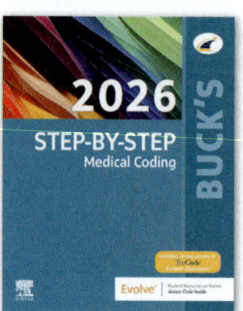

Buck's Step-by-Step Medical Coding, 2026 Edition
ISBN: 978-0-443-38073-0

Also available:
Buck's Workbook for Step-by-Step Medical Coding, 2026 Edition
ISBN: 978-0-443-35063-4

Buck's Medical Coding Online for Step-by-Step Medical Coding, 2026 Edition
ISBN: 978-0-443-40979-0

Step Two: Practice

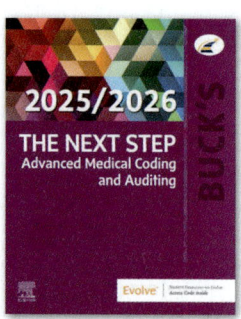

Buck's The Next Step: Advanced Medical Coding and Auditing, 2025/2026 Edition
ISBN: 978-0-443-24880-1

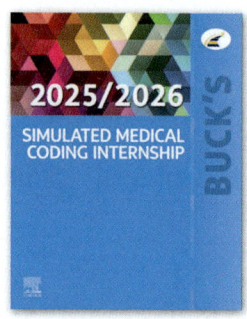

Buck's Simulated Medical Coding Internship, 2025/2026 Edition
ISBN: 978-0-443-26465-8

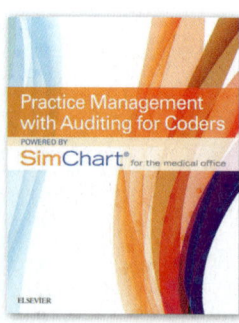

Practice Management with Auditing for Coders Powered by SimChart for the Medical Office
ISBN: 978-0-323-43011-1

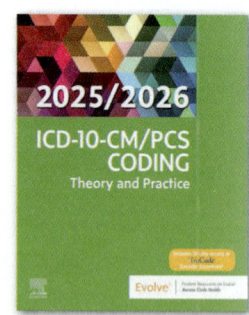

ICD-10-CM/PCS Coding Theory and Practice, 2025/2026 Edition
ISBN: 978-0-443-24893-1